AF670114

Autonomic Innervation of the Heart

Riemer H.J.A. Slart • René A. Tio
Philip H. Elsinga • Markus Schwaiger
Editors

Autonomic Innervation of the Heart

Role of Molecular Imaging

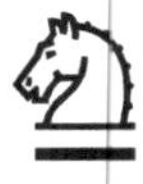
Springer

Editors
Riemer H.J.A. Slart
Nuclear Medicine and Molecular Imaging
University Medical Center Groningen
Groningen
The Netherlands

Philip H. Elsinga
Nuclear Medicine and Molecular Imaging
University Medical Center Groningen
Groningen
The Netherlands

René A. Tio
Thorax center Cardiology
University Medical Center Groningen
Groningen
The Netherlands

Markus Schwaiger
Nuklearmedizinische Klinik
Klinikum Rechts der Isar Technische
Universität München
München
Germany

ISBN 978-3-662-45073-4 ISBN 978-3-662-45074-1 (eBook)
DOI 10.1007/978-3-662-45074-1
Springer Heidelberg New York Dordrecht London

Library of Congress Control Number: 2015930337

Printed on acid-free paper

Springer is part of Springer Science+Business Media (www.springer.com)

Preface

The autonomic innervation of the heart is an integrative part of the physiology of cardiac performance. It is well recognized that cardiac innervation plays an eminent role in the adaptation of cardiac function to daily life. Autonomic innervation of the heart is also known to be an important part of the pathophysiology of various cardiovascular diseases. Arrhythmias have been linked to regional as well as global alterations of electrophysiological properties, which are influenced by autonomic innervations. Cardiac nerves appear to be more sensitive to ischemia as compared to myocytes. Heterogeneity of cardiac innervation as a consequence of regional ischemia may represent an important substrate for the development of arrhythmias in patients with ischemic heart disease. In heart failure, neuronal dysfunction has been linked to the deterioration of function. The ability to predict potentially lethal ventricular arrhythmias promises to help more accurately select patients for implantable cardioverter-defibrillators (ICD), limiting unnecessary devices and identifying additional patients at risk who do not meet current guidelines.

There is a lack of noninvasive methods to access the structure and function of the cardiac autonomic nervous system. A number of techniques, which assess the response to interventions based on temporal changes of heart rate, reflect the overall autonomic tone and can be used to characterize the integrity of neuronal circuits. Since nerve cells are small in comparison to myocytes, direct visualization of cells in vivo appears to be very challenging. In addition, functional assessment of cardiac neurons requires invasive procedures to measure the spillover of neurotransmitters by comparing serum concentrations of catecholamines in arterial and venous blood.

With the advent of specific imaging probes, sympathetic neurons can be identified by their uptake and storage of false neurotransmitters in presynaptic nerve terminals. The uptake of catecholamine analogues is very efficient by presynaptic sympathetic nerve endings, providing high contrast between neuronal and non-neuronal cells. Most imaging probes allow assessment of the integrity of cardiac innervation but fail to provide functional parameters quantifying molecular processes such as transport, storage, and release of neurotransmitters. There are first studies indicating that the washout of MIBG may be related to sympathetic tone; however, since tracer washout is related to physiological and pathophysiological conditions, these measurements may not be very specific for neuronal function. Most recently, new tracers have been introduced, which display kinetics more suitable for quantification of neuronal function. Imaging the postsynaptic α- and β-adrenoceptor density and second messenger systems in the sympathetic nerve ending is a field in exploration. There is also evidence that parasympathetic tone plays a critical role as modulator of the cardiac nervous system in both healthy and diseased hearts and has an impact upon the occurrence of arrhythmias and sudden death. Several radiopharmaceuticals have been used in research trials, and novel tracers are under development for all different target levels of the cardiac innervation system.

In view of recent advances in imaging instrumentation and tracers developed, the available imaging information may provide improved diagnostic and prognostic information in patients with cardiovascular diseases.

This book focuses on the strengths and weaknesses of current techniques to visualize and measure cardiac innervations in vivo. Specially, this book provides a state-of-the-art description of the autonomic innervations of the heart, followed by a methodological discussion of various imaging approaches. Finally, clinical experiences with imaging agents addressing the cardiac innervation are given in various disease groups.

The editors would like to thank all the authors of individual chapters for their excellent contribution. In addition, we appreciate the support by Springer and hope that this book will inspire scientists and physicians, leading to advanced imaging and better care of cardiac patients.

Groningen, The Netherlands — Riemer H.J.A. Slart, MD, PhD
Groningen, The Netherlands — René A. Tio, MD, PhD
Groningen, The Netherlands — Philip H. Elsinga, PhD
Munich, Germany — Markus Schwaiger, MD, PhD

Contents

The Editors

Riemer H. J. A. Slart, MD, PhD, received his medical training at the Medical University in Groningen, the Netherlands. He obtained his PhD in 2005 (new nuclear medicine techniques for the assessment of myocardial viability) at the University of Groningen, the Netherlands. Since 2001, he is member of the permanent medical staff as nuclear medicine physician of the Department of Nuclear Medicine and Molecular Imaging at the University Medical Center Groningen. In 2014, he became part-time clinical professor of Molecular Imaging at the University of Twente, Enschede, the Netherlands. He is involved in cardiovascular imaging with a main focus on myocardial innervation, myocardial perfusion and viability, cardiorenal axis, and atherosclerosis. He is author of over 140 peer-reviewed publications in international journals, 120 abstracts, and 11 book chapters. In 2011, he became discipline leader of Nuclear Medicine and Molecular Imaging for the Center for Medical Imaging Nord-East Netherlands (CMI^{NEN}), and in 2014, he became Board member of the EANM Cardiovascular Committee.

René A. Tio, MD, PhD, is a cardiologist with a broad clinical experience. He received his MD degree at the Erasmus University Rotterdam and earned his Ph.D. degree at the Department of Clinical Pharmacology of the University of Groningen (bradykinin-dependent effects of ACE inhibitors on the heart). After completing his training as a cardiologist, Dr. Tio was appointed to the staff of the catheterization laboratory of the Thoraxcenter at the University Hospital Groningen, where he has worked as an interventional cardiologist for more than 10 years. At present, he is member of the acute cardiac care team and involved in cardiovascular imaging, especially nuclear and molecular imaging. His research focus lies in myocardial perfusion imaging and atherosclerosis. He has published more than 200 peer-reviewed papers.

Philip H. Elsinga, PhD, is an organic chemist by training and obtained his PhD in 1995 at the University of Groningen (promotor Prof W. Vaalburg). He is involved in PET-related radiopharmaceutical research and translation of radiopharmaceuticals to the clinic. His main focus was firstly directed to PET-labeled amino acids, receptor ligands for the beta-adrenergic receptor, and substrates for P-glycoprotein. Later on, his interest broadened to other PET radiopharmaceuticals such as ^{18}F-labeled peptides, sigma receptor antagonists, and artificial amino acids for neuroendocrine tumors. In 2006, he was appointed as guest professor at the University of Ghent, Belgium, and in 2011 as full professor of PET radiochemistry. He is author of >150 peer-reviewed articles. His international activities are (among others) Chairman of the EANM Radiopharmacy Committee, member of Board of Directors of Society of Radiopharmaceutical Sciences, and invited expert for IAEA.

Markus Schwaiger, MD, PhD, received his medical training at the Medical School of the Free University of Berlin, Germany, and completed a fellowship at the division of nuclear medicine, UCLA School of Medicine, Los Angeles. He served as assistant professor of radiological sciences, division of nuclear medicine, UCLA School of Medicine; professor of medicine, division of nuclear medicine, University of Michigan; and professor and director, department of nuclear medicine, Technische Universitaet of Munich, Germany. He is currently dean of the School of Medicine, Technische Universitaet Muenchen, Germany. He has published 764 peer-reviewed publications in international scientific journals, 108 book chapters, and 960 abstracts and has been invited to give 596 presentations.

Abbreviations

[^{11}C]-D2-PHEN	[^{11}C]-(−)-α,α-Dideutero-phenylephrine
[^{11}C]-EPI	[^{11}C]-(−)-Epinephrine
[^{11}C]-GMO	*N*-[^{11}C]-Guanyl-(−)-*meta*-octopamine
[^{11}C]-mHED	[^{11}C]-*meta*-(−)-Hydroxyephedrine
[^{11}C]-MHPG	[^{11}C]-*meta*-Hydroxyphenethylguanidine
[^{11}C]-PHEN	[^{11}C]-(−)-Phenylephrine
[^{11}C]-PHPG	[^{11}C]-*para*-Hydroxyphenethylguanidine
[^{123}I]	Iodine-123
[^{123}I]-MIBG	[^{123}I]-Metaiodobenzylguanidine
[^{123}I]-MIBG	Iodine-123 metaiodobenzylguanidine
[^{131}I]-RIBA	[^{131}I]-*O*-Iodobenzyltrimethylammonium iodide
[^{18}F]-4F-MHPG	4-[^{18}F]-Fluoro-*met*a-hydroxyphenethylguanidine
[^{3}H]-NE	[^{3}H]-Labeled norepinephrine
[^{99m}Tc]	Technetium-99m
6-OHDA	6-Hydroxydopamine
AA	Serum amyloid A protein type of amyloidosis
AAAD	Aromatic l-amino acid decarboxylase
AADC	Aromatic amino acid decarboxylase
AC	Adenylate cyclase
ACE	Angiotensin-converting enzyme
ACEI	Angiotensin-converting enzyme inhibitor
ACh	Acetylcholine
ACLS	Advanced cardiac life support
ADH	Aldehyde dehydrogenase
ADR	Aldehyde reductase
AF	Atrial fibrillation
AHA	American Heart Association
AL	Immunoglobulin light chain type of amyloidosis
AMP	Adenosine monophosphate
ANS	Autonomic nervous system
APD	Action potential duration
AR	Adrenoceptor
ARB	Angiotensin receptor blocker

ARI	Activation recovery interval
ARIC	Atherosclerosis Risk in Communities
ARVC/D	Arrhythmogenic right ventricular cardiomyopathy/dysplasia
ARVD/C	Arrhythmogenic right ventricular dysplasia/cardiomyopathy
ATP	Adenosine triphosphate
ATRMI	Autonomic Tone and Reflexes After Myocardial Infarction
ATTR	Transthyretin type of amyloidosis
AUC	Area under the curve
BET	Bacterial endotoxin tests
BGO	Bismuth germanate
BMC	Bone marrow cell
BNP	Brain natriuretic peptide
BNP	B-type natriuretic peptide
BRS	Baroreflex sensitivity
BS	Brugada syndrome
C6-hNET	Cloned human NET (cells)
CAD	Coronary artery disease
CAG	Coronary angiography
cAMP	Cyclic adenosine 3′,5′-monophosphate
cAMP	Cyclic adenosine monophosphate
CAN	Cardiac autonomic neuropathy
CBD	Corticobasal degeneration
CG	Chromogranins
cGMP	Cyclic guanine monophosphate
cGRPP	Current good radiopharmacy practice
CHD	Coronary heart disease
CHF	Chronic heart failure
CI	Confidence interval
CKD	Chronic kidney disease
CMV	Cytomegalovirus
CNS	Central nervous system
CO	Cardiac output
COMT	Catechol-*O*-methyltransferase
CRP	C-reactive protein
CRS	Cardiorenal syndromes
CRT	Cardiac resynchronization therapy
CSNS	Cardiac sympathetic nervous system
CT	Computed tomography
CV	Cardiovascular
DA	Dopamine
DAG	Diacylglycerol
DAT	Dopamine transporter
DCM	Dilated cardiomyopathy
DDC	DOPA-decarboxylase
DLB	Dementia with Lewy bodies

DM	Diabetes mellitus
DMI	Desipramine
DMSO	Dimethyl sulfoxide
DOMA	Dihydroxymandelic acid
DOPA	Dihydroxyphenylalanine
DOPAC	Dihydroxyphenylacetic acid
DOPEG	Dihydroxyphenylglycol
DSM-V	The Diagnostic and Statistical Manual of Mental Disorders (version 5)
DβH	Dopamine-β-hydroxylase
EANM	European Association of Nuclear Medicine
ECG	Electrocardiogram
EF	Ejection fraction
EMA	European Medicine Agency
EMT	Extraneuronal monoamine transporter
eNOS	Endothelial isoform of NO synthase
EP	Electrophysiological
EP	Electrophysiology
EPHESUS	Eplerenone Post-Acute Myocardial Infarction Heart Failure Efficacy and Survival Study
Epi	Epinephrine
EPS	Electrophysiological studies
ERP	Effective refractory period
ESRD	End-stage renal disease
FAP	Familial amyloid polyneuropathy
FDA	Food and Drug Administration
FDG	Fluorodeoxyglucose
FHS	Framingham Heart Study
FNE	Fluoronorepinephrine
FP-CIT	[123I]-*N*-ω-Fluoropropyl-2β-carbomethoxy-3β-(4-iodophenyl) nortropan
GAD	Generalised anxiety disorder
GAP43	Growth-associated protein 43
GCP	Good clinical practice
GDP	Good distribution practice
GFR	Glomerular filtration rate
GI	Gastrointestinal
GMP	Good Manufacturing Practice
GRPP	Guidelines on good radiopharmacy practice
GSO	Gadolinium oxyorthosilicate
H/L	Heart to lung
H/M	Heart-to-mediastinum ratio
HCM	Hypertrophic cardiomyopathy
HD	Hemodialysis
HDL	High-density lipoprotein
HER2	Human epidermal growth factor receptor type 2

HF	Heart failure
HF	High frequency
HLA	Human leukocyte antigen
HLA	Horizontal long axis
HMG-CoA	3-Hydroxy-3-methylglutaryl-coenzyme A
HMR	Heart to mediastinum ratio
HP	Heart period
HPLC	High-performance liquid chromatography
HR	Heart rate
HRV	Heart rate variability
HTX	Heart transplantation
HTX	Heart transplant surgery
IBI	Inter-beat intervals
IBZM	[123I]-(S)-2-Hydroxy-3-iodo-6-methoxy-*N*-[1-ethyl-2-pyrrodinyl)-methyl]benzamide
ICC	Interstitial cells of Cajal
ICD	Implantable cardioverter defibrillator
ICN	Intracardiac neurons
ID	Injected dose
IDC	Idiopathic dilated cardiomyopathy
IDH	Intradialytic hypotension
IEC	Independent ethics committee
IHD	Ischaemic heart disease
IL-6	Interleukin-6
ILVT	Idiopathic left ventricular tachycardias
IMP	Investigational medicinal product
IMPD	Investigational medicinal product dossier
INA	Integrated nerve activity
IP3	Inositol trisphosphate
IPKI	Isoquinolinesulfonamide protein kinase inhibitor
IVF	Idiopathic ventricular fibrillation
IVT	Idiopathic ventricular tachycardias
JCS	Japanese Circulation Society
JSNM	Japanese Society of Nuclear Medicine
LA	Left atrium
LABDA	Low-amplitude burst discharge activity
LAD	Left anterior descending (artery)
LBBB	Left bundle branch block
LBD	Lewy body diseases
LDL	Low-density lipoprotein
LE	Low energy
LEHR	Low-energy high-resolution
LF	Low frequency
LOR	Line of response
LP	Late ventricular potentials

LQTS	Long QT syndrome
LSO	Lutetium oxyorthosilicate
LV	Left ventricular
LVAD	Left ventricular assist device
LVEF	Left ventricular ejection fraction
MA	Marketing authorization
mAChR	Muscarinic acetylcholine receptor
MAO	Monoamine oxidase
MBF	Myocardial blood flow
MCE	Major cardiac event
ME	Medium energy
mHED	Metahydroxyephedrine
MI	Myocardial infarction
MIBG	Metaiodobenzylguanidine
MPI	Myocardial perfusion imaging
MQNB	Methylquinuclidinylbenzilat
MRA	Mineralocorticoid receptor antagonists
MRI	Magnetic resonance imaging
MSA	Multiple system atrophy
MTA	Microvolt T-wave alternans
MTD	Maximum tolerated dose
MUGA	Multi-gated radionuclide ventriculography
MUGA	Multiple gated acquisition
MVO2	Myocardial oxygen consumption
nAChR	Nicotinic acetylcholine receptor
NADPH	Nicotinamide adenine dinucleotide phosphate
NE	Norepinephrine
NET	Norepinephrine transporter
NGF	Nerve growth factor
NHP	Nonhuman primate
NIDDM	Non-insulin-dependent diabetes mellitus
NMS	*N*-Methylscopolamine
nNOS	Neuronal nitric oxide synthase
NO	Nitric oxide
NOAEL	No-adverse-effect level
NPV	Negative predictive value
NRI	Net reclassification improvement
NSX	Nisoxetine
nTS	Nucleus of the solitary tract
NYHA	New York Heart Association
OCT	Organic cation transporters
OCT3	Organic cation transporter 3
OR	Odds ratio
P	P wave
PAF	Pure autonomic failure

PAPS	Adenosine-3′-phosphate-5′-phosphosulfate
PAR	Population attributable risks
PD	Parkinson disease
PDE	Phosphodiesterases
PDE4	Phosphodiesterase-4
PET	Positron emission tomography
PET/CT	Positron emission tomography/computed tomography
PHEN	Phenylephrine
PKA	Protein kinase A
PKC	Protein kinase C
PLC	Phospholipase C
PMNT	Phenylethanolamine methyltransferase
PSNS	Parasympathetic nervous system
PSP	Progressive supranuclear palsy
PTSD	Post-traumatic stress disorders
PVI	Pulmonary vein isolation
QA	Quality assurance unit
QC	Quality control
QNB	3-Quinuclidinyl benzilate (or quinuclidin-3-yl benzilate)
QP	Qualified person
RA	Right atrium
RAAS	Renin-angiotensin-aldosterone system
RAS	Renin-angiotensin system
RBBB	Right bundle branch block
RBC(s)	Red blood cell(s)
RBX	Reboxetine
RCSD	Regional cardiac sympathetic denervation
RI	Retention index
RMSSD	Root-mean-square successive RR-interval difference
ROC	Receiver Operating Characteristic
ROI	Region of interest
RPP	Rate-pressure product
RR	R-wave to R-wave
RRT	Renal replacement therapy
RV	Right ventricle
RVOT	Right ventricular outflow tract tachycardia
RWMA	Regional wall motion abnormalities
SA	Short axis
SAECG	Signal-averaged ECG
SAP	Serum amyloid P component
SCA	Sudden cardiac arrest
SCD	Sudden cardiac death
SD	Standard deviation

SDNN	Standard deviation of normal RR intervals
SDNN	Standard deviation of normal to normal (NN) interval
SE	Standard error
SHFM	Seattle Heart Failure Model
SLC	Solute carrier transporters
SNARE	Soluble *N*-ethylmaleimide-sensitive factor attachment protein receptor
SNC	Sympathetic nerve chain
SNS	Sympathetic nervous system
SOP	Standard operating procedures
SPECT	Single-photon computed emission tomography
SROC	Summary receiver operating characteristic
SSRP	Small-scale radiopharmaceuticals
STEMI	ST-segment elevation myocardial infarct
STZ	Streptozotocin
SUV	Standardized uptake value
TAC	Time–activity curve
TBP	Tributyl phosphate
TFA	Trifluoroacetic acid
TH	Tyrosine hydroxylase
TMR	Transmyocardial laser revascularization
t-SNARE	t-Soluble *N*-ethylmaleimide-sensitive factor attachment protein receptor
TTE	Transthoracic echocardiography
TTR	Transthyretin
TUI	Time urgency/impatience
Tyr	Tyrosine
UDPGA	Uridine 5′-diphosphoglucuronic acid
VF	Ventricular fibrillation
VLA	Vertical long axis
VLF	Very low frequency
VMAT	Vesicular monoamine transporter
VMAT2	Vesicular monoamine transporter 2
VOI	Volume of interest
V_R	Volume of reaction
VS	Vagal stimulation
VT	Ventricular tachycardia
WBC	White blood cell count
WR	Washout rate
βAR	β-Adrenergic receptors

The Autonomic Nervous System of the Heart

1

Irma Battipaglia and Gaetano A. Lanza

Contents

Abstract

The *autonomic nervous system* (ANS) is the part of the nervous system that controls the visceral functions of the body, which are totally or largely independent of voluntary control of the individual. This part of the nervous system consists of autonomic regions in the central nervous system and of peripheral nerves. According to anatomical and functional characteristics, the ANS is classically divided into two main sections: the sympathetic and the parasympathetic systems. The former division promotes a so-called "fight-or-flight" response, while the parasympathetic autonomic system promotes a "rest and

I. Battipaglia, MD
Department of Cardiological Sciences, Università Cattolica del Sacro Cuore, Rome, Italy

G.A. Lanza, MD (✉)
Department of Cardiological Sciences, Università Cattolica del Sacro Cuore, Rome, Italy
e-mail: g.a.lanza@rm.unicatt.it

R.H.J.A. Slart et al. (eds.), *Autonomic Innervation of the Heart: Role of Molecular Imaging*, DOI 10.1007/978-3-662-45074-1_1

digest" response of the organism. The heart receives nerve fibers from both the sympathetic and the parasympathetic divisions, which variably contribute to the control of heart rate (chronotropism), contractile strength of the heart (inotropism), conductivity (dromotropism) and excitability (bathmotropism) of myocardial cells, as well as of coronary vascular tone and myocardial blood flow. The sympathetic system promotes an increase in heart rate and a positive inotropic response in order to increase cardiac output. On the contrary, the parasympathetic (vagal) system induces bradycardia and reduces myocardial contractile strength, thus resulting in decreased cardiac output.

Abbreviations

ANS	Autonomic nervous system
CNS	Central nervous system
GI	Gastrointestinal
MBF	Myocardial blood flow
nTS	Nucleus of the solitary tract
PET	Positron emission tomography
SNC	Sympathetic nerve chain

The *autonomic nervous system* (ANS) plays an outstanding role in the regulation of heart function. In this chapter, we will briefly review the anatomy and basic function of the cardiac ANS. A full understanding of the topic, however, presumes a sufficient knowledge of the whole structure of the ANS.

1.1 Overview of the ANS

The ANS is the part of the nervous system that controls the visceral functions of the body, which are usually below the level of consciousness, and therefore totally or largely independent of the voluntary control of the individual, including heart activity, respiratory function, digestion, gland secretory activity, organ and vessel motility, pupillary dilation, micturition, and sexual arousal.

The ANS is constituted by autonomic regions in the central nervous system and by peripheral nerves. The former consist of brainstem nuclei and bundles of visceral nerve fibers in the spinal cord, which have motor (efferent) and sensory (afferent) functions; the latter are represented by nerve fibers and ganglia.

The transmission of efferent autonomic impulses occurs through a sequential two-neuron pathway: a preganglionic (or presynaptic) neuron and a postganglionic (or postsynaptic) neuron. Preganglionic neurons origin from autonomic centers in the brain or spinal cord and synapse onto postganglionic neurons, which are located in peripheral ganglia, from where they innervate the target organ (Burt 1993).

According to anatomical and functional characteristics, the ANS is classically divided into two main sections: the sympathetic and the parasympathetic ANS.

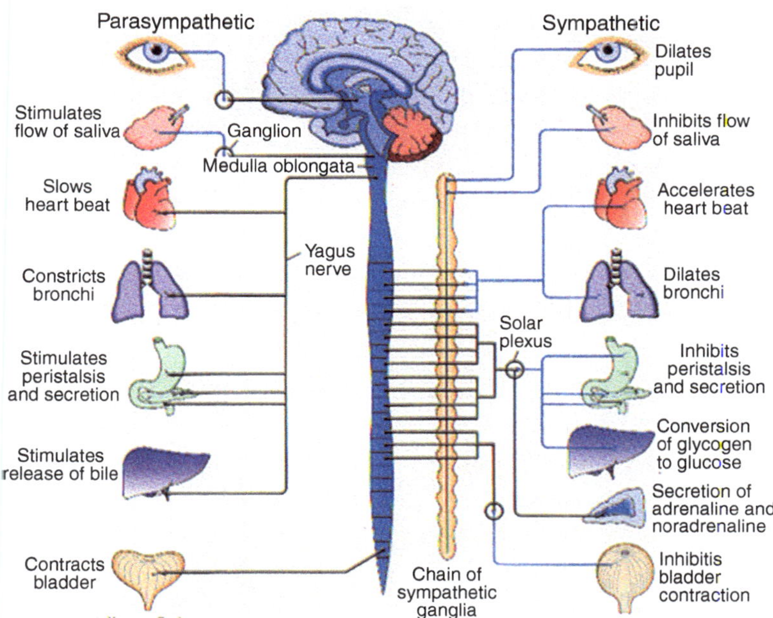

Fig. 1.1 Scheme of the sympathetic and parasympathetic nervous system (see text for description)

1.1.1 The Sympathetic ANS

A scheme of the sympathetic ANS is illustrated in Fig. 1.1. The sympathetic ANS division has a thoracolumbar "outflow," i.e., the cell bodies of the efferent preganglionic neurons are located in the intermediolateral columns of the thoracic and lumbar segments (from T1 to L2–L3) of the spinal cord. Preganglionic neurons are type B myelinated nerve fibers (<3 μm) that leave the spinal cord through the anterior roots of the respective thoracic and lumbar spinal nerves and reach the *sympathetic nerve chain* (SNC) through small white rami communicantes (Fig. 1.2).

The SNC runs on either side of the anterior face of vertebral bodies, extending from the cranium base to the coccyx and includes paravertebral ganglia along its course, specifically, 3 cervical ganglia, 11 or 12 thoracic ganglia, and 5 lumbar, 4 sacral, and 1 coccyx ganglia, which are interconnected by intermediate cords and contain the bodies of postganglionic sympathetic neurons (Fig. 1.1).

Preganglionic axons coming from a given spinal segment and nerve may terminate onto a postganglionic neuron located in the corresponding segmental ganglion or may instead travel either up or down along the SNC, synapsing onto a postganglionic neuron located in another SNC paravertebral ganglion.

Some sympathetic preganglionic fibers do not synapse in paravertebral ganglia but from SNC arrive to some specific *prevertebral ganglia* in the lumbar region (celiac, aorticorenal, and mesenteric ganglia) or ganglia located very proximal to

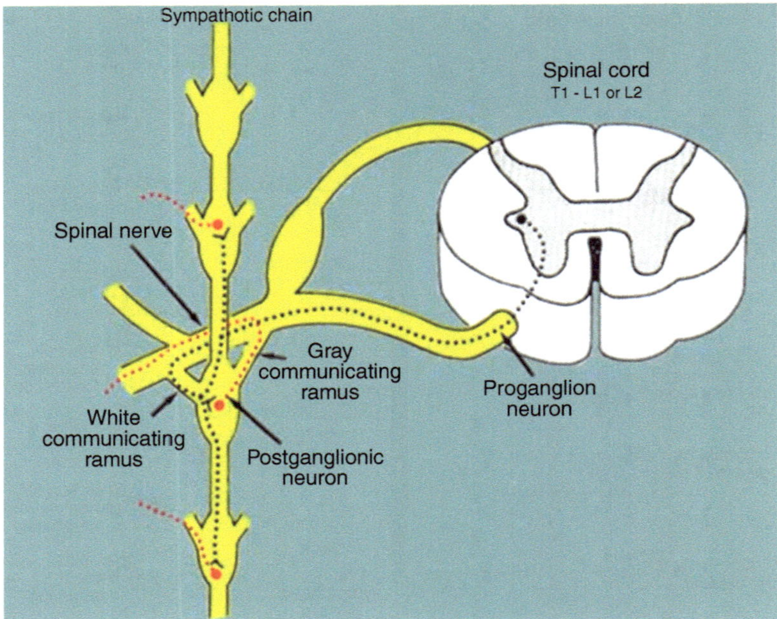

Fig. 1.2 Nerve connections between the spinal cord, spinal nerves, sympathetic nervous chain, and peripheral sympathetic nerves

target organs (*peripheral ganglia*). Finally, the SNC also sends out peripheral nerves that reach the target organs following the course of vessels (*perivascular branches*).

Postganglionic neurons are small nonmyelinated C fibers (0.3–1.2 μm) that reach the target organs by various ways. Some achieve somatic structures of the body (skin, muscles, bones) through spinal nerves that they reach from the SNC by gray rami communicantes (Fig. 1.2); some from cervical and high thoracic ganglia directly achieve cranial structures through peripheral nervous branches; similarly, visceral thoracic and abdominal organs receive sympathetic innervation from postganglionic fibers originating from sympathetic (cervical, thoracic, and splanchnic) ganglia.

1.1.2 The Parasympathetic ANS

A scheme of the parasympathetic ANS is illustrated in Fig. 1.1. The parasympathetic ANS division has craniosacral "outflow," i.e., the preganglionic efferent neurons leave the central nervous system through cranial nerves (III, VII, IX, X) or together with the anterior roots of sacral spinal nerves (mainly S2–S3, but also S1 and S4). Cell bodies of cranial parasympathetic preganglionic neurons are located in some nuclei of the brainstem, whereas those of sacral neurons are located at the base of the intermediolateral portion of the anterior horns of the gray substance of the respective spinal segments.

Parasympathetic postganglionic neurons have cell bodies located in parasympathetic ganglia, which are always found peripherally, next to, or also within, the target organs, and are always reached by preganglionic parasympathetic fibers through somatic nerves.

It is worth noting that 75 % of all parasympathetic nerve fibers are situated in the vagus nerve (X cranial nerve). Vagal fibers mostly originate from the *dorsal motor nucleus* and, in part, from the *ambiguous nucleus*. The vagus nerve sorts out of the central nervous system through the jugular foramen at each side and travels down until the abdomen, giving branches to thoracic and upper abdominal organs.

1.1.3 Afferent ANS Fibers

As for the somatic sensitive system, signals from visceral organs are transmitted by *primary sensory neurons*. The afferent fibers originated from visceral organs travel in sympathetic and parasympathetic nerves and transmit information to the central nervous system about activities of the organ or the occurrence of tissue injury, the latter through nociceptive fibers. These signals also generate autonomic reflexes which allow regulation of organ functions. Some of these signals (e.g., pain signals) can be transmitted to cortical centers and become conscious.

Nociceptive fibers are mainly associated with sympathetic nerves. Their cell bodies are located in spinal ganglia, achieved through the SNC and rami communicantes, and they end in the posterior roots of the spinal cord, where they synapse on "second-order" nociceptive neurons. Nociceptive visceral fibers are much less numerous than nociceptive somatic fibers and usually end at more levels in the spinal cord, thus generating less specific and localized pain sensation.

Afferent primary sensory fibers associated with parasympathetic nerves are more involved in regulatory reflexes of system/organ activities. Again, they are mainly associated with the vagus nerve, but several visceral cranial afferent fibers travel with the glossopharyngeal or facial nerves and pelvic fibers with pelvic nerves. The cell bodies of these afferent fibers are located in ganglia associated with these parasympathetic nerves. Primary sensory neurons then project onto "second-order" visceral sensory neurons located in the medulla oblongata, in the *nucleus of the solitary tract*, and other nuclei.

1.1.4 The Enteric ANS

It is worth noting that enteric ganglia diffused inside the wall of the digestive tube collectively contain as many neurons as the entire spinal cord, including local sensory neurons, motor neurons, and interneurons, and is able to act as a largely autonomous part of the ANS. For this reason, the enteric ANS is often considered as a third, independent part of the ANS.

1.2 Function of the ANS

A description of the functions of the ANS is beyond the scope of this chapter, and therefore some general concepts only are discussed here.

The sympathetic and parasympathetic systems are generally thought to act in opposition to each other. However, their effects in most organs should be better considered as complementary in nature rather than antagonistic, with most visceral functions resulting from the balance of the influence of the two ANS branches (Guyton and Hall 2006). Furthermore, some viscera (e.g., visceral vessels, liver, spleen) only receive sympathetic innervations, and in other cases sympathetic and parasympathetic nerves have synergic effects (e.g., increase of salivary gland secretion).

Overall, however, the sympathetic ANS is typically activated in conditions of stress and is responsible for the so-called "fight-or-flight" response, which is characterized by enhanced heart rate and contractility, dilation of coronary vessels, bronchiole dilation and increased alveolar oxygen exchange, increased blood flow to skeletal muscles, and reduction of blood flow to the gastrointestinal tract and skin.

The parasympathetic ANS, instead, predominates in basal conditions, defining the so-called "rest and digest" status, which is characterized by dilation of blood vessels and accelerated peristalsis of the gastrointestinal tract, together with reduction of cardiac and respiratory activities.

The peripheral effects of sympathetic and parasympathetic systems are mediated by the release from nerve endings of specific chemical neurotransmitters, which act on specific receptors on cell membranes of target organs.

The neuromediator released by peripheral sympathetic fibers and therefore responsible for their effects is *norepinephrine*, while *acetylcholine* is the neuromediator released by parasympathetic nerve fibers (Fig. 1.3). Together with these primary neuromediator, both sympathetic and parasympathetic nerve fibers can variably release other substances, mainly neuropeptides, which can contribute to the final effects of nerve stimulation. Examples of these substances include neuropeptide Y, galanin, and dynorphin in noradrenergic fibers, and vasoactive intestinal peptide, calcitonin gene-related peptide, and substance P in cholinergic fibers (Jänig 2006). The exact role of most of these co-released substances, however, remains to be defined.

It is also worth noting that postganglionic sympathetic fibers for sweat glands and for skeletal muscle vessels release acetylcholine and that acetylcholine is also

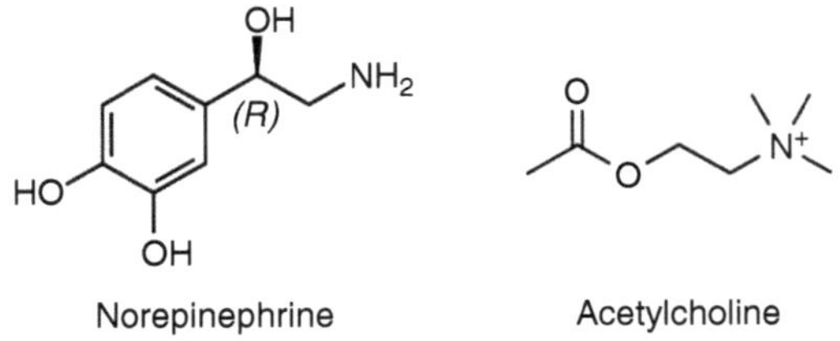

Fig. 1.3 Chemical structure of the sympathetic (norepinephrine) and parasympathetic (acetylcholine) neurotransmitters

Norepinephrine

Acetylcholine

the neurotrasnmitter of both sympathetic and parasympathetic signals by preganglionic neurons in the respective ganglia.

Norepinephrine exerts its effects through binding and activation of adrenergic receptors on target cells. Two main classes of adrenergic receptors have been described, the α- and β-receptors (Ahlquist 1948). The α-adrenergic receptors present two main types α1- and α2-receptors. Similarly, two main types of β-adrenergic receptors have been found, β1- and β2-receptors, although a third type (β3) has recently been found to also play some relevant physiological role (Bylund et al. 1994).

Acetylcholine binding (cholinergic) receptors are also divided into two main classes, based on their response to the alkaloids nicotine and muscarine. Nicotinic receptors can roughly be grouped in two main classes, muscular and neuronal receptors. Five different types of muscarinic receptors have been described, named M1 to M5, with M2 and M3 being the receptors mainly located in the heart and bronchi, respectively (Goyal 1989).

1.3 The ANS of the Heart

1.3.1 Anatomy

The heart receives abundant nerve fibers from both the sympathetic and the parasympathetic ANS.

Preganglionic sympathetic neurons for the heart have their cell bodies in the lateral horns of the spinal cord, at the level of the first 4–5 thoracic segments, and they synapse onto postganglionic nerve fibers located in paravertebral cervical and thoracic ganglia of the SNC, which give origin to *cardiac cervical nerves* (superior, medium, and inferior) and *cardiac thoracic nerves* (from the 2nd to the 4th–5th thoracic ganglia) (Fig. 1.4).

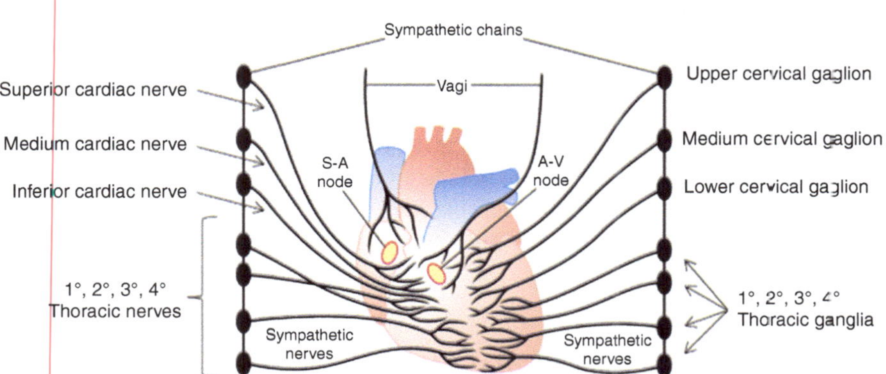

Fig. 1.4 Scheme of the sympathetic and parasympathetic (vagal) innervations of the heart (Modified from Guyton and Hall (2006))

The *superior cardiac nerves* origin, on each side, from the inferior portion of the superior cervical ganglia. They go down to the heart following a different way: the right nerve runs behind the anonymous artery and the aortic arch; the left nerve follows the left common carotid artery. The *medium cardiac nerves*, the biggest among cardiac nerves, derive from the medium cervical ganglia and can reach the cardiac plexus directly, without fusion with other nerve fibers. Finally, the *inferior cardiac nerves* derive from the stellate ganglia and directly arrive to the cardiac plexus.

The efferent parasympathetic preganglionic nerve fibers originate in the medulla oblongata and reach the heart through the two vagal nerves. The postganglionic efferent neurons reside in the inferior ganglia of the vagus nerves or in the cardiac plexus.

The *cardiac plexus* is situated at the base of the heart, in front of the tracheal bifurcation, and below and behind the aortic arch. It consists of the confluence of various, both sympathetic and vagal, cardiac nerves and of a variable number of little parasympathetic ganglia, among which the most remarkable and constant is Wrisberg's ganglion, which is located between the tracheal bifurcation and the pulmonary artery division. Some little parasympathetic ganglia are also located inside the myocardial walls, mainly at atrial level.

The cardiac plexus can be divided into a superficial part, which lies in the concavity of the aortic arch, and a deep part, situated between the aortic arch and the trachea. The two parts are closely connected and provide autonomic innervation to the sinoatrial node, atrioventricular node, atrial and ventricular myocardium, as well as large and small vessel walls.

Afferent nerve fibers from the heart mainly travel in sympathetic cardiac nerves. Many nervous sensory receptorial units, which may consist of either free ending terminations or encapsulated nervous endings, can easily be detected in the heart, especially at subendocardial level and at the level of vena cava and pulmonary veins mergers, interatrial septum, and atrioventricular valve limbs. Cell bodies of sympathetic-sensitive neurons are situated in the first 4–5 spinal thoracic ganglia. Second-order sympathetic sensory fibers originated in the spinal cord cross the median line and ascend in the ventral spinothalamic tract to end in the posteroventral nucleus of the thalamus.

Afferent vagal fibers have also been detected in the heart and play a role primarily in mediating some cardiac reflexes (Gibbins et al. 2003). Stretch receptors present in the atria contribute to minimize changes in arterial pressure following changes in blood volume (Di Carlo and Bishop 2001); their stimulation causes a reflex inhibition of vagal activity and an increase in heart rate (Bainbridge reflex). Stimulation of stretch receptors in the left ventricle can, instead, typically result in vagal-mediated hypotensive and bradycardic responses (Jarisch-Bezold reflex) (Guyton and Hall 2006).

1.3.2 Function of the ANS of the Heart

The autonomic innervation of the heart considerably contributes to the regulation and control of cardiac functions and activities, including heart beat rate (chronotropism), conductivity of the electrical signal (dromotropism) and excitability (bathmotropism), and contractile strength (inotropism) of myocardial cells. Furthermore, the ANS also plays a relevant role in the regulation of coronary vascular motility and myocardial blood flow (MBF).

As in the whole body, the sympathetic and parasympathetic sections of the ANS have also antagonistic effects on most heart functions. Of note, however, they do not necessarily have comparable effects and influence on the various parts of the heart. Instead, some cardiac activities are mainly influenced by one of the two sections, depending on differences in their distribution to the heart.

Thus, sympathetic activation significantly increases myocardial contractility in all heart chambers, whereas vagal activation significantly inhibits atrial contractility, but has poor effects on ventricular cardiomyocytes, due to the poor distribution of vagal fibers to the ventricles. Vagal stimulation, however, can mitigate the increased inotropism resulting from increased β-stimulation of the heart.

1.3.2.1 Effects of the Sympathetic ANS

Overall, the sympathetic division has an excitatory effect on most heart function. The heart is indeed a major target organ in the "fight-or-flight" response associated with sympathetic activation in physical or stressful conditions, as well as in all conditions that require an increase in cardiac output.

Thus, the sympathetic ANS promotes an increase in heart rate (up to 200 bpm and more in young adults), by speeding up the depolarization current rate of the cells of the sinus node. This effect is accompanied by an increase in the velocity of conduction and a reduction of the functional refractory period in the conduction system of the heart, in particular of the AV junction, besides an increase in myocardial contractility to as much as double of normal, with a consequent increase of stroke volume. Furthermore, sympathetic activation also enhances cardiac electrical activation and contractility of both atrial and ventricular myocardial cells.

It is important to stress that conditions associated with activation of the adrenergic ANS also lead to catecholamine release by the adrenal gland (mainly adrenaline) which determines blood-borne-related adrenergic effects on the whole heart.

The effects of catecholamines on myocardial cells are mainly mediated by β1-receptors.

In the healthy human heart, indeed, β1-adrenoceptors are predominant (β1 to β2 ratio = 3:1) and are distributed in all cardiac regions. β2-Adrenoceptors are instead mainly concentrated in the ventricles and atria, where they are functionally linked to inotropic responses. The presence of β3-adrenoceptor in the human heart, on the other hand, is still a matter of debate (Lefkowitz et al. 1984). A summary of adrenergic receptors involved in mediating sympathetic effects on the heart is reported in Table 1.1.

1.3.2.2 Effects of the Parasympathetic (Vagal) ANS

In opposition with sympathetic activity, the parasympathetic (vagal) division of the ANS has inhibitory effects on most heart function. Thus, the sinus node activity is

Table 1.1 Main effects of sympathetic and vagal ANS on the heart and coronary arteries

Target organs	Sympathetic effects		Vagal effects	
	Receptor type (adrenergic)	Effect	Receptor type (muscarinic)	Effect
Heart				
SA node	β1, β2	Heart rate increase	M2	Heart rate decrease
Atria	β1, β2	↑Contractility	M2	↓Contractility
		↑Conduction velocity		↑Conduction velocity
AV node and conduction system	β1, β2	↑Conduction velocity	M2	↓Conduction velocity: AV block
Ventricles	β1, β2	↑Contractility	–	
		↑Conduction velocity		
		↑Automatism		
		↑Ventricular foci excitability		
Coronary arteries	α1, α2	Constriction	M3	Mild dilation
	β2	Dilation		

slowed down, resulting in bradycardia and sinus pauses or blocks; similarly, electrical conduction through the AV node is significantly delayed and can even be blocked. On the other hand, vagal activation has no relevant effects on intraventricular conduction.

Vagal fibers are, indeed, mainly distributed to the atria and not much to the ventricles, even if a strong vagal stimulation can decrease the strength of heart muscle contraction by about 20 %. The effects of vagal activation on atrial cells, on the other hand, are characterized by a reduction of contractile activity but an increase in conduction speed due to a reduction in action potential duration, which can favor some reentrant tachyarrhythmias.

The effects of the vagus nerve on the heart are mediated by cholinergic M2 receptors, whereas its mild direct vasodilating effect on coronary arteries is mediated by M3 receptors (Table 1.1).

1.3.2.3 Sympatho-vagal Balance

As discussed about the general function of the ANS, in rest conditions the heart is mainly under the influence of vagal activity. Thus, sinus node discharge (i.e., heart rate) and AV nodal conduction are substantially determined by the level of vagal activation.

In fact, in rest conditions, the sympathetic nerve fibers to the heart discharge continuously at a slow rate, determining a pumping force just of 30 % above that without any sympathetic stimulation; accordingly, inhibition of sympathetic ANS activity at rest only induces a modest depression of myocardial contractility. Similar considerations apply to sinus node firing.

During exercise or stress arousal, instead, vagal activity is progressively suppressed and sympathetic drive enhances, thus resulting in a predominant sympathetic cardiac stimulation. Thus, adrenergic inhibition in these conditions may significantly blunt the increase in heart rate and contractile force.

1.4 ANS Regulation of Coronary Blood Flow

The ANS in the heart also considerably contributes to the regulation of coronary artery tone and, even more, of MBF, together with biochemical and physical factors.

The ANS influences MBF both in a direct and in an indirect way (Crea et al. 2013). The latter depends on the fact that, as discussed above, the activity of the ANS is a major determinant of heart rate and myocardial contractility, and therefore of myocardial oxygen consumption, which, in turn, is the fundamental determinant of MBF. Thus, any increase in sympathetic activity leads to an increase in cardiac metabolism, which results in a local release of vasodilator substances and, eventually, in MBF. The opposite is achieved through inhibition of adrenergic activity and/or increase in vagal activity.

The direct effect of sympathetic stimulation on coronary vascular tone and MBF depends on the balance between α- and β-adrenergic receptors located in coronary vessels walls. Specifically, smooth muscle cells of coronary vessels mainly contain α_1-receptors and β_2-receptors. Stimulation of α_1-receptors results in coronary vasoconstriction; instead, β_2-stimulation mediates coronary vasodilation. Smaller coronary arteries mainly contain β_2-adrenergic receptors, whereas epicardial larger coronary arteries mainly have α_1-adrenergic receptors. The final physiologic effect of sympathetic activation is a mild to moderate vasodilation and increase in MBF.

On the other hand, while the indirect effect of vagal stimulation of the heart is vasoconstriction, due to the reduced myocardial oxygen consumption, the very limited direct effect of parasympathetic stimulation on coronary vessels is a mild vasodilation, which is likely mediated by a release of NO from endothelial cells (Pelc et al. 1988).

References

Ahlquist RP (1948) A study of the adrenotropic receptors. Am J Physiol 153:586–600

Burt AM (1993) Textbook of neuroanatomy. WB Saunders Company, Philadelphia

Bylund DB et al (1994) International Union of Pharmacology nomenclature of adrenoceptors. Pharmacol Rev 46:121–136

Crea F et al (2013) Coronary microvascular dysfunction. Springer, Milan

Di Carlo SE, Bishop VS (2001) Central baroreflex resetting as a means of increasing and decreasing sympathetic outflow and arterial pressure. Ann N Y Acad Sci 940:324–337

Gibbins IL et al (2003) Functional organization of peripheral vasomotor pathways. Acta Physiol Scand 177:237–245

Goyal RK (1989) Muscarinic receptor subtypes. Physiology and clinical implications. N Engl J Med 321:1022–1029

Guyton AC, Hall JE (2006) Textbook of medical physiology. Elsevier Saunders, Philadelphia

Jänig W (2006) The integrative action of the autonomic nervous system. Cambridge University Press, Cambridge, 2006

Lefkowitz RJ et al (1984) Mechanisms of membrane-receptor regulation: biochemical, physiological and clinical insights derived from studies of the adrenergic receptors. N Engl J Med 310:1570–1579

Pelc LR et al (1988) Muscarinic receptor subtypes mediating myocardial blood flow redistribution. J Cardiovasc Pharmacol 11:424–431

Electrophysiology and Pathophysiology of the Autonomic Nervous System of the Heart

2

Carlo de Asmundis, Guy Van Camp, and Pedro Brugada

Contents

C. de Asmundis, MD, PhD (✉)
Heart Rhythm Management Centre, Universitair Ziekenhuis Brussel, Vrije Universiteit Brussel, Laarbeeklaan 101, Brussel 1090, Belgium
e-mail: carlodeasmundis@me.com; carlo.deasmundis@uzbrussel.be

G. Van Camp, MD, PhD
Department of Cardiology, Universitair Ziekenhuis Brussel, Vrije Universiteit Brussel, Laarbeeklaan 101, Brussel 1090, Belgium

P. Brugada, MD, PhD
Cardiovascular Division, Heart Rhythm Management Centre, Universitair Ziekenhuis Brussel, Vrije Universiteit Brussel, Laarbeeklaan 101, Brussel 1090, Belgium

R.H.J A. Slart et al. (eds.), *Autonomic Innervation of the Heart: Role of Molecular Imaging*, DOI 10.1007/978-3-662-45074-1_2

Abstract

The autonomic nervous system has an important role in the genesis, maintenance, and interruption of arrhythmias. Characterisation of the extrinsic and intrinsic cardiac nervous systems dates back to studies from the 1930s and ranges from recognition of anatomic relationships at the gross anatomic level to discovery of chemoreceptors, mechanoreceptors, and ganglionated plexuses lining specific regions along the veins, arteries, and cardiac chambers. However, with the increasing recognition of anatomic and functional relationships between the nervous system and the heart, also comes a litany of new questions. Specifically, studies to date have revealed the large degree of complexity. Furthermore, the clinical correlation of ex vivo cell-based and isolated perfusion models of the heart has been limited due to anatomic accessibility in recording simultaneous neuronal and cardiac electrophysiologic activity during in vivo electrophysiology studies. Partly because of these limitations, the study of autonomic cardiac electrophysiology remains in its early stages, with several studies pointing towards potential novel and elegant methods of treating electrophysiologic disease, but much remains to be done to translate these findings into clinical practice. In this chapter, we will briefly discuss anatomic aspects of the extrinsic and intrinsic cardiac nervous systems, how these various ganglia and nerves may integrate in modulating cardiac electrophysiology, and their relationships to a variety of electrophysiologic diseases. We will also discuss both current and future avenues of research as they relate to the fundamental understanding of how the cardiac-autonomic interface may offer itself to novel therapeutic targets for treating electrophysiologic diseases.

Abbreviations

ACEi	Angiotensin-converting enzyme inhibitors
ACLS	Advanced cardiac life support
AF	Atrial fibrillation
ANS	Autonomic nervous system
APD	Action potential duration
ARI	Activation recovery interval
BRS	Baroreflex sensitivity
cAMP	Cyclic adenosine monophosphate
EF	Ejection fraction
ERP	Effective refractory period
FHS	Framingham heart study
HRV	Heart rate variability
ICC	Interstitial cells of Cajal

ICD	Implantable cardioverter defibrillator
LAD	Left anterior descending artery
MI	Myocardial infarction
MIBG	Metaiodobenzylguanidine
NADPH	Nicotinamide adenine dinucleotide phosphate (NADPH)
PKA	Protein kinase A
PVI	Pulmonary vein isolation
SCD	Sudden cardiac death
VF	Ventricular fibrillation
VS	Vagal stimulation
VT	Ventricular tachycardia

2.1 Sympathetic and Parasympathetic Effects on Cellular Electrophysiology

How sympathetic and parasympathetic activation differentially affect local cellular electrophysiology and how these effects translate into broader clinical disease are not entirely clear. As discussed earlier, there are complex interconnections between separate ganglia, with different ganglia often having different effects on heart rate, nodal function, or even the likelihood of stimulating AF. Whether these different effects represent relative differences in density of sympathetic vs. parasympathetic nerves, or local differences in electrophysiology representing a greater predilection towards the generation of premature depolarisations in certain target areas over others, are unclear (Zipes 1994; Schwartz 1984; Janse et al. 1985; Hou et al. 2007a, b; Scherlag et al. 2005a, 2006; Ghias et al. 2009; Asirvatham and Kapa 2009; Saito et al. 2000; Tan et al. 2006; Po et al. 2009). It is known that activation of sympathetic and parasympathetic nerves may differentially affect cellular effective refractory periods, with sympathetic activation shortening refractoriness and thus enhancing the potential for early and delayed after depolarisations and parasympathetic activation prolonging refractoriness and thus increasing the potential for other focal trigger(s) to take over as the dominant trigger(s). Thus, it would seem that the most likely source of arrhythmia is either through increased susceptibility to "abnormal" triggers (such as those in the pulmonary veins felt to be responsible for the genesis of AF which may take over in the setting of prolonged atrial refractoriness during periods of increased parasympathetic tone) or through triggered activity (such as from heightened sympathetic nerve activity which may lead to a shortening of the effective refractory period and thus a predilection towards premature contractions that may trigger an arrhythmia) (Patterson et al. 2005; Zhou et al. 2007; Dizon et al. 2009). It is also known that local conduction may be improved during periods of heightened sympathetic stimulation or slowed during periods of parasympathetic stimulation. Although these local cellular effects of sympathetic and parasympathetic stimulation are well known, the ways in which the interplay translates into the onset and propagation of clinically significant arrhythmias are not entirely clear, and data support at a singular mechanism at the clinical level is not available.

Research is needed to better elucidate how the interplay between the sympathetic and parasympathetic systems modulates local and global cardiac electrophysiology during the onset of clinically significant arrhythmias. Furthermore, how this interplay is modulated and impacts the relative importance of autonomic tone in arrhythmogenesis in the presence or absence of structural heart disease is not entirely clear. For example, as stated previously, it would seem that post-heart transplant AF is possible despite total cardiac denervation (Paul et al. 2006; Cao et al. 2000a, b; Ren et al. 2008; Scott et al. 2008; Schwartz et al. 1991, 2004; Wilde et al. 2008; Lopshire et al. 2009; Antzelevitch and Shimizu 2002; Antzelevitch 2002; Noda et al. 2002). However, this AF most likely reflects graft rejection. Thus, all clinical dysrhythmias may not be a reflection of abnormalities in autonomic tone, and it is possible that the presence of concurrent structural disease may increase the susceptibility to autonomic fluctuations. These relationships remain to be elucidated and require further research before we can fully define to what degree autonomic tone may act as a primary mediator of cardiac dysrhythmias (Schwartz et al. 1991; Brugada and Brugada 1992; Miyazaki et al. 1996; Matsuo et al. 1999).

2.2 Electrophysiologic Effect of Abnormal Autonomic Tone

The intricacies of the anatomy and physiology of the cardiac nervous system are key to unravelling the complex associations with electrophysiologic disease (Zipes 1994; Schwartz 1984). Relationships between autonomic tone and electrophysiologic disease may be seen in ventricular arrhythmias, atrial fibrillation (AF), and channelopathies associated with an increased risk of sudden death (Saito et al. 2000; Tan et al. 2006; Po et al. 2009; Paul et al. 2006; Chen et al. 2001; Cao et al. 2000a, b; Ren et al. 2008; Scott et al. 2008; Schwartz et al. 2004; Wilde et al. 2008; Issa et al. 2005b; Lopshire et al. 2009).

2.2.1 Ventricular Arrhythmias

Sympathetic hypersensitivity has been shown in areas of denervation, which may be related in part to nerve sprouting. Other sympathetic and electrical phenomena following myocardial injury include an upregulation of nerve growth factor, a heterogeneous distribution of sympathetic innervation, and electrical heterogeneity with areas of denervation, hyperinnervation, and normal nerve density. Two discoveries by Chen and colleagues are perhaps most noteworthy (Chen et al. 2001). One is that nerve growth factor infusion and stellate ganglion stimulation following MI increase nerve density and ventricular arrhythmias, with increased burst frequency discharge of the stellate ganglion prior to the onset of ventricular tachycardia/ventricular fibrillation (VT/VF) in dogs. More recently, they have shown that infusion of nerve growth factor into the stellate ganglion prolongs the QT interval and prolongs ventricular arrhythmias. A relationship has been established between the hyperinnervation that occurs following myocardial injury and ventricular arrhythmias. Using immunocytochemical staining in explanted native hearts of transplant recipients, Chen and colleagues demonstrated co-localisation of Schwann cells, sympathetic nerves, and nerve axons, as well as regional cardiac hyperinnervation, with the most abundant nerve sprouting in the areas bordering myocardial injury and normal myocardium (Stanton et al. 1989). In addition, they demonstrated positive tyrosine hydroxylase staining of cardiac nerves in areas around coronary arteries in patients with coronary disease and idiopathic dilated non-ischaemic cardiomyopathy. At the origin of ventricular tachycardia (prior to transplant), nerve sprouting was shown by staining for S100 protein and tyrosine hydroxylase. The authors hypothesised that nerve sprouting may give rise to ventricular arrhythmia and sudden cardiac death, in which MI results in nerve injury, followed by sympathetic nerve sprouting and regional myocardial hyperinnervation (Paul et al. 2006; Chen et al. 2001; Cao et al. 2000a, b; Ren et al. 2008; Scott et al. 2008; Schwartz et al. 2004; Wilde et al. 2008; Issa et al. 2005b). The ANS, in particular, sympathetic activation, is known to play a significant role in sudden cardiac death mediated by ventricular tachyarrhythmias. The mechanism by which autonomic tone mediates the risk of ventricular tachycardia or fibrillation is not entirely clear, though several theories exist. Furthermore, most studies done on autonomic tone in ventricular tachyarrhythmias rely on animal and cellular models, and thus it is not readily apparent how these results may extend to humans. The association between elevated sympathetic tone and the risk of ventricular tachyarrhythmias has been well recognised in studies during sleep. Up to 15 % of sudden cardiac death occurs at night and is felt to be at least partly related to rapid eye movement sleep-related surges in sympathetic nerve activity. Furthermore, in patients with comorbidities including coronary artery disease, myocardial infarction, and diabetes, there is a notable decrease in vagus nerve activity during sleep that may lead to unopposed sympathetic activity and consequently a higher risk of ventricular tachyarrhythmias. These findings further highlight the potential role maladaptation of the ANS may play in the onset and propagation of ventricular tachyarrhythmias (Antzelevitch 2002; Schwartz et al. 1991; Brugada and Brugada 1992; Miyazaki et al. 1996; Matsuo et al. 1999; Wichter et al. 2002). The role of denervation and nerve sprouting in mediating the relationship between the cardiac nervous system, myocardial infarction, and ventricular tachyarrhythmias is one prevailing theory of why some patients may be at higher risk of ventricular tachyarrhythmias after a myocardial infarction. Using [^{123}I]-MIBG nuclear studies to image the distribution of cardiac sympathetic nerves, there appears to be decreased activity in areas of infarction when compared with normal areas of the heart. Also, those patients with decreased uptake appear to have a greater incidence of ventricular tachyarrhythmias. It is possible that after infarction, there is nonhomogeneous distribution of sympathetic nerves amid the remaining viable myocardium, particularly in border zones, which may be sources of premature impulses (i.e. premature ventricular contractions) that can initiate tachyarrhythmias. Another theory is that some patients may develop heterogeneous sympathetic innervation due to sprouting of new nerves in previously denervated areas, with these new nerves summarily suppressing both I(to) and I(K1) channels, thereby decreasing heart rate variability and raising susceptibility to ventricular fibrillation. New nerve growth has been demonstrated in work on explanted hearts with an increased density of nerves seen around areas of myocardial injury. How these changes in innervation relate to the nearby ganglia, whether the same ganglia that provided the original inputs to the areas of ischaemia are still "in control," and whether new nerve growth equates to changes in sympathetic tone, however, are unclear. One therapeutic manoeuvre that may reduce risk of ventricular tachyarrhythmias is cervical sympathectomy (Matsuo et al. 1999; Wichter et al. 2002; Walsh and Kass 1991; Terrenoire et al. 2005; Duan 2009). However, whether cervical sympathectomy in patients with ischaemia may reduce the risk of ventricular tachyarrhythmias, similar to patients with congenital sudden cardiac death syndrome, is unclear. Other therapies have focused on alternate ways of either suppressing sympathetic tone or enhancing parasympathetic tone to the heart. One such therapy is spinal cord stimulation, which may chronically enhance cardiac parasympathetic tone while inhibiting sympathetic tone. Acute spinal cord stimulation has been shown to reduce the occurrence of ventricular tachyarrhythmias in ischaemic dog models. Future therapies may focus on attempting to inhibit nerve growth (i.e. prevention of nerve sprouting and resultant hyperinnervation) or to ablate ganglia and thereby attain regional cardiac denervation. These relationships between altered sympathetic tone, changes in sympathetic innervation, and risk of ventricular tachyarrhythmias also raise multiple potential targets for sudden cardiac death risk assessment. Specifically, whether nuclear studies, such as those using [^{123}I]-MIBG, or autonomic studies such as baroreflex sensitivity and heart rate variability, may play a role in predicting those most at risk for ventricular tachyarrhythmias is unclear. Another factor that needs to be taken into account is how markers that represent more global aspects of cardiac autonomic tone (i.e. heart rate variability, baroreflex sensitivity, etc.) may relate to local or regional pathology in the heart. For example, it is known that global changes in depolarisation-repolarisation, characterised by prolongation in the QT interval, occur during stellate ganglion stimulation. However, whether similar changes occur more locally with regional ganglia stimulation or secondary to heterogeneity in sympathetic innervation in such a way as not to be apparent on electrocardiography is unclear. Thus, future methods of sudden cardiac death risk assessment may have to rely not only on global measures of autonomic tone but also the development of novel methods of assessing regional autonomic innervation (Harvey et al. 1990; Vyas et al. 2006; Ward and Sanders 2001; Daniel 2001; Kostin and Popescu 2009; Nguyen et al. 2009; Cao et al. 2000a, b; Chialvo et al. 1990; Taggart et al. 2003).

2.2.2 Atrial Fibrillation

Pulmonary vein isolation (PVI) is an established means of treating AF. The discovery of the effectiveness of PVI arose from data demonstrating that AF could emerge spontaneously from triggered activity in the pulmonary vein ostia. However, later studies have demonstrated that other regions in the atria, including the superior vena cava, the vein of Marshall, and other cardiac structures, such as the atrial appendages, could serve as substrates for the initiation and propagation of AF. The role of the pulmonary veins in the onset and propagation of AF has led to several studies into the potential structural and autonomic cues that may place patients with pulmonary vein-mediated AF at risk for dysrhythmias. The role for the autonomic nervous system (ANS) in the pathogenesis of AF was first recognised by Coumel et al. in 1978. Although AF was initially thought of principally as a sympathetically mediated phenomenon, it has been found to be either sympathetically or parasympathetically (vagally) mediated. The potential role for the parasympathetic nervous system in inducing AF has been implicated in the higher incidence of AF during sleep, when there is a profound parasympathetic dominance. The role of the ANS, particularly enhanced vagal responses, in the onset of AF during sleep has been further supported by studies in patients with sleep apnoea, in whom a higher predilection towards AF is seen. Interestingly, the relative incidence of sympathetic – predominant and parasympathetic – predominant AF appears to be dependent on comorbidities. In other words, lone and nocturnal AF appear to be associated with increased vagal tone, whereas paroxysmal AF in the setting of organic heart disease or the postoperative state appears to be associated with increased sympathetic tone (Po et al. 2009; Chiou et al. 1997; Marron et al. 1995; Scherlag et al. 2005a, b; Patterson et al. 2005; Zhou et al. 2007; Dizon et al. 2009). The situation is made even more complex by some prevailing theories that both the sympathetic and parasympathetic systems may play a role in inducing AF, with increased sympathetic drive converting to a vagal predominance immediately before AF onset. To understand how the interplay between the ANS and AF may occur, an understanding of the anatomy of the human pulmonary veins is also important. The pulmonary veins are characterised by highly anisotropic musculature, which could predispose to reentrant electrical phenomena. Interestingly, there is also a high density of nerves near the venous ostia when compared with the remainder of the left atrium and higher up along the pulmonary veins. These nerves appear to originate in the cardiac ganglionated plexuses along the middle and dorsum of the right atrium, and the nerve endings appear to penetrate mostly at the root of the veins, an average of 5 mm away from the junction of the left atrium. Therefore, one could surmise that successful PVI may not just be a function of effective electrophysiologic isolation of the pulmonary veins, but also of achieving lesions sufficiently low enough so as to disrupt the pulmonary vein neural interface. Physiologically, the presence of autonomic innervations into the pulmonary veins may be suggested by the slowing of the heart rate during pulmonary vein ablation. In fact, the usual response during ablation is one of bradycardia rather than tachycardia, even though the intrinsic cardiac nervous system is made up of a complex network of both sympathetic and parasympathetic fibres. Some theories behind which this reflex bradycardia is seen include complex extracardiac neural pathways, paracrine mechanisms due to ganglion cells being mostly cholinergic, and the wider distribution of adrenergic than cholinergic nerves resulting in a greater bradycardic than tachycardic impulse with ablation. These associations between the ANS and AF are furthered by studies that have suggested that direct stimulation of ganglionated plexuses may induce AF upon an atrial premature stimulus. Also, ablation of the same plexuses may reverse the refractory period change and abolish the ability to induce AF during pulmonary vein stimulation. These findings have led to studies on the potential role of ganglionic ablation, either as a standalone measure or coupled with PVI, to treat AF. Ganglion ablation has been suggested to result in preservation of sinus rhythm in as many as 50–84 % of patients over a short follow-up period. Also, autonomic denervation may result in fewer recurrences of AF, especially when ablation is done in areas that elicit marked vagal responses (Stanton et al. 1989; Paul et al. 2006; Chen et al. 2001; Cao et al. 2000a, b; Ren et al. 2008). The role of autonomic denervation in the prevention of AF is further highlighted in one recent study by Dizon et al. This study demonstrated that AF is fairly uncommon in heart transplant recipients, only occurring in the setting of myocardial dysfunction and graft rejection. However, AF is relatively common after lung transplantation. In this study, patients receiving double lung transplant had each of the donor lung's pulmonary veins with the associated donor atrial cuffs sutured to each of two atriotomies made in the recipient's left atrium. However, those receiving orthotopic heart transplant had the recipient's pulmonary veins with atrial cuff sutured to a single atriotomy in the donor's left atrium. Thus, although focal connections of the pulmonary veins to an atrial cuff exist in both cases, it should be surgically isolated from the remainder of the recipient's heart, creating the effective equivalent of a PVI. These findings suggest that it is not PVI as much as cardiac autonomic denervation seen with heart transplant but not with double lung transplant that affords a protective effect against postoperative AF. One major hurdle to performance of ganglion ablation is determining where the ganglia are located. Various manoeuvres, including high-frequency electrical stimulation and complex fractionated electrograms, have been studied as methods of identifying locations of ganglia. In the former, elicited parasympathetic responses are sought to correlate with the presence of a ganglionated plexus, since even though the ganglia are composed of both sympathetic and parasympathetic elements, parasympathetic effects are usually realised faster than sympathetic effects. In the latter, fractionated electrograms, which may correlate with proximity to the pulmonary veins, are sought during mapping, although their relationship to activity of the intrinsic nervous system and their reproducibility are unclear. Another hurdle is the complex crosstalk that may exist between ganglia composing the intrinsic cardiac nervous system. For example, inducibility of AF at selected sites, whether close to the pulmonary veins or at more peripheral atrial locations, may depend on whether the extrinsic cardiac nerves or intrinsic cardiac ganglia are stimulated. Furthermore, ablation of left vs. right ganglionated plexuses may have different effects on the ability to induce AF. Thus, while the intrinsic cardiac nervous system, partly mediated by signals received from the extrinsic cardiac nerves and partly by more local signals received from the heart, may play an integral role in the inducibility and propagation of AF, ways to use the data most appropriately are still unclear. Furthermore, it is unclear whether one specific anatomic model may be used to guide future ablative therapies or if a more patient-specific, map-guided approach may be most appropriate. Some have attempted to simply ablate every ganglion and every pulmonary vein, although the long-term effects of this approach are unclear. Furthermore, given the evidence of extensive crosstalk and handedness between ganglionated plexuses, any approach involving ablation of all ganglia would necessarily have to also involve extensive ablation throughout both the left and right atria, making procedures significantly longer and more complicated (Cao et al. 2000b; Scott et al. 2008; Schwartz et al. 2004; Wilde et al. 2008; Issa et al. 2005b; Lopshire et al. 2009; Zhou et al. 2001; Antzelevitch and Shimizu 2002; Antzelevitch 2002; Noda et al. 2002; Brugada and Brugada 1992; Miyazaki et al. 1996).

2.2.3 Long QT Syndrome

The long QT syndrome is characterised by prolongation in the QT interval with resulting propensity to develop polymorphic ventricular tachycardia and consequent sudden death. The syndrome is heterogeneous in that it may result from genetic abnormalities in any number of potassium and sodium channels or channel – associated anchoring proteins. The primary arrhythmogenic substrate is theorised to be early after depolarisation-induced triggered activity resulting from increased dispersion of repolarisation. Patients with long QT syndrome are known to have a high sensitivity to autonomic stimulation. However, there is some variability in terms of the degree and duration of response to triggers like sympathetic activation depending on the long QT syndrome type and thus, the type of channel and current affected For example, there may be more prominent and prolonged effects from sympathetic stimulation in long QT type 1 (characterised by an abnormality in KCNQ1 and the I_{Ks} current) than in long QT type 2 (characterised by an abnormality in KCNH2 and the I_{Kr} current). The role of the ANS in long QT syndrome is furthered by the potential role for left cardiac sympathectomy in treating these patients (Antzelevitch and Shimizu 2002; Antzelevitch 2002; Noda et al. 2002; Schwartz et al. 1991). Left cardiac sympathetic denervation has been demonstrated to significantly reduce the incidence of aborted cardiac arrest and syncope in high-risk long QT patients, although it does not entirely prevent sudden cardiac death over the long term. The primary role for sympathetic denervation in these patients may lie in those with recurrent syncope or with recurrent ventricular tachyarrhythmias, in particular in those with electrical storms with implanted defibrillators. The observation that nerve growth factor infused into the left stellate ganglion prolongs the QT interval and prolongs ventricular arrhythmias, resulting in an inordinate risk of sudden death, is fascinating in the context of recent findings of a circadian variation in duration of the QT interval. In measuring QT intervals in 3,700 men without ventricular arrhythmias, we found that the QT interval peaked in winter (between October and January), with a 6-ms difference between the longest and shortest QT intervals. This increase in the QT interval in winter coincides with an increase in the incidence of sudden death, which occurs in many regions of the world regardless of climate. Whether or not this increase in sudden death in winter is related to a longer QT interval is supposition, but the potential interaction deserves further exploration (Brugada and Brugada 1992; Miyazaki et al. 1996; Matsuo et al. 1999; Wichter et al. 2002). A similar surge in sudden death in winter was observed in patients who were eligible for an implantable cardioverter defibrillator (ICD) but did not receive one, as opposed to those who did receive an

ICD, which suggests that the mechanism responsible for the increase in sudden death in winter is ventricular tachyarrhythmia that can be prevented by an ICD. How sympathetic hyperinnervation promotes cardiac arrhythmias is speculative, but increased density of sympathetic nerve endings could promote the release of sympathetic neurotransmitters during sympathetic excitation. The autonomic remodeling is associated with heterogeneous electrical remodeling of cardiomyocytes, resulting in prolongation of action potentials in hyperinnervated regions. Further, acute release of sympathetic neurotransmitters probably accentuates the heterogeneity of excitability and refractoriness, likely contributing to arrhythmia susceptibility (Wichter et al. 2002; Walsh and Kass 1991; Terrenoire et al. 2005; Zhang et al. 1992; Duan 2009; Harvey et al. 1990).

2.2.4 Brugada Syndrome

The Brugada syndrome is characterised by abnormalities in sodium channel function leading to an increased risk of ventricular fibrillation and sudden death, particularly during rest. Many of the tests used to elicit electrocardiographic changes associated with Brugada syndrome (e.g. beta-blockers and parasympathomimetic agents) suggest a role for the ANS. Prior studies have suggested that an imbalance between sympathetic and parasympathetic tone may play a role in the natural history of the Brugada syndrome. One case–control study in particular suggested that in patients with Brugada syndrome, there was presynaptic sympathetic dysfunction of the heart as determined by [^{123}I]-MIBG single-photon emission computed tomography. The authors of this study proposed that this lack of sympathetic drive may affect protein phosphorylation and spatial heterogeneity of transient calcium currents, leading to clinically significant arrhythmias, which may be more profound during periods of parasympathetic dominance, such as during sleep (Brugada and Brugada 1992; Miyazaki et al. 1996; Matsuo et al. 1999; Wichter et al. 2002; Terrenoire et al. 2005; Duan 2009).

2.2.5 Pathophysiology Effect of Sympathetic Innervation in Myocardial Infarction and Heart Failure

It has been known for decades that sympathetic activation can trigger malignant arrhythmias, whereas vagal activity may exert a protective effect (Fig. 2.1). Transmural myocardial infarction (MI) causes denervation and death of sympathetic fibres within the scar. Areas of dense scar do not respond to either sympathetic nerve stimulation or norepinephrine infusion. In the early 1980s, in a canine model of MI, sites apical (distal) to the infarct were shown to demonstrate an abnormal response to sympathetic stimulation. Although non-infarcted sites proximal to the infarct showed effective refractory period (ERP) shortening with both sympathetic (stellate ganglia) stimulation and norepinephrine infusion, sites within non-infarcted myocardial sites distal (apical) to the infarction did not show homogenous

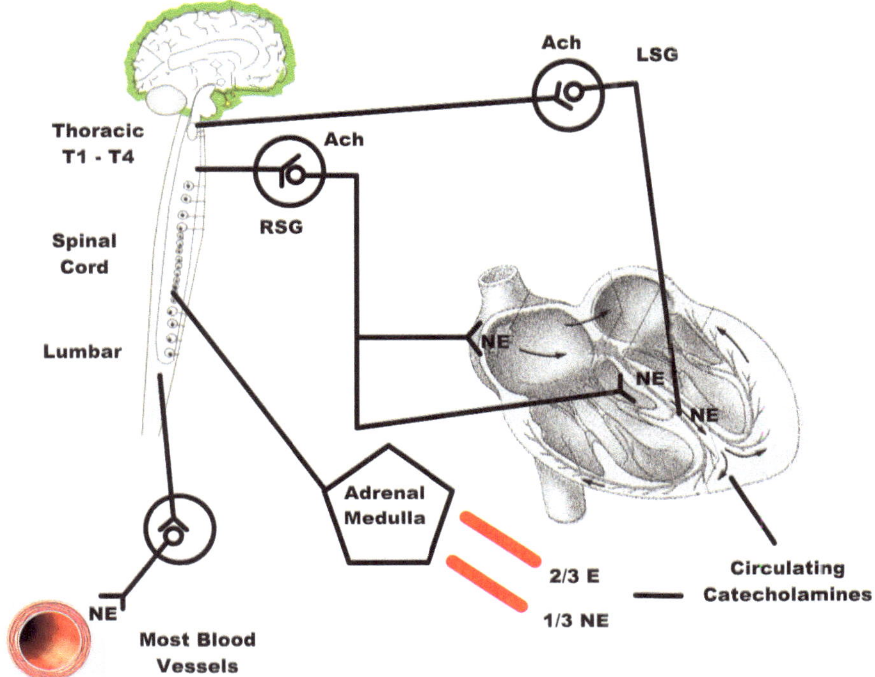

Fig. 2.1 Cardiac sympathetic control

ERP shortening with sympathetic nerve stimulation. Yet, most of these non-infarcted sites showed ERP shortening with norepinephrine infusion, and a few showed ERP shortening with stimulation of either the left or the right stellate ganglion, but not both. Furthermore, these non-infarcted areas showed denervation supersensitivity, defined as an exaggerated shortening of ERP to both norepinephrine and isoproterenol infusions, compared with normal myocardium basal to the infarct. Interestingly, the cellular mechanisms for this exaggerated response did not involve detectable differences in β-adrenergic receptor density or α subunit of the stimulatory G protein density or affinity in the apical vs. basal areas. Myocardial infarction produced loss of efferent sympathetic innervation in non-infarcted apical sites as early as 5–20 min after coronary occlusion, with more significant loss occurring over the following 3 h. Hence, disruption of neurotransmission, likely due to disruption of sympathetic fibres that run along the coronaries, can lead to a heterogeneous response in ERP even in areas of viable non-infarcted myocardium situated apical to the infarct. Furthermore, the innervation of these areas is also heterogeneous because not all sites appeared to be sympathetically denervated. The denervated sites, although no longer responsive to nerve stimulation, demonstrated denervation supersensitivity to infusion of β agonists. Interestingly, they show evidence of norepinephrine depletion on histologic and histo-fluorescent catecholamine analysis, although they appear to be histologically normal. These studies were confirmed by

Yoshioka et al. (2000) in rabbits with regional denervation due to application of phenol. Activation recovery interval (ARI), a surrogate of ERP, was used in these studies to show that norepinephrine infusion shortened ARI in 98 % of denervated regions, with increase in both shortening and dispersion of ARI in more severely denervated regions. On the other hand, left stellate ganglion stimulation shortened ARI in only 30 % of denervated areas with similar increase in dispersion seen in more severely denervated areas. Surprisingly, left stellate ganglion stimulation prolonged ARI in the other 70 % of denervated areas, with no correlation to severity of denervation. The importance of these studies was in demonstrating that transmural MI cannot only alter the substrate for ventricular arrhythmias by creating a scar but can disrupt innervation to histologically normal myocardium distal to the infarct, leading to a no uniform electrophysiologic response early in the stages of acute ischaemia. The heterogeneous response to left or right sympathetic nerve stimulation, an exaggerated response to circulating catecholamines, and reduced protection from vagal denervation all contribute to the genesis of ventricular arrhythmias in both acute and chronic MI. Further insight into the mechanistic basis of noradrenergic nerve terminal abnormalities in heart failure was gained from rapid ventricular pacing-induced heart failure models of dogs. A diffuse decrease in myocardial norepinephrine content and elevated blood norepinephrine levels were observed in failing ventricles. This was also likely due to loss of noradrenergic nerve terminals similar to MI models as evidenced by a reduction in catecholaminergic histo-fluorescence and tyrosine hydroxylase immunostained profiles. Interestingly, similar reduction abnormalities could be produced in normal dogs subjected to 8 weeks of chronic norepinephrine infusion, even without elevated filling pressures, providing evidence that chronically elevated levels of norepinephrine, which is often seen in humans with heart failure, could lead to cardiac noradrenergic nerve abnormalities similar to those found in failing myocardium. As with heart failure, abnormal sympathetic innervation has also been observed in diabetic patients using [^{11}C]-metahydroxyephedrine, a norepinephrine analogue, and positron emission, with maximal denervation affecting distal myocardial segments. Patients with poor glycaemic control have a more heterogeneous hydroxyephedrine uptake, with increased retention in the proximal myocardial segments and much more extensive decrease in retention in distal segments. Following studies showing acute denervation due to MI and heart failure, evidence of nerve sprouting and heterogeneous hyperinnervation was shown in chronic infarction and heart failure models. [^{123}I]-MIBG studies had shown both sympathetic denervation and reinnervation in injured myocardium in both ischaemic and non-ischaemic cardiomyopathy in humans. A consequence of peripheral nerve injury resulting in wallerian degeneration is regeneration via nerve sprouting. The axonal regeneration is slow but accelerates to reach a constant rate by the third day after injury and is triggered by NGF produced by the surrounding myocardium. Excessive and uncontrolled regeneration could lead to hyperinnervation of the myocardium. Vracho et al. demonstrated abnormal patterns of neurilemma proliferation in the scars of a human myocardium. These studies were confirmed by Cao et al. who showed local increases in sympathetic nerves in the periphery of necrotic tissues and in perivascular regions of the hearts of 53 patients with heart failure who underwent cardiac transplantation by using immunochemical staining for S-100 protein, neurofilament protein, and tyrosine hydroxylase on explanted hearts. These changes were scattered in a "swarm-like" pattern at the junction between necrotic and surviving myocardium and were significantly higher in patients with history of ventricular arrhythmias than those without. These border zones of infarcts have been shown to be frequent sites of origin of inducible ventricular tachycardia and ventricular fibrillation (VF) 1 week after left anterior descending artery (LAD) occlusion in dogs. Multiple areas of regional denervation were seen in areas of necrosis or fibrosis in the explanted human hearts, as previously reported. The role of NGF in promoting nerve sprouting has also been studied in animal models of infarction. NGF infusion to the left stellate ganglion results in nerve sprouting in normal dogs. In infarct models of dogs caused by LAD ligation and complete AV block created to induce remodeling, greater sympathetic nerve sprouting occurs with NGF infusion into the left stellate ganglion compared with dogs without an NGF infusion pump. Furthermore, although all dogs show spontaneous VT after MI, spontaneous VT reappeared approximately 2 weeks later in the group with the NGF infusion with higher frequency and showed a diurnal variation, with peak incidence in the morning to early afternoon. Sudden cardiac death due to ventricular fibrillation appeared only in the NGF infusion group (Chen et al. 2001; Cao et al. 2000a, b; Ren et al. 2008; Scott et al. 2008; Schwartz et al. 2004; Wilde et al. 2008; Issa et al. 2005b; Lopshire et al. 2009; Zhou et al. 2001; Antzelevitch and Shimizu 2002; Antzelevitch 2002; Noda et al. 2002; Brugada and Brugada 1992; Miyazaki et al. 1996). However, even dogs without NGF infusion or AV block had evidence of nerve sprouting by 50 days postinfarction. Therefore, NGF infusion accelerates and intensifies the magnitude of nerve sprouting, resulting in higher incidence of sudden cardiac death. Furthermore, NGF infusion to the left stellate ganglion resulted in nerve sprouting in normal dogs but did not cause ventricular arrhythmias or SCD. A differential response of QTc and ventricular arrhythmia was seen when the left vs. the right stellate ganglia were infused with NGF. Infusion into the left stellate ganglion causes sympathetic nerve sprouting on immunocytochemical staining in the left ventricle, with resulting QTc prolongation and sudden cardiac death in 50 % of the experimental dogs. Right stellate ganglion NGF infusion, on other hand, results in right ventricular nerve sprouting, shortened QTc interval, and no sudden cardiac death. The mechanism of cardiac nerve sprouting due to NGF has been studied in dog models of MI. Transcardiac NGF increased immediately after MI, whereas expression of NGF and growth-associated protein 43 was increased within 3.5 h after MI. These changes were more pronounced at the infarcted than non-infarcted sites, fourfold higher than the non-infarcted control group. However, cardiac nerve sprouting and sympathetic hyperinnervation were more pronounced at the non-infarcted than infarction sites, peaking 1 week after MI. Persistent elevation of NGF levels in the aorta and the coronary sinus was seen 1 month after MI. Furthermore, NGF and GAP 3 levels increased in the left stellate ganglion of these dogs 3 days after MI, without a concomitant increase in mRNA, indicating possible retrograde transportation of these proteins to the left stellate ganglion, which then triggers nerve sprouting in non-infarcted left ventricular sites. Further evidence that sympathetic nerve sprouting is arrhythmogenic stems from studies of hypercholesterolaemic rabbits compared with normal controls (Scott et al. 2008; Schwartz et al. 2004; Wilde et al. 2008; Issa et al. 2005b; Lopshire et al. 2009; Zhou et al. 2001; Antzelevitch and Shimizu 2002; Noda et al. 2002; Antzelevitch 2002; Brugada and Brugada 1992; Miyazaki et al. 1996; Matsuo et al. 1999; Wichter et al. 2002; Walsh and Kass 1991; Terrenoire et al. 2005; Zhang et al. 1992; Duan 2009; Vyas et al. 2006). Rabbits fed with a high-cholesterol diet for 8 weeks had significantly higher densities of growth-associated protein 43 (a protein associated with axonal growth cone) and tyrosine hydroxylase, indicating nerve sprouting and sympathetic hyperinnervation. They also showed longer QTc intervals, more QTc dispersion, longer action potential duration, increased heterogeneity of repolarisation, and higher peak calcium current density. Furthermore, significantly higher episodes of ventricular fibrillation, both spontaneous and induced, occurred in the hypercholesterolaemic rabbits, indicating a lower vulnerability to fibrillation. Cardiac nerve sprouting appears to be highly plastic and has been shown in other models of heart failure including rapid pacing where dogs with the most hyperinnervation have the highest risk of sudden cardiac death, in stem cell transplantation and radiofrequency ablation. Heart failure is also known to cause spatially heterogeneous remodeling of cardiomyocytes, with further remodeling of cardiac ion channels, including Ca, K, Cl, and Ca transporters and enzymes in the border zones surrounding the infarct. Specifically, an increase in L-type Ca current density and decrease in potassium current densities are observed in heart failure. I_{Ks} and I_{Kr} are also responsible for the increased sudden cardiac death seen in LQT1 and LQT2. Furthermore, epinephrine may induce torsade, whereas left sympathectomy and β-blockers are antiarrhythmic in LQT1. These studies suggest that sympathetic activation is arrhythmogenic if I_{Ks} is abnormal or downregulated. Furthermore, over-expression of NGF in adult transgenic mice results in further decrease in density of at least two other potassium currents, I_{to} and I_{Kur}. Thus, in areas of hyperinnervation with higher concentration of norepinephrine and neuropeptide Y, sympathetic stimulation could result in prolongation, instead of shortening of action potential duration, accentuating pre-existing heterogeneity of excitability and refractoriness and contributing to arrhythmia susceptibility. Furthermore, superimposed upon prolongation of action potential duration and increased I_{CaL} density, sympathetic stimulation can lead to intracellular Ca overload-induced triggered activity, potentiating the risk spontaneous ventricular arrhythmias. Therefore, an interaction between areas of denervation, regional nerve sprouting (neural remodeling) in the left ventricle, and electrical remodeling due to heart failure all combine to create a high yield substrate for ventricular tachycardia, fibrillation, and sudden cardiac death (Hamdan et al. 2002; Adamson et al. 2003; Zhang et al. 2009; Schwartz et al. 2008; De Ferrari et al. 2011; Hauptman et al. 2012; Krum et al. 2009; Esler et al. 2010; Schlaich et al. 2009).

2.2.6 Effect of Sympathetic Stimulation on Action Potential Duration Restitution

Substantial evidence links enhanced sympathetic activation with ventricular arrhythmias and sudden cardiac death. Destabilisation of ventricular wave fronts leading to degeneration ventricular tachycardia into ventricular fibrillation appears to be related to the restitution properties of action potential duration. Restitution is described as the change in APD in response to the preceding diastolic interval, and steeply sloped restitution curves with large changes in APD for relatively small changes in diastolic interval over a wide range of diastolic intervals have been associated with complex unstable dynamic rhythms. Sympathetic stimulation with epinephrine in porcine models increases the slope of ventricular APD restitution curves. This was confirmed in humans in whom stimulation with both adrenalin and isoproterenol increased the steepness of the slope of APD restitution curves, further demonstrating the known effects of adrenergic stimulation in facilitating ventricular fibrillation (Taggart et al. 1990, 2003; Schwartz et al. 1988a, b; Hohnloser et al. 1994; Rosenshtraukh et al. 1994).

2.3 Cardiac Parasympathetic Nervous System Dysfunction as Manifested by Baroreflex Sensitivity and Heart Rate Variability

As mentioned earlier, the loss of protective vagal reflexes is associated with ventricular arrhythmias in heart failure and MI. Depressed baroreflex sensitivity (BRS) and heart rate variability (HRV), reflections of parasympathetic innervations, have been associated in humans and animal models of MI with a greater susceptibility to ventricular fibrillation during and after ischaemic episodes. Heart rate variability primarily reflects tonic vagal activity, whereas BRS measures predominantly reflex vagal activity in response to stressors. Middle-aged healthy men with high resting heart rates (>75 beats per minute) had a 3.8-fold increase in the risk of SCD compared with those with low basal heart rates (<60 beats per minute), with the risk of SCD increasing linearly with increasing resting heart rates over 23 years of follow-up, suggesting that high parasympathetic tone is protective against SCD (Ferrara et al. 1987; Schwartz et al. 1984; Issa et al. 2005b; Mannheimer et al. 1993).

2.3.1 Heart Rate Variability

Beat to beat, heart rate is not completely regular and is based in part on the autonomic innervation of the sinus node. This can serve as non-invasive marker of autonomic input to the heart, and the analysis can be accomplished in time or frequency domains. High frequencies are thought to represent the parasympathetic component of the autonomic nervous system, whereas low frequencies are mediated by both the sympathetic and parasympathetic nervous system and are affected by BRS. Very-low frequencies are influenced by many factors including the renin–angiotensin system and thermoregulation. This measurement is limited by its inherent use of sinus node innervation as a surrogate for ventricular parasympathetic innervation. In dog models of MI, Hull et al. (1990) showed that dogs who developed ventricular fibrillation had a significant decrease in all measures of HRV, demonstrating a high sensitivity and specificity of HRV in predicting susceptibility to ventricular arrhythmias. These studies were further confirmed by Adamson et al. who also showed that low-risk dogs recovered HRV after MI, whereas high-risk dogs continued to have depressed HRV parameters. Similar results were obtained in humans. Twenty-four-hour Holter recordings in post-MI patients showed that depressed HRV was a significant predictor of mortality after adjusting for clinical and demographic features, including ejection fraction (EF) (Farrell et al. 1991). These studies were further confirmed by other in post-MI patients, showing that impaired HRV was an independent predictor of cardiac mortality only within 6 months of MI and seemed to improve over time. That HRV improves over time is consistent with the decreasing risk of SCD after MI over a similar period. One of the largest of these trials involved 808 patients who underwent HRV analysis using 24-h Holter monitors 11 ± 3 days post-acute MI. In univariate analysis, HRV below 50 ms imposed a hazard relative risk of 5.3, compared with patients with HRV above 100 ms, and remained a significant predictor of mortality after adjusting for clinical and demographic characteristics, other Holter features, and ejection fraction during a mean follow-up of 31 months. Of note, decreased HRV parameters have also been reported in patients with idiopathic dilated cardiomyopathy with history of sudden cardiac death compared with those without a history of ventricular tachyarrhythmias (Odemuyiwa et al. 1994; Kleiger et al. 1987; Schwartz et al. 1988b; La Rovere et al. 1998).

2.3.2 Baroreflex Sensitivity

The arterial baroreceptor control of the heart is generally studied using three techniques: (1) increasing blood pressure with vasoconstrictors such as phenylephrine and analysing heart rate response, this method is used most commonly; (2) lowering blood pressure with vasodilators such as nitroprusside to test reflex sympathetic tone; and (3) direct stimulation of carotid baroreceptors with neck suction. Just as in HRV, BRS was shown to be reduced after MI and to predispose to ventricular fibrillation first in dog MI models. These studies were carried forward to humans, where BRS was found to be lower in patients after MI than in control subjects, but the reduction was transient and appeared to return to baseline levels within 3 months, similar to the improvement seen in HRV and decreasing risk of SCD. The potential prognostic value of BRS was established in several human studies showing that a severely depressed BRS (<3 ms/mmHg) was associated with high mortality due to a high risk of arrhythmic events. The largest of these was the Autonomic Tone and Reflexes After Myocardial Infarction (ATRMI) study, a multicentre prospective trial of 1,028 patients who underwent HRV and BRS analysis within 1 month after MI. During 21 months of follow-up, low values of either heart rate variability (SDNN <70 ms) or BRS (<3.0 ms/mmHg) carried a significant multivariate risk of cardiac mortality (3.2 [95 % CI, 1.42–7.36] and 2.8 [95 % CI, 1.24–6.16], respectively). The association of low standard deviation of normal RR intervals (SDNN) and BRS further increased risk with the 2-year mortality being 17 % when both were low and 2 % when both were well preserved (SDNN >105 ms, BRS >6.1 ms/

mmHg). In patients with EF above 35 % after MI, depressed BRS (<3.0 ms/mmHg) has identified, independently of age and EF, a subgroup of patients at long-term high risk of cardiovascular mortality (HR, 11.4 [95 % CI, 3.3–39]) who may benefit from more aggressive preventive strategies. Of note, BRS is improved in patients with MI who receive thrombolytic therapy or revascularisation compared with those treated conservatively (Taggart et al. 2003; Schwartz et al. 1988a).

2.4 Parasympathetic Modulation of Sudden Death: BRS Versus HRV

Although both HRV and BRS have been shown to be abnormal in heart failure and in post-myocardial infarction patients, the correlation between the two is only moderate ($R=0.63$). This is consistent with the fact that HRV and BRS are different measures of parasympathetic activity, with HRV measuring tonic vagal activity over a 24-h period, whereas BRS is equivalent to a vagal response or variability stress test. Furthermore, BRS in some studies has been a stronger predictor of ventricular tachyarrhythmias than HRV, suggesting that measurements of the dynamic nature of the parasympathetic system may provide superior prognostic information. The underlying mechanisms of the protective effects of the parasympathetic nervous system are not well understood. Loss of vagal innervation, similar to sympathetic innervation, occurs as early as 5–20 min after coronary occlusion. Vigorous vagal activation during acute myocardial ischaemia has been shown to be protective against ventricular fibrillation in anaesthetised cats. Vagal stimulation in these animals after coronary artery ligation increases ventricular repolarisation by increasing levels of pertussis toxin – sensitive G protein – and reduces the risk of ventricular fibrillation. This reduction in risk is no longer observed if vagal stimulation is blocked by atropine or pertussis toxin. The antifibrillatory effects of vagal activation is confirmed by the prevention of ventricular fibrillation during acute ischaemia in dogs susceptible to sudden cardiac death by direct stimulation of the right vagus. In animal studies, direct muscarinic and vagal nerve stimulation with carbacholine, cyclic guanine monophosphate (cGMP), neostigmine, or oxotremorine or even indirect increase with exercise have been shown to reduce the incidence of ventricular tachyarrhythmias in dog infarct models of sudden cardiac death. Based on these studies, low-dose scopolamine was used in humans and was shown to increase HRV and BRS in healthy and in post-MI patients. Endurance exercise training in healthy human subjects also leads to an increase HRV in healthy subjects, suggesting increases in vagal tone. Whether these changes translate into improved mortality and decreased risk of ventricular arrhythmias remains unclear. Post-myocardial infarction dogs treated with low-dose scopolamine compared with controls continued to have a high risk of sudden cardiac death and recurrent ventricular fibrillation despite improvement in HRV parameters. Thus, interventions that improve vagal tone may not provide antifibrillatory effects and those that improve reflex tone may prove to be better targets for reducing the risk of ventricular arrhythmias. Until the cellular mechanisms of the protective effects of vagal innervation are understood, targeting the parasympathetic nervous system in ischaemic cardiomyopathy and prevention of sudden cardiac death will prove difficult (Farrell et al. 1991; Odemuyiwa et al. 1994; Kleiger et al. 1987; Schwartz et al. 1988b).

2.5 Clinical Methods of Assessing Autonomic Innervation in the Heart

One of the limitations in studies of the ANS and its relationship to cardiac electrophysiology has been the limited options available to study autonomic innervation of the heart. Specifically, determining where ganglia are located via an interventional approach or calculating nerve density at the neural-myocardial interface depends on surrogate markers that may not always be reproducible or offer the degree of fine-tuned data needed during ablation procedures. The most commonly used methods include nuclear imaging of sympathetic innervation, high-frequency stimulation, and complex fractionated electrograms (Taggart et al. 2003; Schwartz et al. 1988a). However, each has its limitations and has not been rigorously correlated with anatomic–pathologic studies which would be the gold standard for determining where ganglia are located and the density of sympathetic innervation. In turn, the ex vivo and open heart animal studies that have been done to date need to be translated into clinically useful electrophysiologic mapping procedures. To achieve this, either advances in available catheters or mapping systems or the development of novel agents that can highlight locations of ganglionated plexuses may be needed. Both the sympathetic and parasympathetic nervous systems are intricately involved in the modulation of cardiac excitability and arrhythmias. Neural remodeling with decrease in parasympathetic input, along with heterogeneous sympathetic denervation followed by hyperinnervation in addition to the observed structural remodeling of the diseased heart, creates the electrophysiologic substrate necessary to initiate and maintain arrhythmias. Only by a better understanding of the cellular and electrophysiologic mechanisms underlying normal innervation and neural remodeling will the prevention of sudden cardiac death become feasible (Sanderson et al. 1994; Eliasson et al. 1996; Issa et al. 2005a; Nademanee et al. 2000).

2.6 The Future of Therapeutic Approaches in Neurocardiology

The future of therapeutic approaches in neurocardiology lies both in novel treatment as in applying scientific integrative medical ideas that takes into account concurrent chronic degenerative and vascular disorders and interactions of multiple drug and nondrug treatments. In this respect, vagal stimulation, exercise training, electrical neurostimulation, music therapy, and renal denervation have become interesting options in the treatment of angina pectoris, heart failure, hypertension, and

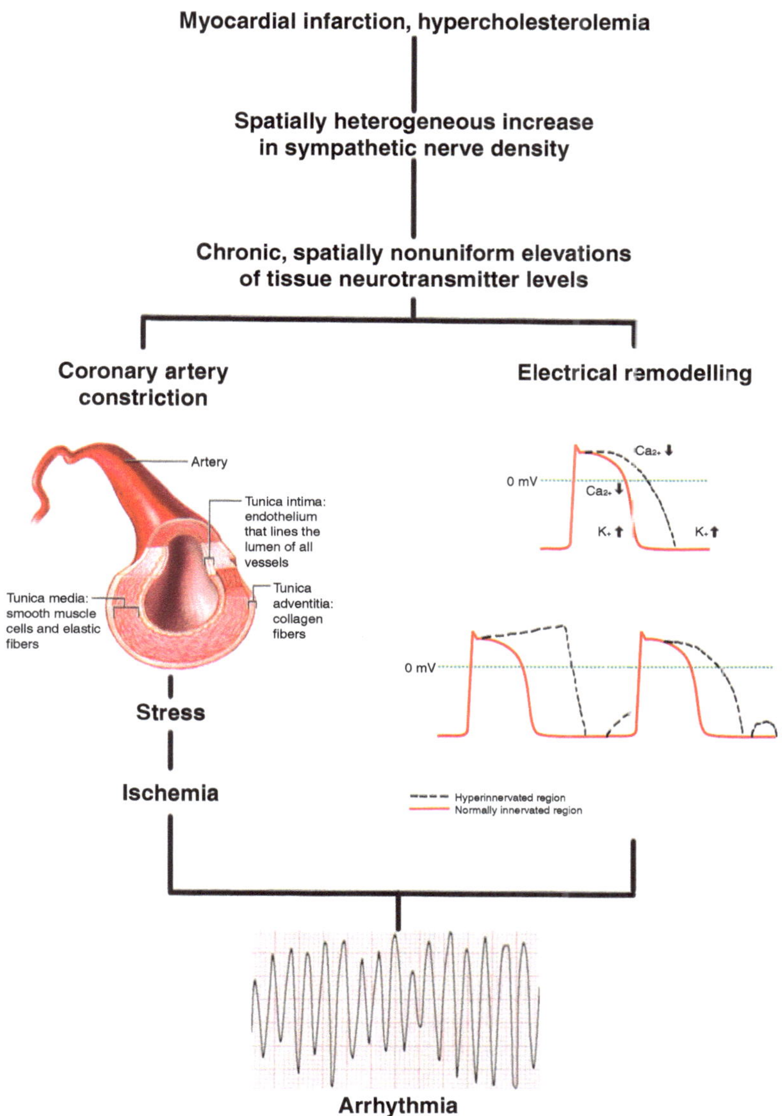

Fig. 2.2 Factors contributing to arrhythmogenesis in hearts with heterogeneous sympathetic innervation

arrhythmias. As sympathetic tone is known to be increased and parasympathetic innervation decreased in cardiomyopathy patients, interventions that aim to reduce sympathetic tone and, therefore, increase parasympathetic tone should reduce the risk of sudden cardiac death and ventricular tachyarrhythmias (Fig. 2.2). This has, in fact, been shown to be true.

2.6.1 Selective Sympathetic Blockade

In 1983, Schwartz et al. showed that the incidence of ventricular fibrillation was decreased from 66 % to zero by performing left stellectomy in post-MI dogs. Issa et al. demonstrated that thoracic spinal cord stimulation at T1–T2 segments reduced the incidence of ventricular tachyarrhythmias in a canine model of ischaemic cardiomyopathy from 59 to 23 % when applied during myocardial ischaemia. Furthermore, they observed a simultaneous decrease in heart rate and reduced systolic blood pressure, consistent with the antisympathetic effects of spinal cord stimulation. In a similar model, intrathecal clonidine, which is known to cause centrally mediated bradycardia and hypotension because of its sympatholytic effects when delivered via a catheter at T2–T4 spinal segments, also significantly reduced the occurrence of ventricular tachycardia and fibrillation during transient myocardial ischaemia. The report of sympathetic blockade in humans compared survival in a group of 49 patients with recurrent ventricular fibrillation (electrical storm) early after MI treated with standard advanced cardiac life support (ACLS) protocol vs. sympathetic blockade. Sympathetic blockade was established using left stellate ganglionic blockade in six patients and infusions of either propranolol or esmolol in 21 patients without antiarrhythmic therapy as recommended by ACLS. The 1-week and 1-year mortality were significantly higher in the group undergoing standard ACLS protocol, compared with the sympathetic blockade group (82 % vs. 22 % at 1 week, 95 % vs. 33 % at 1 year, respectively). Successful treatment of recurrent ventricular tachycardia, refractory to antiarrhythmic therapy, can be achieved by neuraxial modulation at the level of the spinal cord. The benefit of thoracic epicardial anaesthesia was reported in a patient with ischaemic cardiomyopathy and recurrent ventricular arrhythmia refractory to intubation and sedation, with the use of 0.25 % bupivacaine at T1–T2 interspace, reducing the number of ICD shocks from 86 in 48 h to zero (Sanderson et al. 1994).

Inhibiting sympathetic activity pharmacologically reduces the incidence of sudden cardiac death in patients with heart failure. In the Eplerenone Post-Acute Myocardial Infarction Heart Failure Efficacy and Survival Study (EPHESUS), the aldosterone inhibitor eplerenone was associated with a clear reduction in sudden cardiac arrest in patients with acute MI complicated by left ventricular dysfunction. Beta-blockers and angiotensin-converting enzyme inhibitors have had the same effect. These findings indicate that adverse electrophysiologic consequences from sympathetic stimulation may contribute to the development of a proarrhythmic substrate and that antagonizing sympathetic activation can reduce the extent of adverse electrical remodeling to reduce the risk of sudden cardiac death (Nademanee et al. 2000).

2.6.2 Medical Therapies Modulating Cardiac Autonomics

As mentioned above, β-blockers, but also angiotensin-converting enzyme inhibitors (ACEi), angiotensin receptor blockers, aldosterone antagonists, statins, and fish oil have been shown to decrease risk of SCD in ischaemic cardiomyopathy and significantly improve mortality. These classes of drugs have also been shown to modulate the autonomic nervous system to decrease sympathetic tone and/or increase parasympathetic tone.

Angiotensin II in the nucleus solitaire decreases baroreceptor reflex-evoked vagal bradycardia. Microinjection of angiotensin II into the nucleus of the solitary tract in rats significantly attenuates vagal output to the heart. This can be reversed with losartan, suggesting that ACEI and angiotensin receptor blockers may increase parasympathetic output to the heart, decreasing the risk of ventricular tachyarrhythmias. In humans, parasympathetic dysfunction, as measured by abnormal response to Valsalva manoeuvre and respiratory sinus arrhythmia, correlates with severity of heart failure. Treatment of non-ischaemic cardiomyopathy patients with enalapril for 4 weeks reverses these autonomic abnormalities. In experimental rat models of ischaemic cardiomyopathy, rats treated with the spironolactone derivative, canrenone, had decreased myocardial norepinephrine content (suggesting decreased hyperinnervation) and increased VF threshold. These antisympathetic effects were augmented if the rats also received ramipril concomitantly. As with ACEIs and aldosterone antagonists, statins also improve mortality in cardiomyopathy patients. Pliquette et al. showed that in rabbits with pacing-induced heart failure, statin therapy with simvastatin normalises sympathetic outflow and cardiovascular reflex regulation and showed a beneficial dose-dependent effect on baroreceptor sensitivity. The underlying mechanism for the beneficial effects of statin therapy in modulating the autonomic nervous system was further elucidated by recording renal sympathetic nerve activity and studying the effect of statins on angiotensin II type I gene expression and nicotinamide adenine dinucleotide phosphate (NADPH) oxidase activity (a downstream protein activity by angiotensin II receptor activation) in the rostral ventrolateral medulla of rats. Simvastatin therapy significantly reduced angiotensin II-induced pressor and sympathoexcitatory responses, decreased baseline renal sympathetic nerve activity, and increased baroreceptor control of heart rate. Furthermore, simvastatin downregulated mRNA and protein expression of angiotensin II type I receptor and NADPH oxidase subunits in the medulla of heart failure rabbits. Lee et al. once more demonstrated hyperinnervation in rats with MI as shown by an increase in tyrosine hydroxylase and myocardial norepinephrine levels. But they subsequently went on to show that rats treated with pravastatin had lower arrhythmic scores in programmed electrical stimulation studies than controls not treated with a statin or treated with a K-channel blocker. Pravastatin seemed to mediate its antiarrhythmic effects by increasing K_{ATP} activity, as blocking of these potassium channels with the K-channel blocker glibenclamide reversed the beneficial effects of pravastatin. Fish oil has been shown to specifically decrease risk of sudden cardiac death in cardiomyopathy and post-MI patients. In elderly nursing home residents, supplementation with 2 g of fish oil significantly improved both high- and low-frequency components of HRV and SDNN, suggesting that fish oil can decrease sympathetic tone and increase parasympathetic response (Mannheimer et al. 1993; Sanderson et al. 1994; Eliasson et al. 1996; Issa et al 2005a; Nademanee et al. 2000; Hjalmarson 1997).

2.6.3 Effect of Resynchronisation Therapy on Sympathetic Activity

Biventricular pacing has been shown to result in hemodynamic improvement in patients with depressed ejection fraction and intraventricular conduction delay. In patients with cardiomyopathy, biventricular pacing resulted in decreased sympathetic nerve activity along with improvement in blood pressure compared with intrinsic conduction in patients with left ventricular dysfunction and intraventricular conduction delay. Furthermore, in 50 patients implanted with biventricular pacemakers and randomised to therapy-on ($n=25$) vs. therapy-off ($n=25$), HRV was significantly improved in patients receiving resynchronisation therapy despite a lack of difference between mean atrial cycle length. Therefore, improvement in ventricular performance via resynchronisation therapy shifts the cardiac autonomic balance towards a more favourable profile of less sympathetic and more parasympathetic activation (Esler et al. 2010).

2.6.4 Vagal Function Mortality and Cardiovascular Risk

There are multiple measures that can be used to index activity of the vagus nerve. Resting HR, by virtue of being under tonic inhibitory control via the vagus, is a simple, inexpensive, and non-invasive measure of vagal function. The HR change following cessation of exercise is another measure that has been used to characterise vagal function. The decrease in HR after termination of exercise has been termed HR recovery and standardised methods have been developed for its assessment. Measures of heart rate variability (HRV) in both the time and frequency domains have also been used successfully to index vagal activity. In the time domain, the standard deviation of the inter-beat intervals (IBI), the percentage of IBI differences greater than 50 ms, and the mean square of the successive differences in IBIs (MSD) have been shown to be useful indices of vagal activity. In the frequency domain, both low-frequency (LF: 0.04–0.15 Hz) and high-frequency (HF: 0.15–0.40 Hz) spectral power have been used as indices of vagal activity. Whereas there is little contention concerning HF power reflecting primarily parasympathetic influences, LF power has been shown to reflect both sympathetic and parasympathetic influences. However, it is commonly reported that LF and HF are highly and significantly correlated. For example, we have recently reported that LF and HF power were positively correlated in both European American ($r=0.61$) and African-American ($r=0.69$) youths. Even larger correlations have been found between LF and HF in some large epidemiological studies ($n=11{,}654$; $r=0.76$). Thus, LF power often reflects substantial parasympathetic influence. This is not surprising given that parasympathetic influences are present over the whole range of the HRV spectrum, whereas the sympathetic influences roll off at about 0.15 Hz. In addition, measures of baroreflex sensitivity (an index of the responsiveness of the cardiovascular system to changes in blood pressure) have also been shown to be useful indicators of vagal function. The literature linking these different indices to morbidity and mortality is extensive. Importantly, whereas there are some differences among studies, the consensus is that lower values of these indices of vagal function are associated prospectively with death and disability. We will review some of these studies here to illustrate the range and power of the association between vagal function and cardiovascular disease and mortality. The studies related to mortality are listed in Table 2.1 and the studies related to risk factors are listed in Table 2.2. However, we should be clear that this is illustrative and not exhaustive.

The evidence for an association between reduced vagal function and mortality appears to be quite strong. Most of these studies examined the association after controlling for other known risk factors such as diabetes and hypertension. However there is also evidence to suggest that reduced vagal function leads to such risk factors. Thus, those studies that control for those known risk factors for which there exists evidence that reduced vagal function might lead to those risk factors may in fact be underestimating the role of vagal function in death and disease.

The National Heart, Lung, and Blood Institute of the US National Institutes of Health lists eight risk factors for heart disease and stroke (http://www.nhlbi.nih.gov/hbp/hbp/hdrf.htm). Six of these factors are considered to be modifiable. Three of these modifiable risk factors are associated with what could be called biological factors. They are high blood pressure (hypertension), diabetes, and abnormal cholesterol. Three others listed as modifiable could be considered lifestyle factors and are tobacco use (smoking), physical inactivity (exercise), and overweight (obesity). Two factors are considered as non-modifiable. These are age and family history of early heart disease or stroke. It is interesting to note that there is at least some data to suggest that each of these risk factors is associated with decreased vagal function (Sanderson et al. 1994; Eliasson et al. 1996; Issa et al. 2005a; Nademanee et al. 2000; Hjalmarson 1997; Pitt et al. 1999; Pliquett et al. 2003a, b). In the following, we will briefly review some of that evidence.

2.6.4.1 Hypertension

Perhaps the single most important risk factor for CVD is hypertension or high blood pressure. Numerous studies have documented the association between cardiac autonomic function and hypertension. This association has been found in both cross-sectional and prospective analyses. In one of the earlier studies, Liao et al. (1996) examined both the cross-sectional and prospective association between 2 min of supine HRV and hypertension in a stratified random sample of 2,061 black and white men and women from the Atherosclerosis Risk in Communities (ARIC) study. In the cross-sectional analyses, HF power adjusted for age, race, gender, smoking, diabetes, and education was significantly lower in the hypertensive group (both treated and untreated) than in the normotensive group. During the 3-year follow-up period, only 64 individuals developed hypertension. However, baseline HF power was inversely related to the development of hypertension. After adjustment for age, race, gender, smoking, diabetes, and education, the lowest quartile of HRV had a 2.44-fold greater risk of hypertension than those in the highest quartile. The association between HRV and hypertension was also investigated in the Framingham

Table 2.1 Studies of vagal function and mortality

Studies (1st AU)	Subject and sample size	Measures employed	Controlled variables	Relative risk
Habib et al. (1999)	Over 30,000 men and women	HR	Gender and ethnicity	Threefold greater risk if HR > 90 bpm Relative those with HR < 60 bpm
Cole et al. (1999)	*N* = 2,428; 63 % men	HR recovery	Age, sex, the use or nonuse of medications, the presence or absence of myocardial perfusion defects on thallium scintigraphy, standard cardiac risk factors, resting heart rate, the change in heart rate during exercise, workload achieved	Unadjusted: not stated Adjusted: 4.0 [CI, 3.0–5.2]; $P < 0.001$
Cole et al. (2000)	*N* = 5,234 Gender not reported	HR recovery	Age, gender, chronotropic response to exercise, habitual exercise, smoking, resting blood pressure, resting HR, cholesterol level, education, and income	Unadjusted: not stated Adjusted: 2.58 [CI, 2.06–3.20]
Nishime et al. (2000)	*N* = 9,454; 77 % men	HR recovery	Resting systolic blood pressure considered as a continuous variable, body mass index; use of non dihydropyridine calcium channel blockers, and lipid-lowering drugs, diabetes, insulin use, known hypercholesterolemia, documentation of total cholesterol value, known prior coronary heart disease, prior myocardial infarction, prior coronary artery bypass graft surgery, reason for test (screening or not), and presence of chronic obstructive pulmonary disease	Unadjusted: 4.16 [CI, 3.33–5.19]; $p < 0.001$ Adjusted: 2.13 [CI, 1.63–2.78]; $p < 0.001$
Shetler et al. (2001)	2,193 men with previous MI	HR recovery		Unadjusted: 2.6 [CI, 2.4–2.8] Adjusted: not stated
Kleiger et al. (1987)	*N* = 808; gender not reported	HRV	Average of normal RR intervals, ventricular premature complex frequency, ventricular pairs or runs	Unadjusted: 2.7 [CI not reported] Adjusted: 5.3 [CI not reported]
Tsuji et al. (1994)	*N* = 736; 40 % men	HRV	Age, sex, history of myocardial infarction or congestive heart failure, presence of complex or frequent ventricular premature beats, and diuretic use	Unadjusted: 1.87 [CI, 1.55–2.26]; $p = 0.0001$ Adjusted: 1.70 [CI, 1.37–2.09]; $p = 0.0001$

Gerritsen et al. (2001)	$N=605$; gender not reported	HRV	Models for subjects with diabetes were adjusted for age, gender, and known diabetes; high-risk subjects were adjusted for age and gender	Unadjusted: 1.69 [CI, 1.02–2.80] Adjusted: 2.25 [CI, 1.13–4.45]
Liao et al. (2002)	$N=11{,}654$; 42 % men	HRV	Baseline age, sex, ethnicity-centre, cigarette smoking status, and mean heart rate	Unadjusted: not stated Adjusted: 2.03 [CI, 1.28–3.23], 1.60 [CI, 1.12–2.27], 1.50 [CI, 0.65–3.42], and 1.27 [CI, 0.84–1.91] for incident MI, incident CHD, fatal CHD, and non-CHD deaths, respectively, comparing lowest quartile to the upper most three quartiles of HF
La Rovere et al. (1998)	$N=1{,}284$ total; 87 % men	HRV	LVEP and VPC	Unadjusted: 5.3 [2.49–11.4]; $p<0.0001$ Adjusted: 3.2 [CI, 1.42–7.36]; $p=0.005$
Camm et al. (2004)	3,717 total; 78 % men	HRV	Age, LVEF, NYHA class, sex, diabetes, beta-blocker use at baseline	Unadjusted: not started Adjusted: 1.46 [CI, 1.10–1.94]; $p=0.009$

Note: *CHD* congestive heart failure, *CI* confidence interval, *HF* high frequency, *HRV* heart rate variability, *LVEP* left ventricular end-diastolic pressure, *MI* myocardial infarction, *NYHA* New York Heart Association Functional Classification, *p* probability, *RR* R to R interval, *VPC* ventricular premature coupling

Table 2.2 Studies of vagal function and cardiovascular risk factors

Risk factors for CVD	Studies	Subject and sample size	Measures employed	Controlled variables	Relative risk
Hypertension	Liao et al. (1996)	$N=2{,}061$; 45 % men	HRV and hypertension	Age, race, gender, current smoking, diabetes, and education	Unadjusted: not stated Adjusted: 1.00, 1.46 [CI, 0.61–3.46], 1.50 [CI, 0.65–3.50] and 2.44 [CI, 1.15–5.20] from the highest to the lowest quartile of HF
Hypertension	Singh et al. (1998)	$N=2{,}042$; 46 % men	HRV and hypertension	Age, BMI, smoking, and alcohol consumption	Unadjusted: not stated Adjusted: LF power: Men 1.38 [CI, 1.04–1.83] $p<0.05$; Women 1.12 [CI, 0.86–1.46] $p=\text{ns}$
Hypertension	Schroeder et al. (2003)	$n=11{,}061$; men and women	HRV, hypertension and blood pressure	Age, sex, race, study centre, diabetes, smoking, education, and BMI	Unadjusted: not stated Adjusted: SDNN: 1.24 [CI, 1.10–1.40]; RMSSD: 1.36 [CI, 1.21–1.54]; RR interval 1.44 [CI, 1.27–1.63]
Diabetes	Liao et al. (1995)	$n=1{,}933$; 44 % men	HRV and fasting glucose	Age, race, and gender	Unadjusted: not stated Adjusted: mean HF: diabetics: 0.78, non-diabetics: 1.27, $p<0.01$ Adjusted among non-diabetics: inverse relationship between serum insulin and HF lowest quartile to highest quartile of insulin: 1.34 and 1.14, respectively
Diabetes	Singh et al. (2000)	$n=1{,}918$; 57 % men	HRV and blood glucose levels	Age, sex, heart rate, body mass index, antihypertensive and cardiac medications, systolic and diastolic blood pressures, smoking, and alcohol and coffee consumption	Unadjusted: $r=-0.21\pm$; $p<0.05$ Adjusted: $r=-.05\pm$; $p<0.0001$

Diabetes	Carnethon et al. (2003)	$n = 8,185$; gender not reported	Autonomic dysfunction (high HR and low HRV) and development of type diabetes	Age, race, sex, study centre, education, alcohol drinking, current smoking, prevalent coronary heart disease, physical activity, and BMI	Unadjusted: not stated Adjusted: LF lowest to highest quartile 1.2 [CI, 1.0–1.4]
Diabetes	Panzer et al. (2002)	$n = 5,190$; 61 % men	Fasting glucose and HR recovery	Age, gender, BMI, resting blood pressure, antihypertensive treatment, cholesterol, education, and alcohol consumption	Unadjusted: not stated Adjusted: impaired HR recovery more common in diabetics RR = 1.61 [CI, 1.35–1.92] and in those with impaired fasting glucose RR = 1.34 [CI, 1.2–1.5]
Cholesterol	Christensen et al. (1999)	47 men with heart disease and 38 healthy men	Vagal tone and cholesterol	Plasma lipids, lipoproteins, age and BMI	Unadjusted: inverse correlation between total cholesterol and LDL, respectively. Healthy men: $r = -0.38$, $p < 0.05$ and $r = -0.22$, ns; 1.34 [CI, 1.20–1.50]; Men with IHD: $r = -0.38$, $p < 0.05$ and $r = -0.37$, $p < 0.05$ Adjusted: Men with IHD: inverse correlation between total cholesterol and SDNN: $r = -0.43$, $p < 0.01$ Adjusted: Healthy men: inverse correlation between total cholesterol and SDNN: $r = -0.28$, $p < 0.05$
Cholesterol	Kupari et al. (1993)	$n = 88$; 47 % men	Short-term HRV and cholesterol	Physical activity, smoking and alcohol consumption	Unadjusted: not stated Adjusted: inverse correlation between RMSSD and LDL [$\beta = -0.22$; $p = 0.008$]; and total spectral power and LDL [$\beta = -0.25$; $p = 0.007$]

(continued)

Table 2.2 (continued)

Risk factors for CVD	Studies	Subject and sample size	Measures employed	Controlled variables	Relative risk
Cholesterol	Wannamethee and Shaper (1994)	$n=5{,}597$; 100 % men	HR and cholesterol	Age, BMI, smoking, physical activity, alcohol consumption, social class and FEV1	Unadjusted: correlations between HR and triglyceride levels ($r=0.15$, $p<0.0001$); cholesterol ($r=0.07$, $p<0.0001$); HDL cholesterol ($r=-0.04$; $p<0.01$) Adjusted: correlations remained significant between HR and Triglycerides $p<0.05$; cholesterol $p<0.05$
Cholesterol	Bonaa and Arnesen (1992)	$n=19{,}152$; 51 % men	HR and cholesterol	Age, BMI, square of BMI, height, physical activity, cigarettes, and coffee	Unadjusted: not stated Adjusted: HR > 89 bpm vs. HR < 60 bpm for non-HDL: Men = 14.5 % higher non-HDL; Women = 12.5 % higher non-HDL; For triglycerides: Men = 36.3 % higher; Women = 22.2 % higher
Smoking	Yotsukura et al. (1998)	$n=20$; 100 % men	Vagal tone and smoking	Within-subject design	HRV increased after smoking cessation: with withdrawal syndrome (Pre vs. Post): LF = 31.9 ± 7 and 39.4 ± 9.6 years; HF = 18.0 ± 6.0 and 23.7 ± 6.8 years; RMSSD = 40.8 ± 13.3 and 46.0 ± 18.2 years; without withdrawal syndrome: LF = 30.5 ± 4.9 and 36.3 ± 5.0*; HF = 17.3 ± 6.0 and 19.8 ± 2.9; RMSSD = 40.0 ± 14.4 and 46.5 ± 12.9; *$p<0.05$ vs. smoking; *$p<0.01$ vs. smoking

Smoking	Nabors-Oberg et al. (2002)	$n=16$; 50 % men	HRV and smoking	Within-subject design	HF: Baseline = 896 (1,346) vs. Cigarette 1 = 338 (687), $p<0.05$
Smoking	Hayano et al. (1990)	Study I: $n=9$; 100 % men; Study II: $n=81$; 100 % men	Vagal tone and smoking	Within-subject design	Study I: HF decreased after 3 min of smoking ($p=0.0061$); Study II: ≤30 years: HF lower in heavy smokers compared to moderate and non-smokers; >30 no difference in older group among the three smoking groups
Smoking	Minami et al. (1999)	$n=42$; 100 % men	Vagal tone and smoking cessation	Within-subject design	Smoking period vs. nonsmoking period: LF = 5.28 ± 0.11 vs. 5.76 ± 0.11, $p<0.0001$; HF = 4.37 ± 0.17 vs. 5.00 ± 0.16; $p<0.0001$
Physical inactivity	Rossy and Thayer (1998)	$n=40$; 52 % men	Vagal tone and habitual exercise	BMI	Positive relationship between indices of vagal tone and fitness: HP; (t (36) = 2.25, $p=0.015$, rpb = 0.35), % BB50 (t (36) = 3.02, $p=0.0025$, rpb = 0.45), SD (t (36) = 1.78, $p=0.04$, rpb = 0.28), MSD (t (36) = 1.93, $p=0.03$, rpb = 0.31), and HF (t (36) = 1.80, $p=0.04$, rpb = 0.29)
Physical inactivity	Rennie et al. (2003)	$n=3,328$; 70 % men	Physical activity and vagal tone or HR	Smoking and high alcohol intake	Unadjusted: not stated Adjusted: LF Men; [284.6, 332.0, 337.0, 342.4] $p<0.01$; LF Women; [233.5, 246.9, 233.5, 243.2, 0.88]; $p=0.88$; HF Men; [104.8, 118.3, 116.3, 125.2] $p<0.05$; HF Women; [133.8, 146.9, 129.8, 141.0] $p=0.61$; for total physical activity quartile low through high

(continued)

Table 2.2 (continued)

Risk factors for CVD	Studies	Subject and sample size	Measures employed	Controlled variables	Relative risk
Obesity	Petretta et al. (1995)	$n=20$; 10 women, 10 control subjects	BMI and HRV	Age matched controls	Unadjusted: Correlation between BMI and HRV: total power [$r=-0.62$; $p<0.05$], ultra low ($r=-0.59$; $p<0.01$), very low ($r=-0.64$; $p<0.005$), low ($r=-0.61$; $p<0.005$) HF ($r=-0.53$; $p<0.05$) Adjusted: not stated
Obesity	Riva et al. (2001)	$n=37$; boys and girls	BMI and HRV	Gender-matched controls	HRV lower in obese compared to controls: RMSSD; control = 56.7 ± 14.4; obese = 44.1 ± 15.8, <0.05
Obesity	Nagai et al. (2003)	$n=84$; boys and girls	ANS activity and the state and development of obesity	Age	Unadjusted: not stated Adjusted: Obese vs. non-obese; HF: 5.84 ± 0.15 vs. 6.34 ± 0.07, $p<0.01$
Obesity	Rabbia et al. (2003)	$n=50$ obese and $n=12$ controls; 46 % men	HRV and paediatric obesity	Sex-matched controls	Adjusted: recently Obese vs. non-obese; HF: 6.21 ± 0.5 vs. 6.78 ± 0.4, $p<0.05$
Obesity	Karason et al. (1999)	$n=84$; 54 % men	Weight loss in the obese on HRV	Age, sex, smoking, and antihypertensive treatment	Unadjusted: not stated Adjusted: Obese vs. non-obese: LF: Baseline: Obese = 19 ± 6, Non-obese = 27 ± 8, $p<0.001$; HF: Baseline: Obese = 8.5 ± 3.7, Non-obese = 11.7 ± 5.7; $p<0.019$
Age	Antelmi et al. (2004)	$n=653$; 45 % men	Age and vagal tone	Mean HR	Decrease per increase in age decade in ms: HF = 2.1; RMSSD = 3.6; LF = 2.9

Family history/ genetics	Piccirillo et al. (2000)	$n=91$; 53 % men	Family history or CVD risk factors and reduced vagal tone	Age, gender, BMI, SBP, anxiety, sodium, and potassium	HRV lower in family history positive compared to family history negative. HF: FH+= 35±2 vs. FH−=42±3, $p<0.05$
Family history/ genetic	Pitzalis et al. (2001)	$n=87$; men and women	Family history of HT and HRV	Age and gender	FH+vs. FH−: heart rate (RR interval, 766±64 vs. 810±93 ms, $p<0.05$), and HRV [the SDDN; 147±29 vs. 171±33 ms, $p<0.05$]
Family history/ genetics	Maver et al. (2004)	$n=105$; 40 % men	Family history of HT and vagal function	HR	Family history of hypertension associated with lower HRV. HF power: partial regression coefficient=−0.049 (s.e. = 0.01), $p<0.00001$
Family history/ genetics	De Angelis et al. (2001)	$n=40$; 100 % men	Family history of diabetes and vagal function	Not stated	FH+vs. FH− : HF (3,034.6±530.9 vs. 3,366.8±570.7, $p<0.05$)
Family history/ genetics	Lindmark et al. (2003)	$n=27$; 52 % men	Family history of type 2 diabetes and vagal function	Age, BMI, gender	Total power and HF lower in FH+vs. FH−; no means provided. Insulin sensitivity correlated with HF ($r=0.49$, $p=0.013$)
Coronary artery occlusion	Huikuri et al. (1999)	$n=305$; 100 % men	Vagal function and coronary artery occlusion	Minimum HR, demographic and clinical variables, smoking, BP, glucose, lipids, and lipid-modifying therapy	Unadjusted: not stated Adjusted: Association between HRV and change in minimal luminal diameter: SDNN ($b=0.24$, $p=0.0001$)
Inflammation	Janszky et al. (2004)	$n=121$; 100 % women	Coronary heart disease and HR and inflammatory markers	Age, menopausal status, BMI, smoking, education, diabetes, and participation in rchabilitation	Unadjusted: Correlation between HRV and inflammatory markers. IL-6 and LF: $r=-0.27$, $p=0.003$; IL-6 and SDNN: $r--0.26$, $p-0.004$ Adjusted: IL-6 and SDNN: $\beta=-0.20$, $p=0.05$

(continued)

Table 2.2 (continued)

Risk factors for CVD	Studies	Subject and sample size	Measures employed	Controlled variables	Relative risk
Psychosocial factors	Rosengren et al. (2004)	$n=24,767$; sex matched controls (Inter Heart Study)	Psychosocial risk factors and risk of acute Myocardial infarction	Geographic region, age, sex, and large number of potential confounders	Unadjusted: not stated Adjusted: Subjects with myocardial infarction (MI) vs. subjects without MI: Work stress: 1.38 (99 % CI, 1.19–1.61) for several periods of work stress and 2.14 (1.73–2.64) for permanent stress at work. Home stress: 1.52 (99 % CI, 1.34–1.72). General stress: 1.45 (99 % CI, 1.30–1.61) for several periods and 2.17 (1.84–2.55) for permanent stress. Financial Stress: 1.33 (99 % CI, 1.19–1.48). Stressful life events in past year: 1.48 (1.33–1.64). Depression: 1.55 (1.42–1.69)

Psychosocial factors	Yan et al. (2003)	n = 3,156; 44 % men (Cardia Study)	Psychosocial risk factors and risk of acute myocardial infarction	Hypertension risk factors and each of the psychosocial factors of TUI, ASC, hostility, depression, and anxiety in 5 separate logistic regression models	Unadjusted: not stated Adjusted: For TUI: 1.51 [CI, 1.21–2.03] for a score of 1; 1.47 [CI, 1.08–2.02] for a score of 2; and 1.84 [CI, 1.29–2.62] for a score of 3 to 4 (p for trend = 0.001). Compared with the lowest quartile group, the adjusted OR for hostility was 1.06 [CI, 0.76–1.47] for quartile 2; 1.38 [CI, 1.00–1.91] for quartile 3; and 1.84 [CI, 1.33–2.54] for quartile 4 (p for trend <0.001). No consistent patterns were found for ASC, depression, or anxiety
Psychosocial factors	Yusuf et al. (2004)	n = 27,098; 76 % men in cases (Inter Heart Study)	Psychosocial risk factors and risk of acute myocardial infarction	Age, sex, smoking, and geographic region	Unadjusted: not stated Adjusted: Psychosocial index and risk of acute myocardial infarction. OR = 2.67 [99 % CI, 2.21–3.22]
Psychosocial factors	Kang et al. (2004)	n = 169; 100 % men	Job stress on HRV	Not stated	Unadjusted: For lower strain + normal: SDNN = 39.6 (11.3); Lower strain + metabolic syndrome: SDNN = 35.9 (10.2); High strain + Normal: SDNN = 35.1 (9.8), High strain + metabolic syndrome; SDNN = 31.1 (8.4); p = 0.04

(continued)

Table 2.2 (continued)

Risk factors for CVD	Studies	Subject and sample size	Measures employed	Controlled variables	Relative risk
Psychosocial factors	Thayer et al. (1996)	$N=34$; 35 % men	Generalised anxiety Disorder (GAD) and worry were examined using measures of heart period variability	Age, gender, ethnicity, and education	GAD vs. Control: HF power: GAD=606 (SD=700) and Control=1,599 (SD=1,918); F (1.36)=6.03, $p<0.05$

Note: *RMSSD* root-mean-square successive RR-interval difference, *SDNN* standard deviation of normal to normal (NN) interval, *HF* high frequency, *LF* low frequency, *VLF* very low frequency, *HRV* heart rate variability, *HR* heart rate, *SD* standard deviation, *GAD* generalised anxiety disorder, *PAR* population attributable risks, *TUI* time urgency/impatience, *OR* odds ratio, *CI* confidence interval, *MI* myocardial infarction, *IHD* ischaemic heart disease, *HDL* high-density lipoprotein, *LDL* low-density lipoprotein, *HP* heart period

Heart Study (FHS). Again both cross-sectional and prospective analyses were performed. Singh et al. (1998) examined the association between the first 2 h of ambulatory HR recordings and hypertension in 931 men and 1,111 women from the FHS. Cross-sectional analyses indicated that after adjustment for age, BMI, smoking, and alcohol consumption, several measures of both time and frequency domain indices of HRV were significantly lower in hypertensive men and women than in normotensives. During the 4-year follow-up period, 119 men and 125 women developed hypertension. These analyses showed that low LF power was associated with the development of hypertension in men but not in women. In a recent report, the association between HRV, hypertension, and blood pressure was examined in 11,061 men and women from the ARIC study. HRV was assessed by 2 and 6 min recordings separated by 9 years. Consistent with previous reports HRV adjusted for age, race, study centre, diabetes, smoking, education, and BMI was lower at baseline among those persons with hypertension. Importantly among the 7,099 persons without hypertension at baseline, the lowest quartile of HRV as indexed by RMSSD adjusted for relevant covariates was associated with a hazard ratio for the development of hypertension 9 years later of 1.36 compared to those in the highest quartile. These findings from large, epidemiological studies provide strong evidence that vagal tone as measured by HRV is lower in persons with hypertension than in normotensives even after adjustment for a range of covariates. Importantly, these studies suggest that decreases in vagal tone may precede the development of this critical risk factor for CVD (Sanderson et al. 1994).

2.6.4.2 Diabetes

In the first population-based study to examine the relationship among vagal tone, serum insulin, glucose, and diabetes, Liao et al. (1995) investigated 154 diabetic and 1,779 nondiabetic middle-aged men and women in the ARIC study. Two-minute supine resting HR recordings were used to compute HF power as an index of vagal tone while fasting insulin, glucose, and diagnosed diabetes were used to index diabetes and diabetes risk. Consistent with previous cross-sectional studies, these researchers found that diabetics had lower vagal tone than non-diabetics after adjustment for age, race, and gender. In the non-diabetics, an inverse relationship was found between HF power and fasting insulin and fasting glucose. However, after adjustment only the relationship between HRV and insulin remained significant. This was the first study to examine the relationship between HRV and insulin and glucose in a general population and suggests that reduced vagal tone may be involved in the pathogenesis of diabetes. Singh et al. (2000) examined the relationship between HRV and blood glucose levels in 1,919 men and women from the FHS. The first 2 h of ambulatory HR recordings were used to calculate a number of time and frequency domain indices of HRV. Fasting glucose levels were used to classify individuals as having normal or impaired fasting glucose, as well as to identify those with diabetes (in addition to those with diabetic diagnosis). Several indices of HRV including LF and HF power were inversely associated with fasting glucose levels and were significantly reduced in diabetics and those with impaired fasting glucose compared to those with normal fasting glucose levels. The association between reduced HRV and diabetes remained significant after adjustment for age, gender, HR, BMI, antihypertensive and cardiac medications, blood pressure, smoking, and alcohol and coffee consumption. The prospective association between autonomic dysfunction, indexed by high HR and low HRV, and the development of diabetes was examined by Carnethon et al. (2003) in 8,185 middle-aged men and women from the ARIC study. During the 8-year follow-up period, 1,063 persons developed type 2 diabetes. Compared to those in the highest quartile of LF power, those in the lowest quartile had a 1.2-fold greater risk of developing diabetes after adjustment for age, race, gender, study centre, education, alcohol use, smoking, heart disease, physical activity, and BMI. Those with HR in the highest quartile had 1.6 greater risk of diabetes than those in the lowest HR quartile with similar results for analyses restricted to those with normal fasting glucose. The association between fasting glucose and HR recovery was investigated in 5,190 healthy men and women enrolled in the Lipid Research Clinics Prevalence study (Cao et al. 2000a). Exercise testing was done and the HR drop 2 min after exercise cessation was examined using a cutoff of <42 bpm as an indication of an abnormal response. Fasting glucose was an independent predictor of an abnormal HR recovery response across diabetic and nondiabetic participants and remained a significant predictor after controlling for age, gender, BMI, resting HR, resting blood pressure, antihypertensive treatment, cholesterol, education, and alcohol consumption. Over the 12-year follow-up, abnormal HR recovery was a significant predictor of all-cause mortality across the range of fasting glucose levels, and the combination of abnormal HR recovery and impaired fasting glucose was associated with a 2.4 greater risk of mortality (Hjalmarson 1997).

2.6.4.3 Cholesterol

To date few studies have examined the relationship between vagal tone and cholesterol. Christensen et al. (1999) examined the association between 24 h HRV and cholesterol in 47 men with heart disease and 38 healthy men. In both groups, total cholesterol and low-density lipoprotein (LDL) were inversely associated with 24 h HRV. The association between HRV and cholesterol remained significant in both groups after adjustment for age and BMI. In a random sample of 41 men and 47 women without heart disease, Kupari et al. (1993) investigated the association between short-term HRV and cholesterol. RMSSD was inversely related to LDL cholesterol in both men and women after adjustment for other factors including physical activity, smoking, and alcohol consumption. The cross-sectional association between HR and cholesterol was examined in a sample of 5,597 men without heart disease. HR was positively correlated with total cholesterol and LDL and negatively associated with high-density lipoprotein (HDL) after adjustment for age, BMI, smoking, alcohol consumption, and social class. In a very large study of 9,719 men and 9,433 women, Bonaa and Arnesen (1992) examined the association between HR and cholesterol. In both men and women, total cholesterol and non-HDL were positively associated with HR, whereas HDL was inversely associated with HR after adjustment for age, BMI, smoking, and alcohol consumption (Esler et al. 2010; Schlaich et al. 2009).

2.6.4.4 Lifestyle-Related Risk Factors: Smoking, Physical Inactivity, and Overweight

Smoking, physical inactivity, and being overweight are lifestyle-related risk factors for CVD. Perhaps the single most controllable risk for CVD is smoking. Both acute and chronic smoking have been associated with decreased vagal tone. For example, we recently reported that vagally mediated HRV as indexed by HF power and approximate entropy (ApEn: an index of complexity derived from nonlinear dynamical systems theory with higher numbers associated with greater complexity) were reduced after smoking one cigarette and remained reduced upon the smoking of two more cigarettes at 30 min intervals in a controlled smoking paradigm. Hayano et al. (1990) reported that both acute and chronic smoking were associated with decreased vagal tone. Importantly, Minami et al. (1999) showed that indices of vagal tone increased after 1 week of smoking cessation in a group of habitual male smokers. Moreover, in a study that examined the time course of the increase in vagal tone with smoking cessation, Yotsukura et al. (1998) reported that indices of vagal tone increased within 24 h of smoking cessation and remained elevated for the 1 month follow-up period in a group of male habitual smokers. Thus, smoking and smoking cessation have immediate but reversible effects on vagal tone. A large number of cross-sectional as well as training studies have examined the effects of habitual exercise on cardiovascular function. The single most replicable effect of aerobic training on cardiac function is a decreased resting HR. Whereas there is some ongoing debate about the nature of the autonomic nervous system changes that accompany regular physical activity, numerous studies have implicated increased vagal tone in the salubrious effects of exercise. This is true in both cross-sectional and training studies. For example, we have reported in a cross-sectional study that habitual physical activity is associated with greater levels of vagally mediated HRV in both men and women. In 2,334 men and 994 women from the Whitehall II study of British civil servants, moderate and vigorous physical activity were associated with greater vagal tone (in men) and lower resting HR (in men and women) compared to those that reported low levels of physical activity after adjustment for age, smoking, and alcohol consumption. Taken together numerous studies report that physical inactivity, an important lifestyle risk factor for CVD, is associated with decreased vagal tone. Importantly, it also appears that the increased physical activity may decrease resting HR and increase vagal tone. Numerous studies have also documented that vagal function is reduced in overweight and obese individuals. In a study of 10 women with early onset familial obesity and 10 nonobese women, several indices of HRV were reduced in the obese women. In addition, BMI was inversely related with several measures of HRV including HF power. Several studies of obesity in children and adolescence have also found that vagal function is reduced in obese individuals compared to nonobese individuals. In all of these studies, several indices of vagal function such as HF power were reduced in the obese individuals. In a study that examined the effect of weight loss in obese persons on HRV, Karason et al. (1999) studied 28 obese patients referred for gastroplasty, 24 obese patients using a lifestyle dietary modification approach, and 28 nonobese persons. At baseline, both obese groups had reduced HF values relative to the nonobese participants. After 1-year follow-up, those persons that had undergone gastroplasty had an average weight loss of 28 % and showed evidence of increased vagal function as indicated by increased HF power. Taken together these studies of lifestyle-related risk factors all indicate that decreased vagal function is associated with poor risk factor profiles. Importantly, they also indicate that modification of the risk profile towards lower risk is accompanied by increased vagal function (Zhang et al. 2009; Schwartz et al. 2008; De Ferrari et al. 2011; Hauptman et al. 2012; Krum et al. 2009; Esler et al. 2010; Schlaich et al. 2009).

2.6.4.5 Non-modifiable Risk Factors: Age and Family History

Whereas the exact mechanism is still open to debate, numerous studies have shown that increasing age is associated with decreasing vagal tone. Given this fact age is often used as a covariate in large epidemiological studies such as ARIC, FHS, and the Whitehall study. In those studies that have specifically investigated the relationship between age and cardiac function, consistent evidence supports decreasing vagal tone with increasing age. For example, Antelmi et al. (2004) investigated the association between age and vagal tone in 292 men and 361 women aged from 14 to 82 years. They found that RMSSD decreased on average 3.6 ms per decade. Numerous studies report that family members of persons with CVD risk factors such as hypertension or diabetes also have reduced vagal tone. Piccirillo et al. (2000) examined 61 normotensive men and women with a family history of hypertension and 30 normotensive that were negative for family history of hypertension. Spectral analysis of HR and blood pressure variabilities were used to estimate baroreflex sensitivity. Vagal tone as indexed by baroreflex sensitivity and HRV was reduced in those positive for family history compared to those negative for family history of hypertension. Pitzalis et al. (2001) investigated several indices of vagal function including HRV in 45 normotensive men and women with a family history of hypertension and 42 men and women without a family history of hypertension. Again, those with a positive family history compared to those with a negative family history had reduced HRV but no difference in baroreflex sensitivity. Recently, Maver et al. (2004) studied 59 normotensives with a positive family history of hypertension and 46 normotensives negative for family history. Several indices of vagal function including HRV and baroreflex sensitivity were examined. Those with a positive family history of hypertension had lower vagal function as indexed by HF power and baroreflex sensitivity compared to those that were negative for family history of hypertension. These studies suggest that decreased vagal function is evident in persons with a family history of hypertension. Similar results have been found in persons with a family history of diabetes. De Angelis et al. (2001) studied 20 glucose normo-tolerant individuals with a family history of non-insulin-dependent diabetes mellitus (NIDDM) and 20 glucose normo-tolerant individuals without a family history of NIDDM. One-hour recordings of HR were used to calculate several indices of HRV using spectral analysis. Results showed that family history positive individuals had reduced vagal tone compared to those that were family history negative for NIDDM. In a recent study, Lindmark et al. (2003) examined 13 healthy persons with a family history of type 2 diabetes and 14 persons with a negative family history of diabetes. HRV was analysed during a number of conditions including rest and controlled breathing. The results indicated that total spectral power and HF power were lower during controlled breathing in those with a positive family history compared to those with a negative family history of diabetes. Again, these results indicate that decreased vagal function is evident in persons with a positive family history of diabetes compared to those with a negative family history. Taken together these findings suggest that autonomic imbalance, especially decreased vagal function, may be associated with the development of these known risk factors for cardiovascular disease and death. In addition, data suggests that decreased vagal function is associated with degree of coronary artery occlusion and plaque rupture. Recent data also suggest that decreased vagal function is associated with increased markers of inflammation.

2.6.4.6 Emerging Risk Factors: Inflammation and Psychosocial Factors

Inflammation is now thought to play a major role in cardiovascular disease. Importantly, evidence linking decreased vagal function with increased inflammation is quickly accumulating. Tracey (2002) has described the cholinergic anti-inflammatory pathway in which acetylcholine and vagal function tonically inhibits release of proinflammatory cytokines. Clinical evidence in humans is just now starting to become available. In a study of 121 women with coronary heart disease, 24 h recordings of HR were collected and several inflammatory markers examined. Both time and frequency domain indices of HRV were inversely associated with interleukin-6 (IL-6) levels after controlling for age, menopausal status, BMI, smoking, education level, diabetes, and cardiac rehabilitation participation. In a sample of 643 middle-aged and elderly men and women, increased HR and reduced HRV were found to be significant independent predictors of white blood cell count (WBC) and C-reactive protein (CRP) levels after controlling for age and gender. Our group has also found an association between vagally mediated HRV and several inflammatory markers. In a sample of 613 men and women, 24 h RMSSD was inversely associated with WBC and CRP even after controlling for a large number of potential covariates including sympathetic nervous system activity as indexed by norepinephrine. Psychosocial factors such as stressful life events, general stress, hostility, depression, and anxiety are also emerging as risk factors for CVD. Although a detailed examination of the evidence for decreased vagal function in these risk factors is beyond the scope of this chapter, we and others have shown previously that these psychological states and dispositions are associated with decreased vagal function.

In summary, emerging risk factors for CVD and mortality such as inflammation and psychosocial factors are also associated with decreased vagal function. Together with the decreased vagal function associated with the established risk factors, a unified picture of autonomic imbalance and decreased vagal inhibitory cardiac control is developing. In the next section, we show that this decreased vagal inhibitory control is associated with dysregulation in a neural network that is thought to underlie autonomic, affective, and cognitive regulation. As such this set of neural structures may provide the central nervous system concomitants of the autonomic imbalance that tie together the diverse cardiovascular risk factors and provide a pathway via which psychosocial factors may 'get under the skin' to confer risk for a wide range of disorders leading to increased morbidity and mortality.

2.6.5 Vagal Stimulation with Heart Diseases

A significant series of experimental and clinical studies have demonstrated the close association between reduced vagal reflexes and increased sudden and non-sudden cardiovascular mortality. Subsequently, evidence was provided that, also among chronic heart failure (HF) patients, depressed BRS is associated with a poorer outcome. At the same time, the encouraging results with experimental and clinical attempts to increase cardiac vagal activity led to a few experimental studies with vagal stimulation (VS) in different models for HF. Schwartz et al. performed a pilot study for VS in HF patients, and then in 2011 they reported the results of a small-size multicentre clinical trial. The 6-month and 1-year results are encouraging for feasibility and safety and appear to have a favourable clinical effect. An ongoing large clinical trial will provide a definitive assessment of the efficacy and usefulness of chronic VS in HF patients. From these data they concluded that chronic vagal stimulation is safe and tolerable in symptomatic patients with congestive heart failure with marked clinical subjective improvements associated with objective long-lasting favourable changes. The preservation of these effects at 1-year follow-up strongly argues against a major role of a possible placebo effect. Several mechanisms of action may have contributed to the beneficial effects of vagal stimulation in patients with heart failure (Gao et al. 2005; Hamdan et al. 2002). The modest changes in heart rate are unlikely to have played an important role in mediating the clinical effects, and two studies in heart failure models found beneficial effects of vagal stimulation in the absence of any heart rate change. Heart rate-independent effects may include antiadrenergic effects at ventricular level due to sympathetic–parasympathetic interaction, antiapoptotic effects, and the anti-inflammatory reflex postulated by Tracey. In a model of ischaemia reperfusion in rats, vagal stimulation markedly reduced infarct size and markers of inflammation without changes in heart rate. From this small multicentre study, we concluded that it was time to design a controlled clinical trial with an adequate patient population aimed at definitely assessing whether or not chronic vagal stimulation may usefully represent a novel non-pharmacological approach to the treatment of symptomatic patients with heart failure. This is now being done with the ongoing trial called INOVATE-HF, which aims at enrolling up to 650 patients from 80 sites and to randomise them in a 3:2 ratio in order to receive either active treatment or standard optimal medical therapy. Overall, this sequence of experimental and clinical studies, not unmindful of the role of the autonomic nervous system in heart failure, seems to represent a good example of translational cardiology (Adamson et al. 2003).

2.6.6 Renal Denervation

Our better understanding of the interplay between the kidney and sympathetic nervous system elucidates the importance of the sympathetic nervous system in blood pressure control and the pathogenesis of hypertension. In addition, the desirable results of sympathetic denervation in animal models and in patients who have undergone nephrectomies, together with the recognition of the favourable location of the sympathetic fibres and their exquisite sensitivity to radiofrequency, have resulted in the development of catheter-based radiofrequency ablation of the renal sympathetic nervous fibres. In a human feasibility, safety, and efficacy trial (Symplicity-1 [Catheter-based renal sympathetic denervation for resistant hypertension: a multicentre safety and proof-of-principle cohort study]), 45 patients with drug-resistant hypertension underwent bilateral application of radiofrequency to the renal arteries. A significant blood pressure reduction at 1-month follow-up of 14 and 10 mmHg (systolic and diastolic, respectively) was followed by a sustained response with a pronounced systolic and diastolic blood pressure reduction of 27 and 17 mmHg, respectively, at 12 months. Antihypertensive medication was adjusted in 13 patients at follow-up with a reduction in the number of antihypertensive medications in nine patients and an increase in four. Importantly, a significant blood pressure reduction remained even after excluding those four patients from the analysis whose antihypertensive medications were intensified. In 13 % of patients, no favourable blood pressure response occurred. In 10 patients who underwent renal norepinephrine spillover measurements, a significant reduction in renal norepinephrine spillover was shown, confirming the intended reduction in sympathetic drive to the kidney. In addition, total body norepinephrine spillover decreased significantly, lending support to the hypothesis that, by a reduction in afferent renal sympathetic signalling, the overall sympathetic tone can be reduced. In one patient, renal norepinephrine spillover, total body norepinephrine spillover, the plasma renin level, and muscle sympathetic activity decreased after renal denervation. In addition, the cardiac muscle mass assessed by cardiac magnetic resonance imaging decreased by 15 g. Registry data, including patients from Symplicity-1 who have completed 24-months follow-up ($n = 18$), demonstrate a sustained blood pressure reduction (33/14 mmHg). More recently, in the Symplicity HTN-2 (renal sympathetic denervation in patients with treatment-resistant hypertension) trial, 106 patients with resistant hypertension were randomised to catheter-based therapy in addition to conventional antihypertensive medications, vs. antihypertensive medications only, in a 1-to-1 fashion. The transcatheter techniques were similar to the previously described study. The primary endpoint was systolic blood pressure at 6-month follow-up. There was a significant difference in blood pressure changes from baseline between patients treated with catheter-based renal sympathectomy (reductions of 32/12 ± 23/11 mmHg) and those treated medically (0/1 ± 21/10 mmHg), with a mean blood pressure difference of 33/11 mmHg between the groups at 6 months. A systolic blood pressure improvement of at least 10 mmHg was observed in 84 % of patients in the interventional group and in 35 % in the medically treated control group. On 24-h ambulatory blood pressure monitoring, a significant blood pressure reduction was seen in patients who underwent renal sympathectomy (11/7 ± 15/11 mmHg), whereas the blood pressure was unchanged in patients with medically managed hypertension only. Importantly, the blood pressure reduction measured by 24-h ambulatory monitoring was less pronounced than that reported during office visits. Seven patients developed transient bradycardia requiring atropine administration. The renal function and urine–albumin–creatinine ratios remained unchanged at follow-up in both groups. The importance of the renal sympathetic nervous system activity in hypertension and its modulation are well established. Several aspects deserve further exploration. First, it has become apparent that this procedure does not cause universal blood pressure lowering. The reason for the response variability remains to be determined. One potential cause may be incomplete denervation. It is also possible that renal sympathetic activity has a subordinate role in the genesis and maintenance of hypertension in subsets of hypertensive patients with normal renal sympathetic tone. The renal sympathetic tone is not uniformly increased. Instead, there appears to be variability in renal efferent sympathetic nerve activity in hypertensive patients. For example, in patients older than 60 years, though skeletal muscle sympathetic activity is increased, renal norepinephrine spillover is frequently normal, whereas in patients with the metabolic syndrome, renal and overall sympathetic overactivity is frequently very pronounced. Thus, it would be very important to identify parameters that may predict the response to renal denervation and help in patient selection. Second, the sympathetic nervous system activity appears to be of most importance in the earlier stages of hypertension (Zhang et al. 2009; Schwartz et al. 2008). Early modification of sympathetic nervous system activity in these patients may bring a curative treatment for essential hypertension within reach. Thus, trials, including patients with milder forms of hypertension are warranted. Exploration of the impact of renal denervation in patients with secondary forms of hypertension, such as primary hyperaldosteronism that cannot be treated with surgical intervention, should also be considered. Third, obesity and insulin resistance are frequent companions of hypertension. Sympathetic overactivity has been observed with obesity, insulin resistance, and the metabolic syndrome, and improvements in glucose metabolism and insulin resistance have been reported after renal sympathetic denervation. A compromised skeletal muscle microcirculation has been suggested to be present in patients with hypertension. Sympathetic denervation may enhance skeletal muscle blood flow mediated by a reduction in adrenergic $\alpha 1$-receptor stimulation, increased skeletal muscle-capillary density, and a change in muscle fibre types, thereby potentially improving glucose uptake in the skeletal muscle. In addition, a decrease in glucagon secretion and gluconeogenesis and reduced activity of the renin–angiotensin system may contribute to the beneficial effects of renal denervation on glucose metabolism and insulin resistance. Although our current understanding of the preceding findings is far from complete, given the high incidence of cardiovascular events in patients with insulin resistance and impaired glucose metabolism and the favourable impact of reduced sympathetic drive, lower event rates after renal denervation are conceivable. Studies to this effect evaluating the impact of sympathetic denervation on diabetes control and cardiovascular events are ongoing (De Ferrari et al. 2011). In addition, further exploration of the impact of renal sympathectomy on the development of diabetic nephropathy is warranted as increases in glomerular filtration of up to 25–50 % have been described early in the course of (type 1) diabetes, perhaps contributing to the development of glomerulosclerosis and diabetic nephropathy, and prevention of glomerular hyperfiltration has been reported after renal sympathetic denervation in an animal model. Similarly, moxonidine, a central sympathetic inhibitor has been associated with a reduction in microalbuminuria in patients with (type 1) diabetes. Further supporting a potentially protective effect on renal function beyond that expected due to blood pressure reduction, the natural decline in estimated glomerular filtration rate expected depending on blood pressure at any given time was smaller than predicted at early follow-up, even after taking the blood pressure reduction into account, after renal denervation in 153 hypertensive patients (including those enrolled in Symplicity-1). However, in a small number of patients who completed later (up to 24 months) follow-up, the reduction in estimated glomerular filtration rate was more pronounced than that observed in a study examining the effect of ramipril, telmisartan, or both on renal function. Given these findings, further studies of the long-term impact on renal hemodynamic and function, particularly comparing renal denervation in a controlled fashion to conventional medical therapy, are warranted before a final statement regarding either a protective, neutral, or harmful effect can be made. Fourth, the impact of renal denervation on the reno-renal reflex particularly in conditions affecting only one kidney is not clear (Hauptman et al. 2012). For example, whether during urinary obstruction of one kidney a compensatory diuresis of the contralateral kidney can be expected in the same magnitude as would occur in the absence of renal denervation remains to be determined. Fifth, the autonomic nervous system affects nearly every part of the body. Given the myriad effects of an overactive SNS beyond blood pressure control, many of which are detrimental, renal denervation in some conditions associated with sympathetic overactivity requires further investigation. For example, in light of increased sympathetic nervous system activity in patients with systolic heart failure, its association with increased mortality, and the well-established benefits of β-adrenoreceptors blockade and modification of the renin–angiotensin system, the concept of renal denervation to reduce overall sympathetic drive in heart failure is intriguing. Along this line, a reduction in left ventricular filling pressures and improved left ventricular systolic function following renal denervation has been shown in animal models of heart failure. Similarly, a potential benefit in patients with hepatorenal syndrome characterised by sympathetic nervous system overactivity is possible. Lastly, an increased sympathetic drive has been described in patients with sleep apnoea, together with a favourable impact on the apnoea–hypopnea index after catheter-based renal sympathetic denervation. Hypothetically, this may be related to a reduction in fluid shifts to the neck with recumbent positioning after renal denervation based on the observation that a greater fluid shift from the lower extremities to the neck occurs in patients with uncontrolled vs. well-controlled hypertension (Krum et al. 2009). The reported improvements in sleep apnoea with aldosterone antagonists further support a potential deleterious effect of excessive nocturnal rostral fluid shifts. Studies examining the mechanism and impact of sympathetic denervation in patients with sleep apnoea are ongoing. Finally, it should be mentioned that catheter-based renal denervation is not the only device-based therapy available aiming to reduce the sympathetic nervous tone. Similar to renal sympathetic denervation, baroreceptor stimulation reduces the overall sympathetic nervous system activity and has been shown to lower blood pressure in a safety and feasibility trial. Recently, the results of a phase III trial comparing baroreceptor stimulation to conventional medical therapy in patients with resistant hypertension were published demonstrating a significant blood pressure reduction. However, it failed to meet one of the two primary efficacy endpoints (blood pressure responder rate at 6 months) likely related to an underestimation of blood pressure improvements in the control group. Importantly, as expected with the implantation of any foreign body, some adverse events occurred (4.8 % nerve injury with residual deficit and 2.6 % wound complications) (Esler et al. 2010). Further studies will determine this concept's role in hypertension treatment. We have entered an exciting era with the ability to modulate the sympathetic nervous system and achieve an improvement in blood pressure control with percutaneous renal denervation and potentially beneficial effects on a plethora of other conditions associated with sympathetic overactivity. Renal denervation has become a routine in some countries. Nevertheless, we should maintain our quest to further improve our understanding of the sympathetic nervous system in the pathogenesis of hypertension and some other disorders (Schlaich et al. 2009).

Conclusion

The interaction between the heart and brain becomes increasingly important as the underlying mutual mechanisms become better understood. The specialty that deals with the brain–heart connection has become known as neurocardiology. Neurocardiology refers to (patho)physiological interplays of the nervous and cardiovascular systems. A better understanding of the risks, mechanisms, and treatments is required. The usefulness of imaging the cardiac sympathetic nervous system is increasingly supported by prospective clinical studies. The future success of this molecular imaging technique, however, will depend on careful design of additional trials. But preclinical and clinical use requires a thorough understanding of the underlying biology, which defines the relationship between neuronal tracer kinetics, disease mechanisms, and appropriate study interpretation. Although imaging of the cardiac autonomic nervous system has entered large-scale clinical trials that will ultimately lead to approval as a clinical tool, the basic science behind this methodology remains important. Specifics of the used tracers and preclinical animal models need to be considered for translation. Establishment of quantitative measures for global and regional innervation will be important. The latter can be avoided only if previous knowledge from basic science is appropriately incorporated into translational study design.

References

Adamson PB, Kleckner KJ, Van Hout WL et al (2003) Cardiac resynchronization therapy improves heart rate variability in patients with symptomatic heart failure. Circulation 108:266–269

Antzelevitch C (2002) Sympathetic modulation of the long QT syndrome. Eur Heart J 23:1246–1252

Antzelevitch C, Shimizu W (2002) Cellular mechanisms underlying the long QT syndrome. Curr Opin Cardiol 17:43–51

Asirvatham SJ, Kapa S (2009) Sleep apnea and atrial fibrillation: the autonomic link. J Am Coll Cardiol 54:2084–2086

Brugada P, Brugada J (1992) Right bundle branch block, persistent ST segment elevation and sudden cardiac death: a distinct clinical and electrocardiographic syndrome: a multicenter report. J Am Coll Cardiol 20:1391–1396

Cao JM, Chen LS, KenKnight BH et al (2000a) Nerve sprouting and sudden cardiac death. Circ Res 86:816–821

Cao JM, Fishbein MC, Han JB et al (2000b) Relationship between regional cardiac hyperinnervation and ventricular arrhythmia. Circulation 101:1960–1969

Chen PS, Chen LS, Cao JM et al (2001) Sympathetic nerve sprouting, electrical remodeling and the mechanisms of sudden cardiac death. Cardiovasc Res 50:409–416

Chialvo DR, Gilmour RF Jr, Jalife J (1990) Low dimensional chaos in cardiac tissue. Nature 343:653–657

Chiou CW, Eble JN, Zipes DP (1997) Efferent vagal innervation of the canine atria and sinus and atrioventricular nodes. The third fat pad. Circulation 95:2573–2584

Daniel EE (2001) Physiology and pathophysiology of the interstitial cell of Cajal: from bench to bedside. III. Interaction of interstitial cells of Cajal with neuromediators: an interim assessment. Am J Physiol Gastrointest Liver Physiol 281:G1329–G1332

De Ferrari GM, Crijns HJGM, Borggrefe M et al (2011) Chronic vagus nerve stimulation: a new and promising therapeutic approach for chronic heart failure. Eur Heart J 32:847–855

Dizon JM, Chen K, Bacchetta M et al (2009) A comparison of atrial arrhythmias after heart or double-lung transplantation at a single center: insights into the mechanism of post-operative atrial fibrillation. J Am Coll Cardiol 54:2043–2048

Duan D (2009) Phenomics of cardiac chloride channels: the systematic study of chloride channel function in the heart. J Physiol 587:2163–2177

Eliasson T, Augustinsson LE, Mannheimer C (1996) Spinal cord stimulation in severe angina pectoris— presentation of current studies, indications, and clinical experience. Pain 65:169–179

Esler MD, Krum H, Sobotka PA et al (2010) Renal sympathetic denervation in patients with treatment-resistant hypertension (the Symplicity HTN-2 trial): a randomised controlled trial. Lancet 376:1903–1909

Farrell TG, Bashir Y, Cripps T et al (1991) Risk stratification for arrhythmic events in post-infarction patients based on heart rate variability, ambulatory electrocardiographic variables and the signal-averaged electrocardiogram. J Am Coll Cardiol 18:687–697

Ferrara N, Bonaduce D, Abete P et al (1987) Role of increased cholinergic activity in reperfusion induced ventricular arrhythmias. Cardiovasc Res 21:279–285

Gao L, Wang W, Li YL et al (2005) Simvastatin therapy normalises sympathetic neural control in experimental heart failure: roles of angiotensin II type 1 receptors and NAD(P)H oxidase. Circulation 112:1763–1770

Ghias M, Scherlag BJ, Lu Z et al (2009) The role of ganglionated plexi in apnea-related atrial fibrillation. J Am Coll Cardiol 54:2075–2083

Hamdan MH, Barbera S, Kowal RC et al (2002) Effects of resynchronization therapy on sympathetic activity in patients with depressed ejection fraction and intra-ventricular conduction delay due to ischemic or idiopathic dilated cardiomyopathy. Am J Cardiol 89:1047–1051

Harvey RD, Clark CD, Hume JR (1990) Chloride current in mammalian cardiac myocytes. Novel mechanism for autonomic regulation of action potential duration and resting membrane potential. J Gen Physiol 95:1077–1102

Hauptman PJ, Schwartz PJ, Gold MR et al (2012) Rationale and study design of the increase of vagal tone in heart failure study: INOVATE-HF. Am Heart J 163:954–962

Hjalmarson A (1997) Effects of beta blockade on sudden cardiac death during acute myocardial infarction and the postinfarction period. Am J Cardiol 80:35J–39J

Hohnloser SH, Klingenheben T, van de Loo A et al (1994) Reflex versus tonic vagal activity as a prognostic parameter in patients with sustained ventricular tachycardia or ventricular fibrillation. Circulation 89:1068–1073

Hou Y, Scherlag BJ, Lin J et al (2007a) Ganglionated plexi modulate extrinsic cardiac autonomic nerve input: effects on sinus rate, atrioventricular conduction, refractoriness, and inducibility of atrial fibrillation. J Am Coll Cardiol 50:61–68

Hou Y, Scherlag BJ, Lin J et al (2007b) Interactive atrial neural network: determining the connections between ganglionated plexi. Heart Rhythm 4:56–63

Hull SS Jr, Evans AR, Vanoli E et al (1990) Heart rate variability before and after myocardial infarction in conscious dogs at high and low risk of sudden death. J Am Coll Cardiol 16:978–985

Issa ZF, Ujhelyi MR, Hildebrand KR et al (2005a) Intrathecal clonidine reduces the incidence of ischemia- provoked ventricular arrhythmias in a canine postinfarction heart failure model. Heart Rhythm 2:1122–1127

Issa ZF, Zhou X, Ujhelyi MR et al (2005b) Thoracic spinal cord stimulation reduces the risk of ischemic ventricular arrhythmias in a postinfarction heart failure canine model. Circulation 111:3217–3220

Janse MJ, Schwartz PJ, Wilms-Schopman F et al (1985) Effects of unilateral stellate ganglion stimulation and ablation on electrophysiologic changes induced by acute myocardial ischemia in dogs. Circulation 72:585–595

Kleiger RE, Miller JP, Bigger JT Jr et al (1987) Decreased heart rate variability and its association with increased mortality after acute myocardial infarction. Am J Cardiol 59:256–262

Kostin S, Popescu LM (2009) A distinct type of cell in myocardium: interstitial Cajal-like cells (ICLCs). J Cell Mol Med 13:295–308

Krum H, Schlaich M, Whitbourn R et al (2009) Catheter-based renal sympathetic denervation for resistant hypertension: a multicenter safety and proof-of-principle cohort study. Lancet 373:1275–1281

La Rovere MT, Bigger JT Jr, Marcus FI et al (1998) Baroreflex sensitivity and heart-rate variability in prediction of total cardiac mortality after myocardial infarction ATRAMI (Autonomic Tone and Reflexes After Myocardial Infarction) investigators. Lancet 351:478–484

Lopshire JC, Zhou X, Dusa C et al (2009) Spinal cord stimulation improves ventricular function and reduces ventricular arrhythmias in a canine postinfarction heart failure model. Circulation 120:286–294

Mannheimer C, Eliasson T, Andersson B et al (1993) Effects of spinal cord stimulation in angina pectoris induced by pacing and possible mechanisms of action. Br Med J 307:477–480

Marron K, Wharton J, Sheppard MN et al (1995) Distribution, morphology, and neurochemistry of endocardial and epicardial nerve terminal arborizations in the human heart. Circulation 92:2343–2351

Matsuo K, Kurita T, Inagaki M et al (1999) The circadian pattern of the development of ventricular fibrillation in patients with Brugada syndrome. Eur Heart J 20:465–470

Miyazaki T, Mitamura H, Miyoshi S et al (1996) Autonomic and antiarrhythmic drug modulation of ST segment elevation in patients with Brugada syndrome. J Am Coll Cardiol 27:1061–1070

Nademanee K, Taylor R, Bailey WE et al (2000) Treating electrical storm: sympathetic blockade versus advanced cardiac life support-guided therapy. Circulation 102:742–747

Nguyen BL, Fishbein MC, Chen LS et al (2009) Histopathological substrate for chronic atrial fibrillation in humans. Heart Rhythm 6:454–460

Noda T, Takaki H, Kurita T et al (2002) Gene-specific response of dynamic ventricular repolarization to sympathetic stimulation in LQT1, LQT2 and LQT3 forms of congenital long QT syndrome. Eur Heart J 23:975–983

Odemuyiwa O, Poloniecki J, Malik M et al (1994) Temporal influences on the prediction of postinfarction mortality by heart rate variability: a comparison with the left ventricular ejection fraction. Br Heart J 71:521–527

Patterson E, Po SS, Scherlag BJ et al (2005) Triggered firing in pulmonary veins initiated by in vitro autonomic nerve stimulation. Heart Rhythm 2:624–631

Paul M, Schafers M, Kies P et al (2006) Impact of sympathetic innervation on recurrent life-threatening arrhythmias in the follow-up of patients with idiopathic ventricular fibrillation. Eur J Nucl Med Mol Imaging 33:866–870

Pitt B, Zannad F, Remme WJ et al (1999) The effect of spironolactone on morbidity and mortality in patients with severe heart failure Randomized Aldactone Evaluation Study Investigators. N Engl J Med 341:709–717

Pliquett RU, Cornish KG, Peuler JD et al (2003a) Simvastatin normalizes autonomic neural control in experimental heart failure. Circulation 107:2493–2498

Pliquett RU, Cornish KG, Zucker IH (2003b) Statin therapy restores sympathovagal balance in experimental heart failure. J Appl Physiol 95:700–704

Po SS, Nakagawa H, Jackman WM (2009) Localisation of left atrial ganglionated plexi in patients with atrial fibrillation. J Cardiovasc Electrophysiol 20:1186–1189

Ren C, Wang F, Li G et al (2008) Nerve sprouting suppresses myocardial I(to) and I(K1) channels and increases severity to ventricular fibrillation in rat. Auton Neurosci 144:22–29

Rosenshtraukh L, Danilo P Jr, Anyukhovsky EP et al (1994) Mechanisms for vagal modulation of ventricular repolarization and of coronary occlusion-induced lethal arrhythmias in cats. Circ Res 75:722–732

Saito T, Waki K, Becker AE (2000) Left atrial myocardial extension onto pulmonary veins in humans: anatomic observations relevant for atrial arrhythmias. J Cardiovasc Electrophysiol 11:888–894

Sanderson JE, Ibrahim B, Waterhouse D et al (1994) Spinal electrical stimulation for intractable angina: long-term clinical outcome and safety. Eur Heart J 15:810–814

Scherlag BJ, Yamanashi W, Patel U et al (2005a) Autonomically induced conversion of pulmonary vein focal firing into atrial fibrillation. J Am Coll Cardiol 45:1878–1886

Scherlag BJ, Nakagawa H, Jackman WM et al (2005b) Electrical stimulation to identify neural elements on the heart: their role in atrial fibrillation. J Interv Card Electrophysiol 13(Suppl 1):37–42

Scherlag BJ, Patterson E, Po SS (2006) The neural basis of atrial fibrillation. J Electrocardiol 39:S180–S183

Schlaich MP, Sobotka PA, Krum H, Lambert E, Esler MD (2009) Renal sympathetic-nerve ablation for uncontrolled hypertension. N Engl J Med 361:932–934

Schwartz PJ (1984) Sympathetic imbalance and cardiac arrhythmias. In: Randall WC (ed) Nervous control of cardiovascular function. Oxford University Press, New York, pp 225–252

Schwartz PJ, Billman GE, Stone HL (1984) Autonomic mechanisms in ventricular fibrillation induced by myocardial ischemia during exercise in dogs with healed myocardial infarction. An experimental preparation for sudden cardiac death. Circulation 69:790–800

Schwartz PJ, Vanoli E, Stramba-Badiale M et al (1988a) Autonomic mechanisms and sudden death. New insights from analysis of baroreceptor reflexes in conscious dogs with and without a myocardial infarction. Circulation 78:969–979

Schwartz PJ, Zaza A, Pala M et al (1988b) Baroreflex sensitivity and its evolution during the first year after myocardial infarction. J Am Coll Cardiol 12:629–636

Schwartz PJ, Locati EH, Moss AJ et al (1991) Left cardiac sympathetic denervation in the therapy of congenital long QT syndrome: a worldwide report. Circulation 84:503–511

Schwartz PJ, Priori SG, Cerrone M et al (2004) Left cardiac sympathetic denervation in the management of high-risk patients affected by the long-QT syndrome. Circulation 109:1826–1833

Schwartz PJ, De Ferrari GM, Sanzo A et al (2008) Long term vagal stimulation in patients with advanced heart failure: first experience in man. Eur J Heart Fail 10:884–891

Scott PA, Sandilands AJ, Morris GE et al (2008) Successful treatment of catecholaminergic polymorphic ventricular tachycardia with bilateral thoracoscopic sympathectomy. Heart Rhythm 5:1461–1463

Stanton MS, Tuli MM, Radtke NL et al (1989) Regional sympathetic denervation after myocardial infarction in humans detected non-invasively using I-123- metaiodobenzylguanidine. J Am Coll Cardiol 14:1519–1526

Taggart P, Sutton P, Lab M et al (1990) Interplay between adrenaline and interbeat interval on ventricular repolarization in intact heart in vivo. Cardiovasc Res 24:884–895

Taggart P, Sutton P, Chalabi Z et al (2003) Effect of adrenergic stimulation on action potential duration restitution in humans. Circulation 107:285–289

Tan AY, Li H, Wachsmann-Hogiu S et al (2006) Autonomic innervation and segmental muscular disconnections at the human pulmonary vein-atrial junction: implications for catheter ablation of atrial-pulmonary vein junction. J Am Coll Cardiol 48:132–143

Terrenoire C, Clancy CE, Cormier JW et al (2005) Autonomic control of cardiac action potentials: role of potassium channel kinetics in response to sympathetic stimulation. Circ Res 96:e25–e34

Vyas H, Johnson K, Houlihan R et al (2006) Acquired long QT syndrome secondary to cesium chloride supplement. J Altern Complement Med 12:1011–1014

Walsh KB, Kass RS (1991) Distinct voltage-dependent regulation of a heart-delayed IK by protein kinases A and C. Am J Physiol 261:C1081–C1090

Ward SM, Sanders KM (2001) Physiology and pathophysiology of the interstitial cell of Cajal: from bench to bedside. I. Functional development and plasticity of interstitial cells of Cajal networks. Am J Physiol Gastrointest Liver Physiol 281:G602–G611

Wichter T, Matheja P, Eckardt L et al (2002) Cardiac autonomic dysfunction in Brugada syndrome. Circulation 105:702–706

Wilde AA, Bhuiyan ZA, Crotti L et al (2008) Left cardiac sympathetic denervation for catecholaminergic polymorphic ventricular tachycardia. N Engl J Med 358:2024–2029

Yoshioka K, Gao DW, Chin M et al (2000) Heterogeneous sympathetic innervation influences local myocardial repolarization in normally perfused rabbit hearts. Circulation 101:1060–1066

Zhang JF, Robinson RB, Siegelbaum SA (1992) Sympathetic neurones mediate developmental change in cardiac sodium channel gating through long-term neurotransmitter action. Neuron 9:97–103

Zhang Y, Popovic ZB, Bibevski S et al (2009) Chronic vagus nerve stimulation improves autonomic control and attenuates systemic inflammation and heart failure progression in a canine high-rate pacing model. Circ Heart Fail 2:692–699

Zhou S, Cao JM, Tebb ZD et al (2001) Modulation of QT interval by cardiac sympathetic nerve sprouting and the mechanisms of ventricular arrhythmia in a canine model of sudden cardiac death. J Cardiovasc Electrophysiol 12:1068–1073

Zhou J, Scherlag BJ, Edwards J et al (2007) Gradients of atrial refractoriness and inducibility of atrial fibrillation due to stimulation of ganglionated plexi. J Cardiovasc Electrophysiol 18:83–90

Zipes DP (1994) Autonomic modulation of cardiac arrhythmias. In: Zipes DP, Jalife J (eds) Cardiac electrophysiology: from cell to bedside, 2nd edn. WB Saunders Co, Philadelphia, pp 365–395

Development of Heart Failure and the Role of the Autonomic Nervous System of the Heart

3

S. Pardaens and J. De Sutter

Contents

Abstract

Heart failure is a clinical syndrome that develops in response of a cardiac insult, resulting in a decline of cardiac performance. Several neurohormonal mechanisms are activated in response to the underlying myocardial dysfunction, including the autonomic nervous system. Patients with heart failure are characterized by an abnormally activated sympathetic and altered parasympathetic tone, with also attenuated cardiovascular reflexes and a maladaptive downregulation of adrenergic nerve terminals. During exercise, an inappropriate rise in ventilation occurs as well as an enhanced peripheral vasoconstriction in order to preserve an adequate blood pressure level. Although the activation of these systems can

S. Pardaens, MSc (✉) • J. De Sutter, MD, PhD
Department of internal medicine, Ghent University, Ghent, Belgium
e-mail: sofie.pardaens@ugent.be

R.H.J.A. Slart et al. (eds.), *Autonomic Innervation of the Heart: Role of Molecular Imaging*, DOI 10.1007/978-3-662-45074-1_3

initially compensate for the depressed myocardial function, their long-term activation results in a further impairment of cardiac function leading to progression of heart failure with fatigue and dyspnea being major barriers for exercise tolerance. Medication, in particular beta-blocker and ACE-inhibitor therapy, influences both the sympathetic and parasympathetic tone. The sympathetic tone may also be modulated by cardiac resynchronization therapy whereas vagus nerve stimulation may increase the parasympathetic activity. Through its impact on the periphery, physical exercise is also able to influence both the sympathetic and parasympathetic nervous system..

Abbreviations

$[^{123}I]$-MIBG	Iodine-123 metaiodobenzylguanidine
ANS	Autonomic nervous system
CNS	Central nervous system
CO	Cardiac output
CRT	Cardiac resynchronization therapy
nNOS	Neuronal nitric oxide synthase
NO	Nitric oxide
PSNS	Parasympathetic nervous system
RAAS	Renin-angiotensin-aldosterone system
SNS	Sympathetic nervous system

3.1 Introduction

Heart failure is a clinical syndrome that develops in response of a cardiac insult, resulting in a decline of cardiac performance. Several neurohormonal mechanisms are activated in response to the underlying myocardial dysfunction, including the sympathetic nervous system (SNS) and the renin-angiotensin-aldosterone system axis (RAAS axis). Although the activation of these systems can initially compensate for the depressed myocardial function, their long-term activation results in a further impairment of cardiac function leading to progression of heart failure and cardiac decompensation (Mann and Bristow 2005; Triposkiadis et al. 2009).

As pointed out by Parati and Esler (2012), sympathetic activation occurs subsequently to the development of heart failure and then impacts adversely on clinical outcome. This is in contrast to essential hypertension where SNS activation is already important in the initiation and the maintenance of hypertension. Also, there is now clear evidence that besides sympathetic activation, also reduced vagal function plays a role in the development of heart failure (Bibevski and Dunlap 2011). In this chapter we will briefly review the normal cardiovascular actions of the autonomic nervous system (ANS) and then discuss the pathophysiology and potential therapeutic implications of sympathetic hyperactivity and reduced vagal function in heart failure.

3.2 The ANS and Normal Cardiac Function

In the normal heart, the SNS has different cardiovascular actions, including acceleration of the heart rate, increase in cardiac contractility, reduction of venous capacitance, and constriction of resistance vessels. The cardiac sympathetic nerve fibers are located subepicardially and travel along the major coronary arteries (Triposkiadis et al. 2009; Zipes 2008). The sympathetic outflow to the heart and peripheral circulation is regulated by cardiovascular reflexes. Afferent fibers are carried towards the central nervous system (CNS) by autonomic nerves, whereas efferent impulses travel from the CNS towards different organs. The main reflex responses originate from the aortic arch and carotid baroreceptors (SNS inhibition), cardiopulmonary baroreceptors (including the Bezold-Jarish reflex, SNS inhibition), cardiovascular low-threshold polymodal receptors (SNS activation), and peripheral chemoreceptors (SNS activation) (Malliani et al. 1983). As already summarized by Van Stee (1978), the effect of SNS activation on the periphery is mediated by 4 pathways: (1) norepinephrine-releasing neurons through the right stellate ganglion reaching the sinus and atrioventricular nodes (resulting in an increase in heart rate and shortening of atrioventricular conduction) and through the left stellate ganglion reaching the left ventricle (resulting in an increase in contractile strength), (2) epinephrine released in circulation by the adrenal cortex affecting both the myocardium and peripheral vessels, (3) direct effect on peripheral vessels through local release of epinephrine and norepinephrine, and (4) circulating norepinephrine which can act on multiple locations (e.g., increase in heart rate during exercise in heart transplant recipients). Norepinephrine and epinephrine bind to specific adrenergic receptors, of which there are at least nine subtypes (3 α1-receptor subtypes, 3 α2-receptor subtypes, and 3 β-receptor subtypes). In the human heart, activation of β1- and β2-adrenergic receptors is the most powerful physiologic mechanism to acutely increase cardiac performance and the β-adrenergic receptor density is greatest at the apical myocardium (Leineweber et al. 2002). Approximately 80 % of norepinephrine released by the sympathetic nerve terminals is recycled by the norepinephrine transporter 1, whereas the remainder clears into the circulation (Feldman et al. 2005).

The parasympathetic nervous system (PSNS) affects the cardiovascular system by slowing heart rate through vagal impulses. The parasympathetic fibers run with the vagus nerve subendocardially and are mainly present in the atrial myocardium and less abundantly in the ventricular myocardium (Triposkiadis et al. 2009; Zipes 2008). Acetylcholine released from postganglionic cardiac parasympathetic nerves reduces heart rate by binding to muscarinic cholinergic receptors (primarily M2 subtype) on sinoatrial nodal cells (Brodde et al. 2001; Katona et al. 1977). Parasympathetic-mediated changes in heart rate are initiated primarily in the CNS or originate from activation or inhibition of sensory nerves. Stimulation of arterial baroreceptors, trigeminal receptors, and subsets of cardiopulmonary receptors with vagal afferents reflexively increases cardiovagal activity and decreases heart rate. In contrast, stimulation of pulmonary stretch receptors with vagal afferents and subsets of visceral and somatic receptors with spinal afferents reflexively decrease cardiovagal activity and increase heart rate (Chapleau and Sabharwal 2011). Importantly, the PSNS and the SNS are often working interactively with opposing resulting effects.

3.3 Heart Failure and Sympathetic Hyperactivity

3.3.1 Pathophysiology

Patients with heart failure are characterized by an abnormally activated sympathetic and altered parasympathetic tone, with also attenuated cardiovascular reflexes and a maladaptive downregulation of adrenergic nerve terminals (Himura et al. 1993; Liang et al. 1989). In the early changes of heart failure, there is a selective cardiac change in the autonomic regulation with a decrease in heart rate variability and a selective increase in cardiac norepinephrine spillover in order to preserve cardiac output (CO). Chronic persistent myocardial dysfunction is associated with a more generalized sympathetic hyperactivity. Evidence for this increased sympathetic activity in patients with heart failure includes increased central sympathetic outflow and increased norepinephrine spillover to plasma from activated sympathetic nerve fibers and consequently increased plasma norepinephrine levels. Besides the increased muscle sympathetic nerve activity and norepinephrine spillover, patients with heart failure and reduced ejection fraction may also have a decreased neuronal density and a decreased neuronal function resulting in decreased norepinephrine concentration within the cardiomyocytes. Compared with myocardium of healthy individuals, the myocardium of patients with chronic left ventricular dysfunction is also characterized by a significant reduction of presynaptic norepinephrine uptake and postsynaptic β1-adrenergic receptor density (Caldwell et al. 2008; Ungerer et al. 1993). This latter phenomenon has been documented in patients after acute myocardial infarction where it contributes to adverse left ventricular remodeling, in patients with heart failure due to dilated cardiomyopathy as well as in patients with hypertrophic cardiomyopathy who develop left ventricular dilatation and heart failure (Choudhury et al. 1996; Merlet et al. 1993; Spyrou et al. 2002). The increase in norepinephrine levels apparently results in a decrease in β1-adrenergic receptor density and a β1-adrenergic receptor desensitization which appears to be a predominantly protective adaptation. The role of cardiac β2- and β3-adrenergic receptors as well as cardiac α1-adrenergic receptors in heart failure has not been fully elucidated yet (Triposkiadis et al. 2009).

3.3.2 Effects During Exercise

3.3.2.1 Hemodynamic Effects

During exercise, cardiovascular and respiratory responses are regulated by the ANS in order to provide a sufficient oxygen supply to the working muscles (Decherchi et al. 2007). The balance between parasympathetic and sympathetic nerve activity is mediated by the interaction between the central command, originating from the central motor areas, and peripheral feedback afferents, including the baroreflex, chemoreflex, and ergoreflex (Decherchi et al. 2007; O'Leary 2006). Sensory input from these cardiovascular afferents is projected to the nucleus tractus solitarius in the medulla oblongata, which plays a pivotal role in integrating and referring this information to other regions of the CNS with an impact on the sympathetic-parasympathetic outflow (Dampney et al. 2002).

Activation of the SNS during exercise normally induces a rise in heart rate and contractility resulting in an increased CO (Triposkiadis et al. 2009). Together with local metabolic vasodilatation, increased CO amplifies the blood flow to the working muscles. Local vasodilatation is, however, partially restrained by an SNS-mediated vasoconstriction in order to maintain an adequate level of blood pressure (Khan and Sinoway 2000).

Baroreceptors, located in the aortic arch and carotid sinuses (Kougias et al. 2010), and ergoreceptors, group III and IV skeletal muscle afferents (Kaufman et al. 1983) are both responsible for these hemodynamic changes. Once activated, the main function of these baroreceptors is to maintain the arterial blood pressure at an adequate level (set point) by increasing or decreasing peripheral vasoconstriction (Kougias et al. 2010). During exercise, a rapid resetting of this set point occurs (towards a higher level) in order to allow a higher arterial pressure and increased blood flow to adjust to the increased metabolic demands (Dampney et al. 2002). Importantly, in a significant number of patients, additional nonbaroreflex-mediated excitatory stimuli, including coexisting sleep apnea, myocardial ischemia, obesity, and inflammation, may elevate the set point for central sympathetic outflow or neurotransmitter release at rest and during exercise.

As metabolites accumulate during exercise and signal insufficient oxygen supply to the exercising muscles, ergoreceptors become activated and provide a rise in arterial pressure and blood flow primarily via an increased ventricular contractility and stroke volume with a resultant increase in CO (Crisafulli et al. 2003, 2006; O'Leary 2006). The effect of the ergoreflex on heart rate has been a matter of debate. Some authors suggested that the ergoreflex has only a minor influence on HR (Piepoli et al. 1995). However, when the mean arterial pressure is elevated, arterial baroreflex should decrease heart rate to lower mean arterial pressure (Nishiyasu et al. 1994). As heart rate remains unchanged, the influence of the ergoreflex on heart rate regulation is thought to be masked by counterregulation of the arterial baroreflex (Iellamo et al. 1999). During severe exercise the ability of the ergoreflex to elicit further increases in CO becomes limited. Pressor responses are then mediated via peripheral vasoconstriction but are smaller in comparison with the contribution of CO regulation (Augustyniak et al. 2001). In normal healthy subjects, ergoreflex activity is buffered by the arterial baroreflex. If this reflex is left unbuffered, then instead of a rise in CO, peripheral vasoconstriction in the active skeletal muscle is induced as a response to ergoreflex activation (Kim et al. 2005b).

Due to a chronic left ventricular dysfunction, a catabolic state is seen in heart failure with metabolic changes and chronic underperfusion of the skeletal muscle. A shift from type I to type IIb muscular fibers has been reported with a decrease in oxidative enzyme capacity and a concomitant rise in lactate and lactate dehydrogenase activity (Mancini et al. 1989; Schaufelberger et al. 1997). Skeletal muscle apoptosis has also been described in heart failure and is thought to be triggered by proinflammatory cytokines (Vescovo and Dalla Libera 2006; Vescovo et al. 2000).

This altered muscle metabolism may elicit an accumulation of metabolic byproducts which results in a chronic activation of the ergoreceptors and subsequently sympathetic hyperactivity. Whereas in normal conditions the ergoreflex increases CO, a shift towards peripheral vasoconstriction is seen in heart failure, further limiting blood flow and exacerbating skeletal muscle abnormalities and fatigue complaints (Clark et al. 1996; Hammond et al. 2000). The loss of the CO response likely reflects the impaired ability to increase ventricular function (Augustyniak et al. 2001; Hammond et al. 2000; O'Leary 2006), and the shift towards a peripheral vasoconstriction indicates a reduced baroreflex buffering in pathologic situations (Kim et al. 2005a).

3.3.2.2 Ventilatory Effects

Apart from hemodynamic changes, ergoreceptors are also thought to take part in ventilatory responses during exercise. However, the role of these receptors in modulating ventilation in healthy subjects has been questioned due to conflicting results in the literature (Piepoli et al. 1995, 1999; Scott et al. 2000). On the other hand, in patients with heart failure, an overactive ergoreflex mechanism has been demonstrated resulting in an excessive increase in ventilation and symptoms of breathlessness. A disruption of this reflex has been shown to correlate with several prognostic exercise parameters, including the peak VO_2 and the ventilatory slope (Piepoli et al. 1996, 1999; Ponikowski et al. 2001b).

Chemoreceptors may also play a critical role in the increased ventilatory response in heart failure (Chua et al. 1996; Ponikowski et al. 2001b). According to their location, they are subdivided into central medullary and peripheral carotid afferents with the former being particularly sensitive to changes in CO_2 while the latter are activated in hypoxic conditions (Dampney et al. 2002). In patients with heart failure, enhanced hypoxic and central hypercapnic chemosensitivity has been described (Chua et al. 1996; Ponikowski et al. 1997, 2001b). This hypersensitivity is associated with a higher incidence of arrhythmias and Cheyne-Stokes respiration and indicates a poor prognosis (Ponikowski et al. 2001a).

When the chemoreflex and ergoreflex are combined, the response to ventilation is greater than the sum of the two responses separately, suggesting that their interaction has an additional stimulatory effect on ventilation (Lykidis et al. 2009).

In conclusion, in a generalized sympathetic state which is seen in patients with heart failure, an enhanced peripheral vasoconstriction occurs during exercise in order to preserve an adequate blood pressure level. Consequently, this limits blood flow in the exercising muscle and thereby further exacerbates muscular abnormalities. Concerning the ventilatory aspect, an inappropriate rise in ventilation is seen which is related to the complaints of breathlessness and indicates a poor prognosis. As such, sympathetic hyperactivity contributes to the downward vicious cycle characteristic for heart failure, with fatigue and dyspnea being the major barriers for exercise tolerance.

3.3.3 Therapeutic Implications

3.3.3.1 Medication

Several classes of medication can interact with the SNS and inhibit its activity in patients with heart failure. Chronic beta-blocker therapy has been extensively evaluated in patients with heart failure. Several large scale clinical trials have shown that bisoprolol, carvedilol, metoprolol succinate, and nebivolol reverse left ventricular remodeling, reduce the risk of hospitalization and improve survival in patients with chronic heart failure (McMurray et al. 2012). This protective effect of beta-blockers is multifactorial and related to several factors, including the inhibition of catecholamine cardiotoxic effects, β1-adrenergic receptor upregulation, attenuation of the RAAS-axis, subendocardial coronary flow enhancement, and restoration of the reflex control on the heart and circulation (Adamson and Gilbert 2006; Triposkiadis et al. 2009). A meta-analysis in almost 20,000 patients demonstrated that the cardiovascular risk reduction with beta-blockers in patients with systolic heart failure was predominantly due to heart rate reduction achieved by beta-blockade rather than the type of beta-blockade, the dose of the beta-blockade, the underlying course of heart failure, and many other potential confounders (McAlister et al. 2009). The RAAS axis is upregulated in heart failure, and the resulting angiotensin II and aldosterone production enhances the release and inhibits the uptake of norepinephrine at nerve endings. Because of this interaction with the SNS, a part of the beneficial effect of angiotensin-converting enzyme inhibitors and aldosterone antagonists in heart failure can probably be attributed to their effect on norepinephrine (Adamson and Gilbert 2006). However not all medications that interact with the SNS have shown beneficial effects in patients with heart failure. Prazosin, for example, inhibits the α1-receptor but causes an increase in cathecholamine levels which probably explains a worse outcome in clinical trials (Cohn et al. 1986). Also, moxonidine that acts through both α2- and imidazolidine receptors and causes a marked dose-related reduction in plasma norepinephrine was associated with an increased mortality in clinical trials (Cohn et al. 2003).

3.3.3.2 Device Therapy

Cardiac resynchronization therapy (CRT) is an effective therapy in patients with advanced heart failure and electrical/mechanical dyssynchrony. Several large outcome studies have shown that this device therapy is associated with an improvement of symptoms, quality of life, and survival (McMurray et al. 2012). Cha et al. (2011) recently reported that CRT modulates sympathetic function by upregulating presynaptic receptor function as evidenced by increased iodine-123 metaiodobenzylguanidine ([^{123}I]-MIBG) imaging. Importantly, the reversal of neuronal remodeling in response to CRT appeared to be beyond that achieved by medical therapy. Also, patients with a less impaired presynaptic adrenergic preservation (or a better sympathetic reserve) showed a better response to CRT.

3.3.3.3 Physical Exercise

Physical exercise has been demonstrated to improve exercise tolerance and quality of life and reduce hospitalizations in heart failure (Flynn et al. 2009; O'Connor et al. 2009). There is also limited evidence that exercise reduces mortality. One of the responsible mechanisms for these beneficial effects is the counteraction of the sympathetic hyperactivity. Heart rate variability, beat to beat variations in time of consecutive heartbeats expressed in a normal sinus rhythm, is frequently used to evaluate the ANS (McMillan 2002). Training has been shown to improve heart rate variability, indicating that the ANS and the sinoatrial node respond dynamically to environmental changes (Larsen et al. 2004; Malfatto et al. 2002; McMillan 2002; Murad et al. 2012; Roveda et al. 2003).

Regular exercise reverses sympathetic hyperactivity in favor of exercise tolerance, through its influence on the different receptors which mediate the sympathico-vagal balance.

Training effects have traditionally been attributed to peripheral rather than central adaptations. A (partial) reversal of structural abnormalities in skeletal muscle such as a decreased oxidative capacity, an impaired leg muscle blood flow with endothelial dysfunction, and a glycolytic fiber type distribution has been demonstrated after physical exercise (Hambrecht et al. 1995, 1997, 1998; Sullivan et al. 1988). This reshift towards an aerobic metabolism may result in a decreased ergoreflex activity with a concomitant reduced activation of the sympathetic outflow (Piepoli et al. 1996; Wang et al. 2010, 2012). Another effect of physical exercise is the restoration of the blunted baroreflex sensitivity (Gademan et al. 2007; Iellamo et al. 2011). The baroreflex is known to buffer the ergoreflex-mediated vasoconstriction (Kim et al. 2005b). This buffering mechanism together with a reduced triggering of the ergoreceptors results in an improved skeletal muscle blood flow which has a positive effect on fatigue complaints.

As ergoreflex activity is also known to influence ventilation, a decrease in its activation through physical exercise has a positive impact on the prognostic important ventilatory inefficiency, typically seen in patients with heart failure (Piepoli et al. 1996). Physical exercise also reduces chemoreceptor activity, another mediator of the ventilatory drive (Li et al. 2008).

Through its impact on the periphery, physical exercise is able to influence the ANS thereby dealing with the two main reasons for exercise intolerance, dyspnea, and fatigue.

3.4 Heart Failure and Reduced Vagal Function

3.4.1 Pathophysiology

Dysfunction of the PSNS has been documented extensively in heart failure in both animal studies and humans. Already in 1971, Eckberg et al. (1971) showed that arterial baroreflex control of heart rate was reduced in patients with left ventricular dysfunction. Moreover, altered vagal control of heart rate appears to be present early in the development of left ventricular dysfunction (Kinugawa and Dibner-Dunlap 1995) and is associated with a poor prognosis in patients post myocardial infarction and in heart failure post myocardial infarction (Kleiger et al. 1987; La Rovere et al. 1998). Despite the recognition of a reduced vagal control in heart failure and its association with worse outcomes, the precise anatomical sites and mechanisms of abnormal vagal control are not very clear (Bibevski and Dunlap 2011). The overall (limited) evidence suggests that the anatomical level of dysfunction seems to lie at the level of the ganglion since postganglionic mechanisms are upregulated and functional (Bibevski and Dunlap 2011). Different non-invasive techniques can be used to measure vagal nerve activity including resting heart rate, heart rate variability, baroreflex sensitivity, and heart rate turbulence (for an extensive review, see Chapleau and Sabharwal 2011).

3.4.2 Effects During Exercise

In normal subjects, vagal control results in a reduction in resting heart rate through its inhibitory effect on the SNS and hyperpolarization of the sinus nodal cells. Via a NO pathway, parasympathetic activation can cause vasorelaxation, but vasoconstriction through its action on vascular smooth muscle has also been described (Olshansky et al. 2008). Apart from the bradycardic effect, a negative inotropic effect resulting in a decreased myocardial contractility has been demonstrated after vagal nerve stimulation (Lewis et al. 2001). As such, parasympathetic activity decreases the cardiac work and myocardial oxygen demand (Buch et al. 2002).

Vagal function is blunted in heart failure (Binkley et al. 1991; Kinugawa and Dibner-Dunlap 1995; Nolan et al. 1992) and is thought to originate from a withdrawal of baroreflex activity. As blood pressure falls in heart failure, baroreflex activity is reduced resulting in a decrease in the inhibitory input to adrenergic control (Clark and Cleland 2000). Whereas in normal conditions, baroreceptor activity modulates chemoreceptor (Heistad et al. 1975; Somers et al. 1991) and ergoreflex activation (Kim et al. 2005b), this inhibition is impaired in heart failure, with a resultant increase in ergoreflex-mediated vasoconstriction (Kim et al. 2005a) and a hyperventilatory response during exercise (Chua et al. 1996; Piepoli et al. 1996; Ponikowski et al. 2001b).

3.4.3 Therapeutic Implications

While beta-blockade has found its place as a cornerstone therapy for heart failure that impacts the SNS, far less is known about medication and interventions that augment parasympathetic function.

3.4.3.1 Medication

Since there is a close interaction between the sympathetic and vagal nervous system, medical therapy that influences the SNS may also have an effect on the vagal nervous system. This has been shown both experimentally and clinically for beta-blockers in heart failure. They can augment the vagal nerve control of heart rate by blocking the cardiac sympathetic pre-junctional β2-adrenoreceptor that facilitates norepinephrine release (Kubo et al. 2005). Also, they can increase the density of M2 receptors especially in the endocardial tissues of the left ventricle free wall and change heart rate variability measurements, suggesting increased parasympathetic function (Goldsmith et al. 1997; Xu et al. 2006). Accordingly, studies with ACE inhibitors and angiotensin receptor blockers suggest an additional protective role by their reduction of angiotensin II, which potentiates sympathetic activity and blunts vagal inhibitory action. Also, spironolactone might have sympatholytic effects. In contrast, loop diuretics inducing transient disturbances in fluid balances may cause a greater suppression of parasympathetic tone (for an in depth review of this issue see Desai et al. 2011).

3.4.3.2 Device Therapy

The association between impaired vagal reflexes and increased cardiac mortality raised the possibility that increasing vagal activity could have a protective effect. This has been shown in different animal models by direct electrical stimulation of the right cervical vagus (Li et al. 2004; Sabbah et al. 2010; Zhang et al. 2009). The first human experience of chronic vagal stimulation in patients with heart failure suggests that this treatment is feasible, safe, and tolerable and leads to a subjective clinical improvement (Schwartz et al. 2008). Potential mechanisms of a favorable effect include a heart rate-mediated effect, antiadrenergic effects (that may occur at the central level and at the peripheral level), antiapoptotic effects, increase in NO, and antiinflammatory effects (De Ferrari and Schwartz 2011; Olshansky et al. 2008). Larger clinical trials are currently ongoing to further evaluate the safety and efficacy of vagus nerve stimulation in patients with heart failure (Hauptman et al. 2012).

3.4.3.3 Physical Exercise

Numerous studies have demonstrated that physical exercise increases heart rate variability and baroreflex sensitivity, indicating a restoration of the baroreflex function and the concomitant vagal activity (Adamopoulos et al. 1995; Coats et al. 1992; Iellamo et al. 2011; Kiilavuori et al. 1995; Murad et al. 2012; Radaelli et al. 1996).

These training effects are thought to be related to the mediation of different neuromodulators of the parasympathetic nerve activity. A decrease in neuronal nitric oxide synthase (nNOS) has been shown in heart failure and may be involved in the parasympathetic withdrawal (Nihei et al. 2005). Another modulator is angiotensin II, which is known to inhibit vagal function through its action on the baroreflex function and to facilitate sympathetic activity (Mousa et al. 2008; Townend et al. 1995). Physical exercise increases NO bioavailability and endothelial function and suppresses angiotensin II, thereby improving vagal function (Hambrecht et al. 2000; Kingwell 2000; Mousa et al. 2008).

By restoring baroreflex function, physical exercise limits the detrimental effects of ergoreflex and chemoreflex activity which results in improvements of exercise tolerance in patients suffering heart failure.

References

Adamopoulos S, Ponikowski P, Cerquetani E et al (1995) Circadian pattern of heart rate variability in chronic heart failure patients. Effects of physical training. Eur Heart J 16:1380–1386

Adamson PB, Gilbert EM (2006) Reducing the risk of sudden death in heart failure with beta-blockers. J Card Fail 12:734–746

Augustyniak RA, Collins HL, Ansorge EJ et al (2001) Severe exercise alters the strength and mechanisms of the muscle metaboreflex. Am J Physiol Heart Circ Physiol 280:H1645–H1652

Bibevski S, Dunlap ME (2011) Evidence for impaired vagus nerve activity in heart failure. Heart Fail Rev 16:129–135

Binkley PF, Nunziata E, Haas GJ et al (1991) Parasympathetic withdrawal is an integral component of autonomic imbalance in congestive heart failure: demonstration in human subjects and verification in a paced canine model of ventricular failure. J Am Coll Cardiol 18:464–472

Brodde OE, Bruck H, Leineweber K et al (2001) Presence, distribution and physiological function of adrenergic and muscarinic receptor subtypes in the human heart. Basic Res Cardiol 96:528–538

Buch AN, Coote JH, Townend JN (2002) Mortality, cardiac vagal control and physical training–what's the link? Exp Physiol 87:423–435

Caldwell JH, Link JM, Levy WC et al (2008) Evidence for pre- to postsynaptic mismatch of the cardiac sympathetic nervous system in ischemic congestive heart failure. J Nucl Med 49:234–241

Cha YM, Chareonthaitawee P, Dong YX et al (2011) Cardiac sympathetic reserve and response to cardiac resynchronization therapy. Circ Heart Fail 4:339–344

Chapleau MW, Sabharwal R (2011) Methods of assessing vagus nerve activity and reflexes. Heart Fail Rev 16:109–127

Choudhury L, Rosen SD, Lefroy DC et al (1996) Myocardial beta adrenoceptor density in primary and secondary left ventricular hypertrophy. Eur Heart J 17:1703–1709

Chua TP, Clark AL, Amadi AA et al (1996) Relation between chemosensitivity and the ventilatory response to exercise in chronic heart failure. J Am Coll Cardiol 27:650–657

Clark AL, Cleland JG (2000) The control of adrenergic function in heart failure: therapeutic intervention. Heart Fail Rev 5:101–114

Clark AL, Poole-Wilson PA, Coats AJ (1996) Exercise limitation in chronic heart failure: central role of the periphery. J Am Coll Cardiol 28:1092–1102

Coats AJ, Adamopoulos S, Radaelli A et al (1992) Controlled trial of physical training in chronic heart failure. Exercise performance, hemodynamics, ventilation, and autonomic function. Circulation 85:2119–2131

Cohn JN, Archibald DG, Ziesche S et al (1986) Effect of vasodilator therapy on mortality in chronic congestive heart failure. Results of a Veterans Administration Cooperative Study. N Engl J Med 314:1547–1552

Cohn JN, Pfeffer MA, Rouleau J et al (2003) Adverse mortality effect of central sympathetic inhibition with sustained-release moxonidine in patients with heart failure (MOXCON). Eur J Heart Fail 5:659–667

Crisafulli A, Scott AC, Wensel R et al (2003) Muscle metaboreflex-induced increases in stroke volume. Med Sci Sports Exerc 35:221–228; discussion 229

Crisafulli A, Salis E, Pittau G et al (2006) Modulation of cardiac contractility by muscle metaboreflex following efforts of different intensities in humans. Am J Physiol Heart Circ Physiol 291:H3035–H3042

Dampney RA, Coleman MJ, Fontes MA et al (2002) Central mechanisms underlying short- and long-term regulation of the cardiovascular system. Clin Exp Pharmacol Physiol 29:261–268

De Ferrari GM, Schwartz PJ (2011) Vagus nerve stimulation: from pre-clinical to clinical application: challenges and future directions. Heart Fail Rev 16:195–203

Decherchi P, Dousset E, Jammes Y (2007) Respiratory and cardiovascular responses evoked by tibialis anterior muscle afferent fibers in rats. Exp Brain Res 183:299–312

Desai MY, Watanabe MA, Laddu AA et al (2011) Pharmacologic modulation of parasympathetic activity in heart failure. Heart Fail Rev 16:179–193

Eckberg DL, Drabinsky M, Braunwald E (1971) Defective cardiac parasympathetic control in patients with heart disease. N Engl J Med 285:877–883

Feldman DS, Carnes CA, Abraham WT et al (2005) Mechanisms of disease: beta-adrenergic receptors–alterations in signal transduction and pharmacogenomics in heart failure. Nat Clin Pract Cardiovasc Med 2:475–483

Flynn KE, Pina IL, Whellan DJ et al (2009) Effects of exercise training on health status in patients with chronic heart failure: HF-ACTION randomized controlled trial. JAMA 301:1451–1459

Gademan MG, Swenne CA, Verwey HF et al (2007) Effect of exercise training on autonomic derangement and neurohumoral activation in chronic heart failure. J Card Fail 13:294–303

Goldsmith RL, Bigger JT, Bloomfield DM et al (1997) Long-term carvedilol therapy increases parasympathetic nervous system activity in chronic congestive heart failure. Am J Cardiol 80:1101–1104

Hambrecht R, Niebauer J, Fiehn E et al (1995) Physical training in patients with stable chronic heart failure: effects on cardiorespiratory fitness and ultrastructural abnormalities of leg muscles. J Am Coll Cardiol 25:1239–1249

Hambrecht R, Fiehn E, Yu J et al (1997) Effects of endurance training on mitochondrial ultrastructure and fiber type distribution in skeletal muscle of patients with stable chronic heart failure. J Am Coll Cardiol 29:1067–1073

Hambrecht R, Fiehn E, Weigl C et al (1998) Regular physical exercise corrects endothelial dysfunction and improves exercise capacity in patients with chronic heart failure. Circulation 98:2709–2715

Hambrecht R, Wolf A, Gielen S et al (2000) Effect of exercise on coronary endothelial function in patients with coronary artery disease. N Engl J Med 342:454–460

Hammond RL, Augustyniak RA, Rossi NF et al (2000) Heart failure alters the strength and mechanisms of the muscle metaboreflex. Am J Physiol Heart Circ Physiol 278:H818–H828

Hauptman PJ, Schwartz PJ, Gold MR et al (2012) Rationale and study design of the increase of vagal tone in heart failure study: INOVATE-HF. Am Heart J 163:954–962

Heistad D, Abboud FM, Mark AL et al (1975) Effect of baroreceptor activity on ventilatory response to chemoreceptor stimulation. J Appl Physiol 39:411–416

Himura Y, Felten SY, Kashiki M et al (1993) Cardiac noradrenergic nerve terminal abnormalities in dogs with experimental congestive heart failure. Circulation 88:1299–1309

Iellamo F, Pizzinelli P, Massaro M et al (1999) Muscle metaboreflex contribution to sinus node regulation during static exercise: insights from spectral analysis of heart rate variability. Circulation 100:27–32

Iellamo F, Manzi V, Caminiti G et al (2011) Dose–response relationship of baroreflex sensitivity and heart rate variability to individually-tailored exercise training in patients with heart failure. Int J Cardiol 166:334–339

Katona PG, Lipson D, Dauchot PJ (1977) Opposing central and peripheral effects of atropine on parasympathetic cardiac control. Am J Physiol 232:H146–H151

Kaufman MP, Longhurst JC, Rybicki KJ et al (1983) Effects of static muscular contraction on impulse activity of groups III and IV afferents in cats. J Appl Physiol Respir Environ Exerc Physiol 55:105–112

Khan MH, Sinoway LI (2000) Muscle reflex control of sympathetic nerve activity in heart failure: the role of exercise conditioning. Heart Fail Rev 5:87–100

Kiilavuori K, Toivonen L, Naveri H et al (1995) Reversal of autonomic derangements by physical training in chronic heart failure assessed by heart rate variability. Eur Heart J 16:490–495

Kim JK, Sala-Mercado JA, Hammond RL et al (2005a) Attenuated arterial baroreflex buffering of muscle metaboreflex in heart failure. Am J Physiol Heart Circ Physiol 289:H2416–H2423

Kim JK, Sala-Mercado JA, Rodriguez J et al (2005b) Arterial baroreflex alters strength and mechanisms of muscle metaboreflex during dynamic exercise. Am J Physiol Heart Circ Physiol 288:H1374–H1380

Kingwell BA (2000) Nitric oxide as a metabolic regulator during exercise: effects of training in health and disease. Clin Exp Pharmacol Physiol 27:239–250

Kinugawa T, Dibner-Dunlap ME (1995) Altered vagal and sympathetic control of heart rate in left ventricular dysfunction and heart failure. Am J Physiol 268:R310–R316

Kleiger RE, Miller JP, Bigger JT et al (1987) Decreased heart rate variability and its association with increased mortality after acute myocardial infarction. Am J Cardiol 59:256–262

Kougias P, Weakley SM, Yao Q et al (2010) Arterial baroreceptors in the management of systemic hypertension. Med Sci Monit 16:RA1–RA8

Kubo T, Parker JD, Azevedo ER et al (2005) Vagal heart rate responses to chronic beta-blockade in human heart failure relate to cardiac norepinephrine spillover. Eur J Heart Fail 7:878–881

La Rovere MT, Bigger JT Jr, Marcus FI et al (1998) Baroreflex sensitivity and heart-rate variability in prediction of total cardiac mortality after myocardial infarction. ATRAMI (Autonomic Tone and Reflexes After Myocardial Infarction) Investigators. Lancet 351:478–484

Larsen AI, Gjesdal K, Hall C et al (2004) Effect of exercise training in patients with heart failure: a pilot study on autonomic balance assessed by heart rate variability. Eur J Cardiovasc Prev Rehabil 11:162–167

Leineweber K, Wangemann T, Giessler C et al (2002) Age-dependent changes of cardiac neuronal noradrenaline reuptake transporter (uptake1) in the human heart. J Am Coll Cardiol 40:1459

Lewis ME, Al-Khalidi AH, Bonser RS et al (2001) Vagus nerve stimulation decreases left ventricular contractility in vivo in the human and pig heart. J Physiol 534:547–552

Li M, Zheng C, Sato T et al (2004) Vagal nerve stimulation markedly improves long-term survival after chronic heart failure in rats. Circulation 109:120–124

Li YL, Ding Y, Agnew C et al (2008) Exercise training improves peripheral chemoreflex function in heart failure rabbits. J Appl Physiol 105:782–790

Liang CS, Fan TH, Sullebarger JT et al (1989) Decreased adrenergic neuronal uptake activity in experimental right heart failure. A chamber-specific contributor to beta-adrenoceptor downregulation. J Clin Invest 84:1267–1275

Lykidis CK, Kumar P, Balanos GM (2009) The respiratory responses to the combined activation of the muscle metaboreflex and the ventilatory chemoreflex. Adv Exp Med Biol 648:281–287

Malfatto G, Branzi G, Riva B et al (2002) Recovery of cardiac autonomic responsiveness with low-intensity physical training in patients with chronic heart failure. Eur J Heart Fail 4:159–166

Malliani A, Pagani M, Pizzinelli P et al (1983) Cardiovascular reflexes mediated by sympathetic afferent fibers. J Auton Nerv Syst 7:295–301

Mancini DM, Coyle E, Coggan A et al (1989) Contribution of intrinsic skeletal muscle changes to 31P NMR skeletal muscle metabolic abnormalities in patients with chronic heart failure. Circulation 80:1338–1346

Mann DL, Bristow MR (2005) Mechanisms and models in heart failure: the biomechanical model and beyond. Circulation 111:2837–2849

McAlister FA, Wiebe N, Ezekowitz JA et al (2009) Meta-analysis: beta blocker dose, heart rate reduction and death in patients with heart failure. Ann Intern Med 150:784–794

McMillan DE (2002) Interpreting heart rate variability sleep/wake patterns in cardiac patients. J Cardiovasc Nurs 17:69–81

McMurray JJ, Adamopoulos S, Anker SD et al (2012) ESC guidelines for the diagnosis and treatment of acute and chronic heart failure 2012: The Task Force for the Diagnosis and Treatment of Acute and Chronic Heart Failure 2012 of the European Society of Cardiology. Developed in collaboration with the Heart Failure Association (HFA) of the ESC. Eur J Heart Fail 14:803–869

Merlet P, Delforge J, Syrota A et al (1993) Positron emission tomography with 11C CGP-12177 to assess beta-adrenergic receptor concentration in idiopathic dilated cardiomyopathy. Circulation 87:1169–1178

Mousa TM, Liu D, Cornish KG et al (2008) Exercise training enhances baroreflex sensitivity by an angiotensin II-dependent mechanism in chronic heart failure. J Appl Physiol 104:616–624

Murad K, Brubaker PH, Fitzgerald DM et al (2012) Exercise training improves heart rate variability in older patients with heart failure: a randomized, controlled, single-blinded trial. Congest Heart Fail 18:192–197

Nihei M, Lee JK, Honjo H et al (2005) Decreased vagal control over heart rate in rats with right-sided congestive heart failure: downregulation of neuronal nitric oxide synthase. Circ J 69:493–499

Nishiyasu T, Tan N, Morimoto K et al (1994) Enhancement of parasympathetic cardiac activity during activation of muscle metaboreflex in humans. J Appl Physiol 77:2778–2783

Nolan J, Flapan AD, Capewell S et al (1992) Decreased cardiac parasympathetic activity in chronic heart failure and its relation to left ventricular function. Br Heart J 67:482–485

O'Connor CM, Whellan DJ, Lee KL et al (2009) Efficacy and safety of exercise training in patients with chronic heart failure: HF-ACTION randomized controlled trial. JAMA 301:1439–1450

O'Leary DS (2006) Altered reflex cardiovascular control during exercise in heart failure: animal studies. Exp Physiol 91:73–77

Olshansky B, Sabbah HN, Hauptman PJ et al (2008) Parasympathetic nervous system and heart failure: pathophysiology and potential implications for therapy. Circulation 118:863–871

Parati G, Esler M (2012) The human sympathetic nervous system: its relevance in hypertension and heart failure. Eur Heart J 33:1058–1066

Piepoli M, Clark AL, Coats AJ (1995) Muscle metaboreceptors in hemodynamic, autonomic, and ventilatory responses to exercise in men. Am J Physiol 269:H1428–H1436

Piepoli M, Clark AL, Volterrani M et al (1996) Contribution of muscle afferents to the hemodynamic, autonomic, and ventilatory responses to exercise in patients with chronic heart failure: effects of physical training. Circulation 93:940–952

Piepoli M, Ponikowski P, Clark AL et al (1999) A neural link to explain the "muscle hypothesis" of exercise intolerance in chronic heart failure. Am Heart J 137:1050–1056

Ponikowski P, Chua TP, Piepoli M et al (1997) Augmented peripheral chemosensitivity as a potential input to baroreflex impairment and autonomic imbalance in chronic heart failure. Circulation 96:2586–2594

Ponikowski P, Chua TP, Anker SD et al (2001a) Peripheral chemoreceptor hypersensitivity: an ominous sign in patients with chronic heart failure. Circulation 104:544–549

Ponikowski P, Francis DP, Piepoli MF et al (2001b) Enhanced ventilatory response to exercise in patients with chronic heart failure and preserved exercise tolerance: marker of abnormal cardiorespiratory reflex control and predictor of poor prognosis. Circulation 103:967–972

Radaelli A, Coats AJ, Leuzzi S et al (1996) Physical training enhances sympathetic and parasympathetic control of heart rate and peripheral vessels in chronic heart failure. Clin Sci (Lond) 91(Suppl):92–94

Roveda F, Middlekauff HR, Rondon MU et al (2003) The effects of exercise training on sympathetic neural activation in advanced heart failure: a randomized controlled trial. J Am Coll Cardiol 42:854–860

Sabbah HN, Wang M, Jiang A et al (2010) Right vagus nerve stimulation improves left ventricular systolic function in dogs with heart failure. J Am Coll Cardiol 55:A16–E151

Schaufelberger M, Eriksson BO, Grimby G et al (1997) Skeletal muscle alterations in patients with chronic heart failure. Eur Heart J 18:971–980

Schwartz PJ, De Ferrari GM, Sanzo A et al (2008) Long term vagal stimulation in patients with advanced heart failure: first experience in man. Eur J Heart Fail 10:884–891

Scott AC, Francis DP, Davies LC et al (2000) Contribution of skeletal muscle 'ergoreceptors' in the human leg to respiratory control in chronic heart failure. J Physiol 529:863–870

Somers VK, Mark AL, Abboud FM (1991) Interaction of baroreceptor and chemoreceptor reflex control of sympathetic nerve activity in normal humans. J Clin Invest 87:1953–1957

Spyrou N, Rosen SD, Fath-Ordoubadi F et al (2002) Myocardial beta-adrenoceptor density one month after acute myocardial infarction predicts left ventricular volumes at six months. J Am Coll Cardiol 40:1216–1224

Sullivan MJ, Higginbotham MB, Cobb FR (1988) Exercise training in patients with severe left ventricular dysfunction. Hemodynamic and metabolic effects. Circulation 78:506–515

Townend JN, al-Ani M, West JN et al (1995) Modulation of cardiac autonomic control in humans by angiotensin II. Hypertension 25:1270–1275

Triposkiadis F, Karayannis G, Giamouzis G et al (2009) The sympathetic nervous system in heart failure physiology, pathophysiology, and clinical implications. J Am Coll Cardiol 54:1747–1762

Ungerer M, Bohm M, Elce JS et al (1993) Altered expression of beta-adrenergic receptor kinase and beta 1-adrenergic receptors in the failing human heart. Circulation 87:454–463

Van Stee EW (1978) Autonomic innervation of the heart. Environ Health Perspect 26:151–158

Vescovo G, Dalla Libera L (2006) Skeletal muscle apoptosis in experimental heart failure: the only link between inflammation and skeletal muscle wastage? Curr Opin Clin Nutr Metab Care 9:416–422

Vescovo G, Volterrani M, Zennaro R et al (2000) Apoptosis in the skeletal muscle of patients with heart failure: investigation of clinical and biochemical changes. Heart 84:431–437

Wang HJ, Pan YX, Wang WZ et al (2010) Exercise training prevents the exaggerated exercise pressor reflex in rats with chronic heart failure. J Appl Physiol 108:1365–1375

Wang HJ, Zucker ICH, Wang W (2012) Muscle reflex in heart failure: the role of exercise training. Front Physiol. doi:10.3389/fphys.2012.00398

Xu XL, Zang WJ, Lu J et al (2006) Effects of carvedilol on M2 receptors and cholinesterase-positive nerves in adriamycin-induced rat failing heart. Auton Neurosci 130:6–16

Zhang Y, Popovic ZB, Bibevski S et al (2009) Chronic vagus nerve stimulation improves autonomic control and attenuates systemic inflammation and heart failure progression in a canine high-rate pacing model. Circ Heart Fail 2:692–699

Zipes DP (2008) Heart-brain interactions in cardiac arrhythmias: role of the autonomic nervous system. Cleve Clin J Med 75(Suppl 2):S94–S96

Role of the Autonomic Nervous System in Ventricular Arrhythmias During Acute Myocardial Ischemia and Infarction

4

Richard L. Verrier and Alex Y. Tan

Contents

Abstract

Significant advances have been made in recent years to elucidate the neural mechanisms involved in the genesis of cardiac arrhythmias during acute myocardial ischemia and infarction. The cellular and molecular processes whereby the sympathetic nervous system serves as a trigger for arrhythmia, and those responsible for the protective effect of vagus nerve activity, have been extensively characterized. Mounting evidence supports the importance of neural remodeling following myocardial infarction, which has provided valuable clues regarding factors that impact risk for sudden cardiac death. Promising nerve stimulation strategies including vagus nerve activation and spinal cord stimulation have progressed from animal testing to clinical trials.

R.L. Verrier, PhD, FACC (✉) • A.Y. Tan, MD
Division of Cardiovascular Medicine, Harvard Medical School,
Beth Israel Deaconess Medical Center, Harvard-Thorndike Electrophysiology Institute,
99 Brookline Avenue, RN-301, Boston, MA 02215-3908, USA
e-mail: rverrier@bidmc.harvard.edu

R.H.J.A. Slart et al. (eds.), *Autonomic Innervation of the Heart: Role of Molecular Imaging*, DOI 10.1007/978-3-662-45074-1_4

Abbreviation

ICD Implantable cardioverter defibrillator

4.1 Introduction

Neural influences play a major role in determining whether an acute myocardial ischemic event or myocardial infarction culminates in ventricular fibrillation, the arrhythmia responsible for sudden cardiac death. It has been argued that, in many cases, malignant ventricular arrhythmias in patients with coronary artery disease are in fact the consequence of heterogeneous neural remodeling or "frayed nerves."

During acute myocardial ischemia, powerful cardio-cardiac reflexes are activated that are adaptive with respect to maintaining contractility but have deleterious consequences because of the highly arrhythmogenic impact of heightened catecholamine levels (Malliani et al. 1969). The facts that sudden cardiac death exhibits a circadian pattern of heightened risk in the early morning hours (Muller et al. 1987), that β-adrenergic blockade (Olsson et al. 1992) and left stellectomy (Schwartz et al. 1992, 2004; Wilde et al. 2008; Coleman et al. 2012) reduce sudden cardiac death risk, and that, in 20–30 % of events, intense emotions, particularly anger, have been linked to myocardial infarction (Mittleman et al. 1995) and life-threatening arrhythmias as evidenced by implantable cardioverter defibrillator (ICD) discharge (Lampert et al. 2002) attest to the pivotal role of neural factors in malignant arrhythmias.

New evidence suggests that myocardial infarction profoundly disrupts, or "frays," cardiac nerves, setting the stage for heterogeneous reinnervation, which is conducive to sustained reentrant ventricular arrhythmias (Zhou et al. 2004; Verrier and Kwaku 2004). Thus, the concept has emerged that neural remodeling following myocardial infarction should be considered an important element in risk for sudden cardiac death along with remodeling of the myocardial substrate.

The main goal of this review is to discuss both the enduring and the new concepts that underlie our current understanding of the role of neural influences in myocardial ischemia- and infarction-induced ventricular tachycardia and fibrillation.

4.2 Adrenergic Influences on Cardiac Arrhythmia Vulnerability

Adrenergic inputs constitute an important trigger for ventricular arrhythmias during acute myocardial ischemia and infarction. Demonstration of the triggering role of sympathetic nerve discharge in spontaneous ventricular tachycardia and fibrillation was provided by direct recording of left stellate ganglion nerve activity in ambulatory dogs with chronic myocardial infarction (Fig. 4.1) (Zhou et al. 2008). Such striking surges in sympathetic nerve activity also occur within a few

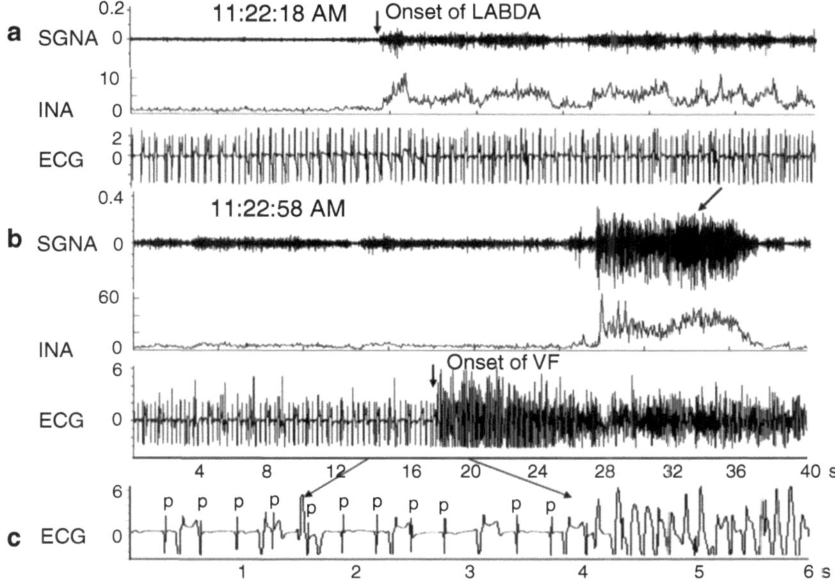

Fig. 4.1 Example of increased left stellate ganglion nerve activity (*SGNA*) preceding ventricular fibrillation (*VF*) and sudden cardiac death (Zhou et al. 2008). (**a**) Increased low-amplitude burst discharge activity (*LABDA*) resulted in accelerated idioventricular rhythm. (**b**) VF occurred approximately 40 s later. Panels (**a**) and (**b**) are continuous. (**c**) A 6-s recording from panel (**b**). *INA* integrated nerve activity in millivolts, *P* P wave, which is dissociated from ventricular activation due to complete AV block (Reprinted with permission from Elsevier)

seconds of experimental left anterior descending coronary artery occlusion (Malliani et al. 1969) and are associated with a fall in ventricular fibrillation threshold (Lombardi et al. 1983), as well as by a marked increase in spontaneous occurrence of ventricular tachycardia and fibrillation and correlated increase in T-wave alternans magnitude (Nearing et al. 1991, 1994). With reperfusion, a second peak in ventricular arrhythmia vulnerability and T-wave alternans occurs, likely provoked by washout of by-products of cellular ischemia (Lombardi et al. 1983; Nearing et al. 1991, 1994; Corbalan et al. 1976). Left stellate ganglionectomy significantly attenuates the surge in vulnerability to ventricular fibrillation during occlusion but enhances its magnitude during reperfusion (Schwartz et al. 1976; Nearing et al. 1991).

4.3 Role of Adrenergic Receptor Activation

Enhanced sympathetic nerve activity increases vulnerability to ventricular arrhythmias in the ischemic heart by complex processes. Multifold direct arrhythmogenic effects on cardiac electrophysiologic function are primarily mediated through β_1-adrenergic receptors. They include derangements in impulse formation, conduction,

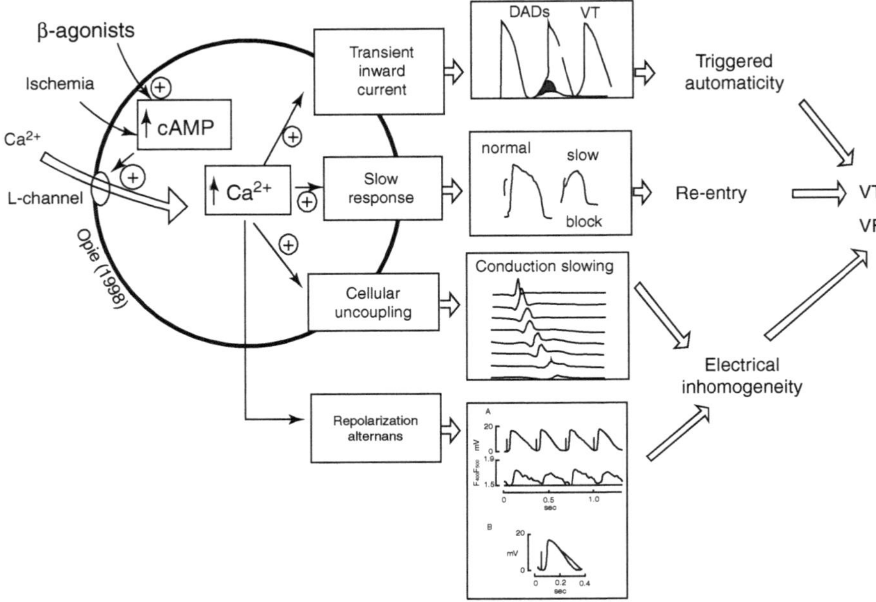

Fig. 4.2 The cardiac β-adrenergic signaling system mediating ventricular arrhythmogenesis. The central pathways include links between cyclic adenosine 3′,5′-monophosphate (*cAMP*), cytosolic calcium, and specific calcium-mediated electrophysiologic abnormalities that predispose to ventricular tachycardia (*VT*) and ventricular fibrillation (*VF*) (Modified from Opie (2004) and used with his permission). The lowest panel is based on Lee et al. (1988), indicating that simulated ischemia results in alternation in calcium transients, which appears to underlie action potential alternans (Reprinted with permission from Lippincott Williams & Wilkins)

repolarization alternans, and heterogeneity of repolarization, with the potential for culmination in ventricular tachycardia and fibrillation (Fig. 4.2) (Opie 2004; Lee et al. 1988). Indirect effects include impairment of oxygen supply–demand ratio resulting from increased cardiac metabolic activity, alpha-adrenergically mediated coronary vasoconstriction, especially in vessels with damaged endothelium, and changes in preload and afterload.

Increased levels of catecholamines stimulate β-adrenergic receptors, which in turn alter adenylate cyclase activity and intracellular calcium flux. These effects are probably mediated by the cyclic nucleotide and protein kinase regulatory cascade, which can alter spatial heterogeneity of calcium transients and consequently provoke T-wave alternans and heterogeneity of repolarization (Verrier et al. 2011).

In the setting of myocardial ischemia, α-adrenergic blockade may alleviate coronary vasoconstriction and reduce platelet aggregability, but in the normal heart, α-adrenergic receptor stimulation or blockade does not appear to affect ventricular electrical stability, as evidenced by the fact that administration of an α-adrenergic agonist such as phenylephrine or methoxamine does not influence excitable properties when the pressor response is controlled to prevent reflex changes in autonomic tone (Verrier et al. 1974; Kowey et al. 1983).

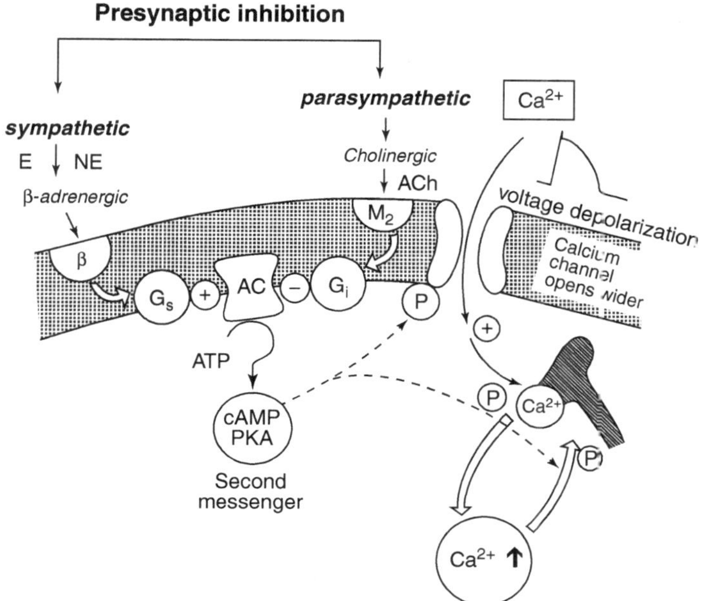

Fig. 4.3 Interaction between parasympathetic and sympathetic systems at a cellular level may involve two opposing cyclic nucleotides, cyclic adenosine 3′,5′-monophosphate (*cAMP*) and cyclic guanosine 3′,5′-monophosphate. Many effects of vagal stimulation can best be explained by the inhibitory effect on the formation of cAMP, including formation of the inhibitory G protein G_i in response to M_2-receptor stimulation (Reprinted from Opie (2004) and used with his permission)

4.4 Sympathetic–Parasympathetic Nerve Interactions

Vagus nerve influences are contingent on the prevailing level of adrenergic tone (Lown and Verrier 1976). When sympathetic nerve activity is augmented by thoracotomy, sympathetic nerve stimulation, myocardial ischemia, or catecholamine infusion, vagus nerve activation exerts a protective effect on ventricular vulnerability. But, vagus nerve stimulation alone is without effect on ventricular vulnerability during β-adrenergic blockade. Levy and Blattberg (1976) termed this phenomenon "accentuated antagonism" (Fig. 4.3) (Opie 2004). The basis for this antagonism of adrenergic effects is presynaptic inhibition of norepinephrine release from nerve endings and muscarinically mediated action at the second messenger level, attenuating the response to catecholamines at receptor sites (Levy and Blattberg 1976). Vagus nerve influences also provide indirect protection against ventricular fibrillation during both myocardial ischemia and reperfusion by reducing excess heart rates, which can otherwise critically compromise diastolic perfusion time to increase the ischemic insult (Zuanetti et al. 1987). However, the beneficial effects of vagus nerve activity may be annulled if profound bradycardia and hypotension ensue.

4.5 Nerve Degeneration and Regrowth in Response to Myocardial Infarction

Myocardial infarction can elicit extensive damage to the afferent and efferent innervation of the heart (Minardo et al. 1988) (Fig. 4.4). The resulting heterogeneous reinnervation, supersensitivity to catecholamines, and loss of antiarrhythmic effects of vagus nerve activity converge to enhance susceptibility to ventricular arrhythmias during the acute phase of myocardial infarction (Table 4.1) (Zipes and Miyazaki 1990).

Chen and coworkers (2001) demonstrated a significant correlation between increased sympathetic nerve density as reflected in immunocytochemical markers and history of ischemia in native hearts of human transplant recipients. In a canine model, they documented increased incidence of ventricular tachycardias and sudden cardiac death following induction of nerve sprouting with nerve growth factor. Episodes of T-wave alternans also occurred (Tsai et al. 2002), consistent with this parameter's capacity to track arrhythmia vulnerability in humans as well as animal models (Verrier et al. 2011). The predisposition to arrhythmias was also linked to immunocytochemical evidence of a heterogeneous pattern of sympathetic nerve reinnervation (Zhou et al. 2004; Verrier and Kwaku 2004) (Fig. 4.5), prompting the

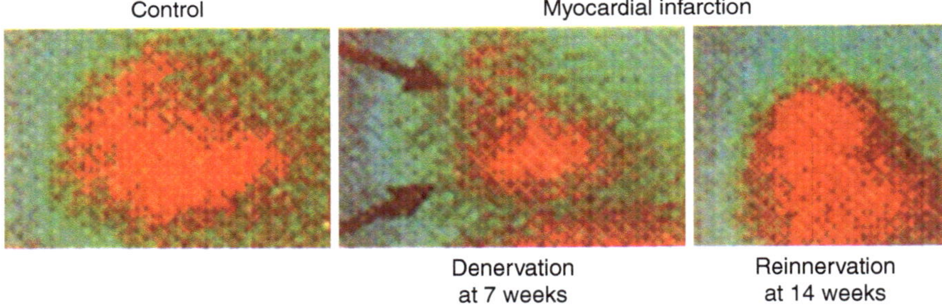

Fig. 4.4 MIBG scintigraphic images of sympathetic innervation before and after myocardial infarction in dogs (Minardo et al. 1988). Left panel: Left lateral preoperative metaiodobenzylguanidine (MIBG) image showing homogeneous uptake. Middle panel: MIBG images obtained 7 weeks after latex injection showing anteroapical defect (*arrow*). Right panel: MIBG images at 14 weeks after latex injection showing homogeneous uptake (Reprinted with permission from Lippincott Williams & Wilkins)

Table 4.1 Autonomic effects of myocardial infarction

Hours: Damage to efferent and afferent autonomic nerve supply
Days, weeks:
Heterogeneous re-innervation (14 weeks)
Denervation supersensitivity (>17 weeks)
Risk for arrhythmias
Desensitization to cardiac pain, due to damage to afferent fibers

From Zipes and Miyazaki (1990)

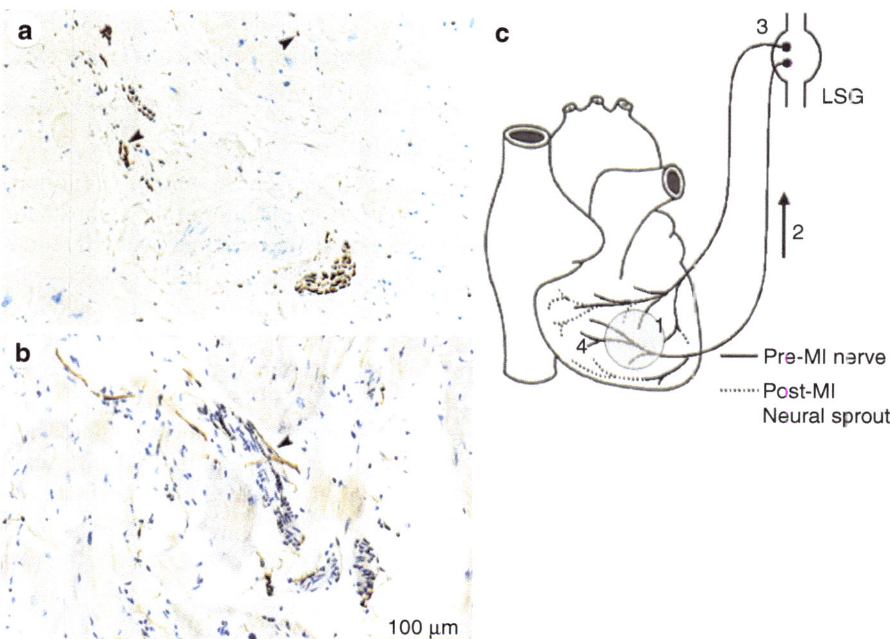

Fig. 4.5 Nerve sprouting after myocardial infarction. Panels (**a**) and (**b**) demonstrate TH-positive nerve fibers (*arrowheads*) in injured areas or around coronary arteries and in a patient with coronary artery disease (Cao et al. 2000). Panel (**c**) signaling of neural remodeling after myocardial infarction (Verrier and Kwaku 2004). Myocardial injury (*shaded area*) results in early local nerve growth factor (NGF) release, presumably from damaged cells, followed by upregulated NGF and growth-associated protein 43 (GAP43) expression, especially in the infarct area (*1*). These signal proteins are then retrogradely transported (*2*) to the nerve cell bodies in the ganglia (*3*) where they stimulate the sprouting of new cardiac nerve endings in the heart (*4*), predominantly in noninfarcted regions, leading to heterogeneous hyperinnervation (Reprinted with permission from Lippincott Williams & Wilkins)

suggestion that the term "neural remodeling" should be employed alongside "myocardial remodeling" in the conceptual framework of the pathophysiology of acute myocardial infarction.

4.6 Nerve Stimulation as an Antiarrhythmic Strategy

Electrical stimulation of the cardiac nerve supply has been reported to reduce ventricular tachyarrhythmias. Spinal cord stimulation, which is both sympatholytic and enhances cardiac vagus nerve tone, is capable of decreasing ischemia-induced arrhythmias in canines (Issa et al. 2005) and T-wave alternans in patients with ischemic cardiomyopathy (Ferrero et al. 2008). Chronic vagus nerve stimulation prevented ventricular fibrillation and sudden cardiac death in conscious dogs with a healed myocardial infarction (Vanoli et al. 1991). In humans, chronic vagus nerve stimulation improves left ventricular function in patients with advanced heart failure (De Ferrari et al. 2011), suggesting the potential for concurrent improvement in mechanical function and reduction in arrhythmia risk.

Conclusion

Our comprehension of the role of the autonomic nervous system has continued to evolve in an intriguing and productive manner. Activation of the sympathetic nervous system is an important factor in the genesis of ischemia- and infarction-induced ventricular arrhythmias. Increased vagus nerve activity is protective by inhibition of norepinephrine release and cyclic nucleotide-mediated antagonism at the adrenergic receptor level. The pattern of local neurocircuitry critically influences heterogeneity of repolarization, a fundamental factor in arrhythmogenesis. Especially important is the neural remodeling that occurs in the post-myocardial infarction period. A number of promising therapeutic approaches based on pharmacologic and electrical targeted neuromodulation to decrease cardiac sympathetic while augmenting vagus nerve tone are being pursued.

References

Cao JM, Fishbein MC, Han JB et al (2000) Relationship between regional cardiac hyperinnervation and ventricular arrhythmia. Circulation 101:1960–1969

Chen PS, Chen LS, Cao JM et al (2001) Sympathetic nerve sprouting, electrical remodeling and the mechanisms of sudden cardiac death. Cardiovasc Res 50:409–416

Coleman MA, Bos JM, Johnson JN et al (2012) Videoscopic left cardiac sympathetic denervation for patients with recurrent ventricular fibrillation/malignant ventricular arrhythmia syndromes besides congenital long QT syndrome. Circ Arrhythm Electrophysiol 5:782–788

Corbalan R, Verrier RL, Lown B (1976) Differing mechanisms for ventricular vulnerability during coronary artery occlusion and release. Am Heart J 92:223–230

De Ferrari GM, Crijns HJ, Borggrefe M et al (2011) Chronic vagus nerve stimulation: a new and promising therapeutic approach for chronic heart failure. Eur Heart J 32:847–855

Ferrero P, Castagno D, Massa R et al (2008) Spinal cord stimulation affects T-wave alternans in patients with ischaemic cardiomyopathy: a pilot study. Europace 10:506–508

Issa ZF, Zhou X, Ujhelyi MR et al (2005) Thoracic spinal cord stimulation reduces the risk of ischemic ventricular arrhythmias in a postinfarction heart failure canine model. Circulation 111:3217–3220

Kowey PR, Verrier RL, Lown B (1983) Effect of alpha-adrenergic receptor stimulation on ventricular electrical properties in the normal canine heart. Am Heart J 105:366–371

Lampert R, Joska T, Burg MM et al (2002) Emotional and physical precipitants of ventricular arrhythmia. Circulation 106:1800–1805

Lee HC, Mohabir R, Smith N et al (1988) Effect of ischemia on calcium-dependent fluorescence transients in rabbit hearts containing indo 1. Correlation with monophasic action potentials and contraction. Circulation 78:1047–1059

Levy MN, Blattberg B (1976) Effect of vagal stimulation on the overflow of norepinephrine into the coronary sinus during cardiac sympathetic nerve stimulation in the dog. Circ Res 38:81–84

Lombardi F, Verrier RL, Lown B (1983) Relationship between sympathetic neural activity, coronary dynamics, and vulnerability to ventricular fibrillation during myocardial ischemia and reperfusion. Am Heart J 105:958–965

Lown B, Verrier RL (1976) Neural activity and ventricular fibrillation. N Engl J Med 294:1165–1170

Malliani A, Schwartz PJ, Zanchetti A (1969) A sympathetic reflex elicited by experimental coronary occlusion. Am J Physiol 217:703–709

Minardo JD, Tuli MM, Mock BH et al (1988) Scintigraphic and electrophysiological evidence of canine myocardial sympathetic denervation and reinnervation produced by myocardial infarction or phenol application. Circulation 78:1008–1019

Mittleman MA, Maclure M, Sherwood JB et al (1995) Triggering of acute myocardial infarction onset by episodes of anger. Circulation 92:1720–1725

Muller JE, Ludmer PL, Willich SN (1987) Circadian variation in the frequency of sudden cardiac death. Circulation 75:131–138

Nearing BD, Huang AH, Verrier RL (1991) Dynamic tracking of cardiac vulnerability by complex demodulation of the T-wave. Science 252:437–440

Nearing BD, Oesterle SN, Verrier RL (1994) Quantification of ischaemia-induced vulnerability by precordial T-wave alternans analysis in dog and human. Cardiovasc Res 28:1440–1449

Olsson G, Wikstrand J, Warnold I (1992) Metoprolol-induced reduction in postinfarction mortality: pooled results from five double-blind randomized trials. Eur Heart J 13:28–32

Opie LH (2004) Heart physiology: from cell to circulation, 4th edn. Lippincott Williams & Wilkins, Philadelphia

Schwartz PJ, Snebold NG, Brown AM (1976) Effects of unilateral cardiac sympathetic denervation on the ventricular fibrillation threshold. Am J Cardiol 37:1034–1040

Schwartz PJ, Motolese M, Pollavini G et al (1992) Prevention of sudden cardiac death after a first myocardial infarction by pharmacologic or surgical antiadrenergic interventions. J Cardiovasc Electrophysiol 3:2–16

Schwartz PJ, Priori SG, Cerrone M et al (2004) Left cardiac sympathetic denervation in the management of high-risk patients affected by the long-QT syndrome. Circulation 109:1826–1833

Tsai J, Cao JM, Zhou S et al (2002) T wave alternans as a predictor of spontaneous ventricular tachycardia in a canine model of sudden cardiac death. J Cardiovasc Electrophysiol 13:51–55

Vanoli E, De Ferrari GM, Stramba-Badiale M et al (1991) Vagal stimulation and prevention of sudden death in conscious dogs with a healed myocardial infarction. Circ Res 68:1471–1481

Verrier RL, Kwaku KF (2004) Frayed nerves in myocardial infarction: the importance of rewiring. Circ Res 94:5–6

Verrier RL, Calvert A, Lown B et al (1974) Effect of acute blood pressure elevation on the ventricular fibrillation threshold. Am J Physiol 226:893–897

Verrier RL, Klingenheben T, Malik M et al (2011) Microvolt T-wave alternans: physiologic basis, methods of measurement, and clinical utility. Consensus guideline by the International Society for Holter and Noninvasive Electrocardiology. J Am Coll Cardiol 44:1309–1324

Wilde AAM, Bhuiyan ZA, Crotti L et al (2008) Left cardiac sympathetic denervation for catecholaminergic polymorphic ventricular tachycardia. N Engl J Med 358:2024–2029

Zhou S, Chen LS, Miyauchi Y et al (2004) Mechanisms of cardiac nerve sprouting after myocardial infarction in dogs. Circ Res 95:76–83

Zhou S, Jung BC, Tan AY et al (2008) Spontaneous stellate ganglion nerve activity and ventricular arrhythmias in a canine model of sudden cardiac death. Heart Rhythm 5:131–139

Zipes DP, Miyazaki T (1990) The autonomic nervous system and the heart: Basis for understanding interactions and effects on arrhythmia development. In: Zipes DP, Jalife J (eds) Cardiac electrophysiology from cell to bedside. WB Saunders, Philadelphia

Zuanetti G, DeFerrari GM, Priori SG et al (1987) Protective effect of vagal stimulation on reperfusion arrhythmias in cats. Circ Res 61:429–435

Tracers for Sympathetic Cardiac Neurotransmission Imaging

5

James T. Thackeray, Jean N. DaSilva, and Philip H. Elsinga

Contents

Abstract

The sympathetic nervous system is the primary extrinsic control of heart rate and contractility and is activated during periods of stress to compensate for increased cardiovascular demand. Signal transduction by the neurotransmitter norepinephrine via postsynaptic β-adrenoceptors and second messenger pathways increases

J.T. Thackeray
Department of Nuclear Medicine, Hannover Medical School, Carl Neuberg Str 1, 30625 Hannover, Germany

J.N. DaSilva
Department of Radiology, Radio-Oncology and Nuclear Medicine, University of Montreal, University of Montreal Hospital Research Centre (CRCHUM), 900 rue Saint-Denis Montreal, QC H2X0A9, Canada

P.H. Elsinga (✉)
Department of Nuclear Medicine and Molecular Imaging, University Medical Center Groningen, University of Groningen, Hanzeplein 1, Groningen 9713 EZ, The Netherlands
e-mail: p.h.elsinga@umcg.nl

R.H.J.A. Slart et al. (eds.), *Autonomic Innervation of the Heart: Role of Molecular Imaging*, DOI 10.1007/978-3-662-45074-1_5

calcium supply in the myocardium, leading to enhanced contractile function. Clinical evidence demonstrates elevated sympathetic tone in cardiovascular disease, resulting in altered expression patterns of multiple proteins involved in sympathetic neuronal transmission. Molecular imaging techniques have been developed targeting these proteins by single-photon emission computed tomography (SPECT) or positron emission tomography (PET). A number of radiotracers have been developed, evaluated, and deployed targeting presynaptic neuronal function (uptake-1 norepinephrine reuptake pathway), postsynaptic α- and β-adrenoceptor density, and second messenger systems (adenylate cyclase/cyclic adenosine monophosphate (cAMP) and phospholipase C/inositol trisphosphate cascades). While the majority of clinical applications to date have utilized analogues of norepinephrine including ^{123}I-metaiodobenzylguanidine ([^{123}I]-MIBG) with SPECT and ^{11}C-meta-hydroxyephedrine ([^{11}C]-mHED) with PET, recent studies have demonstrated added value to multitracer approaches, providing insight not only into neuronal function but also into receptor binding and downstream signaling. In this chapter, the physiology of sympathetic neuronal signaling is discussed with attention to specific targets of current radiotracers in molecular imaging. A summary of the available tracers that have been evaluated in preclinical and clinical settings is provided, with particular attention to those tracers currently utilized in patients.

Abbreviations

AC	Adenylate cyclase
AR	Adrenoceptor
ATP	Adenosine triphosphate
BNP	B-type natriuretic peptide
cAMP	Cyclic adenosine monophosphate
COMT	Catechol-O-methyltransferase
DA	Dopamine
DDC	DOPA-decarboxylase
DOPA	Dihydrxoyphenylalanine
DβH	Dopamine-β-hydroxylase
Epi	Epinephrine
ICD	Implantable cardioverter-defibrillator
IP3	Inositol trisphosphate
IPKI	Isoquinolinesulfonamide protein kinase inhibitor
MAO	Monoamine oxidase
NE	Norepinephrine
NYHA	New York Heart Association
PDE	Phosphodiesterases
PDE4	Phosphodiesterase-4
PET	Positron emission tomography
PKA	Protein kinase A
PKC	Protein kinase C
PLC	Phospholipase C

PMNT	Phenylethanolamine methyltransferase
SNARE	Soluble *N*-ethylmaleimide-sensitive factor attachment protein receptor
SPECT	Single-photon emission computed tomography
TH	Tyrosine hydroxylase
t-SNARE	Target-SNARE
Tyr	Tyrosine
VMAT2	Vesicular monoamine transporter 2

5.1 Introduction

In the last decades, several tracers have been developed to image the sympathetic system in the heart using PET or SPECT. The tracers aim at molecular targets at the presynaptic and postsynaptic side as well as second messenger systems thereby covering the overall signal transduction. This book chapter describes the functionality of the different parts of the sympathetic system followed by a summary of available tracers that have been used in humans.

5.2 Cardiac Sympathetic Nervous System

Cardiac rhythm and contractility is maintained by the intrinsic conduction system comprising pacemaker cells, bundle branches, and Purkinje fibres. The autonomic nervous system provides primary extrinsic control of heart rate and contractility (Armour 2004). The heart is under tonic regulation by the parasympathetic vagus nerve, maintaining homeostatic heart rate and pressure (Johnson et al. 2004). During periods of high-energy demand, acute or chronic stress, signaling of the sympathetic nervous system predominates, contributing to increased heart rate and contractility (Ardell 2004).

5.2.1 Sympathetic Innervation

Sympathetic innervation consists of preganglionic and postganglionic efferent fibres. Preganglionic efferent neurons originate in the locus coeruleus of the pons, projecting to the hypothalamus, cranial nerves, and the intermediolateral tract of the spinal cord (Ardell 2004). Exiting the spinal cord at T1–T5 rami, these efferent neurons synapse within the paravertebral ganglia or at the adrenal gland. Postganglionic fibres project to the heart from the stellate ganglion and other upper thoracic paravertebral ganglia (Pardini et al. 1989). These neurons coalesce with the cardiac extensions of the vagus nerve to form the cardiac neuronal plexus at the base of the heart. From this plexus, sympathetic efferents follow the coronary vasculature to innervate the myocardium, focused at the epicardium, whereas parasympathetic fibres penetrate the outer layers to innervate the endocardium (Denn and Stone 1976). Sympathetic neurons are distributed in a relatively uniform manner throughout the atria and ventricles, with focal innervation at sinoatrial and atrioventricular nodes (Wehrwein et al. 2008).

Terminal release of neurotransmitter occurs from localized swellings of the axons, termed varicosities or boutons, effectively the neuroeffector junctions of the cardiac sympathetic nervous system (Fig. 5.1). Within the varicosity, norepinephrine is stored in neuronal vesicles and synthesized from tyrosine in a series of enzyme-catalyzed reactions: tyrosine is converted to dihydrxoyphenylalanine (DOPA) by tyrosine hydroxylase; DOPA is converted to dopamine by DOPA-decarboxylase; dopamine is converted to norepinephrine by dopamine β-hydroxylase; norepinephrine is converted to epinephrine by phenylethanolamine-N-methyltransferase. Following sympathetic nerve impulse, vesicles dock to the axonal membrane of the varicosity via scaffolding proteins including *t*-soluble *N*-ethylmaleimide-sensitive factor attachment protein receptor (SNARE) complexes (Blanes-Mira et al. 2003; Jung et al. 2008). The contents of the vesicle are released into a synaptic cleft that is wider than in the central nervous system (Woolard et al. 2004).

5.2.2 Neuronal Reuptake

The sympathetic signal is terminated by the active recapture of norepinephrine to the neuron via norepinephrine reuptake transporter (uptake-1). Approximately 80 % of neurotransmitter in the heart is synthesized by local neurons, with relatively low reliance on circulating neurohormones synthesized by the adrenal gland (Kopin and Gordon 1963; Esler et al. 1984). Uptake-1 is a saturable transporter and is dependent on adenosine triphosphate (ATP) and sodium (Jaques et al. 1987). A small proportion of secreted norepinephrine is taken up by post-synaptic, non-saturable, ATP-independent uptake-2 (Russ et al. 1992). Whereas uptake-1 is blocked by non-selective tricyclic antidepressants (e.g. desipramine) or cocaine, uptake-2 is blocked by corticosteroids or sympatholytics (e.g. clonidine) (Salt 1972; Esler et al. 1981; Raffel and Wieland 2001). Following recapture, norepinephrine is packaged into storage vesicles by vesicular monoamine transporter-2 or is subject to break down by monoamine oxidase and catechol-O-methyltransferase. Reduced uptake-1 maximal velocity and expression has been demonstrated in heart failure (Li et al. 2004; Sasano et al. 2008; Matsunari et al. 2010). Binding assays have demonstrated the highest uptake-1 density in the left ventricle with lower binding observed in the right ventricle and atrial tissue (Liang et al. 1989; Wehrwein et al. 2008). Immunoreactivity of uptake-1 is specific to sympathetic nerve fibres, as demonstrated by overlay fluorescence microscopy and colocalization with tyrosine hydroxylase antibodies (Parrish et al. 2008).

As evidenced by electron microscopy and immunoprecipitation studies, uptake-1 exists in two distinct pools: functional membrane-bound uptake-1 associated with large protein scaffolds including syntaxin 1A and SNARE complexes (Geerlings et al. 1998) and non-functional intracellular uptake-1 bound to lipid rafts within the cytosol (Wong and Scott 2004). The expression of uptake-1 is modulated by a variety of factors including short-term internalization of membrane-bound uptake-1 to

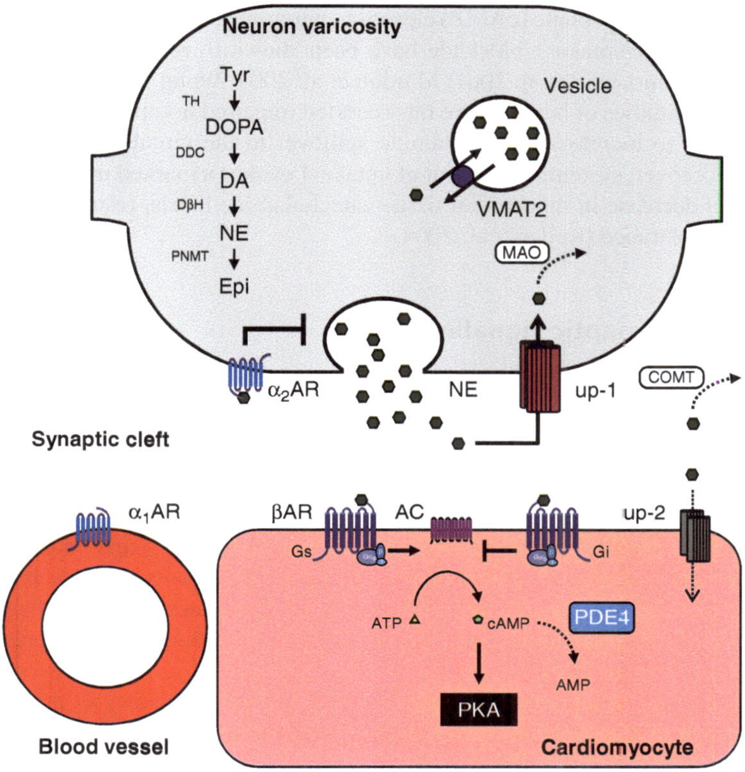

Fig. 5.1 Schematic of sympathetic neuronal transmission in the myocardium. Within the neuronal varicosity, norepinephrine (*NE*) is synthesized in a series of enzyme-catalyzed steps: tyrosine (*Tyr*) is converted to dihydroxyphenylalanine (*DOPA*) by tyrosine hydroxylase (*TH*), DOPA is converted to dopamine (*DA*) by DOPA-decarboxylase (*DDC*), DA is converted to NE by dopamine-β-hydroxylase (*DβH*), and NE is converted to epinephrine (*Epi*) by phenylethanolamine methyltransferase (*PMNT*). NE is packaged in storage vesicles by vesicular monoamine transporter 2 (*VMAT2*). Upon docking to the neuronal membrane, NE is released into the synaptic cleft, where it binds to α-adrenoceptors ($\alpha_{1/2}$AR) or β-adrenoceptors ($\beta_{1/2}$AR). NE binding to α_1AR expressed by vasculature leads to vasoconstriction. NE binding to α_2AR expressed at the neuronal varicosity evokes negative feedback on sympathetic signal transduction. Activation of stimulatory (*Gs*) or inhibitory (*Gi*) βAR leads to activation or inhibition of adenylate cyclase (*AC*), respectively. AC converts adenosine triphosphate (*ATP*) to the second messenger cyclic adenosine monophosphate (*cAMP*), which subsequently phosphorylates protein kinase A (PKA). cAMP is hydrolyzed by phosphodiesterases (*PDE4*) to adenosine monophosphate (*AMP*). Sympathetic signal is terminated by active recapture of NE by presynaptic uptake-1 (*up-1*) or postsynaptic uptake-2 (*up-2*) pathway. NE is metabolized by catechol-O-methyltransferase (*COMT*) or monoamine oxidase (*MAO*) (Adapted from Thackeray et al. (2012))

lipid rafts and longer-term control of gene expression. Chronic KCl depolarization, neurotrophins, and tyrosine hydroxylase cofactors stimulate increased uptake-1 translocation to the neuronal membrane (Ren et al. 2001; Miner et al. 2003; Habecker et al. 2006). By contrast protein kinase C (PKC) activation, cyclic adenosine monophosphate (cAMP) elevation, norepinephrine exposure, and chronic pharmacological uptake-1 blockade have been shown to reduce uptake-1 density and V_{max} (Bryan-Lluka et al. 2001; Mardon et al. 2003; Wong and Scott 2004; Mao et al. 2005). Studies of heart failure rats reported impaired norepinephrine reuptake, contributing to increased catecholamine spillover to the circulation (Backs et al. 2001). Moreover, systemic knockout of uptake-1 evokes a marked increase in circulating and decrease in myocardial tissue catecholamine levels, resulting in cardiac exercise intolerance (Keller et al. 2004).

5.2.3 Postsynaptic Signaling

Sympathetic signaling is conducted postsynaptically by neurotransmitter stimulation of *G* protein-coupled adrenoceptors expressed at the target tissue surface (Fig. 5.1). Adrenoceptors comprise two major subtypes and multiple isoforms. Alpha-adrenoceptors exist in two isoforms: α_1-adrenoceptors which are localized mainly in the vasculature and α_2-adrenoceptors of which the α_{2A}-adrenoceptors are localized on presynaptic neurons. Beta-adrenoceptors are found in three well-characterized isoforms: β_1-adrenoceptors found in the highest quantity in the cardiac and skeletal muscle and adipose tissue, β_2-adrenoceptors found in the greatest concentration in bronchioles, and β_3-adrenoceptors predominantly expressed by adipocytes (Armour 2004).

Both β_1- and β_2-adrenoceptors are coupled to the stimulatory *G* protein (G_s). Dissociation of the α-subunit of G_s activates adenylate cyclase and generates the second messenger cAMP. Subsequent activation of protein kinase A (PKA) phosphorylates a series of proteins involved in Ca^{2+} regulation including ryanadine receptor, sarcoplasmic reticulum Ca^{2+} ATPase, and L-type calcium channels. This signal culminates in an influx of Ca^{2+} which, by binding and inactivating the regulatory protein calmodulin, facilitates the interaction of actin and myosin at the sarcomere and effectively increases the force of cardiomyocyte contraction (Brodde 1991; Wehrens et al. 2006). β_2-Adrenoceptors are also coupled to the inhibitory *G* protein (G_i). The dissociated α-subunit of G_i inhibits adenylate cyclase, resulting in a reduction of cAMP production. This counters the action of G_s stimulation and acts as a regulator of cardiac contractility. Cardiac β_3-adrenoceptors have been shown to contribute to negative inotropic effects in reducing the amplitude and accelerating the repolarization phase of the cardiac action potential in isolated ventricular myocytes (Gauthier et al. 1996). In the healthy human heart, β-adrenergic subtype expression patterns are roughly 62 % β_1, 30 % β_2, and 8 % β_3 adrenoceptors (Bristow et al. 1986).

Continuous stimulation of β-adrenoceptors evokes uncoupling of sympathetic signaling from calcium regulation. Seven day infusion of epinephrine resulted in a decrease in β-adrenoceptor B_{max} by dihydroalprenolol binding assay, and was associated with an earlier shift in phospholipid composition of the sarcolemma (Benediktsdottir et al. 1999). This observation supports the membrane clathrin pit internalization model of β-adrenoceptor internalization and downregulation. Using membrane preparations from failing human hearts post-transplant, Bristow and colleagues demonstrated a 50–56 % reduction in β-adrenoceptor density and a significant attenuation of muscle contractility (Bristow et al. 1982).

5.3 Tracers of the Cardiac Sympathetic Nervous System

The observed changes in sympathetic tone and postsynaptic receptor density have led to the development of molecular imaging probes targeted to the cardiac sympathetic nervous system. Though clinical experiences remain somewhat limited, a number of sympathetic nervous system targeting radiotracers have been routinely synthesized and evaluated over the last 25 years.

5.3.1 Neuronal Tracers

The majority of sympathetic nervous system radiotracers are based on the structure of norepinephrine and other catecholamines, taking advantage of the endogenous reuptake pathway to target sympathetic neurons (Fig. 5.2). This class of tracers includes labelled neurotransmitters (e.g. [^{18}F]-dopamine, [^{11}C]-epinephrine),

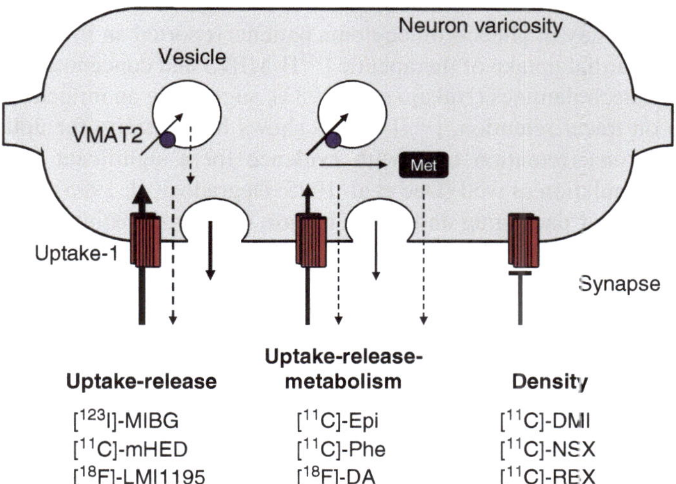

Fig. 5.2 Summary of presynaptic neuronal molecular imaging agents and their differing pharmacologic behaviour. [^{123}I]-MIBG, [^{11}C]-mHED, and [^{18}F]-LMI1195 exhibit high selectivity for uptake-1, with moderate vesicular packaging via VMAT2, moderate passive diffusion across vesicular and neuronal membranes, and active release from vesicles during signal transmission, providing a dynamic picture of norepinephrine uptake and release. By contrast, ^{11}C-epinephrine (*Epi*), [^{11}C]-phenylephrine (*Phe*), and [^{18}F]-dopamine (*DA*) exhibit higher vesicular packaging with less passive diffusion from the neuron, but are susceptible to degradation by monoamine oxidase and catechol-*O*-methyltransferase, providing a complete picture of norepinephrine uptake, release, and metabolism. Experimental tracers [^{11}C]-desipramine (*DMI*), [^{11}C]-nisoxetine (*NSX*), and [^{11}C]-reboxetine (*RBX*) bind to uptake-1, reflecting transporter density alone (Adapted from Raffel and Wieland (2001))

substrate analogues termed "false neurotransmitters" (e.g. [^{123}I]-MIBG, [^{18}F]-LMI1195, [^{11}C]-mHED, [^{11}C]-phenylephrine, [^{11}C]-phenethylguanidines), and uptake-1 inhibitors (e.g. [^{11}C]-methylreboxetine, [^{11}C]-desipramine). The most widely utilized tracers in clinical practice are [^{123}I]-MIBG and [^{11}C]-mHED, with expanding preclinical but limited clinical experience with several other candidate tracers. Each tracer exhibits unique uptake and retention characteristics, providing information on some combination of neuronal reuptake, uptake-1 density, vesicular packaging, vesicular release, and catecholamine metabolism. Chronic sympathetic activation drives a decrease in neuronal reuptake, including internalization and downregulation of uptake-1 and increased synaptic norepinephrine content and spillover. Ideal characteristics of sympathetic neuronal tracers include specificity and selectivity for uptake-1 over other reuptake transporters; high affinity for uptake-1 to minimize competition with endogenous norepinephrine for reuptake; long neuronal retention time potentially with vesicular packaging by vesicular monoamine transporter-2 and/or low lipophilicity; and metabolic stability and resistance to endogenous catecholamine breakdown to facilitate kinetic modelling.

5.3.1.1 [^{123}I]-Metaiodobenzylguanidine

The most widely used radiotracer for evaluation of sympathetic innervation is the SPECT norepinephrine analogue [^{123}I]-MIBG. First developed to image neuroendocrine tumours, early studies identified uptake in the myocardium, prompting further exploration. A study in pheochromocytoma patients reported an inverse correlation between myocardial uptake of therapeutic [^{131}I]-MIBG and concentration of plasma and urinary catecholamines (Nakajo et al. 1983), suggesting an influence of sympathetic tone on tracer retention. [^{123}I]-MIBG shows high affinity for uptake-1 with extended neuronal retention time with evidence for a significant extraneuronal uptake-2 accumulation as well (Dae et al. 1995; Degrado et al. 1995). Uptake is followed by vesicular packaging and active release of neurotransmitter with endogenous catecholamines during sympathetic activation. As such, the rate of [^{123}I]-MIBG washout, in conjunction with early and late measurements of myocardial contrast, provides an estimation of sympathetic tone (Narula and Sarkar 2003). As a non-catechol, [^{123}I]-MIBG is resistant to monoamine oxidase and catechol-O-methyltransferase, rendering it metabolically stable for semi-quantitative imaging. Recent large-scale clinical trials have identified an independent prognostic value for [^{123}I]-MIBG imaging in the identification of heart failure patients at the greatest risk of progression (Bax et al. 2008; Boogers et al. 2010; Kasama et al. 2011).

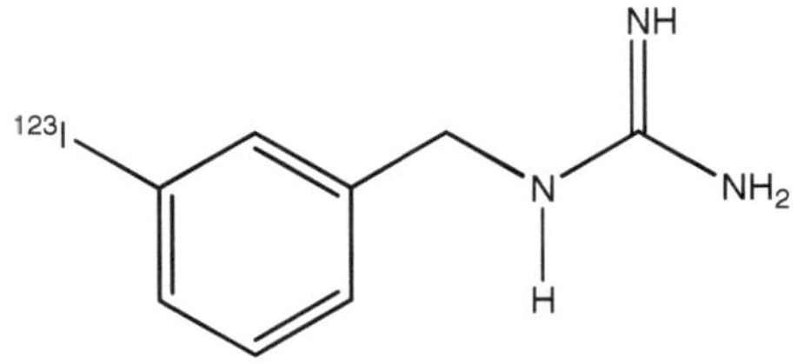

NH

^{123}I

N

NH_2

H

[^{123}I]-m-iodobenzylguanidine

5.3.1.2 [^{11}C]-Meta-Hydroxyephedrine

In PET, the most routinely used radiotracer for sympathetic neuronal imaging is [^{11}C]-mHED. As an analogue of norepinephrine devoid of postsynaptic activity, [^{11}C]-mHED is actively transported by uptake-1 where it is partially packaged to vesicles, released with neurotransmitter, or passively diffused back to the synaptic cleft. [^{11}C]-mHED is not susceptible to monoamine oxidase breakdown. As such, retention of [^{11}C]-mHED reflects complete presynaptic function of the sympathetic neuron. Structure activity relationship experiments identified selectivity of [^{11}C]-mHED for uptake-1 over the dopamine reuptake transporter (1:10) and serotonin reuptake transporter (1:71) (Foley et al. 2002). Synthesis of [^{11}C]-mHED is achieved by the *N*-^{11}C-methylation of metaraminol freebase in high specific activity and yield (Rosenspire et al. 1990; Law et al. 1997). Distribution studies demonstrated high and prolonged retention of [^{11}C]-mHED in tissues with complex adrenergic networks including the heart, adrenal glands, and spleen, with gradual accumulation in the liver. Treatment with selective inhibitors of uptake-1 reduced retention by up to 80–95 % in the heart, with a consequent increase in hepatic activity, reflecting accumulation of metabolites (Rosenspire et al. 1990; Law et al. 1997; Thackeray et al. 2007; Tipre et al. 2008; Law et al. 2010). Myocardial accumulation of [^{11}C]-mHED is reduced by increasing concentrations of true or false neurotransmitters, to a maximal decrease of 90 %, consistent with competition for uptake-1 sites (Degrado et al. 1995; Law et al. 1997; Thackeray et al. 2007; Thackeray et al. 2013). Cardiac sympathetic denervation by phenol or 6-hydroxydopamine established a direct relationship between uptake-1 B_{max} and [^{11}C]-mHED accumulation (Raffel et al. 2006). High-performance liquid chromatography metabolite analysis in guinea pigs and rats established the presence of multiple labelled metabolites in the liver and plasma (~75 % of total activity) by 30 min after injection, but no presence of labelled metabolites in the myocardium (<0.5 % of total activity) (Rosenspire et al. 1990; Law et al. 1997; Thackeray et al. 2007). Similar plasma accumulation was described in human subjects, with a rapid accumulation of [^{11}C]-labelled metabolites in the blood over 10–20 min after injection (Link et al. 1997).

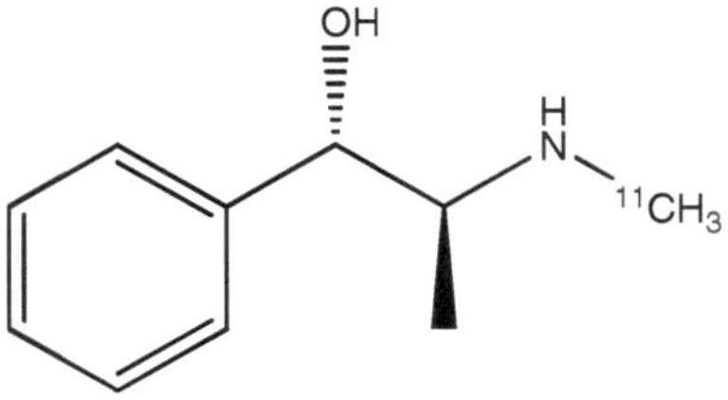

[^{11}C]mHED

5.3.1.3 [^{11}C]-Epinephrine

Epinephrine is an endogenous neurotransmitter synthesized from norepinephrine with high affinity for α-adrenoceptors and a prominent role in peripheral blood pressure homeostasis. Synthesis is carried out by *N*-methylation of norepinephrine, providing

[^{11}C]-epinephrine in high specific activity and radiochemical yield (Nguyen et al. 1997; Tipre et al. 2008). [^{11}C]-Epinephrine has a high affinity for uptake-1 that is effectively blocked by administration of inhibitors (Raffel and Chen 2004; Tipre et al. 2008). Structurally identical to the endogenous neurotransmitter, ^{11}C-epinephrine exhibits more natural physiological behaviour than [^{11}C]-mHED, with a greater proportion of vesicular packaging and susceptibility to monoamine oxidase metabolism (Nguyen et al. 1997; Munch et al. 2000). High vesicular uptake translates to reduced loss of tracer to passive diffusion and a lower overall washout rate of tracer (Raffel and Wieland 2001). Labelled metabolites greatly contribute to the radioactivity signal in the myocardium, necessitating metabolite correction for quantitative imaging.

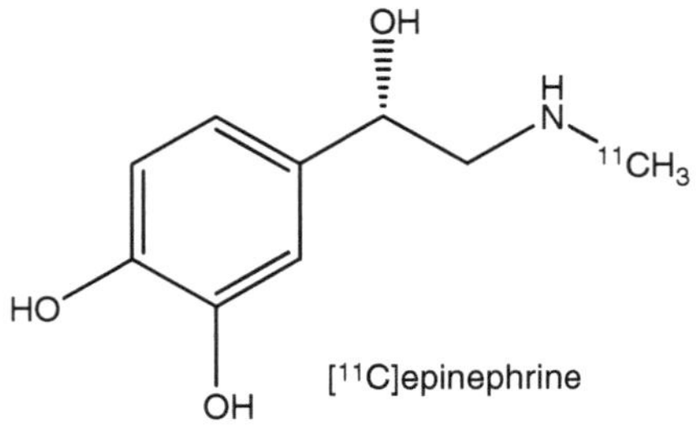

[^{11}C]epinephrine

5.3.1.4 [^{18}F]-LMI1195

More recently, a PET analogue of MIBG has been developed and analyzed, attempting to capitalize on the clinical experience with the iodinated SPECT analogue and the higher spatial resolution of PET. The compound *N*-[3-bromo-4-(3-[^{18}F]fluoropropoxy)-benzyl]-guanidine (LMI1195) which can be easily labelled by direct [^{18}F]-fluorination of a brosylate precursor has undergone preclinical testing, in which cardiac uptake was well defined compared to the liver. Imaging studies in rabbits with desipramine blockade or 6-hydroxydopamine denervation demonstrated a correlation between [^{18}F]-LMI1195 retention and uptake-1 density without a corresponding difference in myocardial blood flow for either model (Yu et al. 2011). The radiotracer has recently entered clinical phase-1 trials, with initial reports of favourable dosimetry (Lazewatsky et al. 2010) and proposed progression to a commercial product.

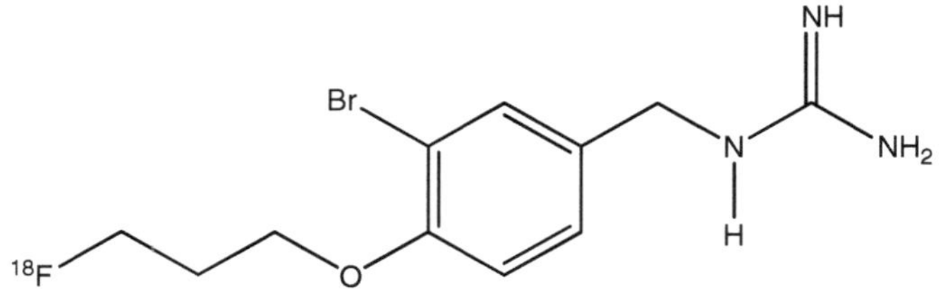

[^{18}F]LMI1195

5.3.1.5 Other Compounds

In addition to these well-characterized compounds, a number of other neuronal radiotracers have been synthesized. [^{11}C]-Phenylephrine exhibits selectivity for uptake-1, but shows a greater membrane permeability than either [^{11}C]-mHED or [^{11}C]-epinephrine, and is highly susceptible to breakdown by monoamine oxidase and catechol-O-methyltransferase, resulting in a high proportion of radiolabelled metabolites (Raffel et al. 1996; Tipre et al. 2008). [^{18}F]-Fluorodopamine has been extensively used in brain imaging studies, demonstrating selective uptake and vesicular packaging, though intraneuronal conversion to [^{18}F]-fluoronorepinephrine and endogenous metabolite generation complicate quantitative image analysis (Raffel and Chen 2004). A series of [^{11}C]-phenethylguanidines have been synthesized and tested in vitro, exhibiting favourable kinetic modelling characteristics including lower uptake-1 transport rate, reduced membrane permeability, and greater vesicular transport, resulting in a more static uptake profile (Raffel et al. 2007). The suitability of [^{11}C]-phenethylguanidines for in vivo imaging has not been fully elucidated. Additionally, a number of tracers based on selective uptake-1 inhibitors have been synthesized to circumvent the complex modelling inherent to labelled true and false neurotransmitters. These include [^{11}C]-nisoxetine, [^{11}C]-desipramine, and [^{11}C]-reboxetine compounds (Haka and Kilbourn 1989; Van Dort et al. 1997; Ding et al. 2005). In vivo experiments with these tracers in the heart have provided mixed results.

5.3.2 Adrenergic Receptor Antagonists

The second major category of sympathetic nervous system radiotracers are labelled adrenoceptor antagonists (Fig. 5.3). The challenge in the design of adrenergic receptor antagonist ligands is to restrict binding to cell membrane receptors, such that tracer binding is sensitive to receptor desensitization, internalization, and downregulation. Therefore, these antagonists should have a hydrophilic character in order to only bind to cell surface functional receptors. Due to altered sympathetic tone to the myocardium in cardiovascular disease, labelled adrenoceptor antagonists facilitate non-invasive longitudinal tracking of the progression of left ventricular remodelling and have been hypothesized to predict patient response to beta-blocker therapy (Tsukamoto et al. 2007; Naya et al. 2009).

5.3.2.1 [^{11}C]-CGP-12177

The best characterized adrenergic receptor antagonist is (*S*)-(3′-*tert*-butylamino-2′-hydroxypropoxy)-benzimidazol-2-[^{11}C]-one ([^{11}C]-CGP-12177). It exhibits a high affinity for β_1- and β_2-adrenoceptors, with lower affinity and partial agonist activity for β_3-adrenoceptors (K_d=0.3, 0.9, 80.0 nM, respectively). Pretreatment with β-adrenergic antagonists propranolol or unlabelled CGP-12177 blocked tracer binding by 80–90 % (Delforge et al. 1991; Van Waarde et al. 1992; Thackeray et al. 2011). Further, the low lipophilicity of the compound ensures binding only to cell surface receptors and not to internalized receptors in the cytosol (van Waarde et al.

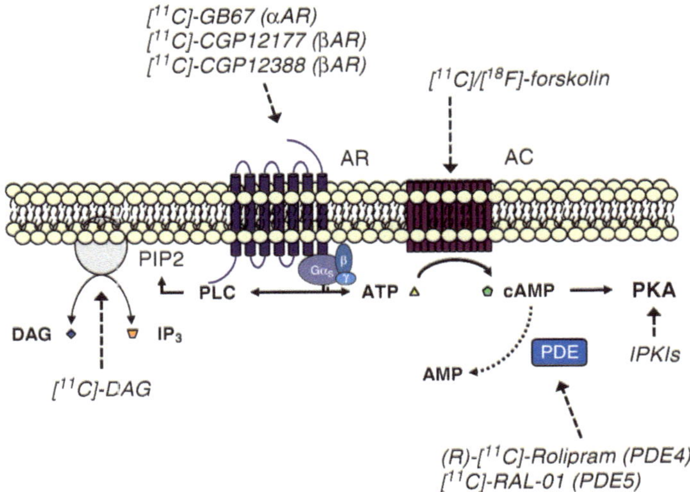

Fig. 5.3 Summary of postsynaptic sympathetic imaging agents and their molecular targets in the adrenergic signaling cascade. [^{11}C]-GB67, [^{11}C]-CGP-12177, and [^{11}C]-CGP-12388 bind to membrane-bound adrenoceptors (*AR*). [^{11}C]-Diacylglycerol (*DAG*) measures the flux of Gq-activated phospholipase C (*PLC*) and phosphatidylinositide-4,5-bisphosphate in converting DAG to inositol trisphosphate (*IP3*). Radiolabelled forskolin measures activity of adenylate cyclase (*AC*) in converting ATP to second messenger cAMP. [^{11}C]-Rolipram and [^{11}C]-RAL-01 target phosphodiesterases (*PDE*) which hydrolyze cAMP to AMP under the regulation of cAMP, providing an indirect index of cAMP levels. Labelled isoquinolinesulfonamide protein kinase inhibitor (*IPKI*) target protein kinase A (*PKA*)

2004). Ex vivo studies in rats demonstrated that chronic treatments with adrenergic receptor agonists decrease the binding potential of [^{11}C]-CGP-12177 due to reduced adrenoceptor B_{max} (Thackeray et al. 2011). Wide deployment of [^{11}C]-CGP-12177 has been limited by the complex synthesis route involving the [^{11}C]-phosgene intermediate. Several institutes experienced laborious procedures in combination with variable-specific activities or radiochemical yields. Recent advances in the generation of [^{11}C]-phosgene have resulted in higher yield reliable production of [^{11}C]-CGP-12177 and more frequent application in basic and clinical settings (Nishijima et al. 2002; Nishijima et al. 2004).

[^{11}C]phosgene

Synthesis of S-[^{11}C]CGP12177

5.3.2.2 [^{11}C]-CGP-12388

The complicated synthesis of [^{11}C]-CGP-12177 was overcome by the use of an alternative labelling approach, generating the analogous (*S*)-4-(3-(^{11}C-isopropylamino)-2-hydroxypropoxy)-2H-benzimidazol-2-one ([^{11}C]-CGP-12388). Instead of using [^{11}C]-phosgene, the labelling synthon [^{11}C]-acetone was used to prepare [^{11}C]-CGP-12388 via a one-pot reductive alkylation reaction. The preparation of [^{11}C]-acetone requires anhydrous trapping of [^{11}C]-CO_2 in a solution of methyl lithium under argon atmosphere. The binding characteristics of [^{11}C]-CGP-12388 are similar to its analogue [^{11}C]-CGP-12177, with selective binding to β_1-, β_2-, and β_3-adrenoceptors with myocardial standardized uptake values of approximately half that of [^{11}C]-CGP-12177. Binding was blocked by administration of propranolol (Elsinga et al. 2001; Momose et al. 2004). Preliminary clinical tests have established good contrast for heart and lung binding of [^{11}C]-CGP-12388, slow generation of labelled metabolites, and low plasma protein binding (de Jong et al. 2005).

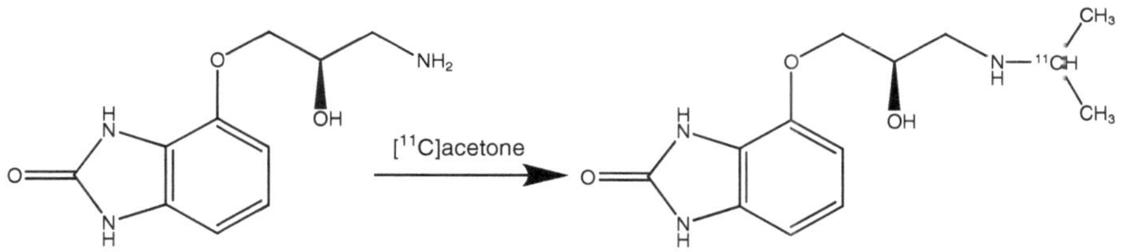

[^{11}C]acetone

Synthesis of *S*-[^{11}C]CGP12388

5.3.2.3 [^{11}C]-GB67

In addition to β-adrenoceptors, evaluation of myocardial α-adrenoceptor density has been thought to provide insight on the progression of cardiovascular disease. The chemical structure of [^{11}C]-GB67 is based on the binding moiety of the selective α_1-adrenoceptor antagonist prazosin. Characterization experiments demonstrated high uptake in the myocardium that was blocked by prior and displaced by subsequent administration of prazosin (Law et al. 2000; Park-Holohan et al. 2008). A compartmental modelling approach evaluated in pigs indicated that specific binding of [^{11}C]-GB67 to myocardial α_1-adrenoceptors accounted for approximately half of the total tracer volume of distribution. Moreover, [^{11}C]-GB67 was metabolically stable, showing no accumulation of labelled metabolites in the cardiac tissue (Law et al. 2000). No studies have yet been carried out in human subjects.

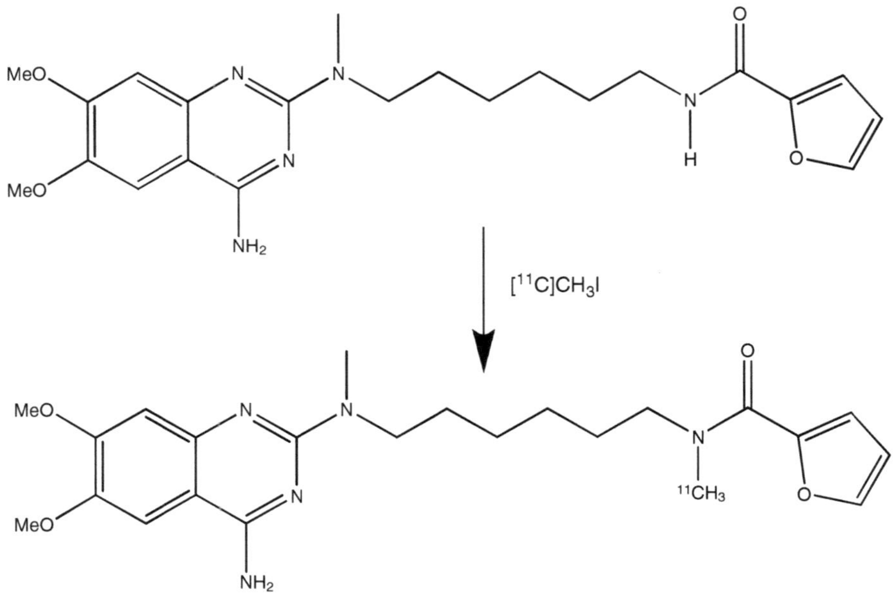

Synthesis of [^{11}C]GB67

5.3.3 Second Messenger Systems

The frequency of β-blocker therapy in the heart failure population limits the utility of adrenoceptor radioligands, as accurate quantitative imaging necessitates discontinuation of this therapy. As such, there has been exploration of the potential to image signal transduction following adrenergic receptor stimulation (Fig. 5.3). While few of these compounds have yet been evaluated in a clinical setting, the preclinical evidence supports long-term development of multitracer studies, including candidate radiotracers of intracellular signaling.

5.3.3.1 (R)-[^{11}C]-Rolipram

Norepinephrine stimulation of G_s-coupled adrenoceptors leads to the activation of adenylate cyclase and the production of the second messenger cAMP and PKA. In the heart, phosphodiesterase-4 (PDE4), under regulation of downstream PKA (via cAMP), hydrolyses cAMP and terminates second messenger signaling (Kenk et al. 2007). The selective PDE4 inhibitor and antidepressant rolipram has been investigated for both brain and heart imaging purposes. Studies in rats have demonstrated selectivity of (*R*)-^{11}C-rolipram for PDE4 in the heart (Lourenco et al. 2006; Kenk et al. 2007), with a favourable metabolite profile for compartmental modelling (Kenk et al. 2008; Thomas et al. 2011; Lortie et al. 2012). In healthy animals, binding of (*R*)-[^{11}C]-rolipram to PDE4 is enhanced by ~30 % following acute localized noradrenergic stimulation by uptake-1 inhibition (Lourenco et al. 2006). This response is diminished or lost in animal models of obesity (Greene et al. 2009) and Adriamycin-induced cardiotoxicity (Kenk et al. 2010), supporting further studies in basic and clinical cardiology.

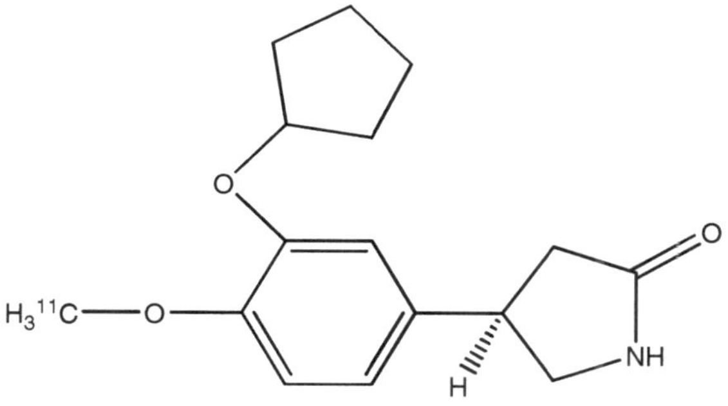

$[^{11}C]$rolipram

5.3.3.2 PKA Imaging Agents

Other radiotracers have been developed to image various components of the PKA signaling axis. Candidate tracers have included $[^{11}C]$- and $[^{18}F]$-forskolin to image adenylate cyclase (Sasaki et al. 1993; Kiesewetter et al. 2000), $[^{11}C]$-RAL-01 an analogue of sildenafil to image phosphodiesterase-5 (Jakobsen et al. 2006), and isoquinolinesulfonamide protein kinase inhibitor analogues to image PKA (Vasdev et al. 2008). Experience with these compounds, particularly in myocardial applications, is limited at present.

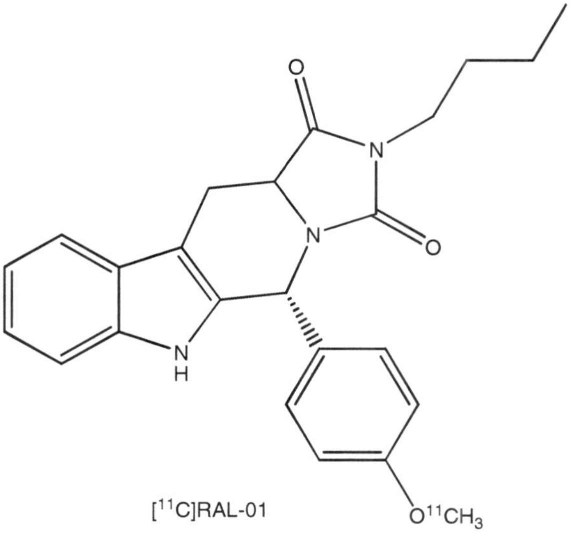

$[^{11}C]$RAL-01

5.3.3.3 [^{11}C]-Diacylglycerol

Norepinephrine and epinephrine stimulation of *G* protein-coupled adrenoceptors leads to the activation of inositol trisphosphate, diacylglycerol, and PKC. The phosphoinositide pathway is involved in ventricular remodelling after infarction. Studies evaluating 1-[1-^{11}C]-butyryl-2-palmitoyl-rac-glycerol ([^{11}C]-DAG) demonstrate metabolism to active intermediates of the phosphoinositide cycle in both the brain and heart (Imahori et al. 1992; Chida et al. 2000). Accumulation of [^{11}C]-DAG was enhanced by cholinergic stimulation and suppressed by angiotensin-converting enzyme inhibitor captopril, suggesting an indirect index of phosphoinositide signaling (Imahori et al. 1992; Kagaya et al. 2002). The myocardium to left atrial chamber (i.e. blood pool) ratio of [^{11}C]-DAG was significantly higher in the left ventricle of patients post-myocardial infarction as compared to healthy controls and correlated with left ventricular dilatation, systolic dysfunction, and plasma B-type natriuretic peptide (BNP) levels (Otani et al. 2005).

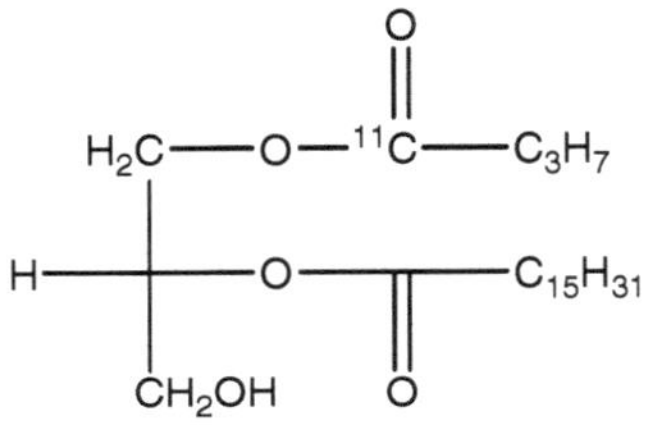

[^{11}C]diacylglycerol

5.4 Future Perspectives

The added value of sympathetic neuronal imaging in cardiovascular disease has been elucidated by prospective clinical trials in recent years. In the ADMIRE HF trial, significantly lower accumulation of [^{123}I]-MIBG was independently associated with progression of heart failure in NYHA class III and IV patients (Jacobson et al. 2010). Substudies have recently demonstrated similar added value in identifying patients at risk for diabetic heart disease (Gerson et al. 2011) and lethal ventricular arrhythmias (Boogers et al. 2010). The ADMIRE HF findings facilitated the US Food and Drug Administration approval of [^{123}I]-MIBG as an imaging agent, which will allow a wider deployment and more routine application of [^{123}I]-MIBG SPECT in stratification of cardiac patient risk. The PAREPET trial identified a prognostic value of regional heterogenous [^{11}C]-HED uptake (denervation) and [^{11}C]-HED/[^{13}N]NH3 mismatch (perfused and denervated) for subsequent ventricular arrhythmia manifesting as sudden cardiac death or implantable cardioverter-defibrillator (ICD) discharge (Fallavollita et al. 2013). The regional abnormalities reported in this study suggest a benefit for PET imaging, in which spatial resolution permits more thorough evaluation of segment innervation. Small-scale trials suggest that postsynaptic β-adrenoceptor imaging may be used to identify patients who will most benefit from targeted β-blocker therapy with carvedilol (Naya et al. 2009). These trials demonstrate the potential for sympathetic neuronal imaging in advanced management of cardiac patients, to identify at-risk patients, and to guide therapeutic interventions in a sophisticated manner.

There remain challenges with the routine application of currently available radiotracers of the sympathetic nervous system. The complex kinetics of neuronal agents, including some combination of reuptake, vesicular storage, metabolism, active release, and passive diffusion, limits the true quantification of sympathetic neuronal integrity. While retention indices, heart to background ratios, or washout rates provide rudimentary data, the accuracy, repeatability, and reproducibility of these measurements can be questionable. Development of novel neuronal tracers with more favourable kinetics, such as the phenethylguanidine series, may overcome some of these challenges and provide more concrete measurements for clinical practice. Second, the majority of PET tracers currently available are labelled with carbon-11, necessitating on-site production for clinical application. Continued development of [^{18}F]-labelled alternatives, particularly [^{18}F]-LMI1195, would overcome these rollout issues to generate a wider clinical relevance. Third, imaging of β-adrenoceptors is complicated by application in a patient population that is frequently treated with chronic β-adrenoceptor blockade. This complication underscores the value of developing novel tracers targeting intracellular second messengers and response elements of the signal cascade. Continued research and development with radiotracers targeting adenylate cyclase, cAMP, PKA, regulatory proteins, and other specific downstream targets not only overcome the complication of β-blockade but also may provide invaluable information on compensatory cardiac function under medical therapy. Alternatively, future tracer development may be targeted upstream of adrenergic signaling, aiming at systems and receptors that modulate sympathetic activity in the heart, such as the renin-angiotensin system or the parasympathetic nervous system. Further development of tracers targeting angiotensin receptors, muscarinic and nicotinic acetycholine receptors, and other targets could contribute to a more complete picture of autonomic regulation of myocardial contractility.

Taken together, while great strides have been made with sympathetic neuronal tracers, many opportunities for molecular imaging remain to be confronted.

Conclusions

Altered sympathetic nervous system signaling is a hallmark characteristic of left ventricular remodelling and progressive cardiovascular disease, including myocardial infarction and ischemia, arrhythmia, cardiomyopathy, and heart failure. Disturbances in myocardial sympathetic neuronal signaling have also been reported in systemic disorders such as diabetes, parkinsonian syndromes, and other neurodegenerative diseases. At present, a wide array of radiotracers is available for the non-invasive evaluation of sympathetic function, with a variety of molecular targets including presynaptic neuronal integrity (uptake-1), vesicular packaging (VMAT2), postsynaptic receptor expression (adrenoceptors), and intracellular second messenger systems (phosphodiesterase, adenylate cyclase). Few of these candidate tracers have yet been established in routine clinical use. As small animal imaging technologies advance, the capacity to identify best candidate tracers within the existing armamentarium will be expedited, potentially accelerating translation from preclinical development to clinical application.

To date, the vast majority of clinical applications have been targeted to the neuron uptake-1 site, using [^{123}I]-MIBG in SPECT and [^{11}C]-mHED in PET. However, clinical studies in recent years have expanded to include non-neuronal targets, providing insight on the regulation of receptors and second messengers of the adrenergic signal cascade. In particular, development and application of β-adrenoceptor antagonists have played a prognostic role in identifying heart failure patients most likely to benefit from beta-blocker therapy. Multitracer studies with novel radiotracers targeting multiple sites of the sympathetic signal cascade provide a more comprehensive understanding of the adaptive and maladaptive changes during the development of disease.

References

Ardell JL (2004) Intrathoracic neuronal regulation of cardiac function. In: Armour JA, Ardell JL (eds) Basic and clinical neurocardiology. Oxford University Press, New York

Armour JA (2004) Cardiac neuronal hierarchy in health and disease. Am J Physiol Regul Integr Comp Physiol 287:R262–R271

Backs J, Haunstetter A, Gerber SH, Metz J, Borst MM, Strasser RH, Kubler W, Haass M (2001) The neuronal norepinephrine transporter in experimental heart failure: evidence for a posttranscriptional downregulation. J Mol Cell Cardiol 33:461–472

Bax JJ, Kraft O, Buxton AE, Fjeld JG, Parizek P, Agostini D, Knuuti J, Flotats A, Arrighi J, Muxi A, Alibelli MJ, Banerjee G, Jacobson AF (2008) 123 I-mIBG scintigraphy to predict inducibility of ventricular arrhythmias on cardiac electrophysiology testing: a prospective multicenter pilot study. Circ Cardiovasc Imaging 1:131–140

Benediktsdottir VE, Curvers J, Gudbjarnason S (1999) Time course of alterations in phospholipid fatty acids and number of beta-adrenoceptors in the rat heart during adrenergic stimulation in vivo. J Mol Cell Cardiol 31:1105–1115

Blanes-Mira C, Pastor MT, Valera E, Fernandez-Ballester G, Merino JM, Gutierrez LM, Perez-Paya E, Ferrer-Montiel A (2003) Identification of SNARE complex modulators that inhibit exocytosis from an alpha-helix-constrained combinatorial library. Biochem J 375:159–166

Boogers MJ, Borleffs CJ, Henneman MM, van Bommel RJ, van Ramshorst J, Boersma E, Dibbets-Schneider P, Stokkel MP, van der Wall EE, Schalij MJ, Bax JJ (2010) Cardiac sympathetic denervation assessed with 123-iodine metaiodobenzylguanidine imaging predicts ventricular arrhythmias in implantable cardioverter-defibrillator patients. J Am Coll Cardiol 55:2769–2777

Bristow MR, Ginsburg R, Minobe W, Cubicciotti RS, Sageman WS, Lurie K, Billingham ME, Harrison DC, Stinson EB (1982) Decreased catecholamine sensitivity and beta-adrenergic-receptor density in failing human hearts. N Engl J Med 307:205–211

Bristow MR, Ginsburg R, Umans V, Fowler M, Minobe W, Rasmussen R, Zera P, Menlove R, Shah P, Jamieson S et al (1986) Beta 1- and beta 2-adrenergic-receptor subpopulations in nonfailing and failing human ventricular myocardium: coupling of both receptor subtypes to muscle contraction and selective beta 1-receptor down-regulation in heart failure. Circ Res 59:297–309

Brodde OE (1991) Beta 1- and beta 2-adrenoceptors in the human heart: properties, function, and alterations in chronic heart failure. Pharmacol Rev 43:203–242

Bryan-Lluka LJ, Paczkowski FA, Bonisch H (2001) Effects of short- and long-term exposure to c-AMP and c-GMP on the noradrenaline transporter. Neuropharmacology 40:607–617

Chida M, Kagaya Y, Imahori Y, Namiuchi S, Fujii R, Fukuchi M, Takahashi C, Tezuka F, Ido T, Shirato K (2000) Visualization of myocardial phosphoinositide turnover with 1-[1-(11) C]-butyryl-2-palmitoyl-rac-glycerol in rats with myocardial infarction. J Nucl Med 41:2063–2068

Dae MW, O'Connell JW, Botvinick EH, Chin MC (1995) Acute and chronic effects of transient myocardial ischemia on sympathetic nerve activity, density, and norepinephrine content. Cardiovasc Res 30:270–280

de Jong RM, Willemsen AT, Slart RH, Blanksma PK, van Waarde A, Cornel JH, Vaalburg W, van Veldhuisen DJ, Elsinga PH (2005) Myocardial beta-adrenoceptor downregulation in idiopathic dilated cardiomyopathy measured in vivo with PET using the new radioligand (S)-[11C] CGP12388. Eur J Nucl Med Mol Imaging 32:443–447

Degrado TR, Zalutsky MR, Vaidyanathan G (1995) Uptake mechanisms of meta-[123I]iodobenzylguanidine in isolated rat heart. Nucl Med Biol 22:1–12

Delforge J, Syrota A, Lancon JP, Nakajima K, Loc'h C, Janier M, Vallois JM, Cayla J, Crouzel C (1991) Cardiac beta-adrenergic receptor density measured in vivo using PET, CGP 12177, and a new graphical method. J Nucl Med 32:739–748

Denn MJ, Stone HL (1976) Autonomic innervation of dog coronary arteries. J Appl Physiol 41:30–35

Ding YS, Lin KS, Logan J, Benveniste H, Carter P (2005) Comparative evaluation of positron emission tomography radiotracers for imaging the norepinephrine transporter: (S, S) and (R, R) enantiomers of reboxetine analogs ([11C]methylreboxetine, 3-Cl-[11C]methylreboxetine and [18F]fluororeboxetine), (R)-[11C]nisoxetine, [11C]oxaprotiline and [11C]lortalamine. J Neurochem 94:337–351

Elsinga PH, Doze P, van Waarde A, Pieterman RM, Blanksma PK, Willemsen AT, Vaalburg W (2001) Imaging of beta-adrenoceptors in the human thorax using (S)-[(11)C]CGP12388 and positron emission tomography. Eur J Pharmacol 433:173–176

Esler M, Jackman G, Leonard P, Skews H, Bobik A, Korner P (1981) Effect of norepinephrine uptake blockers on norepinephrine kinetics. Clin Pharmacol Ther 29:12–20

Esler MD, Jennings GL, Johns J, Burke F, Little PJ, Leonard P (1984) Estimation of 'total' renal, cardiac and splanchnic sympathetic nervous tone in essential hypertension from measurements of noradrenaline release. J Hypertens Suppl 2:S123–S125

Fallavollita JA, Heavey BM, Luisi AJ, Michalek SM, Baldwa S, Mashtare TL, Hutson AD, deKemp RA, Haka MS, Sajid M, Cimato TR, Curtis AB, Cain ME, Canty JA (2013) Regional myocardial sympathetic denervation predicts the risk of sudden cardiac arrest in ischemic cardiomyopathy. J Am Coll Cardiol 63:141–149

Foley KF, Van Dort ME, Sievert MK, Ruoho AE, Cozzi NV (2002) Stereospecific inhibition of monoamine uptake transporters by meta-hydroxyephedrine isomers. J Neural Transm 109:1229–1240

Gauthier C, Tavernier G, Charpentier F, Langin D, Le Marec H (1996) Functional beta3-adrenoceptor in the human heart. J Clin Invest 98:556–562

Geerlings A, Lopez-Corcuera B, Aragon C (2000) Characterization of the interactions between the glycine transporters GLYT1 and GLYT2 and the SNARE protein syntaxin 1A. FEBS Lett 470(1):51–54.

Gerson MC, Caldwell JH, Ananthasubramaniam K, Clements IP, Henzlova MJ, Amanullah A, Jacobson AF (2011) Influence of diabetes mellitus on prognostic utility of imaging of myocardial sympathetic innervation in heart failure patients. Circ Cardiovasc Imaging 4:87–93

Greene M, Thackeray JT, Kenk M, Thorn SL, Bevilacqua L, Harper M-E, Beanlands RS, DaSilva JN (2009) Reduced In Vivo Phosphodiesterase-4 Response to Norepinephrine Challenge in Diet-Induced Obese Rats. Can J Physiol Pharmacol 87:196–202

Habecker BA, Willison BD, Shi X, Woodward WR (2006) Chronic depolarization stimulates norepinephrine transporter expression via catecholamines. J Neurochem 97:1044–1051

Haka MS, Kilbourn MR (1989) Synthesis and regional mouse brain distribution of [11C]nisoxetine, a norepinephrine uptake inhibitor. Int J Rad Appl Instrum B 16:771–774

Imahori Y, Fujii R, Ueda S, Matsumoto K, Wakita K, Ido T, Nariai T, Nakahashi H (1992) Membrane trapping of carbon-11-labeled 1,2-diacylglycerols as a basic concept for assessing phosphatidylinositol turnover in neurotransmission process. J Nucl Med 33:413–422

Jacobson AF, Senior R, Cerqueira MD, Wong ND, Thomas GS, Lopez VA, Agostini D, Weiland F, Chandna H, Narula J (2010) Myocardial iodine-123 meta-iodobenzylguanidine imaging and cardiac events in heart failure. Results of the prospective ADMIRE-HF (AdreView Myocardial Imaging for Risk Evaluation in Heart Failure) study. J Am Coll Cardiol 55:2212–2221

Jakobsen S, Kodahl GM, Olsen AK, Cumming P (2006) Synthesis, radiolabeling and in vivo evaluation of [11C]RAL-01, a potential phosphodiesterase 5 radioligand. Nucl Med Biol 33:593–597

Jaques S Jr, Tobes MC, Sisson JC (1987) Sodium dependency of uptake of norepinephrine and m-iodobenzylguanidine into cultured human pheochromocytoma cells: evidence for uptake-one. Cancer Res 47:3920–3928

Johnson TA, Gray AL, Lauenstein JM, Newton SS, Massari VJ (2004) Parasympathetic control of the heart. I An interventriculo-septal ganglion is the major source of the vagal intracardiac innervation of the ventricles. J Appl Physiol 96:2265–2272

Jung CH, Yang YS, Kim JS, Shin JI, Jin YS, Shin JY, Lee JH, Chung KM, Hwang JS, Oh JM, Shin YK, Kweon DH (2008) A search for synthetic peptides that inhibit soluble N-ethylmaleimide sensitive-factor attachment receptor-mediated membrane fusion. FEBS J 275:3051–3063

Kagaya Y, Chida M, Imahori Y, Fujii R, Namiuchi S, Takeda M, Yamane Y, Otani H, Watanabe J, Fukuchi M, Tezuka F, Ido T, Shirato K (2002) Effect of angiotensin converting enzyme inhibition on myocardial phosphoinositide metabolism visualised with 1-[1-11C]-butyryl-2-palmitoyl-rac-glycerol in myocardial infarction in the rat. Eur J Nucl Med Mol Imaging 29:1516–1522

Kasama S, Toyama T, Sumino H, Kumakura H, Takayama Y, Minami K, Ichikawa S, Matsumoto N, Sato Y, Kurabayashi M (2011) Prognostic value of cardiac sympathetic nerve activity evaluated by [123I]m-iodobenzylguanidine imaging in patients with ST-segment elevation myocardial infarction. Heart 97:20–26

Keller NR, Diedrich A, Appalsamy M, Tuntrakool S, Lonce S, Finney C, Caron MG, Robertson D (2004) Norepinephrine transporter-deficient mice exhibit excessive tachycardia and elevated blood pressure with wakefulness and activity. Circulation 110:1191–1196

Kenk M, Greene M, Thackeray J, Dekemp RA, Lortie M, Thorn S, Beanlands RS, Dasilva JN (2007) In vivo selective binding of (R)-[(11)C]rolipram to phosphodiesterase-4 provides the basis for studying intracellular cAMP signaling in the myocardium and other peripheral tissues. Nucl Med Biol 34:71–77

Kenk M, Greene M, Lortie M, Dekemp RA, Beanlands RS, Dasilva JN (2008) Use of a column-switching high-performance liquid chromatography method to assess the presence of specific binding of (R)- and (S)-[(11)C]rolipram and their labeled metabolites to the phosphodiesterase-4 enzyme in rat plasma and tissues. Nucl Med Biol 35:515–521

Kenk M, Thackeray JT, Thorn SL, Dhami K, Chow BJ, Ascah KJ, Dasilva JN, Beanlands RS (2010) Alterations of pre- and postsynaptic noradrenergic signaling in a rat model of adriamycin-induced cardiotoxicity. J Nucl Cardiol 17:175–176

Kiesewetter DO, Sassaman MB, Robbins J, Elaine MJ, Carson RE, Appel NM, Sutkowski E, Herscovitch P, Braun A, Eckelman WC (2000) Synthesis and evaluation of an 18F analog of forskolin for imaging adenylyl cyclase. J Fluorine Chem 101:297–304

Kopin IJ, Gordon EK (1963) Origin of norepinephrine in the heart. Nature 199:1289

Law MP, Osman S, Davenport RJ, Cunningham VJ, Pike VW, Camici PG (1997) Biodistribution and metabolism of [N-methyl-11C]m-hydroxyephedrine in the rat. Nucl Med Biol 24:417–424

Law MP, Osman S, Pike VW, Davenport RJ, Cunningham VJ, Rimoldi O, Rhodes CG, Giardina D, Camici PG (2000) Evaluation of [11C]GB67, a novel radioligand for imaging myocardial alpha 1-adrenoceptors with positron emission tomography. Eur J Nucl Med 27:7–17

Law MP, Schafers K, Kopka K, Wagner S, Schober O, Schafers M (2010) Molecular imaging of cardiac sympathetic innervation by 11C-mHED and PET: from man to mouse? J Nucl Med 51:1269–1276

Lazewatsky J, Sinusas A, Brunetti J, Heller G, Sparks R, Puretskiy A, Lee LV (2010) Radiation dosimetry of LMI1195, first-in-human study of a novel F-18 labeled tracer for imaging myocardial innervation (Abstract). J Nucl Med 51:1432

Li W, Knowlton D, Van Winkle DM, Habecker BA (2004) Infarction alters both the distribution and noradrenergic properties of cardiac sympathetic neurons. Am J Physiol Heart Circ Physiol 286:H2229–H2236

Liang CS, Fan TH, Sullebarger JT, Sakamoto S (1989) Decreased adrenergic neuronal uptake activity in experimental right heart failure. A chamber-specific contributor to beta-adrenoceptor downregulation. J Clin Invest 84:1267–1275

Link JM, Synovec RE, Krohn KA, Caldwell JH (1997) High speed liquid chromatography of phenylethanolamines for the kinetic analysis of [11C]-meta-hydroxyephedrine and metabolites in plasma. J Chromatogr B Biomed Sci Appl 693:31–41

Lortie M, DaSilva JN, Kenk M, Thorn S, Davis D, Birnie D, Beanlands RS, deKemp RA (2012) Analysis of (R)- and (S)-[(11)C]rolipram kinetics in canine myocardium for the evaluation of phosphodiesterase-4 with PET. Mol Imaging Biol 14:225–236

Lourenco CM, Kenk M, Beanlands RS, DaSilva JN (2006) Increasing synaptic noradrenaline, serotonin and histamine enhances in vivo binding of phosphodiesterase-4 inhibitor (R)-[11C] rolipram in rat brain, lung and heart. Life Sci 79:356–364

Mao W, Iwai C, Qin F, Liang CS (2005) Norepinephrine induces endoplasmic reticulum stress and downregulation of norepinephrine transporter density in PC12 cells via oxidative stress. Am J Physiol Heart Circ Physiol 288:H2381–H2389

Mardon K, Montagne O, Elbaz N, Malek Z, Syrota A, Dubois-Rande JL, Meignan M, Merlet P (2003) Uptake-1 carrier downregulates in parallel with the beta-adrenergic receptor desensitization in rat hearts chronically exposed to high levels of circulating norepinephrine: implications for cardiac neuroimaging in human cardiomyopathies. J Nucl Med 44:1459–1466

Matsunari I, Aoki H, Nomura Y, Takeda N, Chen WP, Taki J, Nakajima K, Nekolla SG, Kinuya S, Kajinami K (2010) Iodine-123 metaiodobenzylguanidine imaging and carbon-11 hydroxyephedrine positron emission tomography compared in patients with left ventricular dysfunction. Circ Cardiovasc Imaging 3:595–603

Miner LH, Schroeter S, Blakely RD, Sesack SR (2003) Ultrastructural localization of the norepinephrine transporter in superficial and deep layers of the rat prelimbic prefrontal cortex and its spatial relationship to probable dopamine terminals. J Comp Neurol 466:478–494

Momose M, Reder S, Raffel DM, Watzlowik P, Wester HJ, Nguyen N, Elsinga PH, Bengel FM, Remien J, Schwaiger M (2004) Evaluation of cardiac beta-adrenoreceptors in the isolated perfused rat heart using (S)-11C-CGP12388. J Nucl Med 45:471–477

Munch G, Nguyen NT, Nekolla S, Ziegler S, Muzik O, Chakraborty P, Wieland DM, Schwaiger M (2000) Evaluation of sympathetic nerve terminals with [(11)C]epinephrine and [(11)C] hydroxyephedrine and positron emission tomography. Circulation 101:516–523

Nakajo M, Shapiro B, Glowniak J, Sisson JC, Beierwaltes WH (1983) Inverse relationship between cardiac accumulation of meta-[131I]iodobenzylguanidine (I-131 MIBG) and circulating catecholamines in suspected pheochromocytoma. J Nucl Med 24:1127–1134

Narula J, Sarkar K (2003) A conceptual paradox of MIBG uptake in heart failure: retention with incontinence! J Nucl Cardiol 10:700–704

Naya M, Tsukamoto T, Morita K, Katoh C, Nishijima K, Komatsu H, Yamada S, Kuge Y, Tamaki N, Tsutsui H (2009) Myocardial beta-adrenergic receptor density assessed by 11C-CGP12177

PET predicts improvement of cardiac function after carvedilol treatment in patients with idiopathic dilated cardiomyopathy. J Nucl Med 50:220–225
Nguyen NT, DeGrado TR, Chakraborty P, Wieland DM, Schwaiger M (1997) Myocardial kinetics of carbon-11-epinephrine in the isolated working rat heart. J Nucl Med 38:780–785
Nishijima K, Kuge Y, Seki K, Ohkura K, Motoki N, Nagatsu K, Tanaka A, Tsukamoto E, Tamaki N (2002) A simplified and improved synthesis of [11C]phosgene with iron and iron (III) oxide. Nucl Med Biol 29:345–350
Nishijima K, Kuge Y, Seki K, Ohkura K, Morita K, Nakada K, Tamaki N (2004) Preparation and pharmaceutical evaluation for clinical application of high specific activity S-(-)[11C]CGP-12177, a radioligand for beta-adrenoreceptors. Nucl Med Commun 25:845–849
Otani H, Kagaya Y, Imahori Y, Yasuda S, Fujii R, Chida M, Namiuchi S, Takeda M, Sakuma M, Watanabe J, Ido T, Nonogi H, Shirato K (2005) Myocardial 11C-diacylglycerol accumulation and left ventricular remodeling in patients after myocardial infarction. J Nucl Med 46:553–559
Pardini BJ, Lund DD, Schmid PG (1989) Organization of the sympathetic postganglionic innervation of the rat heart. J Auton Nerv Syst 28:193–201
Park-Holohan SJ, Asselin MC, Turton DR, Williams SL, Hume SP, Camici PG, Rimoldi OE (2008) Quantification of [11C]GB67 binding to cardiac alpha1-adrenoceptors with positron emission tomography: validation in pigs. Eur J Nucl Med Mol Imaging 35:1624–1635
Parrish DC, Gritman K, Van Winkle DM, Woodward WR, Bader M, Habecker BA (2008) Postinfarct sympathetic hyperactivity differentially stimulates expression of tyrosine hydroxylase and norepinephrine transporter. Am J Physiol Heart Circ Physiol 294:H99–H106
Raffel DM, Chen W (2004) Binding of [3H]mazindol to cardiac norepinephrine transporters: kinetic and equilibrium studies. Naunyn Schmiedebergs Arch Pharmacol 370:9–16
Raffel DM, Wieland DM (2001) Assessment of cardiac sympathetic nerve integrity with positron emission tomography. Nucl Med Biol 28:541–559
Raffel DM, Corbett JR, del Rosario RB, Gildersleeve DL, Chiao PC, Schwaiger M, Wieland DM (1996) Clinical evaluation of carbon-11-phenylephrine: MAO-sensitive marker of cardiac sympathetic neurons. J Nucl Med 37:1923–1931
Raffel DM, Chen W, Sherman PS, Gildersleeve DL, Jung YW (2006) Dependence of cardiac 11C-meta-hydroxyephedrine retention on norepinephrine transporter density. J Nucl Med 47:1490–1496
Raffel DM, Jung YW, Gildersleeve DL, Sherman PS, Moskwa JJ, Tluczek LJ, Chen W (2007) Radiolabeled phenethylguanidines: novel imaging agents for cardiac sympathetic neurons and adrenergic tumors. J Med Chem 50:2078–2088
Ren ZG, Porzgen P, Zhang JM, Chen XR, Amara SG, Blakely RD, Sieber-Blum M (2001) Autocrine regulation of norepinephrine transporter expression. Mol Cell Neurosci 17:539–550
Rosenspire KC, Haka MS, Van Dort ME, Jewett DM, Gildersleeve DL, Schwaiger M, Wieland DM (1990) Synthesis and preliminary evaluation of carbon-11-meta-hydroxyephedrine: a false transmitter agent for heart neuronal imaging. J Nucl Med 31:1328–1334
Russ H, Gliese M, Sonna J, Schomig E (1992) The extraneuronal transport mechanism for noradrenaline (uptake2) avidly transports 1-methyl-4-phenylpyridinium (MPP+). Naunyn Schmiedebergs Arch Pharmacol 346:158–165
Salt PJ (1972) Inhibition of noradrenaline uptake 2 in the isolated rat heart by steroids, clonidine and methoxylated phenylethylamines. Eur J Pharmacol 20:329–340
Sasaki T, Enta A, Nozaki T, Ishii S, Senda M (1993) Carbon-11-forskolin: a ligand for visualization of the adenylate cyclase-related second messenger system. J Nucl Med 34:1944–1948
Sasano T, Abraham MR, Chang KC, Ashikaga H, Mills KJ, Holt DP, Hilton J, Nekolla SG, Dong J, Lardo AC, Halperin H, Dannals RF, Marban E, Bengel FM (2008) Abnormal sympathetic innervation of viable myocardium and the substrate of ventricular tachycardia after myocardial infarction. J Am Coll Cardiol 51:2266–2275
Thackeray JT, Beanlands RS, Dasilva JN (2007) Presence of specific 11C-meta-hydroxyephedrine retention in heart, lung, pancreas, and brown adipose tissue. J Nucl Med 48:1733–1740

Thackeray JT, Parsa-Nezhad M, Kenk M, Thorn SL, Kolajova M, Beanlands RS, Dasilva JN (2011) Reduced CGP12177 binding to cardiac beta-adrenoceptors in hyperglycemic high-fat-diet-fed, streptozotocin-induced diabetic rats. Nucl Med Biol 38:1059–1066

Thackeray JT, Beanlands RS, DaSilva JN (2012) Altered sympathetic nervous system signaling in the diabetic heart: emerging targets for molecular imaging. Am J Nucl Med Mol Imaging 2:319–339

Thackeray JT, Renaud JM, Kordos M, Klein R, deKemp RA, Beanlands RS, DaSilva JN (2013) Test-retest repeatability of quantitative cardiac 11C-meta-hydroxyephedrine measurements in rats by small animal positron emission tomography. Nucl Med Biol 40:676–681

Thomas AJ, DaSilva JN, Lortie M, Renaud JM, Kenk M, Beanlands RS, deKemp RA (2011) PET of (R)-11C-rolipram binding to phosphodiesterase-4 is reproducible and sensitive to increased norepinephrine in the rat heart. J Nucl Med 52:263–269

Tipre DN, Fox JJ, Holt DP, Green G, Yu J, Pomper M, Dannals RF, Bengel FM (2008) In vivo PET imaging of cardiac presynaptic sympathoneuronal mechanisms in the rat. J Nucl Med 49:1189–1195

Tsukamoto T, Morita K, Naya M, Inubushi M, Katoh C, Nishijima K, Kuge Y, Okamoto H, Tsutsui H, Tamaki N (2007) Decreased myocardial beta-adrenergic receptor density in relation to increased sympathetic tone in patients with nonischemic cardiomyopathy. J Nucl Med 48:1777–1782

Van Dort ME, Kim JH, Tluczek L, Wieland DM (1997) Synthesis of 11C-labeled desipramine and its metabolite 2-hydroxydesipramine: potential radiotracers for PET studies of the norepinephrine transporter. Nucl Med Biol 24:707–711

Van Waarde A, Meeder JG, Blanksma PK, Brodde O-E, Visser GM, Elsinga PH, Paans AMJ, Vaalburg W, Lie KI (1992) Uptake of radioligands by rat heart and lung in vivo:CGP 12177 does and CGP 26505 does not reflect binding to ß-adrenoceptors. Eur J Pharmacol 222:107–112

van Waarde A, Vaalburg W, Doze P, Bosker FJ, Elsinga PH (2004) PET imaging of beta-adrenoceptors in human brain: a realistic goal or a mirage? Curr Pharm Des 10:1519–1536

Vasdev N, LaRonde FJ, Woodgett JR, Garcia A, Rubie EA, Meyer JH, Houle S, Wilson AA (2008) Rationally designed PKA inhibitors for positron emission tomography: Synthesis and cerebral biodistribution of N-(2-(4-bromocinnamylamino)ethyl)-N-[11C]methyl-isoquinoline-5-sulfonamide. Bioorg Med Chem 16:5277–5284

Wehrens XH, Lehnart SE, Reiken S, Vest JA, Wronska A, Marks AR (2006) Ryanodine receptor/calcium release channel PKA phosphorylation: a critical mediator of heart failure progression. Proc Natl Acad Sci U S A 103:511–518

Wehrwein EA, Parker LM, Wright AA, Spitsbergen JM, Novotny M, Babankova D, Swain GM, Habecker BA, Kreulen DL (2008) Cardiac norepinephrine transporter protein expression is inversely correlated to chamber norepinephrine content. Am J Physiol Regul Integr Comp Physiol 295:R857–R863

Wong W, Scott JD (2004) AKAP signalling complexes: focal points in space and time. Nat Rev Mol Cell Biol 5:959–970

Woolard J, Bennett T, Dunn WR, Heal DJ, Aspley S, Gardiner SM (2004) Acute cardiovascular effects of sibutramine in conscious rats. J Pharmacol Exp Ther 308:1102–1110

Yu M, Bozek J, Lamoy M, Guaraldi M, Silva P, Kagan M, Yalamanchili P, Onthank D, Mistry M, Lazewatsky J, Broekema M, Radeke H, Purohit A, Cdebaca M, Azure M, Cesati R, Casebier D, Robinson SP (2011) Evaluation of LMI1195, a novel 18F-labeled cardiac neuronal PET imaging agent, in cells and animal models. Circ Cardiovasc Imaging 4:435–443

Imaging the Parasympathetic Cardiac Innervation with PET

6

Dominique Le Guludec, Jacques Delforge, and Frédéric Dollé

Contents

D. Le Guludec (✉)
Department of Nuclear Medicine, Inserm U1148, Laboratory for Vascular Translational Science, Bichat University Hospital, Assistance Publique-Hôpitaux de Paris, University Paris Diderot-Paris 7, 46 rue Henri Huchard, Paris 75018, France
e-mail: dominique.leguludec@bch.aphp.fr

J. Delforge
4 allée du Moulin à Bareau, Briis Sous Forges 91640, France

F. Dollé
CEA, I2BM, Service Hospitalier Frédéric Joliot, 4 place du Général Leclerc, Orsay 91406, France

R.H.J.A. Slart et al. (eds.), *Autonomic Innervation of the Heart: Role of Molecular Imaging*, DOI 10.1007/978-3-662-45074-1_6

Abstract

Parasympathetic tone plays a critical role as modulator of the cardiac sympathetic nervous system the healthy and diseased heart and has a major impact upon the occurrence of arrhythmias and sudden death. Decreased parasympathetic tone is an important prognostic factor in heart failure. Abnormalities of both systems, sympathetic and parasympathetic, have been shown to be either global or regional. This represents a major rationale for the use of imaging techniques to measure autonomic nervous system function, particularly as the other clinical tools such as heart rate variability are of limited value.

Positron emission tomography (PET) imaging with short half-life positron-labeled specific ligands allows this evaluation. However, PET measures the labeled ligand concentration, but the quantification of the receptor density and affinity requires mathematical modeling to simulate the kinetics of the labeled molecule in the tissue, with the use of compartmental analysis and complex protocols. These protocols include injection not only of the tracer but also of pharmacological doses of the cold ligand for co-injection or displacement experiments.

PET imaging with [^{11}C]-methyl-quinuclidin-3-yl benzilate has been validated as an accurate tool to measure muscarinic receptor density and affinity constants in patients with heart failure, including postinfarction patients. A novel ($\alpha_4\beta_2$) nicotinic acetylcholine receptor PET ligand, 2-[^{18}F]-F-A-85380, was also used in patients for evaluation of left ventricular and arterial wall nicotinic receptors.

Although limited today to research centers, PET imaging of the cardiac parasympathetic innervation provides new insight into pathophysiological processes and can be used for the evaluation of new drugs. In the future, it could emerge as a reference for validation of more simple tools and of easier imaging protocols and for early diagnosis, monitoring of treatment, and determination of individual outcome.

Abbreviations

ACh	Acetylcholine
DCM	Dilated cardiomyopathy
DMSO	Dimethyl sulfoxide
ECG	Electrocardiogram
FAP	Familial amyloid polyneuropathy
FDG	Fluorodeoxyglucose
HPLC	High-performance liquid chromatography
mAChR	Muscarinic acetylcholine receptor
MR	See mAChR
MSA	Multiple system atrophy
nAChR	Nicotinic acetylcholine receptor
NMS	N-Methylscopolamine
PET	Positron emission tomography

QNB	3-Quinuclidinyl benzilate (or quinuclidin-3-yl benzilate)
ROI	Region of interest
SD	Standard deviation
SE	Standard error
SPECT	Single-photon emission computed tomography
SPET	See SPECT
SUV	Standardized uptake value
TBP	Tributyl phosphate
TFA	Trifluoroacetic acid
TTR	Transthyretin (gene)

6.1 Introduction

The parasympathetic—or vagal—autonomic nervous system, in balance with the adrenergic system, plays a key role in the regulation of the rate and force of contraction of the heart (Van Zwieten 1991; Brodde et al. 2001). It is involved in the pathophysiology of major cardiac diseases (Olshansky et al. 2008). In the clinical setting, markers of decreased vagal activity are associated with poor prognosis and increased risk of sudden death (Frenneaux 2004; La Rovere et al. 1998; Vanoli and Schwartz 1990; Schwartz et al. 1992; Brack et al. 2013) and represent a target for therapeutic intervention (Townend and Littler 1995; Olshansky et al. 2008).

Previous studies reported that ventricular parasympathetic innervation was spare compared to the sympathetic one. This view is now completely outdated, and modern histological techniques revealed a dense and intricate network of parasympathetic nerves running over the epicardial and endocardial surface of both ventricles with a widespread distribution of muscarinic receptors (mAChR or MR) (Brodde et al. 2001; Kawano et al. 2003; Nenasheva et al. 2013).

The endogenous neuromediator acetylcholine (ACh) is synthesized from choline and acetyl-CoA, taken into storage vesicles by specific transporters, and released into the synapse during parasympathetic stimulation. The parasympathetic signal acts on target tissue via nicotinic and muscarinic receptors, mainly the M_2-MR in the myocardium. MRs are G_i-protein-coupled receptors that mediate the response to acetylcholine released from parasympathetic nerves. There are 5 subtypes of MR (M_1–M_5), 3 of them are found within the heart (M_2, M_3, and M_4). The M_2-MR is the most abundant, found on cardiomyocytes and intracardiac ganglia. They are essential for the physiologic control of cardiovascular function through activation of G-protein-coupled inwardly rectifying potassium channels and indirect effects on adenylate cyclase activity and are of particular interest because of their extensive pharmacological characterization (Stengel et al. 2002). The structure and mode of action of the M_2-MR is still a matter of extensive research (Haga et al. 2012; Miao et al. 2013). Muscarinic receptors were initially defined biochemically as proteins that specifically bind 3-quinuclidinyl benzilate (QNB) and N-methylscopolamine (NMS), this being at the origin of tracers developed for imaging. M_2-MR was more recently described. The location and pathophysiological role of M_3-MR in the cardiovascular system have been extensively studied, and many pathways involved have been uncovered. They are linked with Gq-proteins. Recently, many new findings regarding the relationship between M_3-MR and cardiac diseases have emerged, including cardiac ischemia, pathological cardiac hypertrophy, cardiac arrhythmias, cardiac conduction, and heart failure (Abramochkin et al. 2013; Hang et al. 2013). Finally, the parasympathetic nervous system acts also by the binding of ACh to neuronal nicotinic receptors (nAChR), which are ligand-gated ion channel receptors present in the ventricular myocardium as well as on nerve fibers innervating the blood vessel (Sullivan et al. 1996). Vagal stimulation triggers vascular protection through the cholinergic anti-inflammatory pathway by activating α7 nAChR (Zhao et al. 2013).

Global and regional molecular imaging of parasympathetic function is, as for sympathetic function, of major interest regarding the importance and heterogeneity of neuronal functional alterations in the diseased heart. However, while the myocardial presynaptic and postsynaptic sympathetic innervations were extensively studied with single-photon computed emission tomography (SPECT) and positron emission tomography (PET) tracers on a broad clinical basis, few clinical studies have been conducted to evaluate the parasympathetic system with PET, offering a large field for future research. To date, very few tracers for imaging this parasympathetic pathway achieved a clinical validation. No radiolabeled compounds have been successfully synthesized for non-invasive imaging of the presynaptic parasympathetic innervation, and few tracers are available for PET imaging allowing absolute quantification and tracer kinetics modeling of nicotinic and muscarinic receptors. Ligands based on the structure of vesamicol, a selective antagonist of the vesicular ACh transporters, have been developed for imaging of presynaptic targets, but to date none have been made available for human use (DeGrado et al. 1994). Evaluation of parasympathetic neuronal activity by quantification of the postsynaptic MRs is the most validated technique. In spite of this postsynaptic receptor, PET imaging provides major and new information into mechanisms of heart disease, since it provides non-invasive, repeatable, regional in vivo quantification of autonomic nerve function in the human heart. In particular, it has the potential to evaluate both the sympathetic and parasympathetic balance in a given pathology, providing profound insights into molecular pathophysiology, monitoring of treatment, and determination of individual outcome.

This chapter will summarize the major tools, requirements for accurate quantification, and clinical applications of molecular imaging of the parasympathetic function in patients.

6.2 Radiotracers for PET Imaging

Two radiotracers have been clinically used to date for PET imaging of the parasympathetic innervation, (R, S)-*N*-[^{11}C]-methyl-quinuclidin-3-yl benzilate ([^{11}C]-Me-QNB) and 2-[^{18}F]-fluoro-3-[2(S)-2-azetidinylmethoxy]pyridine (2-[^{18}F]-F-A-85380) (Fig. 6.1).

Fig. 6.1 Chemical structures of (R,S)-*N*-[^{11}C]-methyl-quinuclidin-3-yl benzilate ([^{11}C]-MQNB, (**a**)) and 2-[^{18}F]-fluoro-3-[2(S)-2-azetidinylmethoxy]pyridine (2-[^{18}F]-F-A-85380, (**b**))

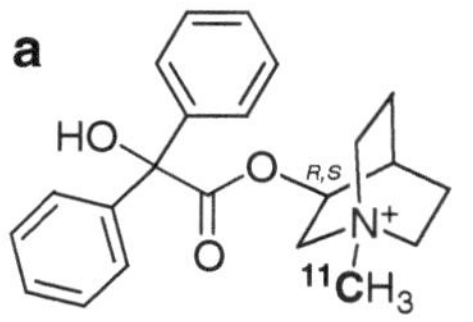

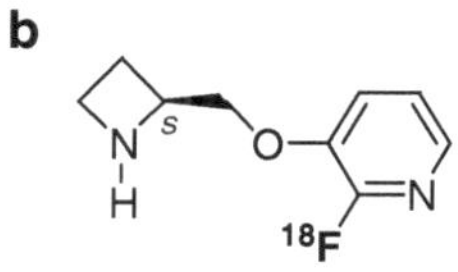

6.2.1 The Radioligands of Interest

6.2.1.1 The MR Antagonist [^{11}C]-MQNB

[^{11}C]-MQNB is an isotopically labeled carbon-11 version of MQNB, a well-known hydrophilic, non-metabolized, and highly specific MR antagonist. This radiotracer of reference for the in vivo imaging of the myocardial MRs using PET and labeled with a short-lived positron emitter (carbon-11, $T_{1/2}$: 20.38 min) (Fig. 6.1a) is derived from QNB (quinuclidin-3-yl benzilate), a structure itself related to the deliriant drugs atropine and scopolamine. It distinguishes itself from the three latter by featuring a quaternary ammonium function, the positive charge of which impairs any brain penetration. Its potential for non-invasive quantification of ventricular MRs was demonstrated and validated in dogs (Delforge et al. 1990a; Valette et al. 1995, 1997) but also in humans (Delforge et al. 1993, 1995). [^{11}C]-MQNB has therefore been used for the assessment of the myocardial MR density and affinity constants in heart transplant patients (Le Guludec et al. 1994), in patients with chronic idiopathic dilated cardiomyopathy (Le Guludec et al. 1997), or in familial amyloid neuropathy patients (Delahaye et al. 1999).

The preparation of [^{11}C]-MQNB includes a carbon-11 methylation reaction (Fig. 6.2), which is by far the most frequently used method for the introduction of this short-lived positron emitter into organic molecules. As such, these processes require first the preparation of a carbon-11-labeled reagent, [^{11}C]-methyl iodide ([^{11}C]-CH_3I) or [^{11}C]-methyl triflate ([^{11}C]-$CH_3O(SO_2)CF_3$ or [^{11}C]-CH_3OTf) (Roeda et al. 2007), both prepared from cyclotron-produced [^{11}C]-carbon dioxide ([^{11}C]-CO_2, produced by the ^{14}N(p,alpha)^{11}C nuclear reaction, Fig. 6.2a, b).

[^{11}C]-MQNB was first synthesized from the corresponding desmethyl precursor (QNB) using [^{11}C]-CH_3I (Fig. 6.2c) (Mazière et al. 1983). No yields were reported, but the conditions include the use of tributyl phosphate (TBP) as solvent and 8 min of reaction at 100 °C. Later on, a more exhaustive study was performed using the same desmethyl precursor (QNB) and solvent (TBP). Decay-corrected yields of about 23 %, based on starting [^{11}C]-CH_3I, were then reported for the conditions mentioned above. Improved conditions that notably include the use of [^{11}C]-CH_3OTf at the same temperature (100 °C) but with reduced heating time (1 min only) were also reported with decay-corrected yields of about 49 %, based on starting [^{11}C]-CH_3OTf. Using the latter conditions, large quantities (important for the above-mentioned multi-injection protocol) of [^{11}C]-MQNB (6.8 ± 1.1 GBq, occasionally

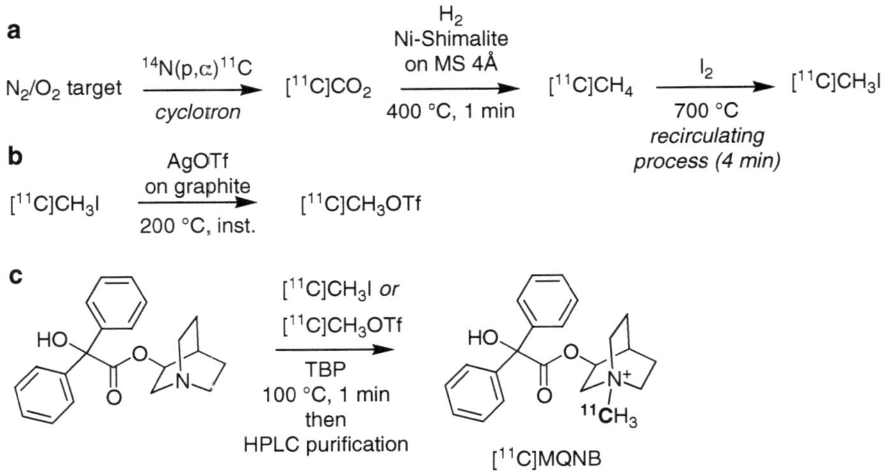

a

N_2/O_2 target — $^{14}N(p,\alpha)^{11}C$, *cyclotron* → [^{11}C]CO_2 — H_2, Ni-Shimalite on MS 4Å, 400 °C, 1 min → [^{11}C]CH_4 — I_2, 700 °C, *recirculating process (4 min)* → [^{11}C]CH_3I

b

[^{11}C]CH_3I — AgOTf on graphite, 200 °C, inst. → [^{11}C]CH_3OTf

c

HO, O, O, N — [^{11}C]CH_3I *or* [^{11}C]CH_3OTf, TBP, 100 °C, 1 min, then HPLC purification → HO, O, O, N^+, $^{11}CH_3$

[^{11}C]MQNB

Fig. 6.2 Carbon-11 production (**a**), [^{11}C]-CH_3I (**a**) and/or [^{11}C]-CH_3OTf (**b**) preparation and radiosynthesis of *N*-[^{11}C]-methyl-quinuclidin-3-yl benzilate ([^{11}C]-MQNB) (**c**)

up to 13 GBq, starting from 55 GBq of [^{11}C]-CO_2) could be synthesized in 28-min, high-performance liquid chromatography (HPLC) purification included (Dollé et al. 2001). Very recently, further optimization of the preparation of [^{11}C]-MQNB was proposed (Gómez-Vallejo et al. 2012) including the use of SepPak® cartridge purification thus replacing the final HPLC purification, and the use of the so-called captive solvent methodology. Complete separation from the precursor QNB is of utmost importance since the latter is a potent MR ligand too that, in contrast to MQNB, enters the brain and may have delirious effects.

6.2.1.2 The Nicotinic Agonist 2-[^{18}F]-F-A-85380

2-[^{18}F]-F-A-85380 (Fig. 6.1b) is a fluorine-18-labeled fluoroanalogue of A-85380, the lead compound of a series of 3-pyridyl ethers developed by Abbott laboratories (Sullivan et al. 1996) as potent and selective ligands for the human $\alpha_4\beta_2$ nAChR subtype. This series not only possesses subnanomolar affinity for brain nAChRs and differentially acts on subtypes of neuronal nAChR but also shows a satisfactory safety profile. Indeed, the structural features of these ligands retain the high potency of epibatidine (a natural compound, isolated from the skin of the Ecuadorian poison frog *Epipedobates tricolor*, also characterized as a very potent high-affinity nAChR agonist) and impart a subtype selectivity not observed with the latter.

2-[^{18}F]-F-A-85380 is probably the most used radiotracer for the in vivo imaging of the nicotinic ($\alpha_4\beta_2$) receptors in the brain using PET and as such a radioligand of reference, despite its slow kinetics demanding very long scanning times and its low signal-to-noise ratio. Its potential for non-invasive quantification of the $\alpha_4\beta_{22}$ nAChR subtype was validated in monkeys and in humans (Bottlaender et al. 2003; Gallezot et al. 2005). A multi-injection protocol, based on mathematical compartmental ligand-receptor modeling and a kinetic approach, was developed in order to analyze

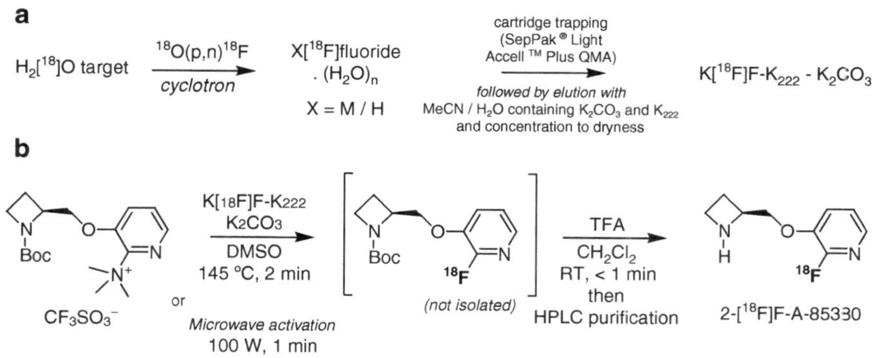

Fig. 6.3 Fluorine-18 production (**a**), K[^{18}F]-F-K$_{222}$ preparation (**a**) and radiosynthesis of 2-[^{18}F]-fluoro-3-[2(S)-2-azetidinylmethoxy]pyridine (2-[^{18}F]-F-A-85380) (**b**)

and fit the PET data. 2-[^{18}F]-F-A-85380 has been extensively used in clinical and preclinical studies on addiction to smoking (Brody et al. 2006; Valette et al. 2003), Alzheimer's disease (Ellis et al. 2008) and Parkinson's disease (Kas et al. 2009), epilepsy (Picard et al. 2006), and normal aging (Ellis et al. 2009). Also it can be used in the assessment of parasympathetic innervation in the human heart, the only non-brain application reported thus far (Bucerius et al. 2006a; b). Please however note that the radiotracer name was misspelled by the authors (2-[^{18}F]-F-A-85380 is the correct nomenclature and not 2-deoxy-2-[^{18}F]-fluoro-D-glucose-A85380).

2-[^{18}F]-F-A-85380 is one of the first reported examples of a radioligand for which the introduction of fluorine-18 was performed using a nucleophilic *hetero*-aromatic radiofluorination reaction (Dollé 2005). These reactions usually involve no-carrier-added (high-specific-radioactivity) [^{18}F]-fluoride as its K[^{18}F]-F-K$_{222}$ complex, the latter nowadays prepared from cyclotron-produced [^{18}F]-fluoride (via the ^{18}O(p,n)^{18}F nuclear reaction), potassium carbonate (K_2CO_3), and Kryptofix®222 (4,7,13,16,21,24-hexaoxa-1,10-diazabicyclo[8.8.8]hexacosane) using a well-established procedure (Fig. 6.3a) (Dollé et al. 2008).

2-[^{18}F]-F-A-85380 was first synthesized in two radiochemical steps from an *N*-Boc-protected nitro-precursor and was obtained in 49–64 % overall decay-corrected radiochemical yield in 105–110-min total synthesis time (Dollé et al. 1998). The nucleophilic *hetero*aromatic substitution with fluorine-18 was performed using K[^{18}F]-F-K$_{222}$ and conventional heating in dimethyl sulfoxide (150 °C for 20 min) or microwave activation (100 W for 1 min), leading to the radiofluorinated intermediate with 70 %, and occasionally up to 90 % radiochemical yield, followed by quantitative trifluoroacetic acid (TFA) removal of the *N*-Boc protective group. This radiochemical two-step process using the same *N*-Boc-protected nitro-precursor was later on simplified, and 2-[^{18}F]-F-A-85380 was obtained with comparable yields but in only 55–60-min total synthesis time (Liu et al. 2002). 2-[^{18}F]-F-A-85380 was also synthesized in two radiochemical steps from the *N-Boc-protected* iodoprecursor but was obtained in only 21 % overall decay-corrected radiochemical yield in 120-min total synthesis time (Horti et al. 1998). Attempts to perform a one-step radiosynthesis from the corresponding non-protected iodoprecursor failed, due to thermal instability of the radiotracer in the rather drastic conditions used (Horti et al. 1998). Nowadays, 2-[^{18}F]-F-A-85380 is still synthesized in two radiochemical steps but from a more reactive, *N*-Boc-protected, trimethylammonium precursor (see Fig. 6.3b). Overall decay-corrected radiochemical yields of 62–68 % were reported with a total synthesis time not exceeding 55 min (Dollé et al. 1999). The nucleophilic *hetero*aromatic substitution with fluorine-18 was performed using K[^{18}F]-F-K_{222} and conventional heating in dimethyl sulfoxide (DMSO) at 145 °C for 2 min (or microwave activation, at 100 W for 1 min). Using the latter conditions, 2-[^{18}F]-F-A-85380 production batches of 3.5–3.7 GBq of >99 % radiochemical purity were routinely obtained in 50–55 min, with specific radioactivities of 111–222 GBq/µmol. Overall decay-corrected radiochemical yields with respect to initial [^{18}F]-fluoride ion were 68–72 %. Later on, this radiochemical two-step process was also simplified and the total synthesis time shortened to only 35 min, notably by replacing the final HPLC purification by a SepPak® cartridge method (Schmaljohann et al. 2004, 2005).

6.3 The Modeling of Ligand-Receptor Interactions

PET measures the labeled ligand concentration, but it does not allow the direct measurement of the receptor concentration and the ligand affinity. To estimate these parameters, a mathematical model must be developed to simulate the kinetic of the labeled molecule in the tissue. These physiological parameters will appear as model parameters which have to be identified from the experimental PET curves, often simultaneously with other model parameters (usually kinetic rate constants).

6.3.1 The Ligand-Receptor Model

6.3.1.1 The Model Structure

The complexity of the model, that is to say, of simulated physiological processes, varies a great deal, depending on the organ, the tracer used, the receptor type, and the available experimental data. However, all the in vivo approaches of the ligand-receptor interactions are based on a mathematical model which includes at least two steps:

1. A transport of the ligand from the blood to a free ligand compartment (a necessary step since the labeled ligand is injected intravenously)
2. A classical ligand-receptor interaction similar to that used in in vitro studies

Thus, one obtains the usual three-compartment model shown in Fig. 6.4.

In this model, $C^*_{\ell}(t)$ is the concentration of free ligand in the blood (usually, the plasma concentration of the ligand non-metabolized and unbound to the proteins). $F^*(t)$ and $B^*(t)$ are the quantities of ligand per unit volume of tissue which are free

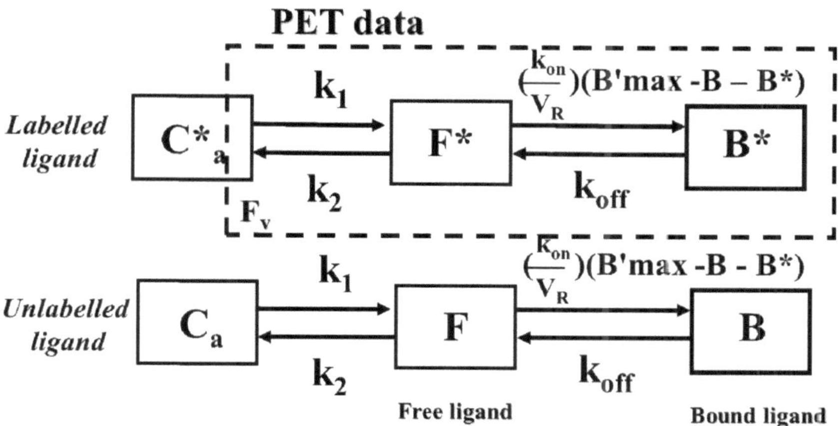

Fig. 6.4 Compartmental ligand-receptor model used in analysis of myocardial tissue data obtained after intravenous injections of [^{11}C]-MQNB. The upper part represents the model describing labeled ligand kinetics (quantities denoted by an *asterisk*) and the lower part the same model associated with the unlabeled ligand. The three compartments represent the free ligand in the plasma, the free ligand, and specifically bound ligand in the tissue, respectively. All transfer probabilities of ligand between compartments are linear except for binding probability which depends on the bimolecular association rate constant and on local concentration of free receptor sites. PET experimental data correspond to the sum of the two tissular compartments and of a fraction F_v of plasma compartment. The unlabeled ligand compartments are not directly observable from PET data, but the concentration of specifically bound ligand ($B(t)$) has an effect on the local concentration of free receptors and consequently on the binding probability of free labeled ligand

in the exchangeable pool and specifically bound to receptor sites, respectively. The PET data correspond to the sum of these two concentrations, plus a fraction of the blood ligand concentration (denoted by F_v and corresponding to the fraction of blood present in the tissue volume).

In some cases, it is needed to introduce a possible nonspecific binding assumed linear, and related to the free ligand compartment. Thus, one obtains a four-compartment model.

6.3.1.2 The Reaction Volume

The reaction volume has been introduced to take into account a possible heterogeneity of the free ligand concentration in the tissue (Delforge et al. 1996). Indeed, the free ligand concentration in the receptor site vicinity may not be equal to the mean free ligand concentration in 1 mL ($F^*(t)$), which is the concentration used in the mathematical model and estimated by modeling the PET data.

Therefore, the reaction volume V_R is defined as the volume in which the free ligand mass present in 1 mL of tissue ($F^*(t)$) would have uniformly distributed with the same concentration as in the vicinity of the receptor sites.

6.3.1.3 The Ligand-Receptor Interactions

The parameter B'_{max} represents the unknown concentration of receptor sites available for ligand binding. At any time t, the concentration of the free receptor sites is equal to $B'_{max}-B^*(t)$, where $B^*(t)$ is the quantity of labeled ligand bound to receptor sites in one mL of tissue.

The probability of binding of a free ligand is given by (k_{on}/V_R) $(B'_{max}-B^*(t))$ where k_{on} is the association rate constant, the concentration of the free ligand in the vicinity of the receptor sites being F^* $(t)/V_R$ by definition of the reaction volume. The equilibrium dissociation rate constant K_d is given by the ratio k_{off}/k_{on}. In vivo, only the product K_dV_R can be estimated.

It is important to mention that the receptor concentration can be separately estimated only if B^* is significant compared to B'_{max}. Indeed, if the receptor occupation is negligible, one can only estimate the product (k_{on}/V_R) (B'_{max}).

6.3.1.4 Influence of the Endogenous Ligand

In most of the quantification studies, the effect of the endogenous ligand is neglected. As a consequence, the estimated parameters can be biased.

However, a previous study (Delforge et al. 2001) shown that, by assuming only the equilibrium state of the endogenous ligand, all model parameters (including B'_{max}) are correctly estimated (without bias), except the estimated apparent affinity which is biased following the same relationship obtained in the in vitro studies (Farde et al. 1995; Endres et al. 1997).

6.3.2 Estimation of the Ligand-Receptor Model Parameters

6.3.2.1 The Multi-injection Approach

The major interest of PET studies of the ligand-receptor interactions is the absolute quantification of both the receptor concentration and the ligand affinity. The best approach, but the more difficult one, is to identify all model parameters from PET data. This complete model identification avoids introducing some simplifying hypotheses, which are difficult to justify without a good understanding of the ligand kinetics and which can lead to bias in the numerical results. Moreover, the complete knowledge of the model parameters is necessary in order to make simulations, which permit detailed studies of the ligand kinetics in each compartment (Delforge et al. 1990b), validation of simplified methods (Delforge et al. 2002), and optimization of experimental protocols (Delforge et al. 1989).

Because of the large number of parameters, the only possibility is to use a protocol including multiple injections of labeled and/or unlabeled ligand.

The injection of unlabeled ligand has no direct effect on the PET data which measures only labeled ligand concentration. However, the kinetics of the unlabeled ligand affects the local concentration of free receptor sites and therefore effects the labeled ligand kinetics. Therefore, the model described in Fig. 6.4 contains two parts: the upper part represents the possible model describing the kinetics of the radioligand (with quantities denoted with a star superscript), and the lower part is associated with the unlabeled ligand kinetics. The two parts of the model have the same structure and the same parameters. However, the quantity of free ligand is now given by $(B'_{max}-B^*)$ where B^* is the receptor concentration occupied by unlabeled ligand.

6.3.2.2 Parameter Estimation

The model parameters are estimated by means of minimization of the usual weighted least-square cost function. For each data set and for each parameter, it is possible to estimate the standard errors (SE) (Delforge et al. 1989). Using the numerical results obtained with different data sets, it is possible to calculate the usual standard deviation (SD) for each model parameter. Usually, SE and SD obtained for a parameter have the same order of magnitude.

6.3.3 The Multi-Injection Experimental Protocols

6.3.3.1 The Experimental Protocols in the Multi-Injection Approach

The experimental protocols used with the multi-injection approach can be very different depending on the kinetic characteristics of the studied molecule and of the practical experimental possibility. This protocol is based on three typical injections performed during a single experiment:

1. A tracer injection with a high specific activity, such as the receptor occupancy remains less than 5 %.
2. A tracer injection with low specific activity, also called a co-injection since the low specific activity is often obtained by a mixture of labeled ligand with high specific activity and an adapted dose of unlabeled ligand. The doses are chosen such as the receptor occupancy is situated between 50 and 70 %.
3. An injection of a large dose of unlabeled ligand, also called displacement injection, to obtain a maximum receptor occupancy, more than 95 % if this is possible.

6.3.3.2 The MQNB Experimental Protocol Used in Animal

The first example of this multi-injection approach is the study of the binding of MQNB to MRs in dog hearts (Delforge et al. 1990a). The first attempts to identify the model parameters from data obtained with a single tracer injection led to disappointing numerical results, since most of the parameters had to be considered unidentifiable.

The possibility of improving parameter estimation using a new experimental design consisting of a first tracer injection followed 30 min later by an injection of the unlabeled ligand (displacement experiment) was then investigated. This second protocol, however, led to two very different numerical solutions (Delforge et al. 1990b). The biologically valid solution was determined by adding a third injection (a co-injection).

A fourth injection (a displacement injection) allowed the identification and estimation of irreversible and nonspecific binding (Delforge et al. 1990b).

6.3.3.3 The MQNB Experimental Protocol Used in Humans

In the first study in humans (Delforge et al. 1993), three kinds of experimental protocols were used in three distinct subsets of subjects.

1. *A three-injection protocol*, which included three injections of [^{11}C]-MQNB and/or MQNB performed: a tracer dose at time 0, unlabeled MQNB (from 0.2 to

0.4 mg) at time 30 min, and a co-injection of [^{11}C]-MQNB and MQNB (from 0.2 to 1 mg) at time 60 min. The total experiment lasted 90 min.

2. *A co-injection protocol* which included only an initial tracer injection followed 30 min afterwards by a simultaneous injection of labeled and unlabeled MQNB (from 0.15 to 0.4 mg, respectively). The total experiment duration was 70 min.
3. A *double-displacement protocol* which involved, after the initial tracer injection, two injections of unlabeled MQNB (0.3 mg) at 30 min and 60 min, respectively. The entire experiment lasted 90 min. This protocol has been used to estimate in human the order of magnitude of the nonspecific binding.

6.3.3.4 Optimization of the Human Experimental Protocol

To set up the best protocol, it is possible to use the experimental design optimization (Delforge et al. 1989). It has been proved that a judicious selection of sampling times, injected ligand doses, injection time, and other degrees of freedom can have a significant effect on parameter estimate uncertainties.

For example, in (Delforge et al. 1993), the uncertainties on B'_{max} have been estimated as a function of the unlabeled MQNB dose for the co-injection and displacement protocol. The simulations prove that the smallest uncertainty on B'_{max} obtained using a co-injection protocol is two times smaller than the best value obtained with the displacement protocol. However, the most important result is that this smallest uncertainty is obtained with the co-injection protocol by using only 0.2 mg of unlabeled ligand dose, whereas the best result with the displacement protocol implies to use about 1 mg. Taking into account the influence of the unlabeled ligand dose on the heart rate, this result is a very strong argument in favor of the co-injection protocol.

However, the three-injection protocol has been used in the first studies on cardiac diseases (Le Guludec et al. 1994; Delahaye et al. 2001) since this protocol gives the best numerical values of parameters. The effect of unlabeled ligand dose on the heart rate can be corrected by a variable blood flow in the model (Delforge et al. 1993).

6.4 Clinical Applications

In recent years, the importance of alterations of cardiac autonomic nerve function in the pathophysiology of heart diseases has been increasingly recognized. Muscarinic cholinergic receptors in balance with β-adrenergic receptors play a key role in the regulation of the rate and force of heart contraction as well as in the pathophysiology of arrhythmias. Changes in receptor's number and affinity have been reported in many clinical conditions including heart failure, arrhythmias, ischemic heart disease, heart transplantation, amyloidosis, and diabetes. These changes are recognized to be predictive of outcome (Frenneaux 2004; La Rovere et al. 1998; Folino et al. 2005; Brack et al. 2013). PET and SPECT imaging have the potential to evaluate both the sympathetic and parasympathetic balance in a given pathology provides profound insights into molecular pathophysiology, monitoring of treatment, and determination of individual outcome. This is of major interest considering the limitations of the other tools such as heart rate variability (Kleiger et al. 2005).

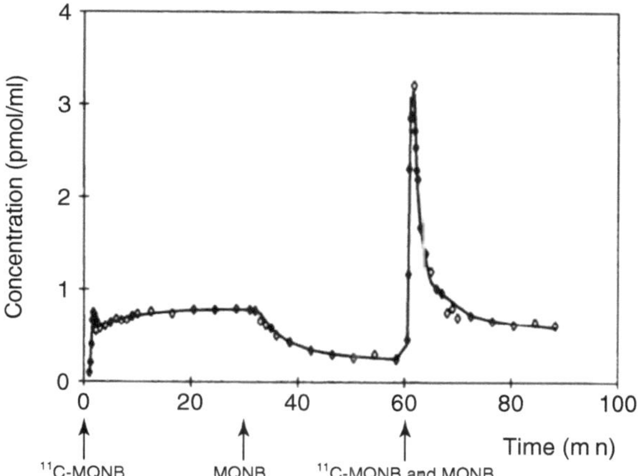

Fig. 6.5 Example of experimental PET data obtained using a three-injection protocol: tracer injection at time 0 (5.2 μg of [^{11}C]-MQNB with a specific activity of 26 MBq/μmol), injection of unlabeled ligand at 30 min (0.25 mg) and coinjection at 60 min(22.7 μg and 1 mg of MQNB, respectively). A comparison is made between the experimental PET data (*open diamonds*) and the model simulation (*solid line*)

6.4.1 Muscarinic Receptors in the Normal Human Left Ventricle

[^{11}C]-MQNB, which is a non-metabolized, hydrophilic antagonist which binds only to the cell surface receptors and is not internalized, offers the opportunity to quantify only the active receptors at the surface of the myocytes in vivo. Using this potential with PET and a mathematical model, the first clinical study aimed to quantify the density and affinity constants in the normal human heart and then to evaluate potential changes in density and/or affinity during pathological conditions.

6.4.1.1 Parameter Estimations

This study was conducted in 11 normal subjects (mean age 32 ± 6 years old), free of any cardiac disease on the basis of clinical electrocardiogram (ECG) and echocardiography examinations. The use of a left ventricular region of interest instead of plasma radioactive concentration measurements was validated in five controls.

Figures 6.5 and 6.6 show examples of experimental curves obtained using three-injection and two-injection protocol, respectively. Fitting the complete mathematical model to experimental data provided values for kinetic rate constants and receptor densities as shown in Table 6.1. The final quality of the fits was satisfactory, as can be seen in Figs. 6.5 and 6.6. A study showed a presence of a small irreversible nonspecific binding, but proved that the fit of the experimental data without nonspecific binding compartment led to small and acceptable bias (Delforge et al. 1993).

Table 6.1 shows that the standard deviations on the model parameters are significantly smaller with the three-injection protocol except for the receptor concentration B'_{max} which is similar. This proves the interest of the optimization of the experimental protocol described in paragraph 6.3.3.4, since it has been optimized in favor of B'_{max}, but as a consequence led to poorer quantification of other parameters.

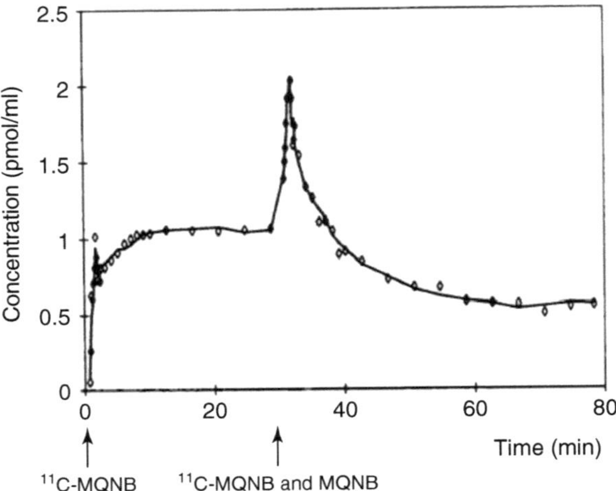

Fig. 6.6 Example of experimental PET data obtained using a coinjection protocol with tracer injection at time 0 (6.5 μg of [^{11}C]-MQNB with a specific activity of 30 MBq/μmol) and injection of labeled and unlabeled ligand at 30 min (8.3 μg and 0.2 mg of MQNB, respectively). A comparison is made between the experimental PET data (*open diamonds*) and the model simulation (*solid line*)

Table 6.1 Model parameters estimated using the three-injection protocol (tracer dose, displacement and co-injection) and using the two-injection protocol (tracer dose and co-injection)

Parameters	Units	Two injections	Three injections
B'_{max}	pmol/mL	25 ± 7	26 ± 7
k_1	min^{-1}	0.46 ± 0.10	0.34 ± 0.06
k_2	min^{-1}	3.9 ± 1.7	2.3 ± 1.1
k_{on}/V_R	mL/(pmol.min)	1.6 ± 1.4	1.3 ± 0.2
k_{off}	min^{-1}	0.29 ± 0.24	0.34 ± 0.08
F_v	–	0.41 ± 0.10	0.48 ± 0.14
$K_d V_R$	pmol/mL	0.36 ± 0.38	0.30 ± 0.06

The receptor concentration was estimated to 26 ± 7 pmol/mL of myocardium. All parameters in this series of normal volunteers are summarized in Table 6.1. No difference in receptor constants was found across left ventricular walls, but one of the limits of the study was the quite rough correction of partial volume effect using echocardiographic thickness measurements, so some minor differences from one wall to the other could have been underestimated.

6.4.1.2 MQNB Images After Tracer Injection

The plateau of [^{11}C]-MQNB concentration observed in the myocardium when the ligand is injected at high specific activity is thus due to a high probability of rebinding and not to an irreversible binding. These findings must be applied cautiously when interpreting PET images if the ligand used displays a high affinity for specific binding sites.

These model parameters also prove that myocardial PET images obtained after a single injection of a high-affinity ligand reflect the myocardial blood flow more than the receptor density (Delforge et al. 1990a, b). The possible changes of concentration observed on the images are mainly the consequence of the local changes of blood flow. As a consequence, to study the distribution of receptor sites in the heart (even with no quantification), it is thus necessary to use an experimental protocol such as a significant part of the receptor sites are occupied (by using low specific activity or by injecting non-labeled ligand).

6.4.1.3 The Reaction Volume Estimation

The volume of reaction V_R is not identifiable from the PET data. Because MQNB is a very hydrophilic molecule, V_R can be considered close to the fraction of extracellular fluid estimated at 0.15 mL/mL tissue (Walker 1986). This value is in agreement with the estimate obtained in the dog study by comparing the $K_d V_R$ value found in vivo by PET (0.072 ± 0.021 pmol/mL tissue) with the K_d value from the in vitro method (0.49 ± 0.06 pmol/mL tissue), which led to a V_R value equal to 0.147 mL/mL (Delforge et al. 1990a).

A third estimate of this parameter can be obtained by assuming that exchanges between plasma and free ligand compartments were passive. In this case, the reaction volume can be estimated from the k_1/k_2 ratio. From the parameter values given in Table 6.1, V_R is estimated by this method at 0.148 mL/mL.

The three estimates of V_R are close to 0.15 mL/mL. By using this value, the equilibrium dissociation constant K_d is estimated at 2.0 ± 0.5 pmol/mL tissue in the normal human myocardium.

6.4.2 Muscarinic Receptors in Heart Denervation

Myocardial denervation can occur in different pathological conditions with different consequences on receptor changes. Denervation generally induces a supersensitivity to agonists that has been lost and an increase in receptor density. However, we will see that the mechanism of denervation can modify these receptor's changes. Heart transplantation induces a surgical parasympathetic denervation at the preganglionic level, in contrast with sympathetic denervation, with no changes in postganglionic nerves. In contrast, denervation observed in patients with familial amyloid polyneuropathy (FAP) is due to amyloid deposition all along the pre- and postganglionic neurons and nerve terminals. PET studies have shown the difference in these two types of denervation in both β-adrenergic receptor and MR changes.

6.4.2.1 Muscarinic Receptors in Heart Transplantation

Myocardial denervation in transplant patients leads to important clinical, physiological and pharmacological alterations such as elevated basal heart rate, silent ischemia, arrhythmias, and difference in drug efficiency (Bristow 1990). Changes in β-adrenergic receptor density have been correlated with an increased total number in dogs but not in patients, suggesting species differences (Vatner et al. 1985). The question of MR changes in transplanted patients was not elucidated.

After determination of normal values, the PET evaluation with [^{11}C]-MQNB was applied to 6 patients 2–7 months (mean 4.7 ± 2.3) after heart transplantation. As expected, the baseline heart rate was significantly higher in patients than controls.

The heart rate remained constant until the end of the procedure in all patients, while it increased significantly in normal volunteers. This discrepancy between controls and patients is explained by the absence of tonic vagal input in patients: the heart rate does not respond to innervation-dependant pharmacological stimulation such as atropine or analogs. So, there was no more difference in heart rate between patients and controls at the end of the procedure. However, no difference in the affinity constants nor in the mean receptor density B'_{max} (24.4 vs. 26.7 pmol/mL) was found between patients and controls. This absence of change in MR density is in agreement with the unchanged sensitivity to MR agonists found in the denervated heart. This may be due to the fact that surgical parasympathetic denervation is preganglionic, in contrast with sympathetic denervation. This is concordant with the persistence of parasympathetic innervation in cardiac allograft tissues.

The only difference between patients and controls in the study was in the volume of reaction (V_R), reflecting an increase in interstitial water volume produced by edema, even in the absence of acute rejection.

6.4.2.2 Muscarinic Receptors in Heart Denervation Observed in Patients With Amyloidosis

FAP is a rare hereditary form of amyloidosis characterized by a progressive sensorimotor polyneuropathy with often severe autonomic neuropathy. It is due to amyloid deposition of a genetic variant transthyretin produced by the liver, with various clinical presentations, as circa 100 mutations have been described. The only effective therapy is liver transplantation which can stop the disease progress, but since a few years new drugs have been proposed that stabilize the abnormal transthyretin and prevent amyloid deposit in the target organs (Adams et al. 2000), and gene therapy is a fast developing therapeutic pathway as well.

Cardiac involvement has been demonstrated as a major prognostic factor, as cardiac deaths are responsible for 40 % of mortality.

Cardiac autonomic neuropathy is the most frequent and earliest manifestation of the cardiac amyloid deposit. Some forms of FAP create pure lesions of cardiac denervation, with sympathetic denervation well demonstrated by MIBG imaging showing a progressive decrease in the tracer uptake (Delahaye et al. 1999, 2006). PET and MQNB were used in a series of 21 patients with genetic transthyretin (TTR) FAP but no left ventricle systolic dysfunction evaluated before liver transplantation (Delahaye et al. 2001). Cardiac β-receptor functional efficiency was studied by heart rate response to intravenous isoproterenol. The mean MR density was significantly higher in patients than in control subjects (B'_{max} 35.5 ± 8.9 vs. 26.1 ± 6.7 pmol/mL, $p < 0.003$), without change in receptor affinity. The increase in heart rate after injection of atropine as well as MQNB was lower in patients compared with control subjects despite a similar basal heart rate, consistent with parasympathetic denervation. Incremental infusion of isoproterenol induced a similar increase in heart rate in patients and control subjects, while cardiac MIBG uptake was markedly decreased in patients compared to controls, suggesting no changes in sympathetic postsynaptic receptor density in spite of presynaptic denervation. The MR density was higher in the septal wall of patients than in the anterior wall and higher in the anterior wall than in the lateral wall, suggesting regional differences, but the wall thickness of patients was higher and more variable.

The absence of increased sensitivity to isoproterenol was consistent with the absence of β-receptor-mediated supersensitivity despite sympathetic denervation.

This difference between muscarinic and β-adrenergic receptor regulation is probably due to the absence of circulating neuromediator for the parasympathetic system. Although myocardial catecholamine release by sympathetic neurons is impaired in patients with FAP, the persistence of catecholamine production by the adrenal glands associated by the lack of reuptake by the sympathetic nerve terminals in the myocardium seems sufficient to maintain the β-receptor stimulation. However, the most accurate way to demonstrate this would be to quantify both muscarinic and β-adrenergic receptors with PET in the same patients.

6.4.3 Muscarinic Receptors in Heart Failure

Congestive heart failure is associated with a marked imbalance of the autonomic nervous system. This includes an increase in sympathetic drive, downregulation of left ventricular β-adrenergic receptors, and selective loss of the myocardial contractile response to β-adrenergic stimulation (Bristow et al. 1990). Cardiac parasympathetic control in patients with chronic heart failure has been less well documented, even though the role of the parasympathetic system is increasingly suspected in heart disease and in the events that characterize its outcome, especially sudden death (Schmitz et al. 1996; Hermosillo et al. 1993; Brack et al. 2013). Several lines of evidence suggest that the parasympathetic receptor-effector system is altered in heart failure. A chronic attenuation of cardiac vagal tone has been inferred from studies of heart rate variability in patients with cardiomyopathy (Binkley et al. 1991; Nolan et al. 1992). Congestive heart failure is associated with decreased stimulated myocardial adenylate cyclase activity, increased amount or functional activity of $G_i\alpha$ regulatory protein G_i-binding protein, attenuated parasympathetic tone, and increased modulation of β-adrenergic inotropic left ventricular stimulation by parasympathetic agonists (Böhm et al. 1990). These data suggest that either the density or affinity of receptors coupling with the inhibitory guanine nucleotide-binding protein, which include MRs, is altered in the failing myocardium (Vatner et al. 1996).

The density and affinity constants of myocardial MRs were evaluated by means of PET with [^{11}C]-MQNB in 20 patients with congestive heart failure due to idiopathic dilated cardiomyopathy (mean left ventricular ejection fraction, 22 ± 9 %) and compared with values in 12 normal subjects (Le Guludec et al. 1997). The mean receptor concentration was significantly higher in patients than in control subjects (B'_{max} 34.5 ± 8.9 vs. 25 ± 7.7 pmol/mL, $p < .005$), with no changes in affinity constants. The change in heart rate after injection of 0.6 mg of non-labeled MQNB was lower in patients than in control subjects (34 ± 20 % vs. 55 ± 36 %, $p < .05$), and receptor density correlated negatively with maximal heart rate in the patients ($r = .45$, $p < .05$).

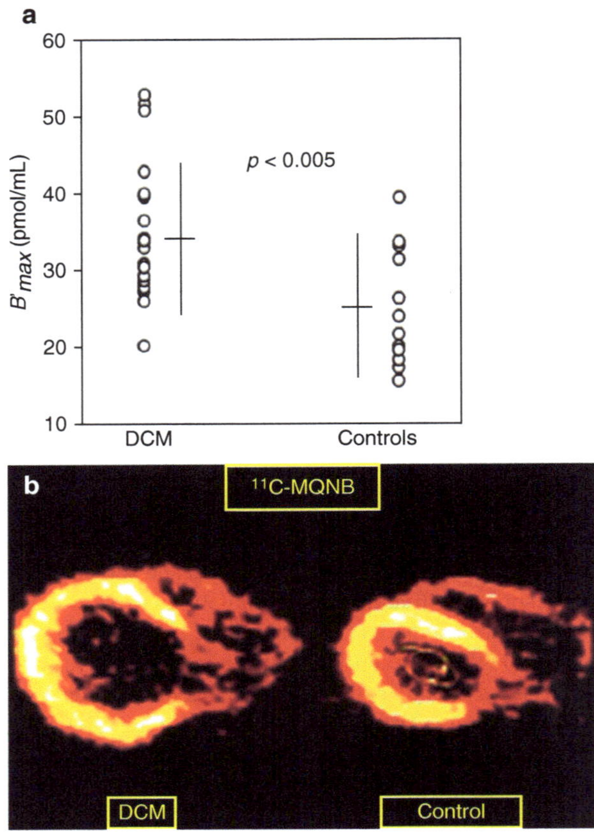

Fig. 6.7 (**a**) Individual ventricular MR concentrations (B'_{max}) in 20 patients with idiopathic DCM and in 12 control subjects, showing a significantly higher mean concentration in patients. (**b**) Tomographic transaxial cross-sectional images of the heart recorded 10 min after intravenous injection of [^{11}C]-MQNB in a control subject (*right*) and a patient with idiopathic DCM (*left*)

This study clearly demonstrated that congestive heart failure is associated with an upregulation of myocardial MRs (Fig. 6.7). This may be an adaptive mechanism to β-agonist stimulation and should increase the number of potential targets for pharmacological intervention.

6.4.4 Muscarinic Receptors in Postinfarct Patients

[^{11}C]-MQNB was used to evaluate the impact of infarction on left ventricular MR density. Myocardial ischemia and infarction drastically alters the autonomous nervous system, and this alteration contributes to the susceptibility of the infarcted regions to the occurrence of arrhythmias and sudden death (Frenneaux 2004; La Rovere et al. 1998; Schwartz et al. 1992). Experimental and clinical data suggest that decreased vagal activity is associated with an enhanced risk of ventricular arrhythmias in patients after myocardial infarction, besides changes in postsynaptic β-adrenergic receptors expression, with a reduction in density in the remote myocardium correlated with remodeling parameters (Ohte et al. 2012). In addition, the

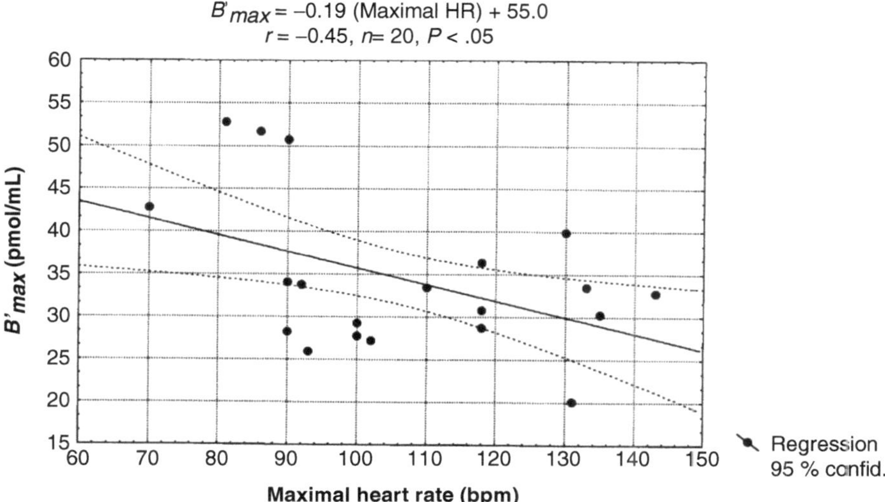

Fig. 6.8 Correlation between the maximal heart rate in patients after intravenous injection of non-labeled MQNB (a MR antagonist equivalent to atropine) and the density of myocardial MRs (B'_{max}) estimated by PET

role of the parasympathetic nervous system in cardioprotection by remote ischemic preconditioning (Mastitskaya et al. 2013; Donato et al. 2013) as well as in prevention of reperfusion injury (Katare et al. 2009) was extensively evaluated.

A group evaluated MR density using [^{11}C]-MQNB PET and a two-injection protocol (injection of labeled MQNB followed by co-injection of unlabeled and labeled tracer) in 11 patients after their first myocardial infarction and in 9 healthy volunteers (Mazzadi et al. 2009). They demonstrated a localized twofold increase in receptor density in the non-infarcted remote myocardium compared with normal regions. The B_{max} was similar in remote and potentially damaged regions, but reduced in damaged regions compared to remote regions. In patients, the mean B_{max} per patient in remote regions was inversely correlated to the heart rate at baseline, but not to the extent of infarction or the time after infarction (Fig. 6.8). This study suggests that the myocardial vagal activity in chronic myocardial infarction is characterized by an upregulation of MRs in remote non-infarcted regions, remaining within normal values in damaged tissue. This upregulation of parasympathetic receptors, resulting in increased endogenous β-blockade due to vagal stimulation, could act as a mechanism attenuating the arrhythmogenic effects of increased and heterogeneous sympathetic activity.

6.4.5 Nicotinic Receptors in the Left Ventricle

The role of the nAChRs in mediating the parasympathetic autonomic control of cardiac function is less known. In a recent study, the assessment of cardiac nAChR distribution with a novel ($\alpha_4\beta_2$) nAChR PET ligand (2-[^{18}F]-F-A-85380), misspelled by the authors, see Sect. 6.2.1.2) was performed in normal controls and neurologic patients (Bucerius et al. 2006a, b). This agent was first used to detect nAChRs in the brain, specifically those containing β2 subunits, showing a reduction in uptake in patients with Parkinson's disease consistent with histopathologic studies. By contrast, smokers presented with an increased neuronal uptake.

Five healthy volunteers without cardiac disease and six patients with either Parkinson's disease or multiple system atrophy without additional overt cardiac disease were evaluated with 2-[^{18}F]-F-A-85380 PET imaging to assess the cardiac parasympathetic innervation and the putative impact of both disorders. Whole-body PET scans were performed 75.4 min ± 6.7 after IV injection of 371.2 ± 58.1 MBq of the tracer. Average count rate density of left ventricle ROIs and a standard ROI in the right lung were measured within three consecutive slices of 10.0 mm thickness. The heart—as well as the lung—tracer uptake was almost constant throughout all subjects leading to a good target-to-background ratio. Heart-to-lung ratios were calculated in each volunteer and patient. These ratio were not different between the volunteer group and patients suffering from Parkinson's disease or multiple system atrophy (MSA) (3.2 ± 0.5 vs. 3.2 ± 0.8 and 2.96 ± 0.7, mean ± SD), respectively.

These first results suggested no impact of either Parkinson's disease or MSA on cardiac nAChRs, according to authors. However, in this study, no mathematical model was used, and it is not evident that a simple activity ratio is accurate to evaluate changes in nAChR density.

6.4.6 Nicotinic Acetylcholine Receptors in the Vascular Wall

It has been demonstrated that nAChRs exist in the vasculature and are stimulated by endogenous ACh or exogenous nicotine. Nicotinic ACh receptors are presents in nerve fibers innervating blood vessels and are activated by either endogenous ACh produced in the vessel wall or by a direct effect of exogenous nicotine (Brüggmann et al. 2002; Egleton et al. 2009). Recent studies have shown that nicotine (the addictive component of cigarettes) binds to the high-affinity cell-surface nAChRs and accelerates the atherogenic process. These receptors are expressed ubiquitously in almost all cells existing in the blood vessels. A recent review summarizes the pro-atherogenic effects of nAChR ligands such as nicotine and tobacco nitrosamines and the contribution of different receptor subunits in plaque growth, progression, and neovascularization (Santanam et al. 2012). This stimulation induces a trophic effect on the endothelium and vascular smooth muscle, enhances cell proliferation and survival, and releases vasoactive and growth factors that maintain vascular homeostasis and repair. Excessive stimulation may contribute to pathological angiogenesis such as that involved in atherosclerotic plaque neovascularization but also tumor progression. This emphasizes the interest for new methods to evaluate density and activity of these receptors in vivo (Cooke 2012).

A recent study used the ($\alpha_4\beta_2$) nAChR PET ligand (2-[^{18}F]-F-A-85380) to evaluate the nAChRs in the vascular wall in healthy volunteers and in patients with neurodegenerative disorders (Bucerius et al. 2012). The uptake of the ligand was quantified in the ascending and descending aorta, the aortic arch, and the carotids in 5 healthy volunteers and 6 patients with either Parkinson's disease or multiple system atrophy. A relative quantification was performed in the same way as [^{18}F]-fluorodeoxyglucose (FDG) PET evaluation is usually performed, i.e., using the maximum target-to-background ratio. The maximal standardized uptake value (SUV), the single hottest segment, and the percent active segments of the ligand uptake in the arteries were also assessed.

Maximum target-to-background ratio uptake values corrected for background activity showed specific tracer uptake in the arterial wall, with significantly higher uptake values in the descending aorta. Comparison between volunteers and the patient group showed lower uptake in the last group when comparing single arterial territories but not when all arterial segments were pooled together. Although this marker may be of high interest, again no mathematical model was used, and it is not evident that a simple activity ratio is accurate to evaluate changes in nAChR density. Additional studies are needed to assess its accuracy in that setting.

Conclusions

There is large evidence that parasympathetic tone plays a critical role as modulator of the cardiac sympathetic nervous system in both healthy and diseased heart and has an impact upon the occurrence of arrhythmias and sudden death. Decreased parasympathetic tone is an important prognostic factor after myocardial infarction or in heart failure patients. Moreover, abnormalities of both systems, sympathetic and parasympathetic, have been shown to be distributed regionally and heterogeneous in many circumstances. This represents a major rationale for the use of imaging to measure autonomic nervous system function. PET imaging together with [^{11}C]-MQNB has been validated as an accurate tool to measure receptor's density and affinity constants. It requires short half-life positron-labeled compound that restrict their use to departments equipped with cyclotrons. The use of compartmental analysis and multi-injection (at least two) protocols is required for adequate quantification of density B_{max} as well as K_d. These requirements make PET imaging evaluation a major tool for pathophysiological studies, but make broad clinical application difficult today. In the future, it could emerge as a reference for validation of more simple tools and easier imaging protocols and for early diagnosis, monitoring of treatment, and determination of individual outcome.

References

Abramochkin DV, Tapilina SV, Sukhova GS (2013) Effect of selective stimulation of muscarinic M3 cholinoceptors on electrical and contractile activity of rat ventricular myocardium. Bull Exp Biol Med 154:295–298

Adams D, Samuel D, Goulon-Goeau C et al (2000) The course and prognostic factors of familial polyneuropathy after liver transplantation. Brain 123:1495–1504

Binkley PF, Nunziata E, Nelson SD et al (1991) Parasympathetic withdrawal is an integral component of autonomic imbalance in congestive heart failure: demonstration in human subjects and verification in a paced canine model of ventricular failure. J Am Coll Cardiol 18:464–472

Böhm M, Gierschik P, Jajobs KH et al (1990) Increase of Giα in human hearts with dilated but not ischemic cardiomyopathy. Circulation 82:1249–1265

Bottlaender M, Valette H, Roumenov D et al (2003) Biodistribution and radiation dosimetry of [18F]fluoro-A-85380 in healthy volunteers. J Nucl Med 44:596–601

Brack KE, Winter J, Ng GA (2013) Mechanisms underlying the autonomic modulation of ventricular fibrillation initiation–tentative prophylactic properties of vagus nerve stimulation on malignant arrhythmias in heart failure. Heart Fail Rev 18:389–408

Bristow MR (1990) The surgically denervated, transplanted human heart. Circulation 82:658–660

Bristow MR, Hershberger RE, Port JD et al (1990) β-Adrenergic pathways in nonfailing and failing human ventricular myocardium. Circulation 82(Suppl I):I12–I25

Brodde OE, Bruck H, Leineweber K et al (2001) Presence, distribution and physiological function of adrenergic and muscarinic receptor subtypes in the human heart. Basic Res Cardiol 96:528–538

Brody AL, Mandelkern MA, London ED et al (2006) Cigarette smoking saturates brain α4β2 nicotinic acetylcholine receptors. Arch Gen Psychiatry 63:907–915

Brüggmann D, Lips KS, Pfeil U et al (2002) Multiple nicotinic acetylcholine receptor alpha-subunits are expressed in the arterial system of the rat. Histochem Cell Biol 118:441–447

Bucerius J, Joe AY, Schmaljohann J et al (2006a) Feasibility of 2-deoxy-2-[18F]fluoro-D-glucose-A85380-PET for imaging of human cardiac nicotinic acetylcholine receptors in vivo. Clin Res Cardiol 95:105–109

Bucerius J, Joe AY, Schmaljohann J et al (2006b) Erratum: Feasibility of 2-deoxy-2-[18F]fluoro-D-glucose- A85380-PET for imaging of human cardiac nicotinic acetylcholine receptors in vivo. Clin Res Cardiol 95:354

Bucerius J, Manka C, Schmaljohann J et al (2012) Feasibility of [18F]-2-Fluoro-A85380-PET imaging of human vascular nicotinic acetylcholine receptors in vivo. JACC Cardiovasc Imaging 5:528–536

Cooke JP (2012) Imaging vascular nicotine receptors: a new window onto vascular disease. JACC Cardiovasc Imaging 5:537–539

DeGrado TR, Mulholland KG, Wieland DM et al (1994) Evaluation of F-18 fluoroethoxybenzovesamicol as a new PET tracer of cholinergic neurons of the heart. Nucl Med Biol 21:189–195

Delahaye N, Dinanian S, Slama M et al (1999) Cardiac sympathetic denervation in familial amyloid polyneuropathy assessed by iodine-123 metaiodobenzylguanidine scintigraphy and heart rate variability. Eur J Nucl Med 26:416–424

Delahaye N, Le Guludec D, Dinanian S et al (2001) Myocardial muscarinic receptor upregulation and normal response to isoproterenol in denervated hearts by familial amyloid polyneuropathy. Circulation 104:2911–6291

Delahaye N, Rouzet F, Sarda L et al (2006) Impact of liver transplantation on cardiac autonomic denervation in familial amyloid polyneuropathy. Medicine 85:229–238

Delforge J, Syrota A, Mazoyer B (1989) Experimental design optimization: theory and application to estimation of receptor model parameters using dynamic positron emission tomography. Phys Med Biol 34:419–435

Delforge J, Janier M, Syrota A et al (1990a) Noninvasive quantification of muscarinic receptors in vivo with positron emission tomography in the dog heart. Circulation 82:1494–1504

Delforge J, Syrota A, Mazoyer B (1990b) Identifiability analysis and parameter identification of an in vivo ligand-receptor model from PET data. IEEE Trans Biomed Eng 37:653–661

Delforge J, Le Guludec D, Syrota A et al (1993) Quantification of myocardial muscarinic receptors with PET in humans. J Nucl Med 34:981–991

Delforge J, Pappata S, Millet P et al (1995) Quantification of benzodiazepine receptors in human brain using PET, [11C]flumazenil, and a single-experiment protocol. J Cereb Blood Flow Metab 15:284–300

Delforge J, Syrota A, Bendriem B (1996) The concept of reaction volume in the in vivo ligand-receptor model. J Nucl Med 37:118–125
Delforge J, Bottlaender M, Pappata S et al (2001) Absolute quantification by positron emission tomography of the endogenous lligand. J Cereb Blood Flow Metab 21:613–630
Delforge J, Mesangeau D, Dolle F, Merlet P, Loc'h C, Bottlaender M, Trebossen R, Syrota A (2002) In vivo quantification and parametric images of the cardiac beta-adrenergic receptor density. J Nucl Med 43:215–226
Dollé F (2005) Fluorine-18-labelled fluoropyridines: Advances in radiopharmaceutical design. Curr Pharm Design 11:3221–3235
Dollé F, Valette H, Bottlaender M et al (1998) Synthesis of 2-[18F]fluoro-3-[2(S)-2-azetidinylmethoxy]pyridine, a highly potent radioligand for in vivo imaging central nicotinic acetylcholine receptors. J Label Compds Radiopharm 41:451–463
Dollé F, Dolci L, Valette H et al (1999) Synthesis and nicotinic acetylcholine receptor in vivo binding properties of 2-fluoro-3-[2(S)-2-azetidinylmethoxy]pyridine: a new positron emission tomography ligand for nicotinic receptors. J Med Chem 42:2251–2259
Dollé F, Hinnen F, Vaufrey F et al (2001) Highly Efficient synthesis of [11C]Me-QNB, a selective radioligand for the quantification of the cardiac muscarinic receptors using PET. J Label Compds Radiopharm 44:337–345
Dollé F, Roeda D, Kuhnast B et al (2008) Fluorine-18 chemistry for molecular imaging with positron emission tomography. In: Tressaud A, Haufe G (eds) Fluorine and health: molecular imaging, biomedical materials and pharmaceuticals. Elsevier, Amsterdam/Boston/Heidelberg/London/New York/Oxford/Paris/San Diego/San Francisco/Singapore/Sydney/Tokyo
Donato M, Buchholz B, Rodríguez M et al (2013) Role of the parasympathetic nervous system in cardioprotection by remote hindlimb ischaemic preconditioning. Exp Physiol 98:425–434
Egleton RD, Brown KC, Dasgupta P (2009) Angiogenic activity of nicotinic acetylcholine receptors: implications in tobacco-related vascular diseases. Pharmacol Ther 121:205–223
Ellis JR, Villemagne VL, Nathan PJ et al (2008) Relationship between nicotinic receptors and cognitive function in early Alzheimer's disease: A 2-[18F]fluoro-A-85380 PET study. Neurobiol Learn Mem 90:404–412
Ellis JR, Nathan PJ, Villemagne VL et al (2009) The relationship between nicotinic receptors and cognitive functioning in healthy aging: an in vivo positron emission tomography (PET) study with 2-[18F]fluoro-A-85380. Synapse 63:752–763
Endres CJ, Kolachana BS, Saunders RC, Su T, Weinberger D, Breier A, Eckelman WC, Carson RE (1997) Kinetic modeling of [11C]raclopride: combined PET-microdialysis studies. J Cereb Blood Flow Metab 17:932–942
Farde L, Hall H, Pauli S, Halldin C (1995) Variability in D2-dopamine receptor density and affinity: a PET study with [11C]Raclopride in Man. Synapse 20:200–208
Folino AF, Tokajuk B, Porta A et al (2005) Autonomic modulation and clinical outcome in patients with chronic heart failure. Int J Cardiol 100:247–251
Frenneaux MP (2004) Autonomic changes in patients with heart failure and in post-myocardial infarction patients. Heart 90:1248–1255
Gallezot JD, Bottlaender M, Grégoire MC et al (2005) In vivo imaging of human cerebral nicotinic acetylcholine receptors with 2-[18F]fluoro-A-85380 and PET. J Nucl Med 46:240–247
Gómez-Vallejo V, González-Esparza M, Llop J (2012) Facile and improved synthesis of [11C]Me-QNB. J Label Compds Radiopharm 55:470–473
Haga K, Kruse AC, Asada H et al (2012) Structure of the human M2 muscarinic acetylcholine receptor bound to an antagonist. Nature 482:547–551
Hang P, Zhao J, Qi J et al (2013) Novel insights into the pervasive role of M(3) muscarinic receptor in cardiac diseases. Curr Drug Targets 14:372–377
Hermosillo AG, Dorado M, Casanova MJ et al (1993) Influence of infarct-related artery patency on the indexes of parasympathetic activity and prevalence of late potentials in survivors of acute myocardial infarction. J Am Coll Cardiol 22:695–706
Horti A, Koren AO, Ravert HT et al (1998) Synthesis of a radiotracer for studying nicotinic acetylcholine receptors: 2-[18F]fluoro-3-(2(S)-azetidinylmethoxy)pyridine (2-[18F]A-85380). J Label Compds Radiopharm 41:309–318

Kas A, Bottlaender M, Gallezot JD et al (2009) In vivo decrease of nigrostriatal nicotinic receptors in Parkinson's disease: A PET study. J Cereb Blood Flow Metab 29:1601–1608

Katare RG, Ando M, Kakinuma Y et al (2009) Vagal nerve stimulation prevents reperfusion injury through inhibition of opening of mitochondrial permeability transition pore independent of the bradycardiac effect. J Thorac Cardiovasc Surg 137:223–231

Kawano H, Okada R, Yano K (2003) Histological study on the distribution of autonomic nerves in the human heart. Heart Vessels 18:32–39

Kleiger RE, Stein PK, Bigger JT Jr (2005) Heart rate variability: measurement and clinical utility. Ann Noninvasive Electrocardiol 10:88–101

La Rovere MT, Bigger JT Jr, Marcus FI et al (1998) Baroreflex sensitivity and heart-rate variability in prediction of total cardiac mortality after myocardial infarction. ATRAMI (Autonomic Tone and Reflexes After Myocardial Infarction) Investigators. Lancet 351:478–484

Le Guludec D, Delforge J, Syrota A et al (1994) In vivo quantification of myocardial muscarinic receptors in heart transplant patients. Circulation 90:172–178

Le Guludec D, Cohen-Solal A, Delforge J et al (1997) Increased myocardial muscarinic receptor density in idiopathic dilated cardiomyopathy: an in vivo PET study. Circulation 96:3416–3422

Liu N, Ding Y-S, Wang T et al (2002) Synthesis of 2-[18F]fluoro-3-[2(S)-2-azetidinylmethoxy] pyridine as a radioligand for imaging nicotinic acetylcholine receptors. Nucl Sci Tech 13:92–97

Mastitskaya S, Marina N, Gourine A et al (2013) Cardioprotection evoked by remote ischaemic preconditioning is critically dependent on the activity of vagal pre-ganglionic neurones. Cardiovasc Res 95:487–494

Mazière M, Berger G, Godot J-M et al (1983) C-11-Methiodide quinuclidinyl benzilate, a muscarinic antagonist for in vivo studies of myocardial muscarinic receptors. J Radioanal Chem 76:305–309

Mazzadi A, Pineau J, Costes N et al (2009) Muscarinic receptor upregulation in patients with myocardial infarction: a new paradigm. Circ Cardiovasc Imaging 2:365–372

Miao Y, Nichols SE, Gasper PM et al (2013) Activation and dynamic network of the M2 muscarinic receptor. Proc Natl Acad Sci U S A 110:10982–10987

Nenasheva TA, Neary M, Mashanov GI et al (2013) Abundance, distribution, mobility and oligomeric state of M2 muscarinic acetylcholine receptors in live cardiac muscle. J Mol Cell Cardiol 57:129–136

Nolan J, Flapan AD, Capwewell S et al (1992) Decreased cardiac parasympathetic activity in chronic heart failure and its relation to left ventricular function. Br Heart J 67:482–485

Ohte N, Narita H, Iida A et al (2012) Cardiac β-adrenergic receptor density and myocardial systolic function in the remote noninfarcted region after prior myocardial infarction with left ventricular remodelling. Eur J Nucl Med Mol Imaging 39:1246–1253

Olshansky B, Sabbah HN, Hauptman PJ et al (2008) Parasympathetic nervous system and heart failure: pathophysiology and potential implications for therapy. Circulation 118:863–871

Picard F, Bruel D, Servent D et al (2006) Alteration of the in vivo nicotinic receptor density in ADNFLE patients: a PET study. Brain 129:2047–2060

Roeda D, Kuhnast B, Hammadi A et al (2007) The Service Hospitalier Frédéric Joliot – contributions to PET chemistry over the years. J Label Compds Radiopharm 50:848–866

Santanam N, Thornhill BA, Lau JK et al (2012) Nicotinic acetylcholine receptor signaling in atherogenesis. Atherosclerosis 225:264–273

Schmaljohann J, Minnerop M, Karwath P et al (2004) Imaging of central nAChReceptors with 2-[18F]F-A85380: optimized synthesis and in vitro evaluation in Alzheimer's disease. Appl Radiat Isot 61:1235–1240

Schmaljohann J, Gündisch D, Minnerop M et al (2005) A simple and fast method for the preparation of n.c.a. 2-[18F]F-A85380 for human use. Appl Radiat Isot 63:433–435

Schmitz W, Boknik P, Linck B et al (1996) Adrenergic and muscarinic receptor regulation and therapeutic implications in heart failure. Mol Cell Biochem 157:251–258

Schwartz PJ, La Rovere MT, Vanoli E (1992) Autonomic nervous system and sudden cardiac death. Experimental basis and clinical observations for post-myocardial infarction risk stratification. Circulation 85:I77–I91

Stengel PW, Gomeza J, Wess J et al (2002) M2 and M4 receptor knockout mice: muscarinic receptor function in cardiac and smooth muscle in vitro. Pharmacol Exp Therap 292:877–885

Sullivan JP, Donnelly-Roberts DL, Briggs CA et al (1996) A-85380 [3-(2(S)-azetidinylmethoxy) pyridine]: In vitro pharmacological properties of a novel, high affinity α4β2 nicotinic acetylcholine receptors ligand. Neuropharmacology 35:725–734

Townend JN, Littler WA (1995) Cardiac vagal activity: a target for intervention in heart disease. Lancet 345:937–938

Valette H, Deleuze P, Syrota A et al (1995) Canine myocardial beta-adrenergic, muscarinic receptor densities after denervation: a PET study. J Nucl Med 36:140–146

Valette H, Syrota A, Fuseau C (1997) Down-regulation of cardiac muscarinic receptors induced by di-isopropylfluorophosphate. J Nucl Med 38:1430–1433

Valette H, Bottlaender M, Dollé F et al (2003) Long-lasting occupancy of central nicotinic acetylcholine receptors after smoking: a PET study in monkeys. J Neurochem 84:105–111

van Zwieten PA (1991) Adrenergic and muscarinergic receptors: classification, pathophysiological relevance and drug target. J Hypertens 9(Suppl):S18–S27

Vanoli E, Schwartz PJ (1990) Sympathetic–parasympathetic interaction and sudden death. Basic Res Cardiol 85(Suppl 1):305–321

Vatner DE, Lavallee M, Amano J, Finizola A, Homcy CJ, Vatner SF (1985) Mechanisms of supersensitivity to sympathomimetic amines in the chronically denervated heart of the conscious dog. Circ Res 57:55–64

Vatner DE, Sato N, Galper JB et al (1996) Physiological and biochemical evidence for coordinate increases in muscarinic receptors and Gi during pacing-induced heart failure. Circulation 94:102–107

Walker JL (1986) Intracellular inorganic ions in cardiac tissue. In: Fozzard H, Haber E, Jennings R, Katz AM, Morgan HE (eds) The heart and cardiovascular system, scientific foundations. Raven Press, New York

Zhao M, He X, Bi XY et al (2013) Vagal stimulation triggers peripheral vascular protection through the cholinergic anti-inflammatory pathway in a rat model of myocardial ischemia/reperfusion. Basic Res Cardiol 108:345

Tracer Application in Cardiovascular Imaging: A Triple Jump

7

F. Michelle de Roo, Koen Hilgerink, Jos G.W. Kosterink, Gert Luurtsema, Herman J. Woerdenbag, and Hendrikus H. Boersma

Contents

F.M. de Roo • K. Hilgerink • J.G.W. Kosterink
Department of Clinical Pharmacy and Pharmacology, University Medical Center Groningen, University of Groningen, 30.001, Groningen 9700 RB, The Netherlands

G. Luurtsema
Department of Nuclear Medicine and Molecular Imaging, University Medical Center Groningen, University of Groningen, 30.001, Groningen 9700 RB, The Netherlands

H.J. Woerdenbag
Department of Pharmaceutical Technology and Biopharmacy, University of Groningen, Groningen, The Netherlands

H.H. Boersma, PharmD, PhD (✉)
Department of Clinical Pharmacy and Pharmacology, University Medical Center Groningen, University of Groningen, 30.001, Groningen 9700 RB, The Netherlands

Department of Nuclear Medicine and Molecular Imaging, University Medical Center Groningen, University of Groningen, 30.001, Groningen 9700 RB, The Netherlands
e-mail: h.h.boersma@umcg.nl

R.H.J.A. Slart et al. (eds.), *Autonomic Innervation of the Heart: Role of Molecular Imaging*, DOI 10.1007/978-3-662-45074-1_7

Abstract

Next to aspects related to the imaging techniques, the quality of the used cardiovascular tracer is of major importance to produce reliable images, leading to accurate diagnoses as well as outcome of research and imaging-correlated treatment. We have built up this chapter on cardiovascular imaging according to the athletic triple jump. Hop, step, and jump are used as metaphors for three subsequent steps in the application of cardiovascular tracers. First, hop addresses general aspects as well as selection criteria of positron emission tomography (PET) and single-photon emission computed tomography (SPECT) tracers for cardiac innervation, myocardial perfusion, and heart failure. Second, step is focusing on the kind of translational as well as good manufacturing practice (GMP) activities needed to produce a clinical grade tracer. Third, jump, in which the relationship between clinical implementation of a radiopharmaceutical and quality management and good clinical practice (GCP) is presented.

Abbreviations

BET	Bacterial endotoxin tests
CAD	Coronary artery disease
cGRPP	Guidelines on current good radiopharmacy practice
COMT	Catechol-O-methyltransferase
EMA	European Medicine Agency
FDA	Food and Drug Administration
GCP	Good clinical practice
GDP	Good distribution practice
GMP	Good manufacturing practice
GRPP	Guidelines on good radiopharmacy practice
HF	Heart failure
IEC	Independent ethics committee
IMP	Investigational medicinal product
IMPD	Investigational medicinal product dossier
MA	Marketing authorization
MAO	Monoamine oxidase
MPI	Myocardial perfusion imaging
MTD	Maximum tolerated dose

NOAEL No-adverse-effect level
PET Positron emission tomography
QA Quality assurance unit
QC Quality control
QP Qualified person
SOP Standard operating procedures
SPECT Single-photon emission computed tomography
SSRP Small-scale radiopharmaceuticals

7.1 Introduction

The current chapter is dedicated to the translation of cardiovascular imaging tracers towards clinical use. It is divided into three parts, according to the three stages (hop, step, jump) of the athletic triple jump. Starting with "Hop," a description of imaging tracers, their selection, development, and validation of cardiovascular tracers is given. Second, the section "Step" describes what kind of regulatory procedures (GMP, toxicology) are needed for the clinical development of the tracer. Finally "Jump" shows how the performance of clinical trials with cardiovascular tracers (first in man and beyond) can take place.

7.2 Hop: Cardiovascular Tracer Selection and Validation

7.2.1 Tracer Selection

For the development of novel tracer molecules in general and cardiovascular imaging pharmaceuticals in particular, the importance of property-directed selection cannot be underestimated. In general, one should look at following features in order to enable feasible tracer design (Elsinga and Dierckx 2014):

- Labeling suitability, design of the molecule, and choice of radionuclide.
- Depending on the interaction between these processes and the involved kinetics of the tracer, the ideal isotope should be found which combines both chemical properties as well as the optimal radionuclide half-life to ensure favorable imaging results.
- Lipophilicity. To avoid too much aspecific binding, the lipophilicity of a molecule should be not too high. Furthermore, there are some exemptions concerning aspecific binding and its relation with lipophilicity. More research is required to further decrease aspecific binding, in order to optimize imaging properties of tracers in general. For cardiovascular tracers overall, their lipophilicity should be low. The latter is correlated to a water/octanol partition coefficient <1. For brain studies, however, a minimum amount of lipophilicity is needed to enable the molecule passing the blood-brain barrier.

- Target binding properties. When the target of a radiopharmaceutical is receptor based, its affinity for the receptor should be high, especially when the receptors are available at low concentrations. Regularly, affinities in the nanomolar range are needed to detect receptors and proteins in an accurate way. For instance, when the density of the target receptor population is low, the affinity of the investigated tracer should be high enough to enable imaging.
- Target binding specificity. It is essential to select a tracer with optimal specificity. In some cases, this may not lead to a very selective tracer, but rather to tracers, which are able to detect an optimal amount of targets for the intended purpose.

7.2.1.1 Selectivity Essentials for Cardiovascular Tracers

Regarding flow tracers, it is essential that hydrophilic molecules are used and isotopes with a very short physical half-life. For receptor-targeted cardiovascular tracers, it must be stressed that the compounds should be generally highly selective for a certain class of receptors, but maybe not too selective to enable adequate imaging quality, e.g., for cardiac innervation imaging.

When implementing transporter substrate tracers, one should be aware that this tracer should have the ability to accumulate in the target tissue. The latter means that the tracer-specific activity can be lower than for the receptor-based tracers (Elsinga and Dierckx 2014). An overview on the available cardiovascular tracers is given in Table 7.1, and a description of these compounds is given in Sect. 7.2.2.

7.2.1.2 Tracer Development Toward Clinical Use

To develop a tracer towards clinical use, often many derivatives of a compound are involved, especially for receptor-targeted tracers, but also for substrate-based tracers. When a lead compound is selected in silico, the compound and some of its nearly related derivates are tested first in vitro and thereafter in vivo using appropriate animal models. When the proof of concept is established, both by binding studies using, e.g., blockers to proof that the tracers reaches the intended target, as well

Table 7.1 Tracers for cardiology applied in humans

Name	Target	Category
[^{13}N]NH3	Perfusion	Flow tracer
[^{15}O]-water	Perfusion	Flow tracer
[^{18}F]-flurpiridaz	Perfusion	Enzyme inhibitor
[^{82}Rb]-rubidiumchloride	Perfusion	Flow tracer
[^{11}C]-CGP-12177	Beta-adrenoceptor	Receptor antagonist
[^{11}C]-CGP-12388	Beta-adrenoceptor	Receptor antagonist
[^{11}C]-MQNB	Muscarinic receptor	Receptor antagonist
[^{11}C]-mHED	Presynaptic NE transport	Transporter substrate
[^{11}C]-palmitate	Fatty acid metabolism	Enzyme substrate
[^{11}C]-acetate	Oxidative metabolism	Enzyme substrate

Adapted from Elsinga and Dierckx (2014)

as by in vivo studies to show that imaging using the new potential radiopharmaceutical is feasible (Elsinga and Dierckx 2014). When both goals are achieved, the tracer can be developed further as a radiopharmaceutical (see Sect. 7.2.6 and onwards). Several animal models can be used for investigation of, e.g., receptor binding properties, as well as perfusion imaging. First, the Langendorf model, exploring a rodent heart for ex vivo perfusion as well as receptor binding/transporter substrate effects can be used for initial suitability testing of novel tracers (Hillman et al. 2014). Second, when ex vivo heart models like these demonstrate the feasibility of the investigated tracer, more complex and sophisticated models can be used for a pilot study, e.g., investigating effects on perfusion and/or innervation using the same tracers, eventually using both a perfusion as well as an innervation tracer. Suitable animal models are mimicking heart failure by induction of blood pressure overload, as caused by aortic constriction in, for instance, murine animal models (Mühlfeld et al. 2013).

7.2.2 Cardiac Innervation Imaging: An Overview on Currently Available Radiopharmaceuticals

The cardiac nervous system in humans is innervated by sympathetic and parasympathetic nerve systems. The main neurotransmitters responsible for this innervation are norepinephrine and acetylcholine. It is known that alterations of this innervation system can lead to various heart diseases, such as arrhythmias and heart failure (Bengel and Schwaiger 2004). Therefore, visualizing innervation of the heart may be an option for diagnosing heart diseases in an early stage. Available tracers for the sympathetic neurons can be divided into two groups, radiolabeled catecholamines and radiolabeled catecholamine analogues. The latter group is resistant to biotransformation by monoamine oxidase (MAO) and catechol-O-methyltransferase (COMT). Differences between the available tracers include their affinity and specificity for uptake-1 (a transport system allowing reuptake into nerve terminals) and the storage of the tracer in vesicles. A limited number of tracers, e.g., [^{123}I]-*N*-methyl-4-iododexetimide, are available for the mapping of parasympathetic neurons, because of the low density of these neurons in the myocardium and the high specificity for acetylcholine in the uptake and storage system (Bengel and Schwaiger 2004; Langer and Halldin 2002; Kassiou et al. 1996).

7.2.3 [^{123}I]-metaiodobenzylguanidine

The most frequently used radiopharmaceutical for visualization of the sympathetic system is [^{123}I]-metaiodobenzylguanidine ([^{123}I]-MIBG), in combination with single-photon emission computed tomography (SPECT) imaging. By processing the patient images obtained after injection of the tracer, it is possible to calculate a heart-to-mediastinum ratio, which is used as an estimation of the uptake of catecholamine throughout the heart (Boersma et al. 2002; Weiland et al. 2010). In addition, the sympathetic tonus can be reflected by measuring the ratio of cardiac uptake between early and delayed images. The latter is also called the washout rate (Bengel and Schwaiger 2004; Bengel 2011). The washout rate and the heart-to-mediastinum ratio indicate norepinephrine release and uptake from and into the nerve terminal. Therefore, [^{123}I]-MIBG is a commonly used tracer for the assessment of sympathetic innervation of the heart in heart failure (Tamaki and Yoshinaga 2011).

7.2.4 [^{11}C]-metahydroxyephedrine

The most frequently used tracer when mapping sympathetic neurons with positron emission tomography (PET) is carbon-11-metahydroxyephedrine (mHED). mHED is a catecholamine analogue and therefore not metabolized by MAO or COMT. It can be produced with sufficiently high specific activity to avoid measurable physiologic effects, and it has low nonspecific binding. When reuptake of the neurotransmitters into the nerve terminals in isolated perfused rat hearts is blocked with desipramine, mHED shows an accelerated washout, indicating that the norepinephrine transporter is responsible for this reuptake. This is also proven by the accelerated washout of mHED when norepinephrine is added to the perfusate. Because of the increased washout in these situations, it is believed that mHED is released from and transported back into sympathetic neurons continually. In contrast with [^{123}I]-MIBG, which has lower uptake in the inferior myocardium, mHED has homogeneous high uptake in the left ventricle throughout all myocardial segments (Bengel and Schwaiger 2004).

7.2.5 Perfusion and Viability Tracers

Perfusion tracers are used to depict myocardial blood flow and are a tool to determine myocardial cell viability. Myocardial perfusion imaging tracers are regularly radiolabeled molecules which are (partially) entrapped within the cardiomyocyte (Candell-Riera et al. 2009; Di Carli et al. 2007). With this nuclear medicine procedure, it is possible to illustrate the function of the heart muscle. This enables the evaluation of several heart conditions from coronary artery disease (CAD) to hypertrophic cardiomyopathy and abnormalities in the motion (using gated PET) of the myocardial wall.

PET myocardial perfusion imaging (MPI) is a very accurate technique in making prognoses in patients with suspected or known CAD. MPI has an average sensitivity and specificity of around 90 % for detection of angiographically significant CAD. PET MPI has proven to be useful as the initial test for detection as well as the extent and location of myocardial ischemia. Imaging with SPECT and PET can be used for detecting obstructive CAD and/or to estimate viability of the myocard. Identifying ischemia in patients with heart failure (HF) is an important step for evaluation and renders prognostic information. According to Canadian HF guidelines, it is recommended to use radionuclide perfusion imaging, SPECT most commonly, for evaluating the presence of infarction, ischemia, and/or viability. The most commonly used and available SPECT tracers are [^{201}Tl], [^{99m}Tc]-tetrofosmin, and [^{99m}Tc]-sestamibi (Paterson et al. 2013).

Comparing PET with SPECT, PET imaging has shown to be a more comprehensive functional and anatomical assessment of the cardiovascular system. For instance, PET has better spatial resolution, higher sensitivity, and ability to measure distribution of tracers in absolute terms as a function of time (Anagnostopoulos et al. 2013).

The most common positron-emitting radiopharmaceuticals for cardiac perfusion imaging are rubidium-82 [^{82}Rb], [^{13}N]NH3, and oxygen-labeled water ([^{15}O]-water). Among these tracers, the most widely used in clinical practice are [^{82}Rb] and [^{13}N]NH3 (Anagnostopoulos et al. 2013).

All three PET tracers have short half-lives (<10 min), making it possible to repeatedly measure at stress and rest. Another major property of current perfusion tracers is they have a high first-pass extraction fraction at different flow rates. Lower extraction occurs at high flow rates, leading to a decrease in accuracy of ischemia detection, representing an error source of underestimation (Rischpler et al. 2012). PET imaging is able to quantify myocardial blood flow and flow reserve. This results in better assessment of the functional importance of CAD in HF. Diagnostic accuracy for PET to detect significant CAD is much higher than SPECT (sensitivity 91 % and specificity 91 %). [^{18}F]-FDG PET imaging is considered one of the gold standards for viability imaging. It has a high accuracy for predicting functional recovery, with a sensitivity of 85–90% (Paterson et al. 2013).

7.2.6 Product Development

Good manufacturing practice (GMP) comprises a defined set of regulations, defining all requirements needed for the correct development and manufacture of a medicinal product under adequately controlled circumstances. According to GMP, new medicinal products need to be thoroughly tested, evaluated and released before it is allowed to administer them to humans (EU-GMP-website).

In most cases, such new medicinal product is classified as an investigational medicinal product (IMP) and is tested during a controlled clinical trial. Then, an ethics committee is involved to review and approve the clinical trial procedure and to ensure the safety of the participating subjects (see Sect. 7.4).

When designing a new radiopharmaceutical, first of all the chemical synthesis of the compound needs to be robust, safe, and reproducible. Furthermore, there is a need to have an accurate quality control (QC) method to warrant correct QC results and thus appropriate release of the tracer before administration (EU-GMP-website, annex 13).

Moreover, the produced radiochemical should be transformed into a radiopharmaceutical. This process is called formulation. Usually, formulation is executed by dilution of the radiochemical dissolved in, for instance, ethanol using water for injections. This, and all requirements sustaining good quality of the radiopharmaceutical, will be discussed in the upcoming paragraphs.

7.3 Step: What Is Needed to Ensure the Clinical Application of a Tracer?

7.3.1 Animal Toxicity Testing

In order to study the toxicity of a newly developed radiopharmaceutical, the biodistribution of the tracer in animals (rodents and non-rodents) has to be investigated. To ensure the efficacious performance of animal experiments, a risk assessment can help to determine the extent of animal studies needed. The biodistribution studies include measurement of plasma levels of the tracer as well as its uptake in different tissues, such as the kidneys or the liver, and the elimination route. Also, the stability of the tracer in the animal plasma has to be determined. Furthermore, it should be investigated which metabolites are formed as well as their excretion via the kidneys and/or gut.

In order to study the acute toxicity of the tracer, it has to be administered in single intravenous doses at different concentrations on day 1 and followed by observation of the animals for 7 days. During this period, it is studied whether there are any clinical signs that might point to toxicity such as changes in body weight, respiratory function, food consumption, eye toxicity, and after termination of the animal: clinical pathology, organ weight, and/or macroscopic/microscopic organ picture. These tests result in the determination of a no-adverse-effect level (NOAEL) and a maximum tolerated dose (MTD). For low-dose radiopharmaceuticals (<100 μg of tested substance in human volunteers), a microdosing approach can be used for toxicity testing, which comprises of single dose toxicity testing at a 1,000-fold dose (ICH M3-website).

7.3.2 Introduction into Good Manufacturing Practice (GMP)

GMP is a quality assurance system which is applied in the pharmaceutical industry. Quality assurance is applied because it is impossible to analyze every (bio)chemical or physical aspect of all pharmaceutical products used before release of a tracer. Because the product quality is the core issue for pharmaceuticals to ensure their efficacy and safety, GMP should be used at every stage of the product life cycle: from the manufacturing of investigational medicinal products, technology transfer, commercial manufacturing to product discontinuation. For pharmaceutical products manufactured by the holder of a manufacturing license, it must be ensured they are fit to their intended use. Authorization for manufacturing is required for all pharmaceutical manufacturers in the European Union, whether the products are sold or used within or outside of the Union, or not.

The final pharmaceutical product must also comply with the requirements of a marketing authorization or an investigational medicinal product dossier (IMPD), and, when applicable, a clinical trial authorization, and does not place patients at an unexpected risk due to inadequate quality or efficacy (EU-GMP-website).

As stated above, GMP ensures that products are consistently produced and controlled to the quality standards appropriate to their intended use and as required by the marketing authorization (MA), clinical trial authorization, or product specification. Both production and quality control are part of GMP. EMA (European Medicine Agency) and FDA (Food and Drug Administration) are the respective regulators in the EU and the USA. These bodies ensure the quality maintenance of all licensed pharmaceuticals. Furthermore, the FDA serves as a pharmaceutical inspectorate as well. Within the EU, inspectors are organized at a national level for each member state.

The basic requirements of GMP are as described below:

1. All manufacturing processes are clearly defined, systematically reviewed in the light of experience and shown to be capable of consistently manufacturing medicinal products of the required quality and complying with their specifications.
2. All necessary facilities for GMP are provided, including:
    - Appropriately qualified and trained personnel
    - Adequate premises and space
    - Suitable equipment and services
    - Correct materials, containers, and labels
    - Approved procedures and instructions, in accordance with the pharmaceutical quality system
    - Suitable storage and transport
3. Instructions and procedures are written in an instructional form in clear and unambiguous language, specifically applicable to the facilities provided.
4. Procedures are carried out correctly, and operators are trained to do so.
5. Records are made, manually and/or by recording instruments, throughout the manufacturing process, to demonstrate that all the steps required by the defined procedures and instructions were in fact taken and that the quantity and quality of the product was as expected.
6. Every change in critical processes is recorded and appropriately validated according to an authorized change control procedure.
7. Any significant deviations are fully recorded, investigated with the objective of determining the root cause and appropriate corrective and preventive action implemented.
8. Records of manufacture, including distribution (which enables to trace the complete history of a batch), are retained in a comprehensible and accessible form.
9. The distribution of the products minimizes any risk to their quality and is performed in accordance with the guidelines concerning good distribution practice (GDP).
10. A system is available to recall any batch of product, from sale or supply.
11. Complaints about products are examined, the causes of quality defects investigated, and appropriate measures taken in respect of the defective products and to prevent reoccurrence (EU-GMP-website).

7.3.2.1 GMP Essentials for Radiopharmaceuticals

The preparation and use of radiopharmaceuticals are regulated by defined EU or FDA guidelines and rules. Within the EU-GMP, annex 3 defines how production of radiopharmaceuticals should take place. Guidelines, such as the EU-GMP intended for the production of medicinal products, should also be used, but it must be taken into consideration that some regulations do not cover special characteristics of radiopharmaceuticals, such as:

- Short shelf life, due to short physical half-life radionuclide
- Small-scale preparations; these are defined as preparations resulting in <25 patient doses. This is typical for radiopharmaceutical production in a hospital
- Low or absent toxicity of final product, due to particular no-carrier-added nature of radiopharmaceuticals or a low dose to be administered to each patient
- Nuclear energy laws regulating some aspects of production requirements, such as protection of the involved staff, which are not covered by GMP

For the production of radiopharmaceuticals, the "guidelines on good radiopharmacy practice (GRPP)" and "guidelines on current good radiopharmacy practice (cGRPP) for the small-scale preparation of radiopharmaceuticals" were developed. These can be used for small-scale preparations at nonindustrial sites such as hospital pharmacies, nuclear medicine departments, and PET centers (Elsinga et al. 2010). Notwithstanding the application of cGRPP, the guidance of, for instance, of EU-GMP annex 3 on radiopharmaceutical production and annex 1 on sterile manufacturing, is currently regarded as mandatory in EU member states. Although national inspectorates will have different interpretations of these rules in their respective countries, most countries in the western world as well as many other states regard radiopharmaceuticals as regular medicinal products up until now (EU-GMP-website). However, in April 2014, the European Parliament has accepted new regulations towards production of radiopharmaceuticals (Anonymous 2014, Publication of the EU-parliament). These will be operational from 2015 onwards. One very important aspect is that for clinical trial use within a specific member state, a GMP license is no longer required. This may implicate that cGRPP will become more important as standard guidance for radiopharmaceutical production within the EU. Nevertheless, this does not mean that the quality of radiopharmaceutical products for clinical trial use should be less well defined after 2015. Furthermore, the policies of inspectorates upon licensed and clinically used radiopharmaceuticals are expected to remain unchanged.

In the USA, the situation is different compared to the EU. As of December 2011, the US legislation on production of radiopharmaceuticals has been amended. In the current situation, each production site for radiopharmaceuticals needs to have a limited license (abbreviated new drug application) for each PET radiopharmaceutical. Furthermore, GMP regulations on PET drugs are given in Chapter <823> of the 32nd Edition of the US Pharmacopeia. Other radiopharmaceuticals need to be licensed or defined as new chemical entity to be part of a clinical trial. However, the

FDA recognizes that many PET tracers have no commercial value and therefore enforces less strict rules compared to otherwise classified pharmaceuticals (FDA-Guidance PET Drugs 2011).

Moreover, when using new radiopharmaceuticals in clinical trials, cGRPP, and the guidelines on good clinical practice should be followed in addition to GMP, and cGRPP guidelines have a main focus on small-scale radiopharmaceuticals (SSRP). In contrast to GMP, cGRPP also applies for the labeling procedures of licensed kit radiopharmaceuticals.

The guidelines on cGRPP and GMP for positron emission tomography (PET) and other locally prepared radiopharmaceuticals are summarized below (Elsinga et al. 2010; EU-GMP-website).

Personnel and Resources

When working with radiopharmaceuticals, personnel needs to be trained in order to acquire necessary practical education, training, regulatory knowledge, and experience with the resources. Furthermore, the entire staff should be trained on the quality control system. Main focus of the training should be on the aseptic techniques of personnel throughout the handling of radiopharmaceuticals for injection. Another primarily important focus is on radiation protection. The extent of radiation exposure should be checked regularly with approved personal dosimeters (Anonymous 2007, cGRPP). Furthermore, extensive training in dealing with accidents is required for the proper maintenance of each radiopharmacy.

For the preparation of small-scale radiopharmaceuticals under a GMP license, there should be at least a qualified person (QP). Furthermore, a responsible person could have most leading tasks related to production and release of radiopharmaceuticals (Elsinga et al. 2010). In the USA, the role of the responsible pharmacist is similar to that of the qualified person in the EU.

Under EU regulations, the QP generally is a licensed pharmacist or educated as biologist or chemist. It is compulsory that the QP has several years of experience working in pharmaceutical manufacturing operations and has knowledge about the specific processes and products to be released. The responsible person has an equivalent academic background to a QP, having at least 2 years practical experience in radiopharmaceutical preparation (Elsinga et al. 2010; EU-GMP-website).

Responsibilities

Depending on the scale of production, the final responsibilities for production and QC may rest with the responsible person, as in the case of small facilities. In general, most sites will work with dedicated staff to perform production and dedicated staff to perform QC.

One of the main responsibilities of the responsible person is reviewing the preparation batch records and records of laboratory control for accuracy and conformance to established specifications. In the EU, the QP is responsible for the final release of an under GMP produced radiopharmaceutical. Licensed kits can be prepared and released under hospital conditions by a pharmacist. In the USA, the latter task is performed by the responsible pharmacist.

Furthermore, in most cases, the QP in cooperation with the responsible person is held responsible for the approval of procedures, specifications, processes, and methods including related SOPs (standard operating procedures).

Quality Assurance

For a radiopharmacy division, mostly operating as a subsection of a nuclear medicine department, it is recommended to establish a quality assurance unit (QA), in order to design and implement a QA system correctly. It is recommended to incorporate the principles of GMP as well as current good radiopharmacy practice (cGRPP) and to consider appropriate risks to justify all items which may differ from standard regulations (Elsinga et al. 2010; EU-GMP-website). The person responsible for QA bears the responsibility to verify if all documentation is written and administrated correctly and to conduct periodic audits. Furthermore, it should be stressed that, although GMP-production of radiopharmaceuticals can be a very fast process, all deviations are to be covered based on predefined risk assessments. The role of QA in defining the risk stratification is essential.

Equipment and Facilities

When working with radiopharmaceuticals, the facilities should be adequate to ensure prevention of cross contamination and mix-up of materials and equipment. In addition, only authorized personnel should have access to work areas and approval for working with open radioactive sources within the room is needed. Spread of radioactivity from controlled areas should be prevented by taking appropriate measures, such as the use of hot cells (see Fig. 7.1). For sterile radiopharmaceuticals, the working area should be provided with a laminar flow workstation delivering HEPA-filtered grade A air. The microbiological quality of workstations and environment should be monitored frequently. The surfaces within the working area should be easy to clean or decontaminate in case of radioactive spill. Sinks for cleaning should be located outside the preparation area (Anonymous 2007, cGRPP).

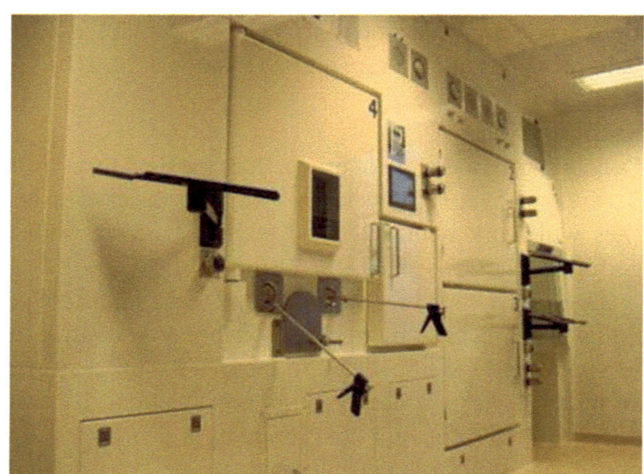

Fig. 7.1 Example of a GMP-clean room for the production of PET radiopharmaceuticals

Nuclear energy laws give guidance to waste management. The latter will not be discussed in this chapter, but it must be stressed that adequate waste management is essential for the effective operation of each radiopharmaceutical production site.

Equipment must be suitable and qualified for its intended purposes. It therefore should be installed and maintained properly and produce valid results (Elsinga et al. 2010).

According to GMP, adequate validation procedures as well as a validation master plan are required. See annex 15 of the EU-GMP for more information (EU-GMP-website).

Furthermore, the QA or QC section is responsible for putting up a system of planned preventive maintenance and calibration of all GMP critical equipment, in order to ensure all equipment for the preparation of radiopharmaceuticals operates accordingly. To ensure this, it is required to keep records and logbooks of performed maintenance and calibration (Anonymous 2007, cGRPP; EU-GMP-website).

When preparing radiopharmaceuticals a variety of equipment is needed, "production equipment" and "quality control equipment" (see Fig. 7.2). Table 7.2 lists all equipment predominantly used for the production and QC of radiopharmaceuticals.

For small-scale radiopharmacies, one room can be used for more than one purpose. With increasing complexity, more measures should be taken to avoid

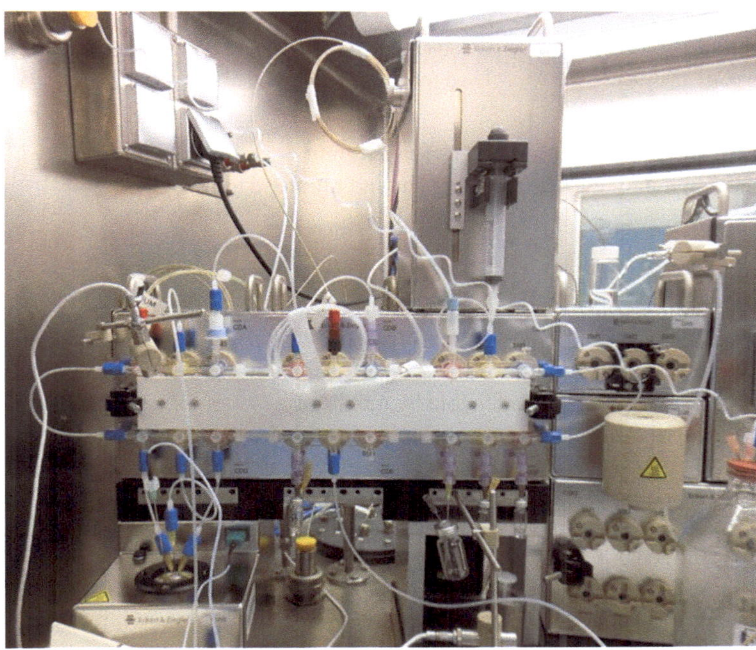

Fig. 7.2 Example of a GMP synthesis module for PET radiopharmaceuticals

Table 7.2 Equipment used for the production and QC of radiopharmaceuticals

Item	Definition
Hot cells	Hot cells are qualified (grades A, B, or C) boxes shielded with lead bricks or lead layers of suitable thickness. Hot cell airtightness and the radiation monitor should be monitored as part of the maintenance. Both for radiation safety reasons and product quality, production of radiopharmaceuticals using high amounts of radiation will take place in hot cells with an appropriate air classification
Analytical weight balance	Precision instrument used for the very accurate measurement of (small) masses. Their use for the preparation of radiopharmaceuticals as well as tracers is essential
Monitoring systems	Temperature, pressure, and humidity of clean rooms, dry heat oven, refrigerator, freezer, and incubator should be recorded. For this automated recording, devices and software can be used
Radiopharmaceutical dispensing systems	Dispensing systems, e.g., located in hot cells can be used to fill all needed syringes before administration to the patients
Modules for radiopharmaceutical production (mainly used for the production of PET tracers)	These modules can be either dedicated to the production of one radiopharmaceutical, or multipurpose modules for the production of several radiopharmaceuticals
Gas chromatography equipment	QC assay equipment
HPLC/UPLC equipment	QC assay equipment
Dose calibrator	Precision instrument used for the accurate measurement of an amount of radiation
Chromatogram scanner	QC assay equipment
Multichannel analyzer	Used for the determination of radiochemical purity

mixing-up and contamination. Areas for different operations should clearly be identified and separated, avoiding mixing-up and unintended use.

Documentation

Quality assurance consists of a documentation system, including different authorized documents such as standard operating procedures (SOP) and records in relevance to any step in the process of radiopharmaceutical preparation. This is in order to ensure that each preparation will be traceable by means of a system of documentation, starting from prescription to the administration of the individual patient doses.

According to GMP, written records should be archived for at least 15 years. However, archiving time may vary between countries according to their own regulations, and as well for other reasons than GMP, such as government archiving laws (Elsinga et al. 2010; EU-GMP-website).

Production and Process Controls

Documenting any deviation from production protocols is necessary to identify trends and to ensure that corrective or preventive action will take place. It is advisable to maintain a deviation system and a change control system. Within this system, all deviant items should be described which are regarded to GMP critical. Furthermore, all correction to the event and preventive actions to ensure reoccurrence is less likely than in the past. A change control system enables documentation of all prospective GMP critical changes in order to assure that these are implemented in an appropriate way (EU-GMP-website).

All relevant production environment parameters like air pressure parameters, room temperatures, and radioactive levels should be monitored, to ensure that all materials are controlled before other necessary tests or verification have been completed. For microbial control, the bioburden of all starting materials should be kept as low as possible. The latter can be achieved by using as much as possible presterilized starting materials. Furthermore, a grade A LAF-hood is preferable as a working environment for the aseptical assembly of, e.g., nonradioactive synthesizer modules.

Most "in-house" manufactured radiopharmaceuticals are passed through a 0.22 μm filter under aseptic circumstances before administration to patient. The used filters must demonstrate compatibility with the products for which they are applied. The membrane filter should be tested for integrity after filtration to ensure that the filter has performed adequately according to its specifications. Even autoclaving a radiopharmaceutical may be an option when chemical stability of the tracer allows this, and the isotope half-life is long enough (>2 h), and the amount of radioactivity produced for the respective batch is large enough to make terminal heat sterilization feasible (Elsinga et al. 2010; EU-GMP-website).

Laboratory Controls

Requirements for laboratory controls by QC of the radiopharmaceutical include information about stability and physical/chemical properties. QC should make use of SOPs for each test as well as for documenting results. It should be assured that starting materials and other components comply with the required quality criteria. Proper labeling is desired to show identity and composition of starting materials and reagents, solutions, and supplies used for testing.

The methods used for testing materials should be validated to prove that they are sensitive, specific, accurate, and reproducible. Furthermore, it is required to keep complete records of all tests, ensuring compliance with previously established specifications.

Any deviation from procedures or specifications should be written down and justified. These deviations should be investigated and documented afterwards. After analysis of materials, results of the tests should be reviewed by QC and released by a designated person responsible for QC (Elsinga et al. 2010; EU-GMP-website).

Starting Materials

For controlling the starting materials, several procedures should be followed, including selection and auditing of vendors, checking receipts of materials, and the release of materials.

It is preferable that only qualified vendors should be used for supplying materials. However, for radiopharmaceuticals, it is not always possible to qualify each supplier at the same level. It has been shown that especially the large suppliers of not-for human use substances are difficult to approach in order to receive a filled out supplier questionnaire. Nevertheless, sometimes starting materials from this kind of companies are needed. In order to be qualified, vendors should show evidence to support their ability to supply materials meeting all quality specifications. Based on a physical or paper audit of the supplier, the vendor can be qualified. The qualification procedure and results should be documented.

All GMP-critical incoming starting materials should be assessed before use and released by a QP or responsible person. When the material meets the specifications, it can be released and used for the intended purpose. Release of materials should be documented, and documents of testing and examination data should also be maintained. When materials are approved, they should be labeled with "Released," when rejected with the label "Rejected." After rejection, materials should be disposed of properly, and these actions should be taken up in records. Released materials should be stored according to the previously defined and documented conditions (Elsinga et al. 2010; EU-GMP-website).

Validation Master Plan

All processes regarding production and analysis of radiopharmaceuticals should be validated. Validation policies are described in the validation master plan (EU-GMP-website, annex 15). When a small-scale radiopharmacy has a history of radiopharmaceutical preparation, validation processes may be carried out using historical batch records. Some of the positron-emitting radionuclides have a short half-life. When validating the process, it should be taken into consideration that the radiopharmaceutical should be released before all QC tests are done. Furthermore, it is recommended that validation includes a careful risk assessment. This is in order to show that the used methods are robust and reliable to justify the pre-release of the radiopharmaceutical. This means that the release will be done before finishing all tests. These actions should be documented and approved by the QP and/or responsible person (Elsinga et al. 2010; EU-GMP-website).

Finished Product Controls

Before a radiopharmaceutical is released, it should be tested to ensure that it meets all predefined acceptance criteria. The acceptance criteria for the analytical methods applied should meet with the criteria defined in monographs of the European Pharmacopoeia or another recognized pharmacopeia (United States Pharmacopeia, Japanese Pharmacopeia). When specific monographs are not available, it is necessary to validate the used analytical methods. For radiopharmaceuticals such as [^{13}N]NH3, which have a short half-life, it is possible to produce several batches on the same day. If a batch of a radiopharmaceutical does not meet the acceptance criteria, it might be reprocessed in this case. However, this is only allowed when the accurate production and process control procedures are followed, to ensure that the finished product complies with the specifications before finally releasing the product. The overall of this procedure should be documented including all conditions in a report describing the deviation. An example of reprocessing could be removing an impurity by passing through a purification column for the second time. Another example is to let it pass through another filter, when the original filter has failed to meet criteria of the integrity test (Elsinga et al. 2010; EU-GMP-website).

Certain radiopharmaceuticals ([^{11}C]- and [^{13}N]-based compounds) may have extremely short shelf lives, due to inherent short half-life of radionuclide, when compared to other drug products. Radiation-related radiolysis may affect the stability of radiopharmaceuticals allowing rapid chemical changes of the compound. Because of these effects, it is needed to evaluate appropriate parameters to ensure and to document the stability under the suggested storage conditions. The radiochemical identity and purity, appearance, and pH are examples of the stability parameters that can be evaluated. Appropriate stability indicating methods should be operational in order to evaluate the stability in a proper manner and to show any signs of degradation and impurities. It is recommended to test the stability of a radiopharmaceutical at the highest radioactive concentration, taking into consideration that the expiry time of a radiopharmaceutical could be altered after adequate testing (Elsinga et al. 2010; EU-GMP-website).

Small-scale radiopharmacies should use appropriate reference standards, when analyzing final products, as identified in the used analytical procedure, SOP or as described in a pharmacopoeia. When small-scale radiopharmacies have established in-house reference standards, data confirming material purity and identity should be established and documented. The supplier of the raw material may also provide data that prove the identity and purity of the reference, for example, in the form of reference spectra (Elsinga et al. 2010; EU-GMP-website).

Testing the sterility of the final product should be conducted as soon as possible after completing the production. It is preferred that a licensed laboratory carries out the test on sterility of the products, using aseptic conditions and techniques, as well as standards complying with the standards of the European Pharmacopoeia (Elsinga et al. 2010; EU-GMP-website).

Sterile radiopharmaceuticals, which are intended for injection, should be tested for the absence of bacterial endotoxins. To measure endotoxins, gel-clot or rapid photometric methods can be used, as described by the European Pharmacopoeia. It is required that results of endotoxin tests comply with the prospectively defined acceptance criteria, before human administration of the product has taken place. However, for radiopharmaceuticals, this is not always feasible due to the limited half-life. Therefore, endotoxin tests should be part of each validation program.

When results of a bacterial endotoxin tests (BET) do not meet the acceptance criteria, a deviation is to be written, and a complete investigation should take place as soon as possible (Elsinga et al. 2010; EU-GMP-website, European Pharmacopoeia, Edition 8.0).

Labeling and Packaging

Labels for products and containers are ideally generated using a computerized system. Most of the labels will be prepared in advance. The QP will conduct a final check to ensure that labels affixed on the container and shield are filled out correctly and completely (Elsinga et al. 2010; EU-GMP-website).

Internal Audits

It is required to have an internal inspection conducted by QA frequently, e.g., every month, to monitor compliance with the QA system. At least two persons from QA should perform an internal audit. When the audit reveals any failures, this should be documented along with appropriate measures to correct them and prevent them from occurring again in the future. Records of all inspections have to be documented and filed (Elsinga et al. 2010; EU-GMP-website).

Records

All records, such as test results and inspection data, should be stored at a location that is accessible and available for further inspection (internal as well as external inspection). It is also allowed to store data electronically, but only when appropriate measurements have been taken regarding protection and backup strategies. It is required to store records for at least 15 years according to EU-GMP as well as according to patient care regulations. However, the length of storage may vary between countries, regions, or states (Elsinga et al. 2010; EU-GMP-website).

7.3.3 Reflection on GMP: What's in It for Us?

Considering all care taken for both safety of the product and safety of personnel, many questions can be raised about the number of measurements in relation to costs and burden to the organization. The first question of many people concerns the burden and the overkill. GMP is often seen as a "paper monster" which only causes burden to the organization and does not add to the safety of the final product.

Of course, it is not the intention of GMP to add more paper than is strictly necessary. The latter is to be assessed with the radiopharmacy organization. GMP aims not only to ensure quality and safety of a product but can be regarded as an awareness creating system. GMP creates awareness for the following situations:

- GMP demands the registration of all deviations. This creates a proper overview on the GMP-related white spots in the organization.
- As all deviations are documented, awareness is increased regarding prevention of a documented event. During the implementation of a deviation system, it is evident that the organization follows a learning curve. Retrospectively, staff members will notice that the issues of concern, about which they were initially unaware, become less abundant over time.
- Deviations exemplify that technical maintenance of the facility is a critical cornerstone in operating a radiopharmacy. It is not only an important source of deviations but also the basis for prevention of such events. Having an accurate SOP on technical maintenance, many pitfalls turn out to be preventable. Unfortunately, it is impossible to give a clear description of a technical maintenance SOP, as the contents may show great variation, depending on the organization.

Another aspect to which GMP may contribute to a large extent is the cooperation with the pharmaceutical industry. Many radiopharmacies and sometimes even pharmaceutical industries are unaware of the fact that they may cause major financial and liability risks to a large pharmaceutical company when they collaborate in a project. This is particularly the case when a radiopharmacy produces radiopharmaceuticals under the sponsorship of a pharmaceutical company. When GMP is inappropriately implemented in a radiopharmacy and deviations are missed, it may, for instance, harm a new pharmaceutical product of the industry. It may even lead to the failure of a new drug product. This is an important reason why (especially) large pharmaceutical companies are extremely cautious in working with external contract partners. The industry's apparent "overkill approach" on GMP is based on these principles. Every radiopharmacy that is selected by a large pharmaceutical company for outsourcing should be fully aware of this and be able to ensure sufficient capacity to meet the contract agreed upon.

7.4 Jump: Good Clinical Practice

When conducting research trials involving human subjects, strict adherence to the rules and principles of good clinical practice (GCP) is necessary. From clinical trials, the safety and efficacy of an IMP can be demonstrated. To guarantee the ethical and scientific soundness of clinical trials, international standards have to be applied (GCP-website).

7.4.1 Principles

Among the most sensitive aspects of clinical trials are the safety, well-being, and rights of the trial subjects. Therefore, the principles of GCP are based on the Declaration of Helsinki (Declaration of Helsinki website 2013). Before a trial with an IMP can be started, it has to be determined whether the benefits for the individual subject and society outweigh the possible risks involved in participating in the trial. Also, a protocol has to be drawn first, according to which the study will be carried out. This protocol needs approval by an independent ethics committee (IEC). If there is already any clinical information about the IMP, the study's approval request should be supported with this information. As well, nonclinical information, such as details of the manufacture process and the pharmaceutical quality of the IMP should be documented. The latter is always necessary to submit. Furthermore, within the EU, an investigational medicinal product dossier should be submitted to the competent authority in the country. This document contains all relevant and available pharmaceutical information concerning the IMP. After approval of the study protocol, the study can be opened by starting patient enrolment. First, the investigator determines whether a subject is eligible for inclusion according to the in- and exclusion criteria of the study protocol. Then, the patient is to be asked to participate in the study and subsequently informed about all possible consequences of study enrolment. Finally, selected trial subjects have to individually and voluntarily give their written informed consent to be included in the study. If the study protocol allows for inclusion of incapacitated subjects, for whatever reason, informed consent can be obtained from a legal representative. Once the study has started, the subject has the right to withdraw its consent and thereby leaving the study.

7.4.1.1 Investigator

The medical care needed during a trial should be provided by qualified physicians. The physicians involved have adequate experience in conducting trials, gained by education and/or training. Personnel releasing prepared radiopharmaceuticals should have adequate experience with the quality systems and be familiar with the regulatory requirements specific for radioactive products. Also, the investigators should be familiar with handling the IMP under conditions as specified in the protocol. Whenever the sponsor of the trial has to monitor the trial or to carry out checks on it, this has to be facilitated by the investigators. If the investigator wishes to delegate any trial-related duties to other qualified investigators, she should make a document containing information such as names, functions, and delegated duties about them, and keep this document updated during the trial. The final responsibility for the study, however, always remains with the coordinating principal investigator. All data gathered during the trial should be stored such that verification is possible, regardless where the study is conducted. However, stored data should be protected if it is possible to identify subjects with this information.

Regarding staff capacity and resources needed to carry out the trials, the investigator should guarantee a sufficient available capacity for the foreseen duration of the trial. Documentation of their names, functions, qualifications, and education is mandatory.

7.4.1.2 Independent Ethics Committee (IEC)

Before a clinical trial can be started, it has to be approved by the IEC. The IEC controls whether the trial meets all requirements they (and they national authorities) have set for it. Their main purpose is to safeguard the rights and dignity of the trial subjects. Depending on national regulations, other issues they take into account include the competence of the investigator to conduct a trial of and the question whether the balance between benefits and risks is equally divided between all subjects. In some countries, such as the Netherlands, also the scientific soundness of a study is evaluated by the IEC. If the requirements are not met, the IEC can request changes, suspend the trial, or deny permission for it. In addition to the IEC, the radiation protection authority must approve the clinical trial when a radiopharmaceutical is involved. Because the IEC has an important role in granting permission for a clinical trial, it needs to have access to all documentation related to the study. This includes trial protocols, informed consent forms, CVs of the investigators, and patient information. For clinical trials involving radiopharmaceuticals, the information is additionally judged based on three basic principles of radiological protection:

- Use of dose limits (dose constraints). For cardiovascular applications, a dose of <10 mSv per scan is regarded as safe for the indication. For certain oncological protocols, higher doses may be allowed, in view of the sometimes shorter life expectancy.
- Justification of activities that could cause or effect radiation exposure.
- Optimization of protection to keep doses as low as reasonably achievable.

The investigator is only allowed to deviate from the protocol without approval from the IEC when there is an immediate hazard potential to the trial subjects. In most cases, the protocols will cover all known hazards in order to create the ability that the patient can always be treated within the protocol. Reasons for inserting changes into the protocol have to be submitted as soon as possible after it has become clear that the change is necessary (GCP-website; Verbruggen et al. 2008).

7.4.1.3 Informed Consent

Informed consent has to be obtained by the investigator. Its purpose is twofold; firstly, the investigator can ensure the IEC that the subjects participating in the trial do this voluntarily, and secondly the investigator can ensure that the research is consistent with the subject's preferences, interests, and values. To ensure that the subjects participating in the study make a rational and voluntary choice, the given information should be clear and set up in such a way that it is fully understandable for the subject.

7.4.2 Trial Design/Type

The trial type determines the trial design. There are several types of trials, which are divided into therapeutic or diagnostic, combined with the disease category to be studied, for example, diagnostic cardiovascular. In clinical trials investigating regular pharmaceuticals, the FDA and EMA require that IMPs are not allowed to have an acute toxic effect in preclinical studies at doses that are a hundred times higher than the anticipated clinical dose. In the first phase of these safety studies, information on pharmacokinetics, biodistribution, and radiation dosimetry is provided. The latter has to be measured for each organ structure as well as for whole-body exposure. In the second phase, the clinical efficacy of diagnostic imaging agents is validated. Parameters like dose, dosing schedule, post injection time to image, image projections and views, and reconstruction algorithms are varied to optimize the images' diagnostic content and the safety profile. The optimal parameters are to be used in the third phase. In this last phase, data is collected and analyzed. These data can be used to support the New Drug Application for its intended clinical use (Rollo et al. 2010).

Conclusions

Many radiotracers are currently under investigation as potential clinical radiopharmaceuticals for indications involving cardiac function and innervation. Before clinical implementation is feasible, all required GMP regulations have to be met. Upon production, release, and administration of the radiopharmaceutical,

GMP adherence is likewise essential. In the near future, the role of cGRPP will become more clear. For the proper conduction of clinical trials using radiopharmaceuticals, GCP regulations are to be followed in order to ensure patient safety and adequate data collection for scientific research.

References

Anagnostopoulos C, Georgakopoulos A, Pianou N, Nekolla SG (2013) Assessment of myocardial perfusion and viability by positron emission tomography. Int J Cardiol 167:1737–1749

Anonymous (2007) Radiopharmacy Committee of the EANM, guidelines on current good radiopharmacy practice (cGRPP) in the preparation of radiopharmaceuticals, version 2 March 2007 URL: http://www.eanm.org/publications/guidelines/gl_radioph_cgrpp.pdf (assessed November 2014)

Bengel FM (2011) Imaging targets of the sympathetic nervous system of the heart: translational considerations. J Nucl Med 52:1167–1170

Bengel FM, Schwaiger M (2004) Assessment of cardiac sympathetic neuronal function using PET imaging. J Nucl Cardiol 11:603–616

Boersma HH, Wensing JW, Kho TL, De Brauw LM, Liem IH, Van Kroonenburgh MJ (2002) Compensatory uptake of I-123 MIBG in the contralateral adrenal gland after removal of a pheochromocytoma. Clin Nucl Med 27:113–116

Candell-Riera J, Romero-Farina G, Aguade-Bruix S, Castell-Conesa J, de Leon G, Garcia-Dorado D (2009) Prognostic value of myocardial perfusion-gated SPECT in patients with ischemic cardiomyopathy. J Nucl Cardiol 16:212–221

Declaration of Helsinki (2013) Website: http://www.wma.net/en/30publications/10policies/b3/index.html. (assessed March 2014)

Di Carli MF, Dorbala S, Meserve J, El Fakhri G, Sitek A, Moore SC (2007) Clinical myocardial perfusion PET/CT. J Nucl Med 48:783–793

Elsinga P, Todde S, Penuelas I, Meyer G, Farstad B, Faivre-Chauvet A, Mikolajczak R, Westera G, Gmeiner-Stopar T, Decristoforo C (2010) Guidance on current good radiopharmacy practice (cGRPP) for the small-scale preparation of radiopharmaceuticals. Eur J Nucl Med Mol Imaging 37:1049–1062

Elsinga PH, Dierckx RAJO (2014) Small molecule PET-radiopharmaceuticals. Curr Pharm Des 20:2268–2274

EU-GMP-website. http://ec.europa.eu/health/documents/eudralex/vol-4/index_en.htm. (assessed March 2014)

FDA-Guidance PET Drugs (2011) Guidance PET drugs, current good manufacturing practice (CGMP). Small entity compliance guide, FDA, Center for Drug Evaluation and Research (CDER) http://www.fda.gov/downloads/drugs/guidancecomplianceregulatoryinformation/guidances/ucm070306.pdf. (assessed November 2013)

GCP-website (Good clinical practices, ICH) http://www.ich.org/products/guidelines/efficacy/article/efficacy-guidelines.html. (assessed March 2014)

Hillman EM, Bernus O, Pease E, Bouchard MB, Pertsov A (2014) Depth-resolved optical imaging of transmural electrical propagation in perfused heart. Opt Express 15:17827–17841

ICH M3-website. Non-clinical safety studies for the conduct of human clinical trials and marketing authorization for pharmaceuticals. http://www.ich.org/products/guidelines/multidisciplinary/article/multidisciplinary-guidelines.html. (assessed November 2014)

Kassiou M, Mardon K, Katsifis AG, Najdovski L, Dikic B, Mattner F, Lambrecht RM, Hicks RJ, Eu P, Loc'h C (1996) Radiosynthesis of [123I]N-methyl-4-iododexetimide and [123I]N-methyl-4-iodolevetimide: in vitro and in vivo characterisation of binding to muscarinic receptors in the rat heart. Nucl Med Biol 23:147–153

Langer O, Halldin C (2002) PET and SPET tracers for mapping the cardiac nervous system. Eur J Nucl Med Mol Imaging 29:416–434

Mühlfeld C, Schipke J, Schmidt A, Post H, Pieske B, Sedej S (2013) Hypoinnervation is an early event in experimental myocardial remodelling induced by pressure overload. J Anat 222:634–644

Paterson I, Mielniczuk LM, O'Meara E, So A, White JA (2013) Imaging heart failure: current and future applications. Can J Cardiol 29:317–328

Regulation (EU) No 536/2014 of the European Parliament and of the Council of 16 April 2014. website: http://eur-lex.europa.eu/legal-content/EN/TXT/PDF/?uri=CELEX:32014R0536&from=EN. (assessed November 2014)

Rischpler C, Park MJ, Fung GS, Javadi M, Tsui BM, Higuchi T (2012) Advances in PET myocardial perfusion imaging: F-18 labeled tracers. Ann Nucl Med 26:1–6

Rollo D, Machado S, Ceschin M (2010) Design of clinical trials. Semin Nucl Med 40:332–337

Tamaki N, Yoshinaga K (2011) Novel iodinated tracers, MIBG and BMIPP, for nuclear cardiology. J Nucl Cardiol 18:135–143

Verbruggen A, Coenen HH, Deverre JR, Guilloteau D, Langstrom B, Salvadori PA, Halldin C (2008) Guideline to regulations for radiopharmaceuticals in early phase clinical trials in the EU. Eur J Nucl Med Mol Imaging 35:2144–2151

Weiland F, Chandna H, Narula J (2010) Myocardial iodine-123 meta-iodobenzylguanidine imaging and cardiac events in heart failure: results of the prospective ADMIRE-HF (AdreView Myocardial Imaging for Risk Evaluation in Heart Failure) study. J Am Coll Cardiol 55:2212–2221

General Principles of PET/CT and Autonomic Innervation of the Heart Including Kinetics and Software

8

Stephan G. Nekolla and Christoph Rischpler

Contents

Abstract

Non-invasive imaging of myocardial innervation using positron emission tomography (PET) and positron emission tomography/computed tomography (PET/CT) is a valuable methodology in cardiac imaging. Although it never entered the clinical arena in an extent as single-photon emission computed tomography (SPECT) imaging for this purpose did, its technical advantages, the excellent properties of the imaging agents, and the availability of tools for quantification combine into an occasionally underrated approach.

S.G. Nekolla (✉) • C. Rischpler
Nuklearmedizinische Klinik und Poliklinik, Technische Universität München, Klinikum rechts der Isar, Ismaningerstrasse 22, Munich D-81675, Germany
e-mail: Stephan.Nekolla@tum.de

R.H.J.A. Slart et al. (eds.), *Autonomic Innervation of the Heart: Role of Molecular Imaging*, DOI 10.1007/978-3-662-45074-1_8

This chapter covers a rather wide range of topics and tries not to repeat information provided in other chapters of this book. Consequentially, the focus is to emphasize where all three elements – imaging technique, tracers, and analysis – have to interact to form a viable workflow.

Abbreviations

BGO	Bismuth germanate
COMT	Catechol-O-methyltransferase
CT	Computed tomography
ECG	Electrocardiogram
EPI	Epinephrine
GSO	Gadolinium oxyorthosilicate
H/M	Heart–mediastinum ratio
HTX	Heart transplant surgery
ID	Injected dose
LOR	Line of response
LSO	Lutetium oxyorthosilicate
LV	Left ventricle
LVEF	Left ventricular ejection fraction
MAO(−A)	Monoamine oxidase (−A)
MR(I)	Magnetic resonance (imaging)
NET	Norepinephrine transporter
PET	Positron emission tomography
PHEN	Phenylephrine
RCSD	Regional cardiac sympathetic denervation
ROI	Region of interest
SCA	Sudden cardiac arrest
SPECT	Single-photon emission computed tomography
SUV	Standardized uptake value
VOI	Volume of interest
VT	Ventricular tachycardia

8.1 PET/CT: A Brief Introduction of Concepts and Methods

8.1.1 Historical Developments

Positron emission tomography (PET) is successfully used in cardiac research applications since the 1980s, and numerous milestone publications have shown the potential of this technique for the characterization of myocardial perfusion, metabolism, and innervation. Since then, PET has developed as a clinical imaging tool but, due to costs and lack of reimbursement in many countries, cardiac PET has never achieved the widespread use which myocardial perfusion single-photon emission computed tomography (SPECT) saw in the same period. However, at least from an oncological point of view, this changed in 2001 when Townsend and Cherry implemented the first hybrid PET/CT system, which combined high-resolution morphological computed tomography (CT) images with lower-resolution but metabolically very specific PET data. From a logistical point of view, another advantage has to be appreciated: the time-consuming acquisition of a transmission data set for attenuation correction using external sources, taking up to 15 min per bed position, was replaced with a scan of few seconds using the CT (Townsend and Cherry 2001). This enabled a higher patient throughput in whole-body, oncological imaging and paved the way for PET/CT's success in today's medical imaging world. Although this success is almost entirely based on tumor imaging, with the clinical availability of PET/CT systems, the interests in cardiac applications using this device also increased.

8.1.2 Technical Principles: The Short Story

PET imaging uses the rapid radioactive decay of positron-emitting isotopes (such as ^{18}F, ^{11}C, ^{13}N, ^{15}O) which are, after their generation in cyclotrons, chemically "inserted" in molecules with high biological relevance (e.g., metabolism, [^{18}F]-deoxyglucose, [^{11}C]-acetate; perfusion, [^{13}N]-NH_3, [^{15}O]-water; and innervation, [^{11}C]-metahydroxyephedrine). These radiopharmaceuticals are injected intravenously in a patient which is positioned inside a PET scanner (Fig. 8.1). Then, the tracer distributes, and during the radioactive decay of their isotopes, positrons are emitted and annihilate within a very short time with electrons under the emission of two 511 keV photons. PET tomographs utilize the near-simultaneous (coincidence) detection of these photons with a ring of detectors. The high-energy photons are detected with dedicated materials which convert them into lower-energy photons which are then in turn detected and amplified (mostly) with photomultiplier tubes. These electrical signals are subsequently processed to estimate the so-called line of response (LOR) along which the decay must have taken place. This is possible since the two annihilation photons travel antiparallel (i.e., they are emitted at an angle of approximately 180°) so that the decay must have taken place somewhere along the LOR. Thus, in contrast to SPECT scanners, where collimators are used to associate a detected event with the direction it came from, PET is using an "electronic collimation" increasing its sensitivity as no photons are lost within heavy collimators (although the needed hardware is clearly more expensive). As shown in Fig. 8.1, the hardware design uses detector rings where the coincidence is determined by using a very short acceptance timing window of typically a few nanoseconds or less for the detection of both events. Fundamentally, three types of events can occur: first, a true coincidence, if indeed the two annihilation photons arrive un-scattered at the two detectors along the LOR. Second, a scattered coincidence when one or both photons from a single positron decay undergo a scatter event in the body but arrive within the time window; obviously, this results in wrong spatial association. Finally, a random coincidence can occur where rays from two unrelated decay events are registered

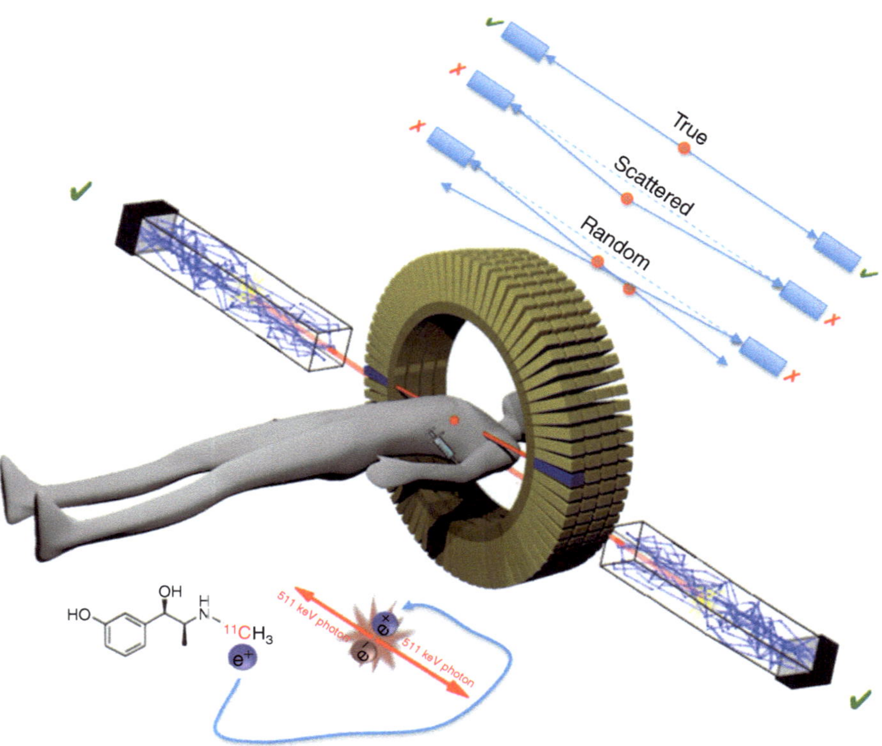

Fig. 8.1 Basic principles of PET imaging: a radioactive tracer such as [^{11}C]-mHED is injected into a patient and emits two 511 keV photons after the positron annihilates with an electron. Those two photons are detected and measured in coincidence mode by dedicated hardware surrounding the patient. Three possibilities exist for such a measurement: true, scattered, and random coincidences

within the time window. Whereas the first possibility results in a "correct" measurement, the two other cases will yield image degradation. Scattered events are of special relevance in cardiac imaging due to relatively high amounts of tracer in the heart and adjacent organs. Originally, PET systems operated in 2-dimensional (2D) mode with interplane septa which reduces scattered photons as coincidence measurements. Basically, in this 2D mode, coincidence measurements are performed only in one plane of the PET camera. Removing the septa and accepting coincidences between scanner planes, however, increase sensitivity and consequentially shorten scan time. This so-called 3D mode has shown many advantages especially in oncological imaging protocols including increased patient throughput (Lartizien et al. 2004; Halpern et al. 2004a). However, it is potentially limited by the counting rate capability of the system and its effectiveness to reject scatter and random coincidences.

Today, the most commonly used detector materials are lutetium oxyorthosilicate (LSO) and gadolinium oxyorthosilicate (GSO) which are both attractive due to their physical properties. Both LSO and GSO are increasingly used instead of bismuth germanate (BGO) in PET/CT systems (Lewellen 2008). LSO and GSO scintillators show a relatively fast light decay time and high light yield (Humm et al. 2003), enabling the use of short coincidence time windows which in turn results in a decreased dead time. Consequently, this improves the count rate capabilities and reduces randoms. Thus, an LSO-based PET/CT scanner (Martinez et al. 2006) shows an approximately 3.8 times higher counting rate than a conventional BGO scanner operating in 2D mode (Brix et al. 1997). In case of [^{13}N]-NH_3 scans, the count rates give rise to a dead time in the range of 25–30 % for both LSO and BGO devices. But as an LSO-based system shows a 5–6 times higher rate of true coincidences, this offers a clear advantage.

In nuclear cardiology, a high counting rate capability is of particular importance as one often faces relatively high tracer concentrations in static imaging and – most importantly – bolus injection techniques with dynamic image acquisition.

Initially, the suitability of 3D tomographs was shown for the practical case of static viability imaging with [^{18}F]-FDG PET imaging (Brogsitter et al. 2005) and [^{82}Rb] PET perfusion imaging (Knesaurek et al. 2003). In a functional extension, Knesaurek et al. demonstrated that cardiac [^{82}Rb] PET allowed the reliable estimation of global functional parameters from PET scanners operating in 2D or 3D mode (Knesaurek et al. 2007). Thus, a very dose-efficient method to clinically relevant parameters in modern PET/CT systems is available.

One advantage of PET is the capability for absolute quantification. For this purpose it must be ensured that – for example, in the case of myocardial flow quantification – the input function, which is usually obtained from a small region of interest (ROI) placed in the left ventricular cavity and which is necessary for tracer kinetic modeling, can be accurately determined (Yoshida et al. 1995; Raylman et al. 1993). Consequently, a high counting rate is of crucial importance because a relatively large amount of the injected radiotracer gets into the field of view early and rapidly after radiotracer application. This might ultimately cause a saturation of the PET scanner and, thus, inaccurate assessment of the input function. Despite these challenges, several studies have proven that accurate, non-invasive myocardial flow quantification using 3D PET is feasible. Lekx et al., for example, showed a moderate to strong correlation of absolute flow values assessed by 2D or 3D [^{82}Rb] PET myocardial perfusion imaging in a canine model (Lekx et al. 2010). In a similar study in humans, an excellent agreement between 2D and 3D acquisition of absolute myocardial blood flow using [^{13}N]NH_3 was demonstrated (Schepis et al. 2007). These studies suggest that – at least for the hard- and software used in those studies – blood flow can be accurately determined using either 2D or 3D PET, while 3D PET offers an obvious advantage: the radiation exposure to the patient can be clearly reduced by a lower administration dose. All these publications used perfusion agents rather than innervation tracers. However, as shown later, dynamic imaging with this category of radiopharmaceuticals is a relevant element in quantification.

With the aim to improve spatial resolution, recent PET/CT systems are equipped with smaller crystals, which is of particular importance in nuclear cardiology in order to decrease partial-volume effects (Parodi et al. 1984). As the enhancement of the spatial resolution from 7.0 to 4.5 mm leads to an increase of about 30 % in count recovery (given an average ventricular wall thickness of about 10 mm), the use of high-resolution PET ameliorates the assessment of regional tracer distribution in the myocardium and allows more accurate quantification of physiologic parameters such as blood flow, metabolism, or innervation.

8.1.3 Attenuation and Scatter Correction

Attenuation correction in PET is the prerequisite for any quantification of the radiotracer's uptake signal. Absolute quantification is the key to improve diagnostic performance, to enable comparisons between serial examinations, and to perform any pharmacokinetic modeling. A large fraction of the 511 keV annihilation photons from the positron decay are actually scattered by the patient's body. Consequentially, they are discriminated due to a lower energy or do not reach the PET detectors at all. To account for these effects and thus compute activity-wise correct PET images, it is necessary to determine an attenuation map with the appropriate attenuation coefficients for 511 keV photons at each voxel. In hybrid PET/CT systems, this is achieved using the information about the tissue electron density provided by the CT and adjusting it for the difference in photon energy (Souvatzoglou et al. 2007). However, as the CT scan is done (a) very fast compared to the PET and (b) either before or after the PET scan, misalignment can occur. Importantly, any misregistration between emission and "transmission" might lead to uptake errors, since the difference in tissue density between the heart and the surrounding lung is high. Clinical studies showed that artifacts due to misalignment can occur in 20–30 % of PET/CT studies, typically in anterolateral or lateral segments of the left ventricle (LV) (Martinez-Moller et al. 2007a). This is a considerable problem in PET studies where clear and strong tracer uptake is seen (such as perfusion or viability) and the presence of artifacts can be appreciated visually. Possible countermeasures for this issue are manual or automatic registration and repeated reconstruction. In the case of the relatively weak truly molecular signals from innervation tracers, this might be more difficult, and substantial caution and quality control steps are required.

In addition to the effects of misalignment, metal implants such as leads, pace makers, or other interventional devices may affect the quantification of PET tracer uptake – although this was only investigated in cardiac PET using flow and metabolism markers (Halpern et al. 2004b; DiFilippo and Brunken 2005). However, these PET artifacts are primarily due to the effects of the metallic components in reconstruction artifacts of the CT and migrate through the overestimating of attenuating tissue into the PET images. The relevance of these artifacts differ depending on their position, and thus, hybrid reading or reviewing also non-attenuation-corrected data is advisable also for innervation tracers.

8.1.4 Technical Developments with Special Relevance to Cardiac PET/CT

Cardiac and respiratory motions both blur the signal from the myocardium and reduce the spatial resolution which can theoretically be achieved. Especially in the presence of weaker molecular signals, this is a potential problem. Cardiac-gated PET imaging is available on all commercial scanners and the implementation works in such a way that, in parallel to the measurement of all coincidence events, the electrocardiogram (ECG) signal using conventional electrodes is recorded and stored together with the

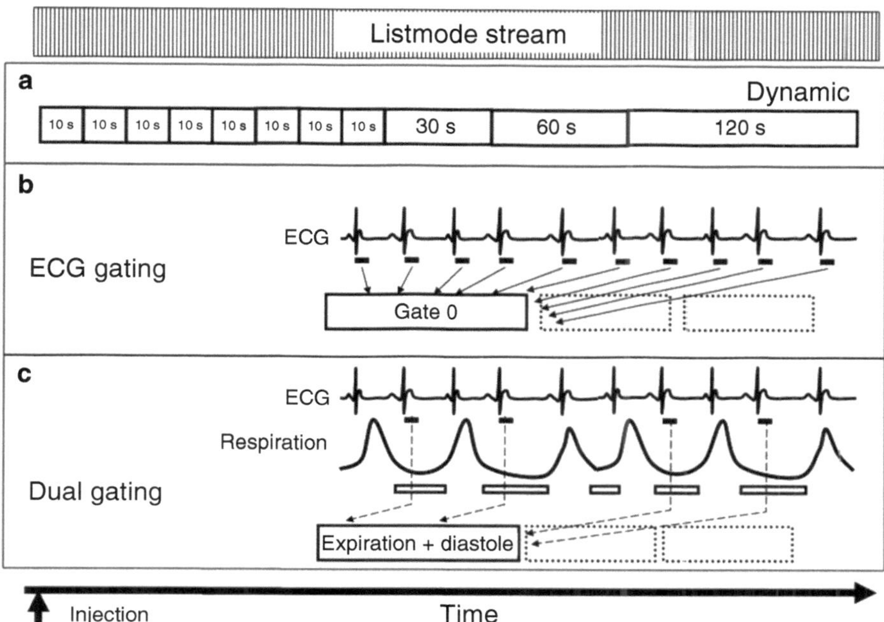

Fig. 8.2 List mode data acquisitions allow a flexible and retrospective generation of image data matching to various criteria. Three examples using the list mode stream are shown here: dynamic (**a**), ECG (**b**), and dual ECG and respiratory gating (**c**). The triggered intervals are indicated as filled (ECG) and open (respiratory) boxes

so-called list mode stream (Fig. 8.2). Thus, the association of a given annihilation event with the state of myocardial contraction is possible for the complete acquisition time. Technically, for retrospective gating, the number of gates after the detected R wave must be specified (forward gating) together with the allowed R–R interval. This R–R interval is selected based on a beat histogram which is shown to the user as part of the reconstruction workflow. Then, the events are sorted into, for example, 8 or 16 sinogram buffers. Finally, the sinograms are normalized and corrected for scatter and attenuation (typically using a non-gated attenuation map as the endocardial/pericardial silhouette is not moving significantly over the contractile cycle), and image reconstruction is performed. In case of cardiac arrhythmias, those beats outside of the allowed R–R interval are rejected or collected in a "bad beat" buffer.

Technically similar, respiratory gating can be performed and gained interest in oncological imaging as the detectability of lung or liver lesions is also degraded by the respiratory motion (Bundschuh et al. 2008; van Elmpt et al. 2011). Instead of the ECG, a detection system such as a pneumatic device is integrated into an elastic belt, which is then fastened around the lower chest of the patient. In magnetic resonance imaging (MRI), this technique is widely used and a standard technique to limit artifacts from respiration. Other implementations are placing optical tracking systems (Buther et al. 2010), bio-impedance systems (Koivumaki et al. 2012),

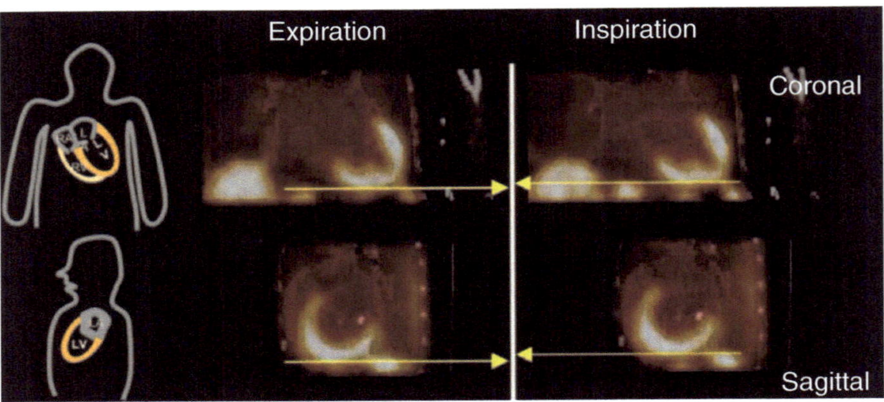

Fig. 8.3 Effects of respiratory gating on the location of the heart cardiac is shown in this [^{13}N] NH3 study. Total acquisition time was 10 min p.i. tracer injection, with the list mode data starting at 2 min until the end of the scan. Acquired list mode data were charted into six respiratory and two cardiac cycles. The images above show end-diastolic frames in end inspiration and end expiration. The *yellow line* marks the most apical position in both respiratory states. The maximal spatial difference is 8 mm. *LA* left atrium, *LV* left ventricle, *RA* right atrium, *RV* right ventricle (Taken with permission from Schwaiger et al. (2005))

pressure/temperature sensors in close proximity to the nose or mouth to directly measure inhalation/exhalation patterns (Boucher et al. 2004), or data-driven methods identifying motion in the PET raw or image data (Buther et al. 2009) (Bundschuh et al. 2007). Independent of the technical design, the frequency distribution of human respiration is significantly different to that of cardiac gating as it is much more irregular and its distribution may vary substantially over the lengths of a PET acquisition as the patients might go from an anxious into a more relaxed state or even fall asleep.

The combination of respiratory and cardiac gating (dual gating) has the potential to improve imaging of the myocardium (Martinez-Moller et al. 2007b; Gigengack et al. 2012), coronaries (Delso et al. 2011), and potentially even nerves. However, most of these findings are still on a rather experimental level. In Fig. 8.2, we demonstrate the processing of a cardiac list mode study. Three examples using the list mode stream are illustrated to generate a variety of data sets all from the same acquisition: dynamic (A), ECG gated (B), and dual ECG and respiratory gating (C). The more nested and complex the trigger criteria are, the longer the histogramming and the reconstruction will naturally take. For instance, as shown in the dual-gating case, the number of events varies according to the frequency of the combinations (e.g., the combination of systole and expiration will happen more often than systole and inspiration). In general, only cardiac gating is performed in a clinical setup; however, the potential of more advanced acquisition schemes can be appreciated although further studies are needed to proof this claim. In Fig. 8.3, the possible effects of respiratory gating in addition to cardiac gating are illustrated on the basis of an example of a [^{13}N]-NH_3 perfusion PET study.

8.1.5 Coregistration in Sequential Imaging: PET/CT

As PET and CT are acquired sequentially, the proper data alignment must be ensured to make synergistic use of them – in addition to the problems mentioned for attenuation correction. Related to different spatial resolutions and the complexity of motion state differences, no final solution to this issue is known, although substantial progress was made in the last decade (Slomka and Baum 2009; Nakazato et al. 2012). The manual alignment of two or more three-dimensional objects which are not only translated but can also be rotated due to different motion states might introduce quite some interobserver variability. As a consequence, it is an obvious prerequisite for routine clinical application that proper quality control steps are implemented as long as no such automated software is available.

8.2 Imaging the Autonomic Innervation with PET and PET/ CT

The core competence of nuclear imaging in comparison to morphological imaging (such as CT) is the access to molecular processes at a cellular level. Radiolabeled catecholamine analogs labeled with radioisotopes such as [^{11}C], [^{18}F] (both for PET), or [^{123}I] (for SPECT) are avidly taken up into the cardiac sympathetic neurons primarily via the uptake-1 mechanism very similar to the process for norepinephrine. Thus, they mark the location of functioning nerve terminals. In particular, those radiotracers that are not metabolized facilitate their detection by imaging means. In consequence, measuring tracer uptake enables the assessment of alterations in cardiac sympathetic nerve function.

In an excellent, recent update to a decade-old review on imaging of autonomic innervation (Thackeray and Bengel 2013), the authors listed the major achievements in this field as follows:

- Increased number of multi-tracer studies evaluating pre- and postsynaptic autonomic signaling and application in disease states.
- Expansion of animal imaging studies in both small and large animal models provides greater insight into the suitability of available tracers in disease.
- Greater interest and evaluation of parasympathetic innervation by muscarinic receptor antagonists.
- Increased evidence and interest in regional inhomogeneous tracer uptake in arrhythmia.
- First large-scale PET clinical trial (PAREPET) evaluating the suitability of autonomic neuronal PET in prediction of arrhythmia.
- Development and evaluation of [^{18}F]-labeled tracers for measuring myocardial innervation, moving toward a commercial product.

Looking back even further, the use of non-invasive imaging to delineate the regional distribution of the autonomic innervation started in the late 1980s with PET as the high detection sensitivity of this imaging modality enabled a methodology which is now known as molecular imaging. In these years, PET was primarily used in research, and due to its rather limited transaxial field of view, its application was most likely and most attractive in neurology and cardiology.

Today, a variety of PET radiotracers for the assessment of the myocardial sympathetic innervation are available. [^{11}C]-metahydroxyephedrine (mHED) is the most widely used PET tracer and represents, like the SPECT tracer [^{123}I]-MIBG, a norepinephrine analog. [^{11}C]-mHED is predominantly taken up into the sympathetic terminals via the noradrenaline transporter. DeGrado showed initially in an isolated rat heart model that this tracer demonstrates a strong uptake in control hearts ($K1 = 2.66 \pm 0.39$ ml/g/min) and a relatively slow mono-exponential washout ($k2 = 0.011 \pm 0.003$ min^{-1}) (DeGrado et al. 1993). Positive features of this radiotracer are that only a small proportion enters the nerve terminal via the nonspecific type 2 transport mechanism (Bengel et al. 2000) and that it is not metabolized by the intraneuronal monoamine oxidase A (MAO-A) or catechol-O-methyltransferase (COMT).

Another PET radiotracer for presynaptic sympathetic imaging is [^{11}C]-epinephrine (EPI). EPI is metabolically degraded by MAO and is considered to be superior to [^{11}C]-mHED, as it traces the entire pathway of catecholamine uptake, metabolism, and vesicular storage. Despite these advantages, EPI has so far mainly been used in preclinical studies (Nguyen et al. 1997). [^{11}C]-phenylephrine (PHEN) is another valuable radiotracer for cardiac neuronal imaging. It is also degraded by the MAO and the consequent metabolite, [^{11}C]-methylamine, is washed out quickly from the nerve terminals. Under normal circumstances, PHEN diffuses out slower from the storage vesicles compared to [^{11}C]-mHED. Therefore, PHEN is considered to be valuable for the assessment of vesicular leakage (Raffel et al. 1999). While [^{11}C]-mHED and PHEN show similar images of the initial uptake with comparable quality and uniformity, the washout of PHEN is – expectedly for a MAO substrate – much faster (Raffel et al. 1996). Using PHEN the storage half-life, which reflects to a certain degree the functional integrity of the cardiac sympathetic innervation, may be calculated.

Even though PHEN and EPI demonstrate interesting features, the majority of human studies have been carried out using [^{11}C]-mHED. In 2008, Sasano and coworkers published results from an animal model where the impaired innervation in the border zone of an infarct gave rise to ventricular tachycardia (VT) (Sasano et al. 2008). PET imaging with [^{13}N]-NH_3 and [^{11}C]-mHED was performed 4–12 weeks post infarction followed by MRI and electro-anatomical mapping a week later (Fig. 8.4).

8.2.1 Recent Developments: [^{18}F]-Labeled Imaging Agents

PET imaging of the autonomic innervation never really left the research domain. The primary reasons were the increasing complexity of regulatory processes and the use of radioisotopes which required an on-site cyclotron.

Meanwhile a new [^{18}F]-labeled perfusion agent was developed (Yalamanchili et al. 2007). The initial success of this approach together with the interest in

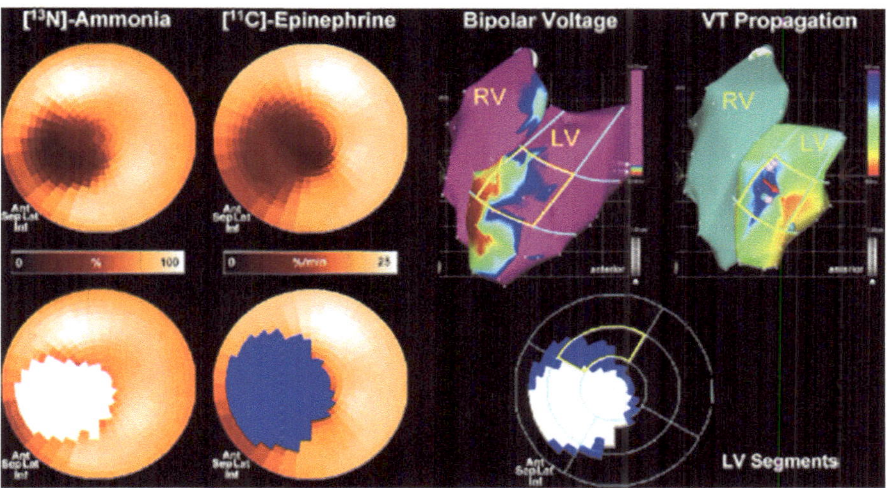

Fig. 8.4 Sample PET polar maps of [13N]NH3 and [11C]-epinephrine (*left panel*) in a pig following myocardial infarction demonstrate regions of perfusion and innervation defects, illustrated in *white* and *blue*, respectively (*lower left panel*). The innervation defect exceeds the perfusion defect in the distal anterior wall (*lower right panel*). Electroanatomical mapping (*upper right panel*) demonstrates reduced voltage in the apex and distal anteroseptal wall. The region of earliest activation of VT (*red arrow*) is localized to the infarct border zone in the distal anterior wall (Sasano et al. (2008), reprinted with permission from Elsevier)

ADMIRE-HF (Jacobson et al. 2010) stimulated the development of an also [18F]-labeled compound acting as substrate for the neuronal norepinephrine transporter (NET) – basically with very similar molecular properties to [123I]-MIBG but utilizing all the advantages of PET, namely, high sensitivity, resolution, and quantification. Yu and colleagues found in cells, rats, rabbits, and nonhuman primates very favorable imaging properties of [18F]-LMI1195 (*N*-[3-bromo-4-(3-18F-fluoro-propoxy)-benzyl]-guanidine) (Yu et al. 2011). In rats, [18F]-LMI1195 cardiac uptake at 15 and 60 min after intravenous administration was 2.36 ± 0.38 and 2.16 ± 0.38 % injected dose per gram tissue (%ID/g), similar to [123I]-MIBG (2.14 ± 0.30 and 2.19 ± 0.27 % ID/g) – but the heart to liver and lung uptake ratios were significantly higher for LMI1195 (see Fig. 8.5). When compared to [123I]-MIBG, the LMI1195 uptake was overall lower but its washout in nontarget organs was faster. This resulted in significantly higher target to nontarget uptake ratios and explains the visually impressive images. The same group investigated then the use of LMI1195 in a rabbit model of myocardial infarction which resulted in substantial myocardial denervation (Yu et al. 2012). The authors specifically addressed the association between regional cardiac sympathetic denervation (RCSD) and reduced NET function in the context of cardiac arrhythmia. The new tracer again showed a high association with NET and its suitability for imaging RCSD in a rabbit model. The myocardial denervation increases cardiac risks to the antiarrhythmic drug, dofetilide, by inducing more QTc prolongation. Using a rat model of infarction, our group confirmed the positive findings of this agent (Higuchi et al. 2013). [18F]-LMI1195 produced high

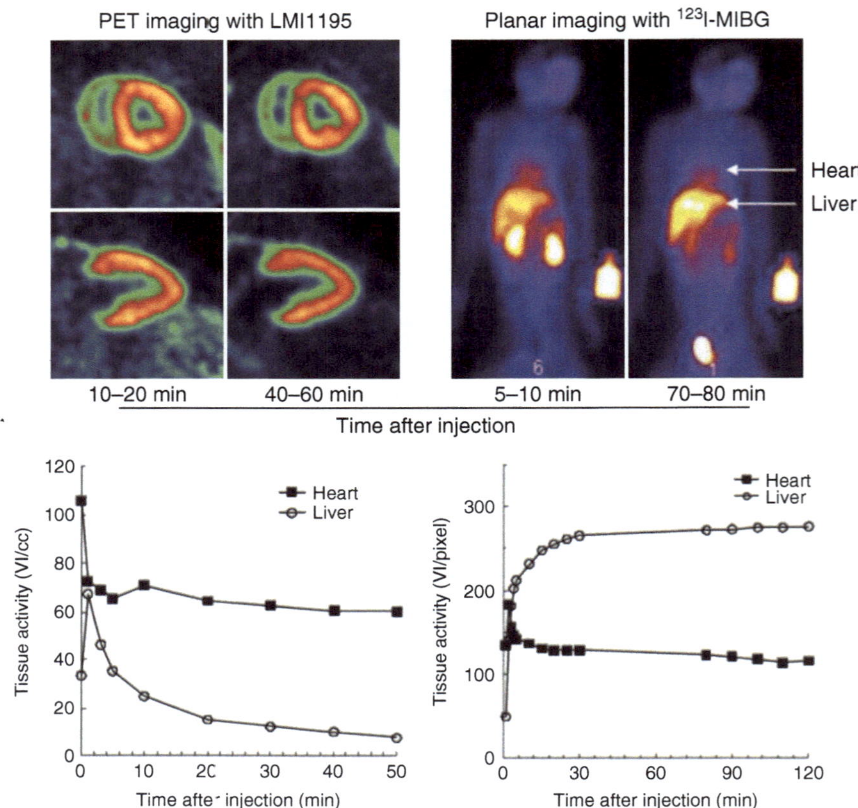

Fig. 8.5 *Left panels*: cardiac PET images of [^{18}F]-LMI1195 in a nonhuman primate (NHP) and the time–activity curve (TAC) calculated from the image dynamic image data. *Right panels*: whole-body planar images of [^{123}I]-mIBG in a NHP and also the TAC. In contrast to the SPECT tracer, the PET compound washed out rapidly from nontarget organs over time (Reproduced from (Yu et al. 2011) by permission)

and sustained heart uptake which enabled the excellent delineation of the LV for 60 min p.i. (Fig. 8.6). Pretreatment with phenoxybenzamine clearly reduced the [^{18}F]-LMI1195 myocardial uptake. In contrast, there was a preserved [^{18}F]-LMI1195 signal post desipramine pretreatment. Thus, in rats, cardiac uptake was significantly inhibited by phenoxybenzamine but not desipramine, suggesting the new agent is a substrate for the uptake-2 mechanism consistent with the fact that in rat myocardium this is the dominant process. The excellent image quality can also be acknowledged in Fig. 8.7, showing high tracer uptake in a rabbit model using a human PET/MR system.

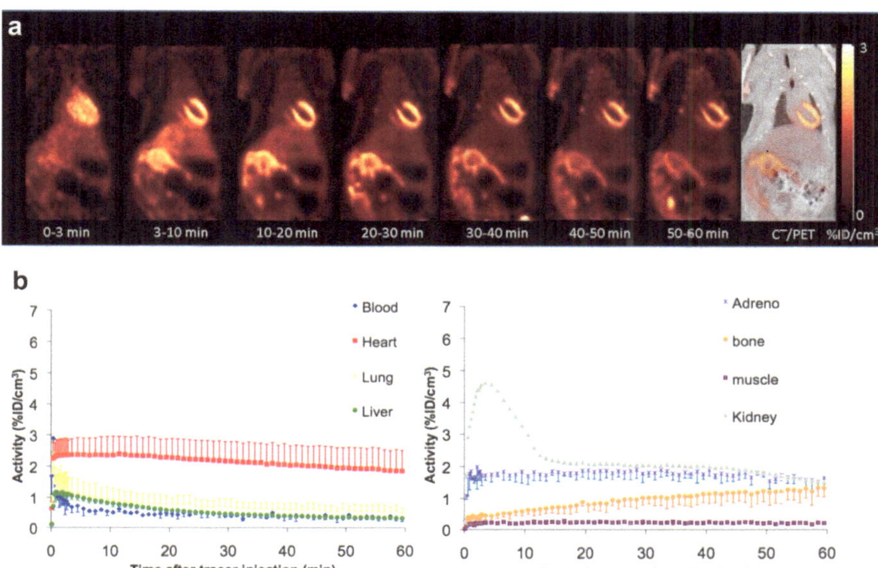

Fig. 8.6 (**a**) Example images in coronal section of a dynamic PET/CT study at different time points after tracer injection showing a healthy rat using the radiotracer [^{18}F]-LMI1195. (**b**) Average time–activity curves of different organs assessed by PET imaging. Stable increase of cardiac [^{18}F]-LMI1195 uptake throughout the whole scan can be observed (Reproduced from (Higuchi et al. 2013) with permission)

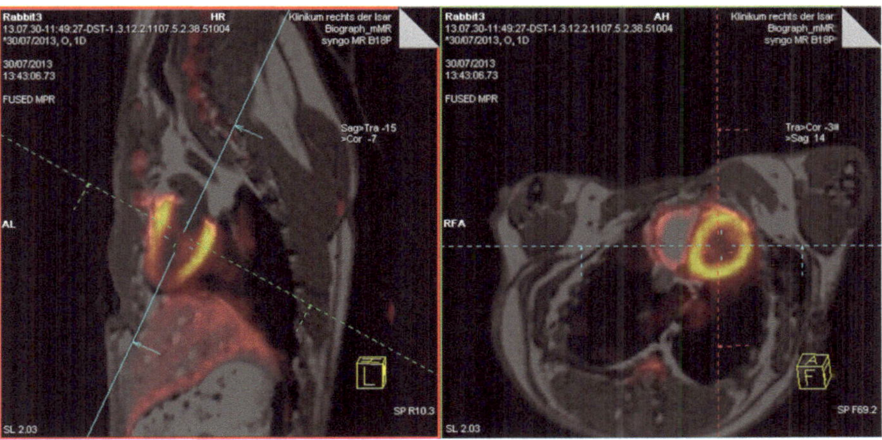

Fig. 8.7 LMI1195 tracer uptake in rabbit model using a fully integrated human PET/MR system. PET data is fused with a high-resolution MPRAGE MR sequence

8.3 From Images to Quantitative Data: Methods and Tools

8.3.1 Looking Back

In the last two decades, imaging hardware has improved in terms of speed and resolution. Reconstruction algorithms creating visually impressive images[1] and new, promising tracers became available. Strangely, the situation differs for the algorithms and software to analyze those images. In order to understand why this is the case, a look at the acquisition protocols helps: whereas on plain PET scanners the acquisition of dynamic and gated data sets was standard in the 1990s, whole-body, oncological imaging was less prominent due to the very long acquisition time which could be as long as 90 min. Today, such an examination is performed in less than 20 min. In contrast, cardiac scans back then routinely took between 30 and 60 min and – as only one bed position was investigated – the dynamic distribution of the tracers was observed and parameters such as myocardial blood flow, metabolic rates of glucose consumption, quantitative retention values, or other physiologically relevant parameters were assessed. Interestingly, this did not change over the years since the required scan time is determined by the characteristics of the tracer rather than the performance of the camera. In other words, the evolution of the throughput on PET scanners differs massively. Consequentially, the focus of the vendors where to invest their (always limited) resources changed accordingly. In parallel, the attention of the industry moved from research to routine application. This resulted in yet another consequence for the analysis software: whereas 20 years ago, basically all vendors' workstations could process dynamic data, this feature disappeared soon after the focus shifted to whole-body imaging. Cheaper computer platform replaced the expensive UNIX workstations and thus the need to re-implement the analysis software naturally lead to a reduction of functionality.[2] A final component to this development is the increasingly complex mechanisms for the development and implementation of software for medical imaging in terms of the regulatory framework. Whereas back then a vendor could implement an algorithm developed by a university partner into their product, this approach is almost impossible today as the university would have to develop by the same mechanism and standards as the industry.[3]

This spectrum of reasons results in today's situation that the availability of advanced analysis tools for kinetic PET studies from the vendors of imaging hardware is almost not existent. There is one exception, namely, the quantification of myocardial blood flow. As perfusion imaging has a very high clinical relevance, tools to process those studies are available primarily from third-party vendors (Saraste et al. 2012; Tahari et al. 2014). Interestingly, those vendors already

[1] The fact that the visual impression is so important comes quite obviously from the dominance of oncological imaging. The potential side effects of introducing changes in image quantification are not too widely investigated although effects on dynamic imaging and thus kinetic analysis exist.

[2] This trend has a name: "de-featuring" of a product.

[3] The development and production of new radiopharmaceuticals suffers from similar problems.

developed a software for SPECT perfusion studies since the 1990s and built on their expertise to expand into this rather new field. Unfortunately, and again due to regulatory issues, those tools are limited to perfusion tracers.

8.3.2 Quantification of Image Data

As discussed in Chap. 9, the quantification of [^{123}I]-MIBG uptake is relatively straightforward (although not undisputed): uptake signals from two regions drawn in planar images result in the so-called heart–mediastinum ratio (H/M). Usually two measurements are performed, namely, after 1.5 and 4 h, which also yields the diagnostic information of tracer washout. However, although planar imaging is logistically and technically easy to perform, PET offers, through superior spatial resolution and sensitivity, access to the regional tracer distribution. As first shown in the assessment of the long-term dynamics of myocardial innervation, advanced image analysis tools showed their value (Fig. 8.8). Using volumetric sampling (Nekolla et al. 1998) and rigid registration (Marinelli et al. 2010), the 3D information is transferred from the flow study to the innervation, thus enabling precise comparison of the two (or more) tracers even in the absence of partial and poor tracer uptake. In these publications, we started with the imaging of the metabolism of the heart after transplant surgery (HTX) (Bengel et al. 1999). In an extension to this project to

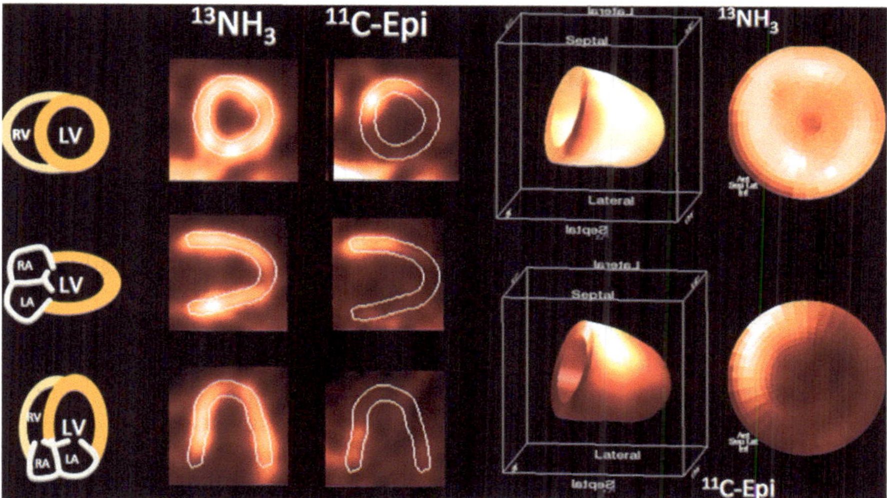

Fig. 8.8 Example of PET innervation imaging (performed with [^{11}C]-epinephrine) in a patient performed after HTX. [^{11}C]-Epi retention can be seen in the basal anteroseptal myocardium indicating sympathetic reinnervation. Perfusion as depicted by $^{13}NH_3$ uptake is normal in the complete LV myocardium. Using volumetric sampling and rigid registration, the 3D sampling information is transferred from the flow study to the innervation, thus enabling precise comparison of the two tracers

characterize the complex myocardial processes after HTX, the visualization and quantification of the myocardial innervation was performed (Odaka et al. 2001). As all myocardial nerves are severed during this operation, their reappearance and the monitoring of their spread over almost one decade after HTX and the integration with cardiac performance are an excellent example of the translational use of molecular imaging and its application in a clinical scenario (Bengel et al. 2001).

Almost a decade later, in the PAREPET trial, regional polar map analysis of normalized tracer uptake [^{11}C]-mHED, [^{13}N]-NH_3, and [^{18}F]-FDG was compared in denervated, infarcted, and viable myocardium in 204 patients at risk for sudden cardiac arrest (SCA) (Fallavollita et al. 2014). Follow-up after 4 years in these patients with ischemic cardiomyopathy revealed that the measurement of regional myocardial denervation with [^{11}C]-mHED is capable to predict mortality from SCA independently of left ventricular ejection fraction (LVEF) and infarct volume assessment.

Assessment of inhomogeneous tracer uptake in arrhythmia (Fallavollita et al. 2010; de Jong et al. 2005) could be a valuable approach where quantification of regional tracer uptake might play a vital role as it offers reproducible, convenient, and routine capable means. Although currently no algorithm is defined, a methodologically similar question is to quantify the dyssynchrony of the mechanical contraction of the LV which is accomplished by the analysis of the phase histogram in gated SPECT and PET studies (Chen et al. 2005; Lehner et al. 2013). Although this might appear very far reaching today, the rapidly moving field of texture analysis in oncologic PET could also offer powerful approaches (Orlhac et al. 2014).

8.3.3 Kinetic Data Analysis

The Gelfand and Thomas of literature on how to process dynamic data grew over three to four decades and is now almost impossible to oversee (examples of extended reviews would be from Bassingthwaighte and others (Bassingthwaighte et al. 2012; Schmidt and Turkheimer 2002; Willemsen and van den Hoff 2002; Wen et al. 2012)). Starting as a domain of nuclear medicine (Gelfand and Thomas 1987), kinetic analysis is now used basically in all modern medical imaging modalities. From a conceptual point of view, 2–3 general approaches are used: the use of compartmental models, their simplifications, and non-compartmental parameters. As a rule of thumb, the first approach requires a good understanding of the different compartments where the tracer is distributed such as blood, interstitial space, and cellular compartments, where the tracer is bound. Specifically in the case of innervations tracers, the cellular compartments would be the axoplasm and the vesicles (Raffel et al. 2013b). All these compartments are connected by rate constants describing the exchange of the tracer between them (Fig. 8.9). Mathematically, this leads to a set of coupled differential equations and the measured blood and tissue activity curves are fitted to the solution of those equations. The results are then the estimates of those rate constants. There is a clear emphasis on “estimates.” This is a very complex numerical operation and the data fed into it are rarely noise-free. From a pragmatic

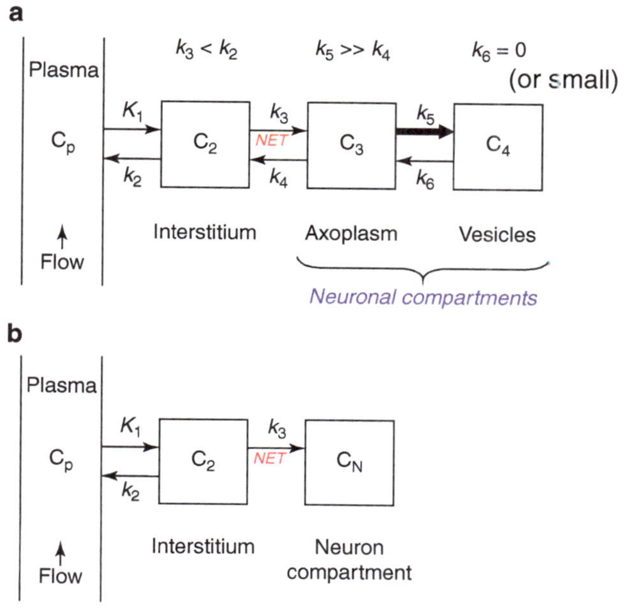

Fig. 8.9 Compartment model description for innervation tracers from Raffel (Raffel et al. 2013b) showing a rather complete (**a**) and a reduced model (**b**) based on the approximations that $k_3 < k_2$, $k_5 >> k_4$, and k_6 small or even zero. Such a reduction of free parameters makes the reliable use of kinetic imaging in a routine setting much more stable and thus likely

point of view, these estimates get less and less reliable the higher the number of compartments get (or deviate in a pathological situation from the theoretical model) as the solution is not unique anymore. In order to reduce complexity, the combination of, for example, axoplasm and vesicles into one neuronal compartment improves the situation if it can be justified from a physiological point of view (Raffel et al. 2013b). However, as an alternative to these more complex but potentially rather variable approaches, the calculation of numerically easier to assess variables such as washout and retention rates has shown value (although they are related to parameters derived from the compartmental models). There are some similarities to the standardized uptake value (SUV) used in oncological PET imaging. This "simplified" value is not undisputed (Huang 2000), but due to methodological advances towards standardization and harmonization, it is not only widely used in clinical reality but also recognized academically as a useful parameter if utilized in a careful manner (Visser et al. 2010; Makris et al. 2013). Especially for [^{11}C]-mHED, a simplified parameter is the so-called retention (Allman et al. 1993) (also called retention fraction, retention index, or fractional uptake rate). This parameter is calculated by the activity found at a defined time point (e.g., 40 min p.i.) and divided by the integral of the arterial input function which is usually derived from the dynamic images (Fig. 8.10). As the tracer uptake of [^{11}C]-mHED in the myocardium is very stable in the first hour p.i., this parameter is in a practical setting very reliable. However, as

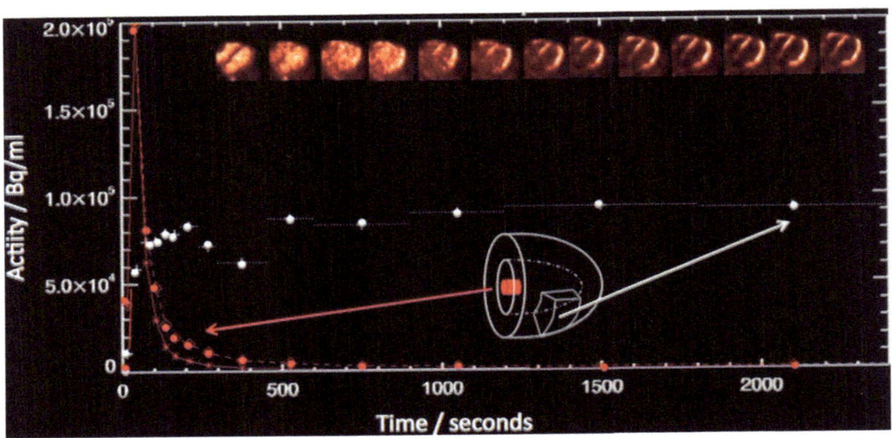

Fig. 8.10 Dynamic PET study with [^{11}C]-mHED in a human. Tissue time–activity curves are shown with *white spheres*, uncorrected blood values with *red spheres*. The *solid red line* marked with *stars* resulted in the use of a population-based metabolite correction. From these data, the retention is calculated as the value in a late frame divided by the integral under the blood curve (i.e., arterial input function). Representative transaxial images for every frame are shown on the *top*. The volume of interest (VOI) for the input function is located in the basal plane; the VOIs for the tissue curves are located within the left ventricular wall

the blood pool always shows residual activity due to circulating metabolites, the blood pool integral increases over time. One method to address this implements a population-based metabolite correction, which effectively suppresses the effect of metabolites on the input function at later time points (Rosenspire et al. 1990; Munch et al. 2000). Thus, standardizing the image acquisition and reconstruction protocol as well as the investigated time interval is required for reproducible measurements – in the very same way as discussed above for the SUV.

Coming back to kinetic modeling – which, with an emphasis on innervation tracers, is described in an excellent review by Raffel and colleagues (Raffel et al. 2013a) – in terms of compartment models, Doze and colleagues showed in their paper one of the most complex implementations of compartmental modeling in cardiac PET using (S)-^{11}C-CGP-12388, a β-adrenoceptor agent to determine receptor density in vivo (Doze et al. 2002). They used a two-tissue compartment model with six free parameters which relies on explicit compartments for describing the kinetics of both labeled and unlabeled radioligands. This model was simultaneously fitted to the dynamic data from a triple-injection protocol (Fig. 8.11). Although technically very demanding, this approach was capable of producing regional estimates of receptor densities.

Another example of addressing systems which are described by complex compartmental models and dual-injection protocols was demonstrated with the following tracer using well-justified approximations: [^{11}C]-CGP-12177 is also a postsynaptic, nonselective β-adrenoceptor antagonist which was first synthetized in the 1990s. The quantification of [^{11}C]-CGP-12177 binding yielding estimates of

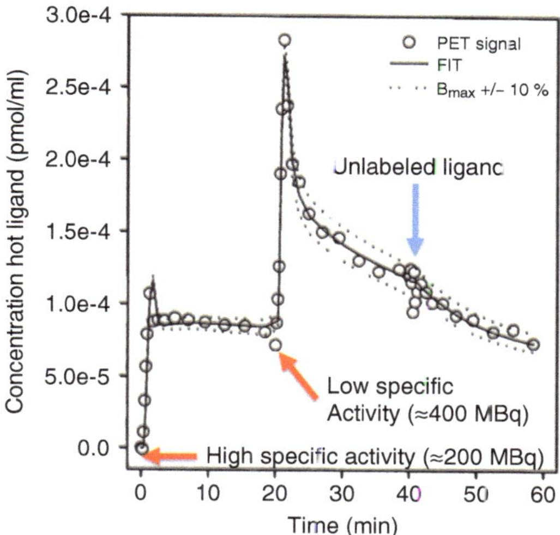

Fig. 8.11 Example of a very complex, triple-injection protocol to determine regional β-receptor density in humans. Measured PET signal (○) and the simulated fit (*solid line*) of volunteer 4 for a large region of the LV (With permission (Doze et al. 2002))

receptor density has been realized using a dual-injection protocol, which utilizes different doses of high and low specific activity. Although logistically not trivial, the concatenation of two dynamic PET scans allowed the generation of those absolute parameters by the use of graphical analysis methods (Logan 2000; Delforge et al. 1991). In 2002, this methodology was further improved and even yielded parametric images (Delforge et al. 2002). It is important to point out that such complex protocols and analysis schemes yield relevant diagnostic information when [^{11}C]-CGP-12177 was used in patients with idiopathic dilated cardiomyopathy (Merlet et al. 1993). In their proof of concept study in ten patients, the authors demonstrated the possibility of repeated measurements of β-receptor concentrations during follow-up, enabling the evaluation of the effects of therapy on β-receptor density in vivo.

8.3.4 Generic Tools for Kinetic Analysis

As the number of applications in oncological and especially neurological imaging tends to outnumber the use in cardiac imaging, those generic software packages offer all the necessary tools to generate time–activity curves for blood and tissue based on typically manually placed regions or volumes of interest (ROIs resp. VOIs). As discussed above, the typical analysis for tracers such as [^{11}C]-mHED is mostly the calculation of retention and washout rates and the use of single tissue compartment models which are used in the other noncardiac applications as well. Although the creation of ROI/VOIs to cover the LV can be tedious, practical experience shows that a pragmatic approach of drawing regions in remote and altered tissue is useful in many circumstances (Magota et al. 2013).

Widely used programs in this setting are JSIM (Butterworth et al. 2013) or PMOD (www.pmod.com). The latter was used in a study by Tipre et al., where the kinetics of 6-18F-fluorodopamine and its uptake by cardiac noradrenergic nerves was determined using ROIs in the heart and other organs (Tipre and Goldstein 2005). The generated time–activity curves were analyzed with respect to uptake, retention, as well as loss of tracer and related to the kinetics of [^{13}N]NH_3 in the same individuals.

8.3.5 Dedicated Tools for Kinetic Analysis in Cardiac Imaging

As is true for general kinetic analysis, research applications require a flexibility which is rarely provided by commercials tools. Consequentially, many imaging centers and research groups developed their own tools for internal use, which are perfectly matched for this task, and much dedication, energy, and enthusiasm were invested. However, as their number is large and referencing is not trivial, we will focus only on the more visible ones, either because they are used not only monocentrically and thus gained a certain acceptance in the research community or because a publication related to innervation puts a significant focus on them.

As mentioned above, there are a variety of dedicated, commercial or semicommercial tools for nuclear cardiac imaging available which allow the processing of dynamic data, although the focus is on blood flow quantification. Nevertheless, those tools offer the advantage that a mostly automatic segmentation of the myocardium and the subsequent generation of a series of time–activity curves enable regional analysis and thus replace the concept of manually defined ROI/VOIs. This concept was used in a study by Thackeray where he investigated the myocardial presynaptic sympathetic neuronal integrity in insulin-resistant diabetic rats using [11C]-mHED (Thackeray et al. 2013). The authors were using the tool FlowQuant®, developed by Rob A. deKemp and colleagues at the University of Ottawa Heart Institute in Canada. Just as an aside: this tool was also used in the aforementioned PAREPET trail (Fallavollita et al. 2014). Another cardiac analysis tool is Carimas, developed at the University of Turku, Finland. Even though it was also designed for multi-tracer flow quantification (Nesterov et al. 2009), it is flexible enough to be used with innervation tracers.

The VU University Medical Center in Amsterdam, the Netherlands, is home of Cardiac VUer, also initially developed for the quantification of [^{15}O]-water PET studies in the heart (Harms et al. 2011).

Katoh and colleagues developed HOQUTO, a tool initially dedicated to PET flow quantification (Katoh et al. 2012) which was also used in PET innervation imaging using [^{11}C]-CGP-12177 and a dual-injection protocol (Naya et al. 2009).

We also devolved an analysis environment, MunichHeart, which allows the regional analysis of any cardiac nuclear imaging study (Nekolla et al. 1998). In difference to the other programs mentioned above, we started with metabolism (Haas et al. 2000) and innervation (Bengel et al. 2001) studies before extending into flow quantification (Ibrahim et al. 2002).

8.4 Summary

Without any doubt, innervation imaging with PET is technically and logistically more challenging than using single-photon technology. However, the availability of excellent PET imaging hardware, an increasing number of clinical studies showing both relevance and practicability, and the potential of [^{18}F]-labeled agents make this technology very attractive.

References

Allman KC, Wieland DM, Muzik O, Degrado TR, Wolfe ER Jr, Schwaiger M (1993) Carbon-11 hydroxyephedrine with positron emission tomography for serial assessment of cardiac adrenergic neuronal function after acute myocardial infarction in humans. J Am Coll Cardiol 22:368–375

Bassingthwaighte JB, Butterworth E, Jardine B, Raymond GM (2012) Compartmental modeling in the analysis of biological systems. Methods Mol Biol 929:391–438

Bengel FM, Ueberfuhr P, Nekolla S, Ziegler SI, Reichart B, Schwaiger M (1999) Oxidative metabolism of the transplanted human heart assessed by positron emission tomography using C-11 acetate. Am J Cardiol 83:1503–1505

Bengel FM, Ueberfuhr P, Ziegler SI, Nekolla SG, Odaka K, Reichart B, Schwaiger M (2000) Non-invasive assessment of the effect of cardiac sympathetic innervation on metabolism of the human heart. Eur J Nucl Med 27:1650–1657

Bengel FM, Ueberfuhr P, Schiepel N, Nekolla SG, Reichart B, Schwaiger M (2001) Effect of sympathetic reinnervation on cardiac performance after heart transplantation. N Engl J Med 345:731–738

Boucher L, Rodrigue S, Lecomte R, Benard F (2004) Respiratory gating for 3-dimensional PET of the thorax: feasibility and initial results. J Nucl Med 45:214–219

Brix G, Zaers J, Adam LE, Bellemann ME, Ostertag H, Trojan H, Haberkorn U, Doll J, Oberdorfer F, Lorenz WJ (1997) Performance evaluation of a whole-body PET scanner using the NEMA protocol. National Electrical Manufacturers Association. J Nucl Med 38:1614–1623

Brogsitter C, Gruning T, Weise R, Wielepp P, Lindner O, Korfer R, Burchert W (2005) 18F-FDG PET for detecting myocardial viability: validation of 3D data acquisition. J Nucl Med 46:19–24

Bundschuh RA, Martinez-Moeller A, Essler M, Martinez MJ, Nekolla SG, Ziegler SI, Schwaiger M (2007) Postacquisition detection of tumor motion in the lung and upper abdomen using list-mode PET data: a feasibility study. J Nucl Med 48:758–763

Bundschuh RA, Martinez-Moller A, Essler M, Nekolla SG, Ziegler SI, Schwaiger M (2008) Local motion correction for lung tumours in PET/CT–first results. Eur J Nucl Med Mol Imaging 35:1981–1988

Buther F, Dawood M, Stegger L, Wubbeling F, Schafers M, Schober O, Schafers KP (2009) List mode-driven cardiac and respiratory gating in PET. J Nucl Med 50:674–681

Buther F, Ernst I, Dawood M, Kraxner P, Schafers M, Schober O, Schafers KP (2010) Detection of respiratory tumour motion using intrinsic list mode-driven gating in positron emission tomography. Eur J Nucl Med Mol Imaging 37:2315–2327

Butterworth E, Jardine BE, Raymond GM, Neal ML, Bassingthwaighte JB (2013) JSim, an open-source modeling system for data analysis. F1000Res 2:288

Chen J, Garcia EV, Folks RD, Cooke CD, Faber TL, Tauxe EL, Iskandrian AE (2005) Onset of left ventricular mechanical contraction as determined by phase analysis of ECG-gated myocardial perfusion SPECT imaging: development of a diagnostic tool for assessment of cardiac mechanical dyssynchrony. J Nucl Cardiol 12:687–695 de Jong RM, Willemsen AT, Slart RH, Blanksma PK, van Waarde A, Cornel JH, Vaalburg W, van Veldhuisen DJ, Elsinga PH (2005) Myocardial beta-adrenoceptor downregulation in idiopathic dilated cardiomyopathy measured in vivo with PET using the new radioligand (S)-[11C] CGP12388. Eur J Nucl Med Mol Imaging 32:443–447

DeGrado TR, Hutchins GD, Toorongian SA, Wieland DM, Schwaiger M (1993) Myocardial kinetics of carbon-11-meta-hydroxyephedrine: retention mechanisms and effects of norepinephrine. J Nucl Med 34:1287–1293

Delforge J, Syrota A, Lancon JP, Nakajima K, Loc'h C, Janier M, Vallois JM, Cayla J, Crouzel C (1991) Cardiac beta-adrenergic receptor density measured in vivo using PET, CGP 12177, and a new graphical method. J Nucl Med 32:739–748

Delforge J, Mesangeau D, Dolle F, Merlet P, Loc'h C, Bottlaender M, Trebossen R, Syrota A (2002) In vivo quantification and parametric images of the cardiac beta-adrenergic receptor density. J Nucl Med 43:215–226

Delso G, Martinez-Moller A, Bundschuh RA, Nekolla SG, Ziegler SI, Schwaiger M (2011) Preliminary study of the detectability of coronary plaque with PET. Phys Med Biol 56:2145–2160

DiFilippo FP, Brunken RC (2005) Do implanted pacemaker leads and ICD leads cause metal-related artifact in cardiac PET/CT? J Nucl Med 46:436–443

Doze P, Elsinga PH, van Waarde A, Pieterman RM, Pruim J, Vaalburg W, Willemsen AT (2002) Quantification of beta-adrenoceptor density in the human heart with (S)-[11C]CGP 12388 and a tracer kinetic model. Eur J Nucl Med Mol Imaging 29:295–304

Fallavollita JA, Banas MD, Suzuki G, deKemp RA, Sajjad M, Canty JM Jr (2010) 11C-meta-hydroxyephedrine defects persist despite functional improvement in hibernating myocardium. J Nucl Cardiol 17:85–96

Fallavollita JA, Heavey BM, Luisi AJ Jr, Michalek SM, Baldwa S, Mashtare TL Jr, Hutson AD, Dekemp RA, Haka MS, Sajjad M, Cimato TR, Curtis AB, Cain ME, Canty JM Jr (2014) Regional myocardial sympathetic denervation predicts the risk of sudden cardiac arrest in ischemic cardiomyopathy. J Am Coll Cardiol 63:141–149

Gelfand MJ, Thomas SR (1987) Effective use of computers in nuclear medicine. McGraw-Hill, New York

Gigengack F, Ruthotto L, Burger M, Wolters CH, Jiang X, Schafers KP (2012) Motion correction in dual gated cardiac PET using mass-preserving image registration. IEEE Trans Med Imaging 31:698–712

Haas F, Augustin N, Holper K, Wottke M, Haehnel C, Nekolla S, Meisner H, Lange R, Schwaiger M (2000) Time course and extent of improvement of dysfunctioning myocardium in patients with coronary artery disease and severely depressed left ventricular function after revascularization: correlation with positron emission tomographic findings. J Am Coll Cardiol 36:1927–1934

Halpern BS, Dahlbom M, Quon A, Schiepers C, Waldherr C, Silverman DH, Ratib O, Czernin J (2004a) Impact of patient weight and emission scan duration on PET/CT image quality and lesion detectability. J Nucl Med 45:797–801

Halpern BS, Dahlbom M, Waldherr C, Yap CS, Schiepers C, Silverman DH, Ratib O, Czernin J (2004b) Cardiac pacemakers and central venous lines can induce focal artifacts on CT-corrected PET images. J Nucl Med 45:290–293

Harms HJ, de Haan S, Knaapen P, Allaart CP, Lammertsma AA, Lubberink M (2011) Parametric images of myocardial viability using a single 15O-H2O PET/CT scan. J Nucl Med 52:745–749

Higuchi T, Yousefi BH, Kaiser F, Gartner F, Rischpler C, Reder S, Yu M, Robinson S, Schwaiger M, Nekolla SG (2013) Assessment of the 18F-labeled PET tracer LMI1195 for imaging norepinephrine handling in rat hearts. J Nucl Med 54:1142–1146

Huang SC (2000) Anatomy of SUV. Standardized uptake value. Nucl Med Biol 27:643–646

Humm JL, Rosenfeld A, Del Guerra A (2003) From PET detectors to PET scanners. Eur J Nucl Med Mol Imaging 30:1574–1597

Ibrahim T, Nekolla SG, Schreiber K, Odaka K, Volz S, Mehilli J, Guthlin M, Delius W, Schwaiger M (2002) Assessment of coronary flow reserve: comparison between contrast-enhanced magnetic resonance imaging and positron emission tomography. J Am Coll Cardiol 39:864–870

Jacobson AF, Senior R, Cerqueira MD, Wong ND, Thomas GS, Lopez VA, Agostini D, Weiland F, Chandna H, Narula J, Investigators A-H (2010) Myocardial iodine-123 meta-iodobenzylguanidine imaging and cardiac events in heart failure. Results of the prospective ADMIRE-HF (AdreView Myocardial Imaging for Risk Evaluation in Heart Failure) study. J Am Coll Cardiol 55:2212–2221

Katoh C, Yoshinaga K, Klein R, Kasai K, Tomiyama Y, Manabe O, Naya M, Sakakibara M, Tsutsui H, deKemp RA, Tamaki N (2012) Quantification of regional myocardial blood flow estimation with three-dimensional dynamic rubidium-82 PET and modified spillover correction model. J Nucl Cardiol 19:763–774

Knesaurek K, Machac J, Krynyckyi BR, Almeida OD (2003) Comparison of 2-dimensional and 3-dimensional 82Rb myocardial perfusion PET imaging. J Nucl Med 44:1350–1356

Knesaurek K, Machac J, Ho Kim J (2007) Comparison of 2D, 3D high dose and 3D low dose gated myocardial 82Rb PET imaging. BMC Nucl Med 7:4

Koivumaki T, Vauhkonen M, Kuikka JT, Hakulinen MA (2012) Bioimpedance-based measurement method for simultaneous acquisition of respiratory and cardiac gating signals. Physiol Meas 33:1323–1334

Lartizien C, Kinahan PE, Comtat C (2004) A lesion detection observer study comparing 2-dimensional versus fully 3-dimensional whole-body PET imaging protocols. J Nucl Med 45:714–723

Lehner S, Uebleis C, Schussler F, Haug A, Kaab S, Bartenstein P, Van Kriekinge SD, Germano G, Estner H, Hacker M (2013) The amount of viable and dyssynchronous myocardium is associated with response to cardiac resynchronization therapy: initial clinical results using multiparametric ECG-gated [18F]FDG PET. Eur J Nucl Med Mol Imaging 40:1876–1883

Lekx KS, deKemp RA, Beanlands RS, Wisenberg G, Wells G, Stodilka RZ, Lortie M, Klein R, Zabel P, Kovacs MS, Sykes J, Prato FS (2010) 3D versus 2D dynamic 82Rb myocardial blood flow imaging in a canine model of stunned and infarcted myocardium. Nucl Med Commun 31:75–81

Lewellen TK (2008) Recent developments in PET detector technology. Phys Med Biol 53:R287–R317

Logan J (2000) Graphical analysis of PET data applied to reversible and irreversible tracers. Nucl Med Biol 27:661–670

Magota K, Hattori N, Manabe O, Naya M, Oyama-Manabe N, Shiga T, Kuge Y, Yamada S, Sakakibara M, Yoshinaga K, Tamaki N (2013) Electrocardiographically gated C-hydroxyephedrine PET for the simultaneous assessment of cardiac sympathetic and contractile functions. Ann Nucl Med 28:187–195

Makris NE, Huisman MC, Kinahan PE, Lammertsma AA, Boellaard R (2013) Evaluation of strategies towards harmonization of FDG PET/CT studies in multicentre trials: comparison of scanner validation phantoms and data analysis procedures. Eur J Nucl Med Mol Imaging 40:1507–1515

Marinelli M, Martinez-Moller A, Jensen B, Positano V, Weismuller S, Navab N, Landini L, Schwaiger M, Nekolla SG (2010) Registration of myocardial PET and SPECT for viability assessment using mutual information. Med Phys 37:2414–2424

Martinez MJ, Bercier Y, Schwaiger M, Ziegler SI (2006) PET/CT biograph sensation 16. Performance improvement using faster electronics. Nuklearmedizin 45:126–133

Martinez-Moller A, Souvatzoglou M, Navab N, Schwaiger M, Nekolla SG (2007a) Artifacts from misaligned CT in cardiac perfusion PET/CT studies: frequency, effects, and potential solutions. J Nucl Med 48:188–193

Martinez-Moller A, Zikic D, Botnar RM, Bundschuh RA, Howe W, Ziegler SI, Navab N, Schwaiger M, Nekolla SG (2007b) Dual cardiac-respiratory gated PET: implementation and results from a feasibility study. Eur J Nucl Med Mol Imaging 34:1447–1454

Merlet P, Delforge J, Syrota A, Angevin E, Maziere B, Crouzel C, Valette H, Loisance D, Castaigne A, Rande JL (1993) Positron emission tomography with 11C CGP-12177 to assess beta-adrenergic receptor concentration in idiopathic dilated cardiomyopathy. Circulation 87:1169–1178

Munch G, Nguyen NT, Nekolla S, Ziegler S, Muzik O, Chakraborty P, Wieland DM, Schwaiger M (2000) Evaluation of sympathetic nerve terminals with [(11)C]epinephrine and [(11)C] hydroxyephedrine and positron emission tomography. Circulation 101:516–523

Nakazato R, Dey D, Alexanderson E, Meave A, Jimenez M, Romero E, Jacome R, Pena M, Berman DS, Slomka PJ (2012) Automatic alignment of myocardial perfusion PET and 64-slice coronary CT angiography on hybrid PET/CT. J Nucl Cardiol 19:482–491

Naya M, Tsukamoto T, Morita K, Katoh C, Nishijima K, Komatsu H, Yamada S, Kuge Y, Tamaki N, Tsutsui H (2009) Myocardial beta-adrenergic receptor density assessed by 11C-CGP12177 PET predicts improvement of cardiac function after carvedilol treatment in patients with idiopathic dilated cardiomyopathy. J Nucl Med 50:220–225

Nekolla SG, Miethaner C, Nguyen N, Ziegler SI, Schwaiger M (1998) Reproducibility of polar map generation and assessment of defect severity and extent assessment in myocardial perfusion imaging using positron emission tomography. Eur J Nucl Med 25:1313–1321

Nesterov SV, Han C, Maki M, Kajander S, Naum AG, Helenius H, Lisinen I, Ukkonen H, Pietila M, Joutsiniemi E, Knuuti J (2009) Myocardial perfusion quantitation with 15O-labelled water PET: high reproducibility of the new cardiac analysis software (Carimas). Eur J Nucl Med Mol Imaging 36:1594–1602

Nguyen NT, DeGrado TR, Chakraborty P, Wieland DM, Schwaiger M (1997) Myocardial kinetics of carbon-11-epinephrine in the isolated working rat heart. J Nucl Med 38:780–785

Odaka K, von Scheidt W, Ziegler SI, Ueberfuhr P, Nekolla SG, Reichart B, Bengel FM, Schwaiger M (2001) Reappearance of cardiac presynaptic sympathetic nerve terminals in the transplanted heart: correlation between PET using (11)C-hydroxyephedrine and invasively measured norepinephrine release. J Nucl Med 42:1011–1016

Orlhac F, Soussan M, Maisonobe JA, Garcia CA, Vanderlinden B, Buvat I (2014) Tumor texture analysis in 18F-FDG PET: relationships between texture parameters, histogram indices, standardized uptake values, metabolic volumes, and total lesion glycolysis. J Nucl Med 55:414–422

Parodi O, Schelbert HR, Schwaiger M, Hansen H, Selin C, Hoffman EJ (1984) Cardiac emission computed-tomography – underestimation of regional tracer concentrations due to wall motion abnormalities. J Comput Assist Tomogr 8:1083–1092

Raffel DM, Corbett JR, del Rosario RB, Gildersleeve DL, Chiao PC, Schwaiger M, Wieland DM (1996) Clinical evaluation of carbon-11-phenylephrine: MAO-sensitive marker of cardiac sympathetic neurons. J Nucl Med 37:1923–1931

Raffel DM, Corbett JR, del Rosario RB, Mukhopadhyay SK, Gildersleeve DL, Rose P, Wieland DM (1999) Sensitivity of [11C]phenylephrine kinetics to monoamine oxidase activity in normal human heart. J Nucl Med 40:232–238

Raffel DM, Chen W, Jung YW, Jang KS, Gu G, Cozzi NV (2013a) Radiotracers for cardiac sympathetic innervation: transport kinetics and binding affinities for the human norepinephrine transporter. Nucl Med Biol 40:331–337

Raffel DM, Koeppe RA, Jung YW, Gu G, Jang KS, Sherman PS, Quesada CA (2013b) Quantification of cardiac sympathetic nerve density with N-11C-guanyl-meta-octopamine and tracer kinetic analysis. J Nucl Med 54:1645–1652

Raylman RR, Caraher JM, Hutchins GD (1993) Sampling requirements for dynamic cardiac PET studies using image-derived input functions. J Nucl Med 34:440–447

Rosenspire KC, Haka MS, Van Dort ME, Jewett DM, Gildersleeve DL, Schwaiger M, Wieland DM (1990) Synthesis and preliminary evaluation of carbon-11-meta-hydroxyephedrine: a false transmitter agent for heart neuronal imaging. J Nucl Med 31:1328–1334

Saraste A, Kajander S, Han C, Nesterov SV, Knuuti J (2012) PET: is myocardial flow quantification a clinical reality? J Nucl Cardiol 19:1044–1059

Sasano T, Abraham MR, Chang KC, Ashikaga H, Mills KJ, Holt DP, Hilton J, Nekolla SG, Dong J, Lardo AC, Halperin H, Dannals RF, Marban E, Bengel FM (2008) Abnormal sympathetic innervation of viable myocardium and the substrate of ventricular tachycardia after myocardial infarction. J Am Coll Cardiol 51:2266–2275

Schepis T, Gaemperli O, Treyer V, Valenta I, Burger C, Koepfli P, Namdar M, Adachi I, Alkadhi H, Kaufmann PA (2007) Absolute quantification of myocardial blood flow with 13N-ammonia and 3-dimensional PET. J Nucl Med 48:1783–1789

Schmidt KC, Turkheimer FE (2002) Kinetic modeling in positron emission tomography. Q J Nucl Med 46:70–85

Schwaiger M, Ziegler S, Nekolla SG (2005) PET/CT: challenge for nuclear cardiology. J Nucl Med 46:1664–1678

Slomka PJ, Baum RP (2009) Multimodality image registration with software: state-of-the-art. Eur J Nucl Med Mol Imaging 36(Suppl 1):S44–S55

Souvatzoglou M, Bengel F, Busch R, Kruschke C, Fernolendt H, Lee D, Schwaiger M, Nekolla SG (2007) Attenuation correction in cardiac PET/CT with three different CT protocols: a comparison with conventional PET. Eur J Nucl Med Mol Imaging 34:1991–2000

Tahari AK, Lee A, Rajaram M, Fukushima K, Lodge MA, Lee BC, Ficaro EP, Nekolla S, Klein R, deKemp RA, Wahl RL, Bengel FM, Bravo PE (2014) Absolute myocardial flow quantification with (82)Rb PET/CT: comparison of different software packages and methods. Eur J Nucl Med Mol Imaging 41:126–135

Thackeray JT, Bengel FM (2013) Assessment of cardiac autonomic neuronal function using PET imaging. J Nucl Cardiol 20:150–165

Thackeray JT, deKemp RA, Beanlands RS, DaSilva JN (2013) Insulin restores myocardial presynaptic sympathetic neuronal integrity in insulin-resistant diabetic rats. J Nucl Cardiol 20:845–856

Tipre DN, Goldstein DS (2005) Cardiac and extracardiac sympathetic denervation in Parkinson's disease with orthostatic hypotension and in pure autonomic failure. J Nucl Med 46:1775–1781

Townsend DW, Cherry SR (2001) Combining anatomy and function: the path to true image fusion. Eur Radiol 11:1968–1974

van Elmpt W, Hamill J, Jones J, De Ruysscher D, Lambin P, Ollers M (2011) Optimal gating compared to 3D and 4D PET reconstruction for characterization of lung tumours. Eur J Nucl Med Mol Imaging 38:843–855

Visser EP, Boerman OC, Oyen WJ (2010) SUV: from silly useless value to smart uptake value. J Nucl Med 51:173–175

Wen L, Eberl S, Fulham M, Feng DD (2012) Recent software developments and applications in functional imaging. Curr Pharm Biotechnol 13:2166–2181

Willemsen AT, van den Hoff J (2002) Fundamentals of quantitative PET data analysis. Curr Pharm Des 8:1513–1526

Yalamanchili P, Wexler E, Hayes M, Yu M, Bozek J, Kagan M, Radeke HS, Azure M, Purohit A, Casebier DS, Robinson SP (2007) Mechanism of uptake and retention of F-18 BMS-747158-02 in cardiomyocytes: a novel PET myocardial imaging agent. J Nucl Cardiol 14:782–788

Yoshida K, Endo M, Fukuda H, Kagaya A, Himi T, Masuda Y, Inagaki Y, Iinuma T, Yamasaki T, Tateno Y (1995) Measurement of arterial tracer concentrations from cardiac PET images. J Comput Assist Tomogr 19:182–187

Yu M, Bozek J, Lamoy M, Guaraldi M, Silva P, Kagan M, Yalamanchili P, Onthank D, Mistry M, Lazewatsky J, Broekema M, Radeke H, Purohit A, Cdebaca M, Azure M, Cesati R, Casebier D, Robinson SP (2011) Evaluation of LMI1195, a novel 18F-labeled cardiac neuronal PET imaging agent, in cells and animal models. Circ Cardiovasc Imaging 4:435–443

Yu M, Bozek J, Lamoy M, Kagan M, Benites P, Onthank D, Robinson SP (2012) LMI1195 PET imaging in evaluation of regional cardiac sympathetic denervation and its potential role in antiarrhythmic drug treatment. Eur J Nucl Med Mol Imaging 39:1910–1919

General Principles of [^{123}I]-MIBG Scintigraphy for the Assessment of the Cardiac Sympathetic Activity: From Planar to SPECT

9

Hein J. Verberne and Arthur J.H.A. Scholte

Contents

Abstract

In patients with heart failure, increased sympathetic activity and cardiac sympathetic dysfunction are present and are related to an unfavorable outcome. In recent years, large-scale clinical trials have documented the benefits of pharmacological therapies aimed at limiting left ventricular remodeling and even reversing this process. These beneficial effects were associated with an increase in

H.J. Verberne, MD, PhD (✉)
Department of Nuclear Medicine, Academic Medical Center, University of Amsterdam, F2-238, 22700, Amsterdam 1100 DE, The Netherlands
e-mail: h.j.verberne@amc.uva.nl

A.J.H.A. Scholte, MD, PhD
Department of Cardiology, Leiden University Medical Center, University of Leiden, Leiden, The Netherlands

R.H.J.A. Slart et al. (eds.), *Autonomic Innervation of the Heart: Role of Molecular Imaging*, DOI 10.1007/978-3-662-45074-1_9

myocardial uptake of [^{123}I]-metaiodobenzylguanidine (MIBG), a radiolabeled norepinephrine analog. However, despite the large number of published studies on cardiac [^{123}I]-MIBG imaging, methodological and analytical limitations have interfered with the unequivocal interpretation of the imaging data. In this chapter, the assessment of myocardial sympathetic innervation with [^{123}I]-MIBG is discussed with emphasis on patient preparation, image acquisition, and analysis. Special attention is given to overcoming the aforementioned possible methodological and analytical limitations. In conclusion, improving the standardization and validation of [^{123}I]-MIBG myocardial scintigraphy and thus reducing variations in obtained results will lead to much more accepted application of the findings to clinical patient management.

Abbreviations

CHF	Chronic heart failure
DAT	Dopamine transporter
EANM	European Association of Nuclear Medicine
EMT	Extraneuronal monoamine transporters
H/M ratio	Heart-to-mediastinum ratio
ICD	Implantable cardioverter defibrillator
JCS	Japanese Circulation Society
JSNM	Japanese Society of Nuclear Medicine
LE	Low energy
LEHR	Low energy, high resolution
ME	Medium energy
MIBG	Metaiodobenzylguanidine
NET	Norepinephrine transporter
OCT	Organic cation transporters
ROI(s)	Region(s) of interest
SCD	Sudden cardiac death
SLC	Solute carrier transporters
SPECT	Single-photon emission computed tomography

9.1 Sympathetic Innervation

The sympathetic nervous system is one of the neurohormonal compensation mechanisms that play a key role in the pathogenesis of heart failure. The cardiac autonomic nervous system consists of two distinct and counter acting forms: sympathetic and parasympathetic innervation. They differ in their major neurotransmitters, norepinephrine, and acetylcholine and exert stimulating or inhibitory effects on target tissues via adrenergic and muscarinic receptors. Both are responsible for electrophysiologic and hemodynamic adaptation of the cardiovascular system to changing demands.

9.1.1 Uptake-1 and Uptake-2

The reuptake of catecholamines from the synaptic cleft is mediated by high-affinity, low-capacity, sodium chloride-dependent transporters present in the outer membrane of the presynaptic nerve endings. This transport system is also known as the uptake-1 mechanism and consists of the norepinephrine transporter (NET) and the dopamine transporter (DAT). In addition to NET, catecholamines are removed from the circulation by a second transport system. This second transport system (i.e., uptake-2) consists of sodium chloride-independent, corticosterone-sensitive, high-capacity extraneuronal monoamine transporters (EMT) (Iversen 1965). Molecular cloning has shown that NET and uptake-2 belong to two different families of transporters. The presynaptic neuronal transporters for norepinephrine and dopamine are both members of the solute carrier family of transporters (SLC6A2 and SLC6A3, respectively) (Chen et al. 2004). Uptake-2 belongs to another subgroup of the SLC transporters (SLC22) and can be placed in the family of organic cation transporters (OCT), which has several members (OCT1, OCT2, and OCT3 or SLC22A1, SLC22A2, and SLC22A, respectively) (Koepsell and Endou 2004). The classical uptake-2 or EMT is most likely to be represented by OCT3 and comes to expression in different organs (i.e., heart, liver, skeletal muscle, placenta, and kidney) (Grundemann et al. 1998; Wu et al. 1998). The OCTs are involved in the absorption, distribution, and elimination of endogenous compounds (i.e., amines) as well as of drugs, toxins, and other xenobiotics (Burckhardt and Wolff 2000; Eisenhofer 2001). Neuronal reuptake by NET is quantitatively most important for the clearance of released catecholamines, accounting for about 90 % of their removal at the presynaptic nerve endings. Although OCT3 has been proposed to be the classical EMT, the three OCTs together are thought to be responsible for the extraneuronal clearance of catecholamines that have escaped from reuptake by NET (Eisenhofer 2001). In general, NET and uptake-2 mechanisms are thought to have similar functions between species. However, small differences in the relative expression of these mechanisms between species have been reported. Due to these differences in distribution (i.e., expression) of uptake mechanisms, results found in experimental animal studies may not exactly reflect the situation in humans.

9.2 From Guanethidine to Metaiodobenzylguanidine

9.2.1 Guanethidine

In the 1960s, guanethidine, a false neurotransmitter, was found to be a sympathetic selective and potent neuron blocking agent and was developed as an antihypertension drug (Short and Darby 1967). Guanethidine acts on the presynaptic sympathetic nerve ending by inhibiting or interfering with the release and/or distribution of norepinephrine, rather than acting on the postsynaptic (i.e., effector cell) by inhibiting the association of norepinephrine with its receptors. In contrast to ganglionic blocking agents, guanethidine suppresses equally the responses mediated by α- and β-adrenergic receptors, but does not produce parasympathetic blockade.

9.2.2 MIBG

The modification of guanethidine into metaiodobenzylguanidine (MIBG) increased the affinity for the presynaptic sympathetic nerve endings (Patel and Iskandrian 2002; Sisson et al. 1987a; Wafelman et al. 1994). The labeling of MIBG with radioactive iodine enabled scintigraphic visualization of the presynaptic sympathetic nerve endings in humans. The first clinical application of the radiolabeled [^{131}I]-MIBG was the visualization of the adrenal medulla and different neural crest-derived tumors such as pheochromocytomas and neuroblastomas (Sisson et al. 1981; Wieland et al. 1980). The striking myocardial uptake, however, made Wieland et al. suggest the potential use of the radiolabeled MIBG for myocardial imaging (Wieland et al. 1980). However, due to the suboptimal imaging characteristics of [^{131}I] and a less favorable radiation burden, radiolabeling of MIBG with [^{123}I] for diagnostic scintigraphic purposes was to be preferred. In 1981 Kline et al. were one of the first to report on the use of myocardial scintigraphy with [^{123}I]-MIBG in five healthy subjects. They concluded that [^{123}I]-MIBG had the potential to provide (semi-) quantitative information on myocardial catecholamine content (Kline et al. 1981).

Much work has been done to elucidate the uptake mechanisms of MIBG in the presynaptic sympathetic nerve endings. MIBG localizes in adrenergic nerve terminals primarily via the NET (see uptake-1 and uptake-2). The affinity (K_m, affinity constant) and capacity (V_m, capacity constant) of the NET for MIBG are similar to those for norepinephrine (K_m of 1.22 ± 0.12 μ*M* for MIBG and 1.41 ± 0.12 μ*M* for norepinephrine, V_m of 64.3 ± 3.3 pmol/10^6 cells/10 min for MIBG and 36.6 ± 7.2 pmol/10^6 cells/10 min for norepinephrine) (Jaques et al. 1984). NET predominates at low concentrations of both catecholamines and MIBG, whereas uptake-2 predominates at higher concentrations (DeGrado et al. 1995). It is therefore to be expected that MIBG administered in tracer amounts will primarily reflect NET activity. Blocking experiments, however, have shown that uptake-2 is responsible for up to 61 % of cardiac MIBG uptake (Dae et al. 1989; Fagret et al. 1993; Rabinovitch et al. 1993; Sisson et al. 1987a, b).

9.3 [^{123}I]-MIBG Myocardial Scintigraphy

In the past two decades, a large number of investigators have demonstrated decreased myocardial [^{123}I]-MIBG uptake in chronic heart failure (CHF) patients and have shown that those with the lowest uptake tend to have the poorest prognosis (Agostini et al. 2008; Jacobson et al. 2010; Verberne et al. 2008). There have also been findings suggesting that abnormalities of myocardial [^{123}I]-MIBG uptake may be predictive of increased risk for ventricular arrhythmia and sudden cardiac death (SCD) and implantable cardioverter defibrillator (ICD) discharge (Arora et al. 2003; Boogers et al. 2010; Paul et al. 2006). One factor that has constrained acceptance of cardiac [^{123}I]-MIBG imaging as a clinical management tool in heart failure has been the variability of technical aspects of the procedure. Although most publications have included the heart-to-mediastinum ratio (H/M) as the measure of myocardial uptake, the methods used to obtain this parameter show considerable variation.

9.3.1 Patient Preparation and Radiation Burden

Data obtained in patients with neuroendocrine tumors have shown that there are several drugs that may or are known to interfere with organ MIBG uptake. In addition drugs that are regarded as standard of care in patients with heart failure, beta-blockers, angiotensin-converting enzyme inhibitors, and/or angiotensin receptor blockers, known to ameliorate functional capacity and prognosis, change (i.e., improve) cardiac [^{123}I]-MIBG uptake. These drugs may therefore influence the outcome of the cardiac [^{123}I]-MIBG scan. It would therefore preferable to temporarily discontinue these drugs. Nevertheless, in patients with heart failure, it is currently regarded unethical to temporarily discontinue these drugs. In contrast and probably more importantly, many studies have demonstrated that cardiac [^{123}I]-MIBG imaging can be performed in patients with optimum medical therapy including beta-blockers, angiotensin-converting enzyme inhibitors, and/or angiotensin receptor blockers. More importantly, these studies showed that cardiac [^{123}I]-MIBG semi-quantitative uptake parameters were able to discriminate between those patients with a poor prognosis and those with a relative preserved prognosis despite the use of possible [^{123}I]-MIBG myocardial uptake interfering drugs (Jacobson et al. 2010; Verberne et al. 2008). Therefore, there is no need to withdraw such medication prior to cardiac [^{123}I]-MIBG imaging. In addition, it might be of importance to stop food containing vanillin and catecholamine-like compounds (e.g., chocolate and blue cheese) since some of these may interfere with the uptake of MIBG (depletion of granules) (Solanki et al. 1992; Wafelman et al. 1994).

The effective dose of [^{123}I]-MIBG is estimated to be 0.013 mSv/MBq (ICRP 1987). This allows for an administered dosage between 185 and 370 MBq of [^{123}I]-MIBG (i.e., 2.4–4.8 mSv). To keep the radiation burden for patients as low as reasonably possible and because [^{123}I]-MIBG is primarily secreted via the kidneys, patients are encouraged to void frequently to facilitate rapid excretion of the radiopharmaceutical. In patients with severe renal impairment, the absorbed radiation dose may be increased and the quality of images decreased due to the delayed elimination of the radiopharmaceutical. In patients with severe renal impairment, cardiac [^{123}I]-MIBG uptake may be impaired. However, Verschure et al. showed that the variability in the semiquantitative [^{123}I]-MIBG myocardial parameters could not be explained by estimates of renal function. Therefore, within the time frame of [^{123}I]-MIBG cardiac imaging (up to 4 h after injection), the semiquantitative [^{123}I]-MIBG myocardial parameters are independent of renal function

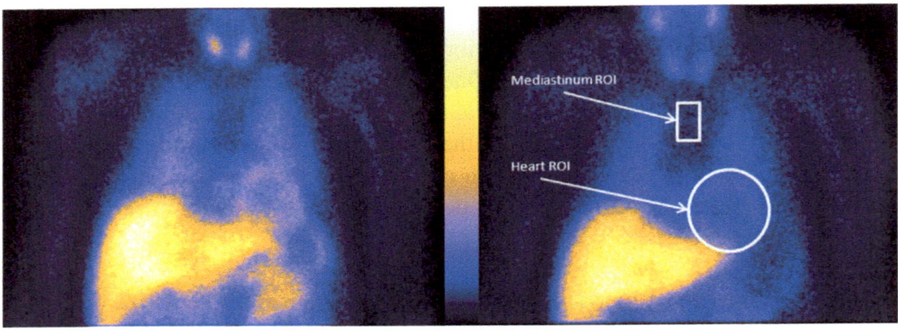

Fig. 9.1 Heart-to-mediastinum ratio quantification of [^{123}I]-MIBG

(Verschure et al. 2012). These findings are in line with a recent publication showing that differences in the rate of renal excretion did not contribute to variability in mediastinal and myocardial counts between early and late planar [^{123}I]-MIBG images (Verberne et al. 2011). This is eminent for clinical practice as renal dysfunction is often present in CHF patients (Aaronson et al. 1997; Flack et al. 1993).

9.3.2 General Procedure for Planar [^{123}I]-MIBG Scintigraphy

In order to block thyroid uptake of free radioactive iodide, either 500 mg potassium perchlorate or 200 mg potassium iodide (10 % solution) is orally administered. Thirty minutes later, approximately 185–370 MBq of [^{123}I]-MIBG is administered intravenously. [^{123}I]-MIBG is internalized by presynaptic nerve endings of postganglionic neuronal cells through the energy-dependent NET. A 15 % energy window is usually used, centered on the 159-keV [^{123}I] photopeak. Anterior planar scintigraphic images are obtained 15 min (early) and 4 h (late) after injection and stored in 128 × 128 or 256 × 256 matrixes.

9.3.3 Semiquantitative Parameters

The commonly used myocardial [^{123}I]-MIBG indices are the heart-to-mediastinum ratio (H/M ratio) and myocardial washout. On anterior planar images, regions of interest (ROIs) are drawn over the heart (H) and the mediastinum (M) (Fig. 9.1). The mean count density (i.e., average counts per ROI) in each ROI is obtained, and the H/M ratio (specific activity/nonspecific activity) is calculated. Myocardial [^{123}I]-MIBG washout is calculated as the difference between the early and late H/M and expressed as a percentage of the early H/M. Another possibility to calculate myocardial [^{123}I]-MIBG washout is to correlate the actual myocardial counts:

$$\left\{\frac{early\,H\,/\,M - late\,H\,/\,M\,*}{early\,H\,/\,M}\right\}\times 100\%$$

$$\left\{\frac{early\,H - late\,H\,*}{early\,H}\right\}\times 100\%$$

$$\left\{\frac{(early\,H - early\,M) - (late\,H - late\,M)\,*}{(early\,H - early\,M)}\right\}\times 100\%$$

* Denotes that the average counts need to be corrected for decay to the moment of the early acquisition.

The early H/M probably reflects the integrity of presynaptic nerve terminals and NET function. The late H/M combines information on neuronal function from uptake to release through the storage vesicle at the nerve terminals. Myocardial [^{123}I]-MIBG washout is an index of the degree of sympathetic drive. This implies that increased sympathetic activity is associated with high myocardial [^{123}I]-MIBG washout and low myocardial [^{123}I]-MIBG delayed uptake.

9.3.4 Impact of ROI Definition

For [^{123}I]-MIBG, there are several ways to define the mediastinal (size and placement) and myocardial ROIs (i.e., myocardium including the left ventricular cavity vs. myocardium excluding the left ventricular cavity). However, there are limited data on the impact of ROI definition on H/M ratios and myocardial washout. Somsen et al. demonstrated in 25 healthy volunteers that [^{123}I]-MIBG semiquantitative parameters using an ROI of the myocardium including the left ventricle showed the lowest interindividual and within-subject variability (Somsen et al. 1996). In a large retrospective study, a uniform analysis with clear definition of the myocardial ROI (variable in size, including the left ventricular cavity) and the mediastinal ROI (fixed size) showed remarkable consistency in interpretation between three blinded image evaluators (Agostini et al. 2008). These findings were corroborated by Veltman et al. in a population of 70 patients with heart failure showing an excellent intra- and interobserver agreement irrespective of the level of experience of the observer. Furthermore, even in patients with a very low late H/M ratio (i.e., $\leq$1.4), the late H/M ratio measurements remained excellent (Veltman et al. 2012). These findings suggest that rigorous and uniform analysis of cardiac [^{123}I]-MIBG semiquantitative parameters minimizes inter- and intraindividual variation. Furthermore, the variation in the assessment of the semiquantitative parameters is relatively uninfluenced by the level of experience of the observer and the disease state of the patient.

9.3.5 Influence of Collimation

The most well-validated influence on the measured late H/M is the collimator type. In addition to the prime emission of 159-keV photons, [^{123}I] emits high-energy photons of more than 400 keV (approximately 2.87 %, main contributor 529 keV (1.28 %)). These high-energy photons lead to penetration of the collimator septa and cause scatter detected in the 159-keV energy window. Septal penetration affects estimation of the H/M ratio in [^{123}I]-MIBG imaging with a low-energy (LE) collimator (Verberne et al. 2005). Regardless, LE collimators are frequently used for imaging [^{123}I]-MIBG (Dobbeleir et al. 1999; Verberne et al. 2008). Medium-energy (ME) collimators have been shown to improve quantitative accuracy in [^{123}I] studies (Dobbeleir et al. 1999; Inoue et al. 2003; Verberne et al. 2005). Therefore, in order to minimize the effects of septal penetration, the ME collimator is preferred. However, the use of ME collimation provides relatively low spatial resolution which may hamper accurate estimation of activity in small regions through a partial volume effect. In brain SPECT imaging with [^{123}I]-labeled agents, collimation with low energy, high resolution (LEHR) is preferred, because high spatial resolution is required, the head and brain tissue lead to a more or less homogeneous scatter, and the regions are mostly equidistant from the gamma camera. In cardiac scintigraphy with [^{123}I]-labeled agents, however, H/M ratios are assessed from counts in relatively large regions, the thorax and abdomen lead to an inhomogeneous scatter, and the myocardium is not equidistant from the gamma camera, especially for SPECT imaging. In cardiac scintigraphy with [^{123}I]-labeled agents, the trade-off between spatial resolution and septal penetration is therefore in favor of low septal penetration. Moreover, as shown by Inoue et al. in a checker phantom, the use of ME collimation in cardiac scintigraphy with [^{123}I] showed contrast accuracy similar to [^{99m}Tc] (Inoue et al. 2003).

While these results would suggest that semiquantitative cardiac [^{123}I]-MIBG imaging might be best performed using ME collimators, there are practical limitations to such a recommendation. Almost all nuclear medicine procedures are now performed on a multi-head gamma camera, and many dedicated dual-head cardiac cameras are not supplied with ME collimators. Despite these considerations, the use of ME collimation in cardiac scintigraphy with [^{123}I] is advocated.

9.3.6 SPECT: Assessment of Regional Cardiac [^{123}I]-MIBG Distribution

Most of the published data on cardiac [^{123}I]-MIBG scintigraphy are related to planar imaging. Although planar imaging seems to be able to discriminate patients who tend to have a poor prognosis from those patients with a relatively good prognosis, information on regional cardiac [^{123}I]-MIBG distribution might even further improve this discrimination. However, only a limited amount of data on cardiac SPECT is available.

SPECT images can be acquired by a single pass of 60 steps at 30 s per step (64×64 matrix), starting at 45° right anterior oblique projection and proceeding anticlockwise to the 45° left posterior oblique projection. The data are reconstructed in short-axis, horizontal long-axis, and vertical long-axis tomograms, and scatter or attenuation correction may be applied. The majority of published studies performed SPECT only 3–4 h after [^{123}I]-MIBG (i.e., late SPECT).

When regional MIBG distribution was observed, factors of physical characteristics of [^{123}I], pharmaceutical dynamics, and relative count distribution in liver, heart, and lungs are related. MIBG distribution in the SPECT study is similar to that of perfusion imaging tracers, but the inferior accumulation is relatively lower in an MIBG study, in particular for aged persons. The Japanese Society of Nuclear Medicine (JSNM) working group for standardization of myocardial SPECT accumulated cardiac [^{123}I]-MIBG data from near-normal subjects. No history of cardiac diseases and subjects with hypertension and diabetes mellitus that required medication were excluded. A characteristic finding of these images (late SPECT) was that the inferior wall had a relatively lower activity, however with a considerable variation in [^{123}I]-MIBG uptake (Matsuo et al. 2009). The heterogeneity of the cardiac [^{123}I]-MIBG distribution is probably not explained as an artifact (i.e., attenuation artifact or reconstruction artifact due to high liver uptake) but is most likely a reflection of variation in physiology (Morozumi et al. 1997). There is data to support this variation in physiology showing that the anterior wall has predominantly sympathetic afferent innervation (Geis and Kaye 1968). However, Minisi et al. showed that sympathetic afferent nerves were equally distributed to the inferoposterior and anterior myocardial wall (Minisi and Thames 1993).

Regional myocardial uptake of [^{123}I]-MIBG can be influenced by underlying diseases and/or medication (see section patient preparation). In patient with myocardial ischemia or a previous myocardial infarction, there can be regional absence of [^{123}I]-MIBG uptake in the area of ischemia or infarct. The interpretation of the cardiac [^{123}I]-MIBG (SPECT) results should therefore always be done in combination with all relevant patient characteristics. In addition the interpretation should be performed, with knowledge of normal variants and potential artifacts.

9.4 Procedure Guidelines

Despite that several studies have shown the prognostic value of semiquantitative parameters of myocardial [^{123}I]-MIBG uptake in patients with CHF, there is no consensus (Cohen-Solal et al. 1999; Kasama et al. 2002; Kyuma et al. 2004; Merlet et al. 1992, 1999; Momose et al. 1999; Nakata et al. 2005; Wakabayashi et al. 2001; Yamada et al. 2003). The lack of consensus is reflected in the absence of [^{123}I]-MIBG in any of the current guidelines regarding heart failure (Bonow et al. 2005; Hunt 2005; Nieminen et al. 2005; Radford et al. 2005; Swedberg et al. 2005). However, recently published guidelines for clinical use of cardiac nuclear medicine of the Japanese Circulation Society (JCS) Joint Working Group state that there is a class I recommendation for the use [^{123}I]-MIBG for the assessment of severity and prognosis of heart failure (JCS Joint Working Group 2012).

Recently a proposal for standardization of [^{123}I]-MIBG cardiac sympathetic imaging has been published by the European Association of Nuclear Medicine (EANM) Cardiovascular Committee and the European Council of Nuclear Cardiology (Flotats et al. 2010). This will further the standardization of procedures for cardiac [^{123}I]-MIBG imaging among individual users and thereby reduce variation in results and increase clinical acceptability and implementation. Given the current data, myocardial [^{123}I]-MIBG planar scintigraphy is preferred with ME collimation without scatter correction, adequate acquisition duration (at least 10 min), and simple but robust analysis of the semiquantitative parameters.

References

Aaronson KD, Schwartz JS, Chen TM et al (1997) Development and prospective validation of a clinical index to predict survival in ambulatory patients referred for cardiac transplant evaluation. Circulation 95:2660–2667

Agostini D, Verberne HJ, Burchert W et al (2008) I-123- m IBG myocardial imaging for assessment of risk for a major cardiac event in heart failure patients: insights from a retrospective European multicenter study. Eur J Nucl Med Mol Imaging 35:535–546

Arora R, Ferrick KJ, Nakata T et al (2003) I-123 MIBG imaging and heart rate variability analysis to predict the need for an implantable cardioverter defibrillator. J Nucl Cardiol 10:121–131

Bonow RO, Bennett S, Casey DE Jr et al (2005) ACC/AHA clinical performance measures for adults with chronic heart failure: a report of the American College of Cardiology/American Heart Association Task Force on Performance Measures (Writing Committee to Develop Heart Failure Clinical Performance Measures) endorsed by the Heart Failure Society of America. J Am Coll Cardiol 46:1144–1178

Boogers MJ, Borleffs CJ, Henneman MM et al (2010) Cardiac sympathetic denervation assessed with 123-iodine metaiodobenzylguanidine imaging predicts ventricular arrhythmias in implantable cardioverter-defibrillator patients. J Am Coll Cardiol 55:2769–2777

Burckhardt G, Wolff NA (2000) Structure of renal organic anion and cation transporters. Am J Physiol Renal Physiol 278:F853–F866

Chen NH, Reith ME, Quick MW (2004) Synaptic uptake and beyond: the sodium- and chloride-dependent neurotransmitter transporter family SLC6. Pflugers Arch 447:519–531

Cohen-Solal A, Esanu Y, Logeart D et al (1999) Cardiac metaiodobenzylguanidine uptake in patients with moderate chronic heart failure: relationship with peak oxygen uptake and prognosis. J Am Coll Cardiol 33:759–766

Dae MW, O'Connell JW, Botvinick EH et al (1989) Scintigraphic assessment of regional cardiac adrenergic innervation. Circulation 79:634–644

DeGrado TR, Zalutsky MR, Vaidyanathan G (1995) Uptake mechanisms of meta-[123I]iodobenzylguanidine in isolated rat heart. Nucl Med Biol 22:1–12

Dobbeleir AA, Hambye AS, Franken PR (1999) Influence of high-energy photons on the spectrum of iodine-123 with low- and medium-energy collimators: consequences for imaging with 123I-labelled compounds in clinical practice. Eur J Nucl Med 26:655–658

Eisenhofer G (2001) The role of neuronal and extraneuronal plasma membrane transporters in the inactivation of peripheral catecholamines. Pharmacol Ther 91:35–62

Fagret D, Wolf JE, Vanzetto G et al (1993) Myocardial uptake of metaiodobenzylguanidine in patients with left ventricular hypertrophy secondary to valvular aortic stenosis. J Nucl Med 34:57–60

Flack JM, Neaton JD, Daniels B et al (1993) Ethnicity and renal disease: lessons from the Multiple Risk Factor Intervention Trial and the Treatment of Mild Hypertension Study. Am J Kidney Dis 21:31–40

Flotats A, Carrio I, Agostini D et al (2010) Proposal for standardization of 123I-metaiodobenzylguanidine (MIBG) cardiac sympathetic imaging by the EANM Cardiovascular Committee and the European Council of Nuclear Cardiology. Eur J Nucl Med Mol Imaging 37:1802–1812

Geis WP, Kaye MP (1968) Distribution of sympathetic fibers in the left ventricular epicardial plexus of the dog. Circ Res 23:165–170

Grundemann D, Schechinger B, Rappold GA et al (1998) Molecular identification of the corticosterone-sensitive extraneuronal catecholamine transporter. Nat Neurosci 1:349–351

Hunt SA (2005) ACC/AHA 2005 guideline update for the diagnosis and management of chronic heart failure in the adult: a report of the American College of Cardiology/American Heart Association Task Force on Practice Guidelines (Writing Committee to Update the 2001 Guidelines for the Evaluation and Management of Heart Failure). J Am Coll Cardiol 46:e1–e82

ICRP (1987) Radiation dose to patients from radiopharmaceuticals. A report of a Task Group of Committee 2 of the International Commission on Radiological Protection. Ann ICRP 18:1–377

Inoue Y, Suzuki A, Shirouzu I et al (2003) Effect of collimator choice on quantitative assessment of cardiac iodine 123 MIBG uptake. J Nucl Cardiol 10:623–632

Iversen LL (1965) The uptake of catecholamines at high perfusion concentrations in the rat isolated heart: a novel catecholamine uptake process. Br J Pharmac Chemother 25:18–33

Jacobson AF, Senior R, Cerqueira MD et al (2010) Myocardial iodine-123 meta-iodobenzylguanidine imaging and cardiac events in heart failure results of the prospective ADMIRE-HF (AdreView Myocardial Imaging for Risk Evaluation in Heart Failure) study. J Am Coll Cardiol 55:2212–2221

Jaques S Jr, Tobes MC, Sisson JC et al (1984) Comparison of the sodium dependency of uptake of meta-lodobenzylguanidine and norepinephrine into cultured bovine adrenomedullary cells. Mol Pharmacol 26:539–546

JCS Joint Working Group (2012) Guidelines for clinical use of cardiac nuclear medicine (JCS 2010). Circ J 76:761–767

Kasama S, Toyama T, Kumakura H et al (2002) Spironolactone improves cardiac sympathetic nerve activity and symptoms in patients with congestive heart failure. J Nucl Med 43:1279–1285

Kline RC, Swanson DP, Wieland DM et al (1981) Myocardial imaging in man with I-123 meta-iodobenzylguanidine. J Nucl Med 22:129–132

Koepsell H, Endou H (2004) The SLC22 drug transporter family. Pflugers Arch 447:666–676

Kyuma M, Nakata T, Hashimoto A et al (2004) Incremental prognostic implications of brain natriuretic peptide, cardiac sympathetic nerve innervation, and noncardiac disorders in patients with heart failure. J Nucl Med 45:155–163

Matsuo S, Nakajima K, Yamashina S et al (2009) Characterization of Japanese standards for myocardial sympathetic and metabolic imaging in comparison with perfusion imaging. Ann Nucl Med 23:517–522

Merlet P, Valette H, Dubois-Rande JL et al (1992) Prognostic value of cardiac metaiodobenzylguanidine imaging in patients with heart failure. J Nucl Med 33:471–477

Merlet P, Benvenuti C, Moyse D et al (1999) Prognostic value of MIBG imaging in idiopathic dilated cardiomyopathy. J Nucl Med 40:917–923

Minisi AJ, Thames MD (1993) Distribution of left ventricular sympathetic afferents demonstrated by reflex responses to transmural myocardial ischemia and to intracoronary and epicardial bradykinin. Circulation 87:240–246

Momose M, Kobayashi H, Iguchi N et al (1999) Comparison of parameters of 123I-MIBG scintigraphy for predicting prognosis in patients with dilated cardiomyopathy. Nucl Med Commun 20:529–535

Morozumi T, Kusuoka H, Fukuchi K et al (1997) Myocardial iodine-123-metaiodobenzylguanidine images and autonomic nerve activity in normal subjects. J Nucl Med 38:49–52

Nakata T, Wakabayashi T, Kyuma M et al (2005) Cardiac metaiodobenzylguanidine activity can predict the long-term efficacy of angiotensin-converting enzyme inhibitors and/or beta-adrenoceptor blockers in patients with heart failure. Eur J Nucl Med Mol Imaging 32:186–194

Nieminen MS, Bohm M, Cowie MR et al (2005) Executive summary of the guidelines on the diagnosis and treatment of acute heart failure: the Task Force on Acute Heart Failure of the European Society of Cardiology. Eur Heart J 26:384–416

Patel AD, Iskandrian AE (2002) MIBG imaging. J Nucl Cardiol 9:75–94

Paul M, Schafers M, Kies P et al (2006) Impact of sympathetic innervation on recurrent life-threatening arrhythmias in the follow-up of patients with idiopathic ventricular fibrillation. Eur J Nucl Med Mol Imaging 33:866–870

Rabinovitch MA, Rose CP, Schwab AJ et al (1993) A method of dynamic analysis of iodine-123-metaiodobenzylguanidine scintigrams in cardiac mechanical overload hypertrophy and failure. J Nucl Med 34:589–600

Radford MJ, Arnold JM, Bennett SJ et al (2005) ACC/AHA key data elements and definitions for measuring the clinical management and outcomes of patients with chronic heart failure: a report of the American College of Cardiology/American Heart Association Task Force on Clinical Data Standards (Writing Committee to Develop Heart Failure Clinical Data Standards): developed in collaboration with the American College of Chest Physicians and the International Society for Heart and Lung Transplantation: endorsed by the Heart Failure Society of America. Circulation 112:1888–1916

Short JH, Darby TD (1967) Sympathetic nervous system blocking agents. 3. Derivatives of benzylguanidine. J Med Chem 10:833–840

Sisson JC, Frager MS, Valk TW et al (1981) Scintigraphic localization of pheochromocytoma. N Engl J Med 305:12–17

Sisson JC, Shapiro B, Meyers L et al (1987a) Metaiodobenzylguanidine to map scintigraphically the adrenergic nervous system in man. J Nucl Med 28:1625–1636

Sisson JC, Wieland DM, Sherman P et al (1987b) Metaiodobenzylguanidine as an index of the adrenergic nervous system integrity and function. J Nucl Med 28:1620–1624

Solanki KK, Bomanji J, Moyes J et al (1992) A pharmacological guide to medicines which interfere with the biodistribution of radiolabelled meta-iodobenzylguanidine (MIBG). Nucl Med Commun 13:513–521

Somsen GA, Borm JJ, Dubois EA et al (1996) Cardiac 123I-MIBG uptake is affected by variable uptake in reference regions: implications for interpretation in clinical studies. Nucl Med Commun 17:872–876

Swedberg K, Cleland J, Dargie H et al (2005) Guidelines for the diagnosis and treatment of chronic heart failure: executive summary (update 2005): The Task Force for the Diagnosis and Treatment of Chronic Heart Failure of the European Society of Cardiology. Eur Heart J 26:1115–1140

Veltman CE, Boogers MJ, Meinardi JE et al (2012) Reproducibility of planar (123)I-meta-iodobenzylguanidine (MIBG) myocardial scintigraphy in patients with heart failure. Eur J Nucl Med Mol Imaging 39:1599–1608

Verberne HJ, Feenstra C, de Jong WM et al (2005) Influence of collimator choice and simulated clinical conditions on 123I-MIBG heart/mediastinum ratios: a phantom study. Eur J Nucl Med Mol Imaging 32:1100–1107

Verberne HJ, Brewster LM, Somsen GA et al (2008) Prognostic value of myocardial 123I-metaiodobenzylguanidine (MIBG) parameters in patients with heart failure: a systematic review. Eur Heart J 29:1147–1159

Verberne HJ, Verschure DO, Somsen GA et al (2011) Vascular time-activity variation in patients undergoing 123I-MIBG myocardial scintigraphy: implications for quantification of cardiac and mediastinal uptake. Eur J Nucl Med Mol Imaging 38:1132–1138

Verschure DO, Somsen GA, van Eck-Smit BL et al (2012) Renal function in relation to cardiac (123)I-MIBG scintigraphy in patients with chronic heart failure. Int J Mol Imaging. doi:10.1155/2012/434790

Wafelman AR, Hoefnagel CA, Maes RA et al (1994) Radioiodinated metaiodobenzylguanidine: a review of its biodistribution and pharmacokinetics, drug interactions, cytotoxicity and dosimetry. Eur J Nucl Med 21:545–559

Wakabayashi T, Nakata T, Hashimoto A et al (2001) Assessment of underlying etiology and cardiac sympathetic innervation to identify patients at high risk of cardiac death. J Nucl Med 42:1757–1767

Wieland DM, Wu J, Brown LE et al (1980) Radiolabeled adrenergic neuron-blocking agents: adrenomedullary imaging with [131I]iodobenzylguanidine. J Nucl Med 21:349–353

Wu X, Kekuda R, Huang W et al (1998) Identity of the organic cation transporter OCT3 as the extraneuronal monoamine transporter (uptake2) and evidence for the expression of the transporter in the brain. J Biol Chem 273:32776–32786

Yamada T, Shimonagata T, Fukunami M et al (2003) Comparison of the prognostic value of cardiac iodine-123 metaiodobenzylguanidine imaging and heart rate variability in patients with chronic heart failure: a prospective study. J Am Coll Cardiol 41:231–238

Preclinical Evaluations of Cardiac Sympathetic Innervation Radiotracers

10

David M. Raffel

Contents

Abstract

Preclinical evaluations of radiotracers designed for imaging cardiac sympathetic innervation have played a key role in the development of this branch of nuclear cardiology. In this chapter, many of the experimental approaches used to characterize the neuronal uptake and retention mechanisms of sympathetic nerve radiotracers are reviewed, from in vitro assays to in vivo imaging studies in animal models. Data from these studies have been critically important in the development of the most optimal radiotracers for cardiac innervation imaging studies in human subjects They have also provided invaluable insights into the underlying neuronal retention mechanisms of each radiotracer, which are essential to understanding observed changes in the myocardial retention and kinetics of the radiotracer in heart diseases.

D.M. Raffel, PhD
Division of Nuclear Medicine, Department of Radiology, University of Michigan Medical School, 2276 Medical Sciences I Building, SPC 5610, Ann Arbor, MI 48109, USA
e-mail: raffel@umich.edu

R.H.J.A. Slart et al. (eds.), *Autonomic Innervation of the Heart: Role of Molecular Imaging*, DOI 10.1007/978-3-662-45074-1_10

Abbreviations

[^{11}C]-D2-PHEN	[^{11}C]-(–)-α,α-dideutero-phenylephrine
[^{11}C]-EPI	[^{11}C]-(–)-epinephrine
[^{11}C]-GMO	*N*-[^{11}C]-guanyl-(–)-*meta*-octopamine
[^{11}C]-mHED	[^{11}C]-*meta*-(–)-hydroxyephedrine
[^{11}C]-MHPG	[^{11}C]-*meta*-hydroxyphenethylguanidine
[^{11}C]-PHEN	[^{11}C]-(–)-phenylephrine
[^{11}C]-PHPG	[^{11}C]-*para*-hydroxyphenethylguanidine
[^{123}I]-MIBG	[^{123}I]-metaiodobenzylguanidine
[^{131}I]-RIBA	[^{131}I]-*o*-iodobenzyltrimethylammonium iodide
[^{18}F]-4F-MHPG	4-[^{18}F]-fluoro-*meta*-hydroxyphenethylguanidine
[^{3}H]-NE	[^{3}H]-labeled norepinephrine
6-OHDA	6-hydroxydopamine
C6-hNET	Cloned human NET (cells)
COMT	Catechol-*O*-methyltransferase
DMI	Desipramine
EMT	Extraneuronal monoamine transporter
HMG-CoA	3-hydroxy-3-methylglutaryl-coenzyme A
HPLC	High-performance liquid chromatography
LAD	Left anterior descending (artery)
MAO	Monoamine oxidase
mHED	(–)-*meta*-hydroxyephedrine
MIBG	Metaiodobenzylguanidine
NET	Norepinephrine transporter
OCT3	Organic cation transporter 3
PAPS	Adenosine-3′-phosphate-5′-phosphosulfate
PET	Positron emission tomography
PHEN	(–)-phenylephrine
RBC(s)	Red blood cell(s)
RI	Retention index
ROI	Region-of-interest
SPECT	Single photon emission computed tomography
STZ	Streptozotocin
UDPGA	Uridine 5′-diphosphoglucuronic acid
VMAT2	Vesicular monoamine transporter 2

10.1 Introduction

Preclinical evaluations of new cardiac radiopharmaceuticals in various experimental models are an essential stage in the development of a successful imaging agent for clinical studies in human subjects. Data from these studies are used to identify which compounds exhibit the most favorable properties for cardiac imaging, such as high heart-to-lung and heart-to-liver ratios. Demonstration of the specificity of a radiotracer's cardiac retention for the particular physiological process being targeted is also a very important goal of these studies. Assessments of the kinetics of a new tracer in heart and plasma can also provide key preliminary information about the suitability of the compound for quantitative analyses by tracer kinetic methods. Studies of the biodistribution of the tracer are frequently used to calculate initial estimates of internal radiation absorbed doses in human subjects. Together, the data from these studies form the scientific foundation supporting the clinical translation of a new cardiac imaging agent. However, even after a new radiopharmaceutical has an established clinical role, more detailed investigations in animal models of disease are often performed to further characterize the robustness of the clinical parameters measured with the agent.

This chapter reviews some of the laboratory studies performed during the development of radiopharmaceuticals targeting presynaptic sympathetic nerve terminals in the heart, which illustrate most of the elements of preclinical evaluations described above. Specific considerations of important differences between animal models are also highlighted, since these factors must be kept in mind when interpreting the results of preclinical studies in different species. The data presented emphasize recent work in our laboratory on radiolabeled phenethylguanidines as novel sympathetic nerve imaging agents with more optimal kinetics for quantifying regional sympathetic nerve density using tracer kinetic analyses.

10.2 Key Characteristics of Sympathetic Nerve Radiotracers

The norepinephrine transporter (NET) is the primary imaging target of most radiotracers developed for imaging cardiac sympathetic neurons. In the heart, NET is exclusively expressed in the outer membrane of presynaptic sympathetic terminal nerve axon varicosities (Fig. 10.1). Transporters are often imaged scintigraphically using radiolabeled inhibitors of the transporter. However, this approach has been largely unsuccessful for imaging cardiac NET due to the high lipophilicity of most selective NET inhibitors. For example, desipramine is a high-affinity NET inhibitor with an equilibrium dissociation constant K_D of ~1.5 nM (Raisman et al. 1982). Yet due to its high lipophilicity ($\log P = 4.9$) (Hansch et al. 1995), [^{11}C]-desipramine was found to have extremely high levels of nonspecific binding in the heart, occluding any specific binding to NET and preventing its use as a positron emission tomography (PET) radiotracer (Van Dort et al. 1997).

A more fruitful approach to imaging cardiac sympathetic nerve terminals has been the use of radiolabeled NET substrates. NET actively transports a large number of structural analogs of the endogenous neurotransmitter norepinephrine (Burgen and Iversen 1965). Thus, after its initial extraction from plasma into interstitium, a radiolabeled norepinephrine analog is transported by NET into the axoplasm of sympathetic nerve varicosities. Once inside the nerve, it interacts with other key processes involved in the neuronal handling of norepinephrine. Most important among these are storage in vesicles by the vesicular monoamine transporter 2 (VMAT2) and metabolism by intraneuronal enzymes, including mitochondrial-bound monoamine oxidase (MAO). Unlike many NET inhibitors, most norepinephrine analogs have very low lipophilicity (log$P$ < 0.5); thus, radiolabeled norepinephrine analogs tend to have very low nonspecific binding to myocytes.

The chemical structure of a given radiolabeled norepinephrine analog will determine its NET transport rate, rate of VMAT2-mediated uptake into vesicles, and whether or not it is vulnerable to metabolism by intraneuronal enzymes such as MAO. A fourth structurally related factor is the lipophilicity of the compound, which influences its diffusion rate across vesicular and neuronal membranes. Together, these four factors predominantly determine the kinetics of the uptake and retention of the tracer by sympathetic nerve terminals. Other important aspects to consider include selectivity of the radiotracer for NET, the rate of tracer metabolism

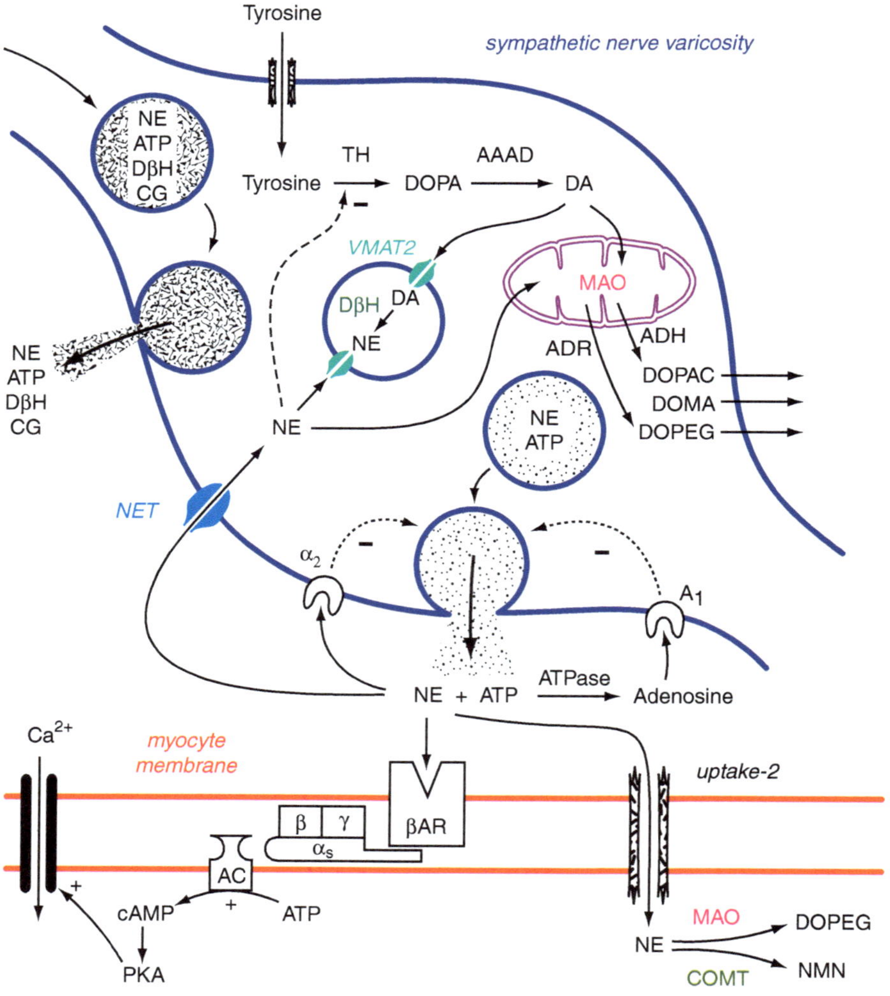

in plasma, and interaction of the tracer with blood components (partitioning into red blood cells, plasma protein binding). It is also important to verify that any radiometabolites formed are inactive (i.e., not actively transported by NET).

In some mammalian species, a second transporter system localized in myocytes, termed "uptake-2," competes with the NET-mediated neuronal reuptake of norepinephrine (Fig. 10.1) (Iversen 1965). As described in detail in Sect. 10.4, evidence strongly suggests that uptake-2 is absent or negligible in human hearts. Therefore, if a new sympathetic nerve radiotracer is a substrate for uptake-2, this is not a roadblock to its further clinical development. However, it is important to be aware of the uptake-2 activity of the compound to properly interpret results from studies in a given animal model. If possible, blocking uptake-2 activity pharmacologically will provide a more accurate picture of the kinetics and imaging properties of the tracer in humans.

Preclinical assessments of a new sympathetic nerve radiotracer are designed to characterize the following aspects of the tracer:

- NET transport rate
- Uptake into vesicles by VMAT2
- Vulnerability to intraneuronal metabolism by MAO or other enzymes
- Lipophilicity (diffusion rates across membranes)

Fig. 10.1 Sympathetic nerve varicosity. Norepinephrine (*NE*) is synthesized from tyrosine, which is actively transported into the varicosity. Tyrosine is converted to dihydroxyphenylalanine (*DOPA*) by tyrosine hydroxylase (*TH*). This is the rate-limiting step in NE synthesis. DOPA is converted to dopamine (*DA*) by aromatic L-amino acid decarboxylase (*AAAD*). DA is stored in vesicles by the vesicular monoamine transporter2 (*VMAT2*) and converted to NE by dopamine-β-hydroxylase (*DβH*). NE is localized in two types of storage vesicles. Large dense-core vesicles (diameter ~85 nm) containing NE, ATP, DβH, and chromogranins (*CG*) originate in the neuron's cell body and are transported along the axon to the varicosities. The more numerous small dense-core vesicles (diameter 30–60 nm) are formed locally. Nerve stimulation causes exocytotic release of vesicular contents. After release, NE binds to postsynaptic β-adrenergic receptors (*βAR*) in the myocyte membrane, which stimulates adenylate cyclase (*AC*) via the stimulatory G protein G_s (β, γ, α_s). Enhanced adenylate cyclase activity increases intracellular levels of cyclic adenosine monophosphate (*cAMP*), which activates protein kinase A (*PKA*), ultimately increasing influx of Ca^{2+} through L-type Ca^{2+} channels. The influx of Ca^{2+} leads to enhanced myocyte contractility. NE can also bind to presynaptic α_2-adrenergic (α_2) receptors to inhibit further release of NE. The majority of released NE is actively transported back into the varicosity by the norepinephrine transporter (*NET*) and stored in vesicles by VMAT2. The NE in the neuronal axoplasm can slow NE synthesis by directly inhibiting TH. NE in axoplasm can also be metabolized by the mitochondrial-bound enzyme monoamine oxidase (*MAO*). The aldehyde produced by MAO oxidation of NE is rapidly metabolized by aldehyde reductase (*ADR*) to form 3,4-dihydroxyphenylglycol (*DOPEG*) or by aldehyde dehydrogenase (*ADH*) to form dihydroxymandelic acid (*DOMA*). DA in axoplasm can also be metabolized by MAO and ADH to form 3,4-dihydroxyphenylacetic acid (*DOPAC*). In some mammalian species, extraneuronal uptake of NE into myocytes (uptake-2) competes with neuronal reuptake as a mechanism for terminating the action of NE. NE is metabolized extraneuronally by enzymes such as catechol-*O*-methyltransferase (*COMT*) to form normetanephrine (*NMN*) or MAO to form DOPEG

- Selectivity for NET in the heart
- Rate of metabolic breakdown in plasma
- Inactivity of radiometabolites at NET
- Interaction with blood components
  - Partitioning into red blood cells
  - Plasma protein binding
- Uptake-2 activity
- Biodistribution and/or animal imaging studies
  - Assess imaging properties and kinetics
  - Radiation dosimetry estimates

This list is not meant to be comprehensive, but knowledge of these parameters for a novel tracer would provide enough information to assess the suitability of the compound for further development.

Defining optimal values for each of these parameters is dependent on the particular aspect of presynaptic function the tracer has been designed to measure. Early radiotracers like [^{123}I]-metaiodobenzylguanidine ([^{123}I]-MIBG) (Wieland et al. 1981) and [^{11}C]-*meta*-(−)-hydroxyephedrine ([^{11}C]-mHED) (Rosenspire et al. 1990) were designed to have fast NET transport rates and resistance to intraneuronal metabolism by MAO and other enzymes with the goal of achieving maximal tracer retention in nerve terminals. [^{11}C]-(−)-Epinephrine ([^{11}C]-EPI) (Chakraborty et al. 1993), like norepinephrine, is metabolized by MAO and is rapidly stored in vesicles, leading to prolonged neuronal retention times (Nguyen et al. 1997). Because of these two properties, PET studies with [^{11}C]-EPI likely provide accurate mapping of the regional distribution of norepinephrine stores in the heart. [^{11}C]-(−)-Phenylephrine ([^{11}C]-PHEN) (Del Rosario et al. 1996), which is also readily metabolized by MAO, was originally designed to be a radiotracer for measuring MAO metabolism rates in sympathetic nerve terminals (Del Rosario et al. 1996). However, preclinical (Raffel and Wieland 1999) and clinical (Raffel et al. 1999) studies with [^{11}C]-PHEN demonstrated that the rate-limiting step in its clearance kinetics was leakage from vesicles rather than MAO metabolism, complicating interpretation of kinetic studies with this tracer.

There are several aspects of cardiac sympathetic function that are of interest to clinicians. The most fundamental of these is "cardiac sympathetic nerve density," the number of functional sympathetic nerve terminals per gram of heart tissue. A related concept is "neuronal integrity," the ability of nerves to recover and store norepinephrine, which depends on the key elements of NET transport, VMAT2 transport, and MAO metabolism all functioning normally. "Sympathetic nerve activity" or "sympathetic outflow" is the rate of nerve impulses being sent to terminal nerve axons. Finally, "sympathetic tone," a combination of sympathetic outflow plus postsynaptic receptor responses and related baroreflex mechanisms, is very important in assessing the functional modulation of cardiac output by the sympathetic nervous system. Current sympathetic nerve radiotracers largely assess the first two of these aspects of sympathetic function, although there is evidence in the literature suggesting that [^{123}I]-MIBG clearance rates are modulated by sympathetic outflow (Sisson et al. 1991).

Recently our laboratory has been investigating radiolabeled phenethylguanidines in an effort to develop a new PET radiotracer with optimal kinetics for accurately quantifying regional sympathetic nerve density using tracer kinetic analysis methods (Raffel et al. 2007). The motivation for these studies has been our dissatisfaction with our attempts to apply standard tracer kinetic analyses to the myocardial kinetics of [^{11}C]-mHED. We hypothesized that the very rapid neuronal uptake of [^{11}C]-mHED, mediated by NET transport, causes it to be a "flow-limited" tracer. A flow-limited tracer exhibits very rapid uptake into its tissue distribution spaces after its initial extraction from plasma into interstitium. The rate of tracer extraction from plasma characterized by the rate constant K_1 (mL/min/g) is equal to $E \cdot F$, where E is the "unidirectional extraction fraction" of the tracer (often close to 1.0) and F is blood flow (mL/min/g). Since blood flow is the rate-limiting step in the net tissue uptake of tracers with these kinetic properties, they are referred to as flow-limited tracers. Because of its flow-limited behavior, cardiac [^{11}C]-mHED retention levels, which are used as surrogate measures of sympathetic nerve density, are insensitive to clinically important levels of cardiac denervation. For example, studies with [^{11}C]-mHED have shown that its cardiac retention does not decline significantly until regional nerve losses are quite high, as much as 40 % of control levels (Ungerer et al. 1998). Since the neuronal uptake rate of [^{123}I]-*meta*-iodobenzylguanidine ([^{123}I]-MIBG) is even faster than that of [^{11}C]-mHED, it is likely that it too is a flow-limited tracer (see Sect. 10.5 for details).

The only way to overcome the flow-limited behavior of [^{11}C]-mHED was to design a new tracer with more optimal kinetic properties. After consideration of the limitations of [^{11}C]-mHED, we sought to develop a new sympathetic nerve tracer with two specific kinetic properties. First, a slower transport rate into neurons by NET was needed, making this the rate-limiting step in the neuronal uptake of the tracer. Second, efficient uptake into norepinephrine storage vesicles by VMAT2 was desired, leading to very long neuronal retention times (provided the compound was not too lipophilic). We predicted that the myocardial kinetics of a tracer with these two kinetic properties could be analyzed using standard kinetic analysis methods to yield quantitative measures of regional sympathetic nerve density. Also, we hypothesized that since NET transport would be the rate-limiting step in the kinetics, the quantitative measures derived from tracer kinetic analysis would be sensitive to low to moderate levels of nerve losses and thus would detect cardiac denervation earlier in its progression than is currently possible with [^{11}C]-mHED.

We chose to study phenethylguanidines because several of these compounds are known to potently deplete cardiac stores of norepinephrine due to their avid retention in storage vesicles (Costa et al. 1962; Fielden and Green 1965; Green et al. 1967). While some phenethylguanidines are inhibitors of MAO at micromolar concentrations (Fielden and Green 1965; Kuntzman and Jacobson 1963), they are not substrates for MAO or other intraneuronal enzymes, so they are metabolically stable inside nerve terminals.

In the following sections on various preclinical studies of sympathetic nerve radiotracers, we include some data from our preclinical studies of radiolabeled phenethylguanidines. At the end of the chapter, we summarize the preclinical studies on phenthylguanethidines as a case study in developing novel sympathetic nerve imaging agents.

10.3 In Vitro Studies

Some of the most fundamental studies of a potential new imaging agent are in vitro assessments of its interactions with the targeted physiological process. A classic example is measurement of the binding affinity of a receptor-binding ligand to its target receptor, characterized by an equilibrium dissociation constant K_d, with units of molarity (M). While the binding affinity of a radiolabeled substrate for NET has some influence on its kinetics in vivo, the more important kinetic parameters are its transport constants K_m and V_{max}.

Transport rates of NET substrates are described by the Michaelis–Menten equation, V_{init} (pmol/min/g) $= [S_o]V_{max}/(K_m + [S_o])$, where $[S_o]$ is the radiotracer concentration (μM) outside nerve varicosities in interstitium, V_{max} is the maximum velocity of transport (pmol/min/g), and K_m is the half-saturation constant (μM). Scintigraphic imaging studies typically use "tracer level" concentrations of substrate, where $[S_o] << K_m$ at all times, simplifying the transport rate equation to $V_{init} = (V_{max}/K_m)[S_o]$. This equation shows that it is the ratio of an NET substrate's transport constants V_{max} and K_m that determines its neuronal uptake rate. Thus, a "neuronal uptake rate constant" $k_{uptake} = V_{max}/K_m$ can be defined for each NET substrate. Furthermore, V_{max} is directly proportional to NET transporter density (e.g., an NET B_{max} value from a binding assay). This is an important point to consider for imaging studies in vivo with radiolabeled NET substrates. In diseases in which cardiac sympathetic denervation occurs, regional NET density decreases, and thus V_{max} will decline in direct proportion to reductions in NET density. Hence, the value of $k_{uptake} = V_{max}/K_m$ will also decline in proportion to the degree of regional NET density deficits. Thus, while information about the binding affinities (K_d) of radiotracers for NET are interesting, accurate measurements of their transport constants K_m and V_{max} for NET transport are more valuable as it is their V_{max}/K_m ratios that determine their neuronal uptake rates.

Our laboratory previously measured binding affinities ($K_i = K_d$) of several NET inhibitors and substrates in competitive inhibition assays using the NET radioligand [^{3}H]-mazindol and NET in purified rat heart membranes (Table 10.1) (Raffel and Chen 2004). NET inhibitors studied included the potent NET inhibitor desipramine (DMI). NET substrates studied included the biogenic amines (norepinephrine, epinephrine, dopamine, and serotonin) and nonradioactive analogs of several sympathetic nerve radiotracers, including metaiodobenzylguanidine (MIBG), (−)-*meta*-hydroxyephedrine (mHED), and (−)-phenylephrine (PHEN). Higher binding affinity for NET is a desirable property for a sympathetic nerve radiotracer since it can compete favorably with endogenous norepinephrine for available NET

Table 10.1 Binding affinities (K_i) of some NET inhibitors and substrates for NET in purified rat heart membranes measured in competitive binding assays with [^{3}H]-mazindol (Raffel and Chen 2004)

NET inhibitors	K_i (nM)
Desipramine	2.76±0.30
(+)-Oxaprotiline	6.42±1.72
(−)-Oxaprotiline	2,877±646
NET substrates	K_i (μM)
para-Iodobenzylguanidine	1.22±0.05
Methcathinone	3.55±0.31
meta-Iodobenzylguanidine (MIBG)	3.95±0.08
Dopamine	4.49±0.22
(±)-Tranylcypromine	5.04±0.29
(−)-*meta*-Hydroxyephedrine (mHED)	20.9±0.1
(−)-Metaraminol	21.8±0.4
(−)-Norepinephrine	34.1±2.2
(−)-Epinephrine (EPI)	53.8±4.7
Guanethidine	66.3±3.5
(−)-*meta*-Octopamine	104.7±13.9
(−)-Phenylephrine (PHEN)	109.2±14.8
Bretylium	209.4±30.1
Serotonin	471.4±16 5

Values are mean ± SD of $n=2$–4 determinations. Hill slopes were close to unity in all cases

transporters. This is likely to be most important in diseases associated with elevated plasma norepinephrine levels, such as congestive heart failure (Cohn et al. 1984). For example, the NET binding affinity of MIBG ($K_i=3.95$ μM) is higher than that of norepinephrine (34.1 μM). However, as described above, uptake rates of sympathetic nerve radiotracers into neurons do not correlate with NET binding affinity but rather with NET V_{max}/K_m ratios.

The transport kinetics of several radiolabeled NET substrates were characterized in vitro using a rat C6 glioma cell line stably transfected with the cloned human NET (C6-hNET cells) (Raffel et al. 2013a). Transport assays with C6-hNET cells (Fig. 10.2) provided highly reproducible measurements of the transport constants K_m and V_{max} for each substrate (Table 10.2). NET binding affinities (K_i) were also measured using competitive inhibition binding assays with [^{3}H]-mazindol and purified membranes from homogenized C6-hNET cells (Table 10.2). Ratios of V_{max}/K_m from the transport kinetics assays are also provided in Table 10.2, as these reflect the relative uptake rates of each NET substrate into sympathetic nerve terminals for tracer level concentrations of substrate (i.e., $[S_o] << K_m$). From examination of the measured V_{max}/K_m ratios, [^{3}H]-norepinephrine has the fastest transport rate at NET, while [^{3}H]-dopamine, [^{11}C]-mHED, and the radiolabeled phenethylguanidine [^{11}C]-*meta*-hydroxyphenethylguanidine ([^{11}C]-MHPG) are transported at rates about one-half the rate of [^{3}H]-norepinephrine. [^{11}C]-(−)-Epinephrine ([^{11}C]-EPI) is

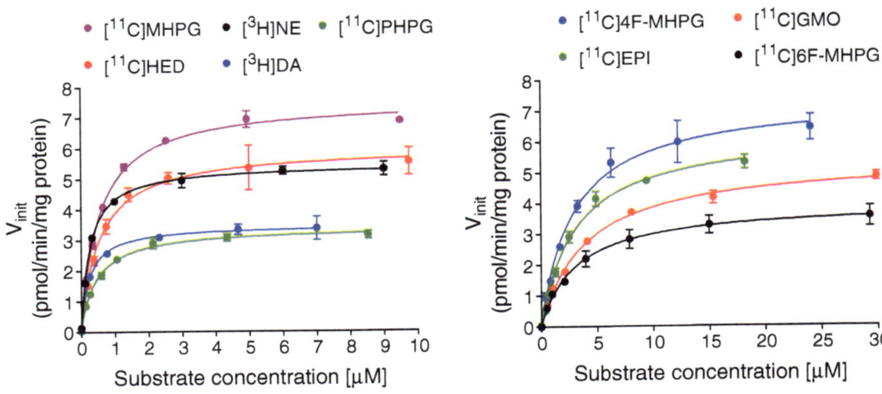

Fig. 10.2 NET transport kinetics assays of biogenic amines and sympathetic nerve radiotracers in vitro with C6-hNET cells. Nonlinear regression analysis yielded estimates of the transport constants K_m and V_{max} for each assay. NET substrates with lower K_m values are shown in the left panel, and those with higher K_m values are plotted in the right panel

Table 10.2 Binding affinities (K_i) and transport constants (K_m, V_{max}) for the cloned human norepinephrine transporter stably expressed in rat C6-glial cells (C6-hNET cells) (Raffel et al. 2013a)

NET substrate	Acronym	K_i (μM)	K_m (μM)	V_{max} (pmol/min/mg protein)	V_{max}/K_m (μl/min/mg protein)
[³H]-(−)-norepinephrine	NE	63.9 ± 2.3	0.28 ± 0.03	5.83 ± 0.49	21.3 ± 2.4
[³H]-dopamine	DA	8.1 ± 0.5	0.24 ± 0.04	2.91 ± 0.47	12.2 ± 1.8
[¹¹C]-(−)-epinephrine	EPI	68.4 ± 7.6	3.16 ± 0.78	6.09 ± 1.04	2.0 ± 0.2
[¹¹C]-(−)-*meta*-hydroxyephedrine	MHED	43.2 ± 1.8	0.48 ± 0.08	5.43 ± 0.71	11.4 ± 1.3
[¹¹C]-*meta*-hydroxyphenethylguanidine	MHPG	4.9 ± 0.5	0.73 ± 0.20	7.83 ± 1.73	11.2 ± 2.8
[¹¹C]-*para*-hydroxyphenethylguanidine	PHPG	1.9 ± 0.2	0.52 ± 0.06	3.31 ± 0.40	6.4 ± 1.1
N-[¹¹C]-guanyl-(−)-*meta*-octopamine	GMO	20.3 ± 2.5	4.43 ± 0.31	5.57 ± 0.30	1.3 ± 0.1
[¹¹C]-4-fluoro-*meta*-hydroxyphenethylguanidine	4F-MHPG	5.6 ± 0.5	2.57 ± 0.35	7.46 ± 0.64	3.0 ± 0.5
[¹¹C]-6-fluoro-*meta*-hydroxyphenethylguanidine	6F-MHPG	17.7 ± 0.5	2.86 ± 0.43	4.06 ± 0.66	1.4 ± 0.3

Values are means ± SD for n = 4–5 assays

transported by NET at a rate approximately one-tenth of the rate of norepinephrine. Another phenethylguanidine, *N*-[¹¹C]-guanyl-(−)-*meta*-octopamine ([¹¹C]-GMO), had the slowest NET transport rate among the compounds studied.

The transport rates of NET substrates measured as V_{max}/K_m ratios in C6-hNET transport assays were found to be highly correlated (r^2 = 0.96) with their uptake rates

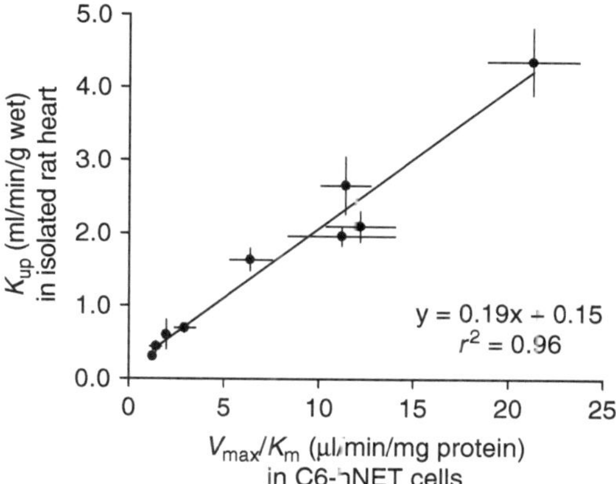

Fig. 10.3 Correlation of measured neuronal uptake rates of NET substrates in isolated rat hearts (K_{up}, mL/min/g wet) with V_{max}/K_m ratios from transport kinetic assays with C6-hNET cells

into sympathetic neurons measured previously in isolated perfused rat hearts (Fig. 10.3) (Iversen 1967; Hellmann et al. 1971; Raffel et al. 2007). This result strongly suggests that the NET transport rates measured in vitro using C6-hNET cells accurately reflect the relative neuronal uptake rates of NET substrates in vivo in the heart.

10.4 Uptake-2

An important factor to consider in animal studies is that some mammalian species have an extraneuronal transporter-mediated uptake pathway in the heart that can confound interpretation of the cardiac kinetics and retention of these tracers (Fig. 10.1). This was defined by Iversen as "uptake-2" to describe the extraneuronal uptake of norepinephrine into myocytes of the isolated rat, while "uptake-1" was used for NET-mediated uptake into neurons (Iversen 1965). The transporter involved in uptake-2 has more recently been called the extraneuronal monoamine transporter (EMT) or the organic cation transporter 3 (OCT3) which is encoded by the solute carrier family 22 member 3 (SLC22A3) gene in humans (Wu et al. 1998; Hayer-Zillgen et al. 2002). The presence or absence of the uptake-2 pathway in the hearts of various animal species is summarized in Table 10.3. In addition to the rat heart, cardiac uptake-2 activity is important in the hearts of mice (Zwart et al. 2001), dogs (Eisenhofer et al. 1992), pigs (Lameris et al. 1999), and cats (Graefe 1981). On the other hand, uptake-2 activity is absent in the hearts of humans (Glowniak et al. 1989; Dae et al. 1992), monkeys (Carr et al. 1979), and rabbits (Graefe et al. 1978). In an important study in this area, scintigraphic imaging studies with [^{131}I]-*o*-iodobenzyltrimethylammonium iodide ([^{131}I]-RIBA), a selective substrate for uptake-2, demonstrated that uptake-2 activity is important in the hearts of pigs, but is absent in monkey and human hearts (Carr et al. 1979). It has been suggested that the physiological purpose of uptake-2 may be to serve as a secondary mechanism for terminating the actions of norepinephrine released from sympathetic nerve

Table 10.3 Extraneuronal uptake (uptake-2) in the hearts of various animal species

Species	Uptake-2 activity?	References
Human	No	Carr et al. (1979)
		Glowniak et al. (1989)
		Dae et al. (1992)
Rat	Yes	Iversen (1965)
		Carr et al. (1979)
Rabbit	No	Graefe et al. (1978)
Dog	Yes	Eisenhofer et al. (1992)
Monkey	No	Carr et al. (1979)
Cat	Yes	Graefe (1981)
Mouse	Yes	Zwart et al. (2001)
Pig	Yes	Carr et al. (1979)
		Lameris et al. (1999)

terminals since uptake-2 transports norepinephrine into myocytes, where it is metabolized by MAO or catechol-*O*-methyltransferase (COMT) (Fig. 10.1). Uptake-2 is also likely to be an important process for limiting the actions of epinephrine and norepinephrine circulating in plasma on the heart (Lightman and Iversen 1969). For example, the well-known "flight-or-fight" response in mammals leads to the release of high amounts of epinephrine and norepinephrine from the adrenal glands into the bloodstream (Kvetnansky et al. 2009). Uptake-2 may play a key role in limiting the time course of cardiac effects of circulating catecholamines during flight-or-fight responses.

Most sympathetic nerve imaging agents have been found to be good substrates for the uptake-2 pathway, including [^{123}I]-MIBG (DeGrado et al. 1995) and [^{11}C]-EPI (Iversen 1965). A noteworthy exception is [^{11}C]-mHED, which is a very poor substrate for uptake-2 (DeGrado et al. 1993). Thus, [^{11}C]-mHED studies in different animal models are easier to interpret since cardiac uptake and retention of [^{11}C]-mHED are exclusively mediated by NET uptake into sympathetic nerve terminals.

The transplanted human heart is denervated due to atrophy of the surgically severed nerves and thus is devoid of uptake-1 activity. Since we know that [^{123}I]-MIBG is a good uptake-2 substrate, the clinical observation that [^{123}I]-MIBG does not localize in the denervated myocardium of recent heart transplant recipients (Dae et al. 1992; Glowniak et al. 1989) is consistent with uptake-2 being negligible in human heart.

10.5 Ex Vivo Studies in Isolated Rat Hearts

The isolated perfused rat heart has proven to be a very valuable model for characterizing the kinetics and neuronal retention mechanisms of sympathetic nerve radiotracers. Iversen's groundbreaking studies of uptake-1 and uptake-2 were done primarily in the isolated rat heart (Iversen 1963, 1965). This system, when combined with external radiodetection of emitted gamma rays or positron annihilation photons from a radiotracer, allows for detailed kinetic studies of the interaction of the tracer with various neuronal components involved in its neuronal uptake and handling. Using pharmacological interventions, it is possible to selectively block key physiological mechanisms that govern a tracer's neuronal uptake and retention, including NET transport, storage in vesicles by the vesicular monoamine transporter (VMAT2), and susceptibility to metabolism by various intraneuronal enzymes such as monoamine oxidase (MAO) (Fig. 10.1). One advantage of this preparation over intact animal studies is the ability to study the kinetics and retention mechanisms of the tracer with the heart under highly controlled conditions, without such complicating factors as tracer metabolism in plasma, partitioning into red blood cells, and effects from the tracer recirculating in the blood stream.

The system we use for studies of sympathetic nerve radiotracers is an isolated working rat heart system (Taegtmeyer et al. 1980) that uses two separate perfusion circuits, each with its own perfusate reservoir, which allows for instantaneous switching of the heart from one perfusion circuit to the other. For positron-emitting radiotracers, a pair of cesium fluoride (CsF) detectors is positioned so that the isolated rat heart is centered between the faces of the two detector crystals (Raffel et al. 1998). Coincidence detection circuitry measures the coincidence count rate between the two CsF detectors as a measure of the total amount of radioactivity in the heart. The typical experimental protocol begins by stabilizing the isolated heart on one perfusion circuit for 20–30 min with normal heart perfusate. After this, the heart is switched to the second perfusion circuit containing the radiotracer at very low concentrations (<10 nM) for 10 min. After the 10 min constant infusion study, the heart is switched back to normal perfusate to characterize the clearance kinetics of the radiotracer. The acquired coincidence count rate data are corrected for random coincidences and radioactive decay. The slope of the linear uptake curve from 1 to 4 min during the constant infusion study is a measure of the neuronal uptake rate of the radiotracer (K_{up}, mL/min/g wet tissue). The clearance kinetics data are fit to multiple exponential clearance components using nonlinear regression analysis (Raffel et al. 1998). Since uptake-2 is an important pathway in the rat heart, it is necessary to block uptake-2 pharmacologically to get a more accurate picture of the interaction of a radiotracer with the sympathetic nerve terminals. We block uptake-2 by adding 54 μM corticosterone to the heart perfusion buffer, based on a reported IC_{50} value of 2.7 μM for inhibition of uptake-2 by this steroid (Salt 1972). Another uptake-2 inhibitor that has been used in isolated rat heart studies is *N*-(9-fluorenyl)-*N*-methyl-*beta*-chloroethylamine (SKF550) at concentrations of 0.4–0.8 μM (DeGrado et al. 1995, 1998). Two examples of the effect of blocking uptake-2 on the kinetics of sympathetic nerve radiotracers in the isolated rat heart are shown in Fig. 10.4. In the first example (Fig. 10.4a), the kinetics of [^{11}C]-MIBG with and without uptake-2 blocked are shown. For the study performed without any uptake-2 inhibitor, the total uptake rate of [^{11}C]-MIBG was $K_{up}=5.09$ mL/min/g wet tissue. Blocking uptake-2 with corticosterone, the neuronal uptake rate was $K_{up}=3.65$ mL/min/g wet tissue. Similar K_{up} values were measured previously in isolated rat hearts for

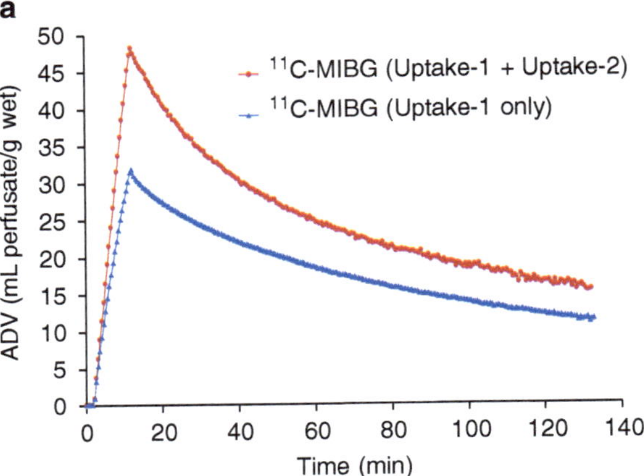

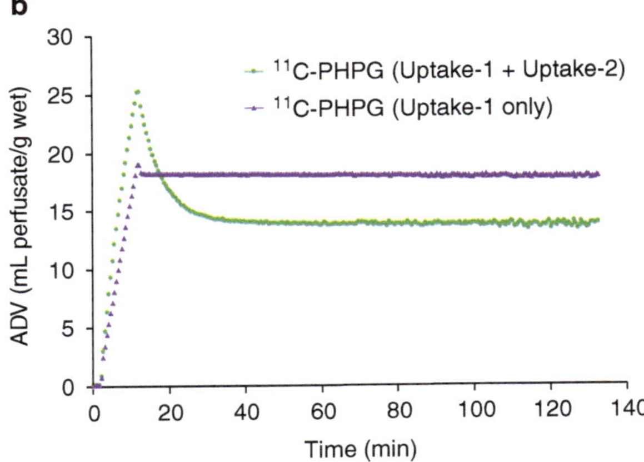

Fig. 10.4 Effect of inhibiting uptake-2 activity on kinetic studies of radiotracer uptake and clearance rates in isolated rat hearts. (**a**) Studies with [^{11}C]-MIBG, (**b**) studies with [^{11}C]-PHPG

[^{123}I]-MIBG, with $K_{up}=4.44\pm0.72$ mL/min/g wet for the total uptake rate and 3.66 ± 0.56 mL/min/g wet for the neuronal uptake rate (DeGrado et al. 1995). For [^{123}I]-MIBG, when uptake-1 was selectively blocked by adding the NET inhibitor DMI to the heart perfusate (50 nM), a K_{up} of 3.22 ± 0.40 mL/min/g wet tissue was measured (DeGrado et al. 1995). What these data show is that uptake-1 and uptake-2 compete with each other during the constant infusion study, with uptake-2 "stealing" a significant fraction of available radiotracer molecules away from uptake-1. When uptake-2 is blocked, the true neuronal uptake rate associated with uptake-1 is measured. Since human hearts lack any significant uptake-2 activity, uptake rate measurements made in isolated rat hearts with uptake-2 blocked more accurately reflect relative neuronal uptake rates in human hearts.

During the clearance phase of the [^{11}C]-MIBG studies, when uptake-2 is not blocked, there is faster efflux of tracer early in the study that clears to reveal a slower clearance rate later in the study. Comparison with the [^{11}C]-MIBG study with

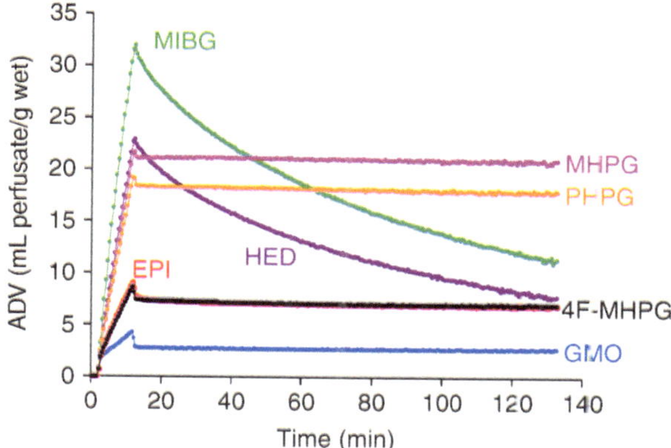

Fig. 10.5 Neuronal uptake and clearance kinetics of several sympathetic nerve radiotracers in isolated rat hearts, with uptake-2 blocked by corticosterone (54 μM) in heart perfusate. The kinetics of [¹¹C]-EPI and [¹⁸F]-4F-MHPG are very similar in this system

uptake-2 blocked indicates that MIBG clears more quickly from the extraneuronal compartment ($T_{1/2}$ ~ 26.6 min) than it does from neuronal spaces ($T_{1/2}$ ~ 127 min). This was also demonstrated by DeGrado and coworkers in their pharmacological blocking studies with [¹²³I]-MIBG in isolated rat hearts. A half-time $T_{1/2} = 21.7 \pm 1.7$ min was measured for clearance from the extraneuronal compartment when uptake-1 was blocked with DMI and $T_{1/2} = 112 \pm 11$ min was measured for [¹²³I]-MIBG clearance from sympathetic nerve terminals when uptake-2 was blocked with SKF550 (DeGrado et al. 1995).

A similar set of uptake-2 blocking studies with [¹¹C]-*para*-hydroxyphenethylguanidine ([¹¹C]-PHPG) are shown in Fig. 10.4b. In this case, the total uptake rate (uptake-1 and uptake-2) was $K_{up} = 2.95$ mL/min/g wet, while with uptake-2 blocked, the neuronal uptake rate was $K_{up} = 1.88$ mL/min/g wet. In this case, since [¹¹C]-PHPG is efficiently stored in norepinephrine storage vesicles inside sympathetic nerve terminals (Raffel et al. 2007), comparing the clearance kinetics of the two studies, the much faster clearance of [¹¹C]-PHPG from the extraneuronal compartment is readily apparent. In the study with uptake-2 blocked, the true neuronal kinetics of [¹¹C]-PHPG are clearly seen (and accurately measured) without the complicating effect of additional uptake into and clearance from extraneuronal spaces.

The neuronal uptake rates and clearance kinetics of several sympathetic nerve radiotracers have been measured in the isolated rat heart with uptake-2 blocked, some of which are shown in Fig. 10.5 and Table 10.4. The relative magnitudes of the measured K_{up} values likely correspond to their relative neuronal uptake rates in human hearts. [¹¹C]-MIBG and [¹¹C]-mHED have the fastest neuronal uptake rates but clear from sympathetic neurons more quickly than the other compounds shown. In general, clearance rates observed in the isolated rat heart are faster than those observed in human hearts because the heart perfusion buffer cannot carry as much oxygen as blood and in response the heart autoregulates its coronary flow rates to more than ten times physiological levels (Ng et al. 1991). [¹¹C]-EPI has a relatively slow neuronal uptake rate but very long neuronal retention times due to efficient storage in vesicles (Nguyen et al. 1997). The four radiolabeled phenethylguanidines

Table 10.4 Neuronal uptake rates (K_{up}) and major clearance half-times ($T_{1/2}$) for several sympathetic nerve radiotracers in isolated rat hearts with uptake-2 blocked

	Acronym	K_{up} (mL/ min/g wet)	$T_{1/2}$ (h)	References
[^{3}H]-(−)-norepinephrine	NE	4.37 ± 0.44	–	Iversen (1971)
[^{11}C]-metaiodobenzylguanidine	MIBG	3.65	2.1	Our lab
[^{11}C]-(−)-*meta*-hydroxyephedrine	mHED	2.35	1.4	Our lab
[^{11}C]-(−)-epinephrine	EPI	0.87	>41	Our lab
[^{11}C]-*meta*-hydroxyphenethylguanidine	MHPG	1.96 ± 0.13	>102	Raffel et al. (2007)
[^{11}C]-*para*-hydroxyphenethylguanidine	PHPG	1.64 ± 0.15	>45	Raffel et al. (2007)
4-[^{18}F]-fluoro-m*eta*-hydroxyphenethylguanidine	4F-MHPG	0.82 ± 0.14	>24	Our lab
N-[^{11}C]-guanyl-(−)-*meta*-octopamine	GMO	0.30 ± 0.02	>152	Raffel et al. (2007)

shown in Fig. 10.5 exhibit a range of neuronal uptake rates, but all have very long neuronal retention times due to sequestration into vesicles (Raffel et al. 2007).

The isolated rat heart has been particularly valuable in understanding differences in the way sympathetic neurons handle different radiotracers. For example, studies with [^{11}C]-mHED showed that blocking NET by adding DMI to the heart perfusate almost completely abolished heart uptake of the tracer during the constant infusion phase of the study, indicating a high selectivity for sympathetic nerve terminals (DeGrado et al. 1993). If DMI (40 nM) was added to the perfusate only during the clearance phase of the study (a DMI "chase" study), the clearance rate was greatly accelerated, from a control clearance $T_{1/2}$ value of 63 ± 17 min to only 3.6 ± 0.9 min. This indicates that during the clearance phase of a control study, a significant amount of [^{11}C]-mHED molecules leaking from the neurons are recovered by the neurons by NET transport (i.e., uptake-1 activity). Also, in hearts isolated from animals injected with the VMAT2 inhibitor reserpine (1 mg/kg i.p., 3 h before heart isolation) to block vesicular storage, a reduction in the neuronal uptake of [^{11}C]-mHED was seen, and the clearance rate was again greatly accelerated to a $T_{1/2}$ ~ 8.0 min (Raffel and Wieland 2001). These results show that VMAT2-mediated uptake of [^{11}C]-mHED into storage vesicles is an important process that increases its neuronal distribution volume and prolongs its neuronal retention.

Isolated rat heart studies of [^{11}C]-PHPG demonstrate that the neuronal handling of this tracer is significantly different from that of [^{11}C]-mHED (Fig. 10.6). In control studies, [^{11}C]-PHPG has a fairly rapid neuronal uptake rate of 1.64 ± 0.15 mL/min/g wet and a very slow clearance rate from nerve terminals ($T_{1/2}$ = 190 h for the study shown). In a DMI-chase study with [^{11}C]-PHPG, there is no acceleration of the clearance rate from nerve terminals, unlike the DMI-chase results seen with [^{11}C]-mHED. On the contrary, binding up NET transporters with high amounts of DMI leads to a complete trapping of [^{11}C]-PHPG in the neurons. This suggests that

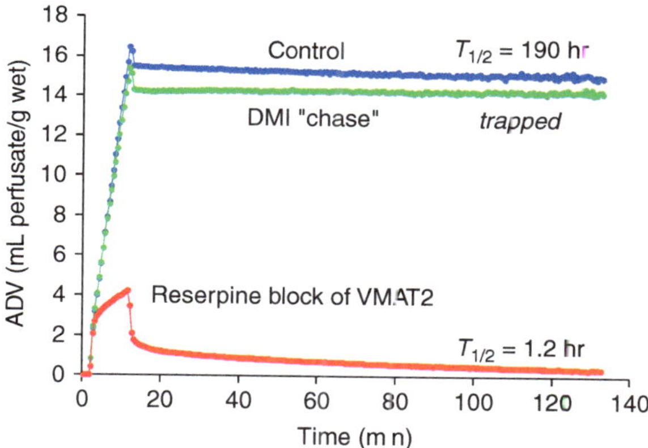

Fig. 10.6 Kinetic and mechanistic studies of [^{11}C]-PHPG in isolated rat hearts under control conditions, during a "DMI-chase" study (where 100 nM DMI was added to heart perfusate during the clearance phase of the study), and a study using reserpine to block VMAT2 transport into norepinephrine storage vesicles

the very slow clearance of [^{11}C]-PHPG from neurons is due to reverse transport by NET from the neuronal axoplasm to interstitium. Inhibition of VMAT2 by reserpine greatly reduced the neuronal uptake of [^{11}C]-PHPG and greatly accelerated its clearance rate, demonstrating that vesicular storage of [^{11}C]-PHPG is the main mechanism involved in its neuronal retention.

The influence of intraneuronal metabolism by MAO on neuronal retention of some has also been investigated for some sympathetic nerve radiotracers. [^{11}C]-PHEN was designed to be a tracer that would be metabolized at the α-carbon of its side chain by MAO to yield the radiometabolite [^{11}C]-methylamine. Since methylamine is a small molecule that easily crosses cell membranes, it was thought that the regional rate of radioactivity efflux from the heart could be used as a measure of neuronal MAO activity (Del Rosario et al. 1996). Studies of [^{11}C]-PHEN in isolated rat hearts showed that inhibition of MAO by adding the MAO inhibitor pargyline (100 μM) to the heart perfusate slowed the efflux of activity from sympathetic nerve terminals from a $T_{1/2}=98.2 \pm 13.7$ to 163.2 ± 13.7 min (Raffel and Wieland 1999). Substitution of deuterium for hydrogen atoms at the α-carbon of the side chain of [^{11}C]-PHEN as a means of inhibiting MAO activity at the tracer level was also studied (Del Rosario et al. 1996). The dideutero analog [^{11}C]-(−)-α,α-dideutero-phenylephrine ([^{11}C]-D2-PHEN) was found to have kinetics almost identical to those of [^{11}C]-PHEN during pargyline inhibition of MAO in the isolated rat heart, with a neuronal efflux $T_{1/2}=140.4 \pm 27.8$ min. However, while the efflux kinetics of [^{11}C]-PHEN were shown to be sensitive to MAO activity, the efflux rate was found to be rate limited by the leakage rate of [^{11}C]-PHEN from vesicles rather than by MAO metabolism (Raffel and Wieland 1999). Since [^{11}C]-EPI has the same side chain as [^{11}C]-PHEN, its metabolism by MAO also forms the radiometabolite [^{11}C]-methylamine (Nguyen et al. 1997). Because of its α-methyl group, [^{11}C]-mHED is not a substrate for MAO metabolism. Similarly, benzylguanidines (e.g., [^{123}I]-MIBG) and phenethylguanidines (e.g., [^{18}F]-4F-MHPG) are not substrates for neuronal enzymes like MAO, although some have been shown to be reversible MAO inhibitors at micromolar concentrations (Kuntzman and Jacobson 1963;

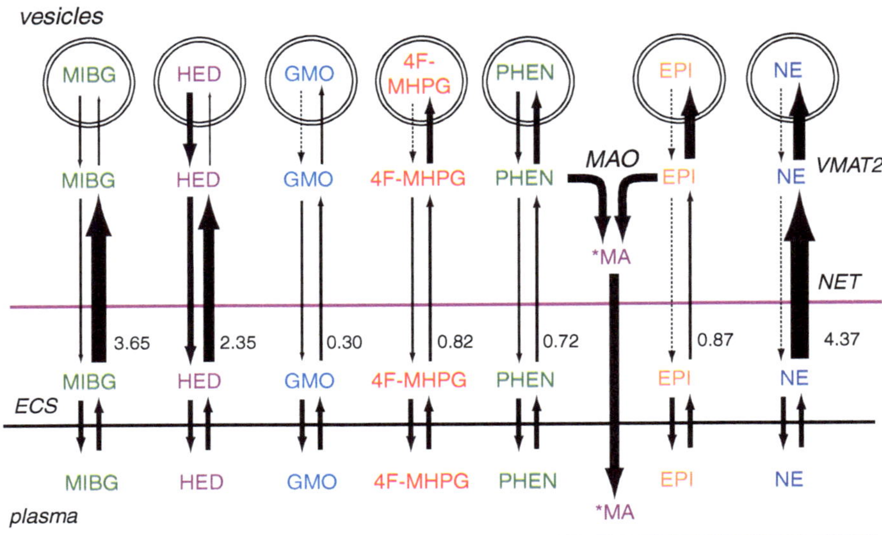

Fig. 10.7 Schematic illustration of neuronal uptake and retention mechanisms of norepinephrine (NE) and several sympathetic nerve radiotracers. *Arrow thicknesses* are drawn in approximate proportion to the magnitudes in uptake and diffusion rates. *NET* norepinephrine transporter, *VMAT2* vesicular monoamine transporter 2, *MAO* monoamine oxidase, **MA* [^{11}C]-methylamine. Neuronal uptake rates measured in isolated rat hearts (K_{up}, mL/min/g wet) are shown next to *arrows* for NET transport. Among the radiotracers, only [^{11}C]-PHEN and [^{11}C]-EPI are metabolized by MAO into [^{11}C]-methylamine, which quickly diffuses from nerve terminals. [^{11}C]-EPI, [^{18}F]-4F-MHPG, and [^{11}C]-GMO have very long neuronal retention times due to efficient storage in vesicles

Fielden and Green 1965). Based on various studies in intact animals and isolated rat hearts, a schematic drawing illustrating differences in the neuronal uptake and retention of some sympathetic nerve radiotracers is shown in Fig. 10.7.

10.6 In Vivo Studies

Several intact animal models have been used for preclinical evaluations of sympathetic nerve radiotracers. Since most of the studies performed in species with significant uptake-2 activity (rat, dog, pig, etc.) have not used pharmacological approaches to block uptake-2, the influence of extraneuronal uptake on a tracer's retention and kinetics should be kept in mind when interpreting the results of these studies. Development of validated uptake-2 blocking strategies that do not interfere with NET-mediated uptake into neurons in intact animal models would be an important contribution to this field.

Radiotracer biodistribution studies are some of the most fundamental in vivo evaluations of sympathetic nerve radiotracers. Biodistribution studies in rodents are frequently used to initially screen new radiotracers for favorable uptake and retention in the heart, along with sufficiently low uptake in the lungs, liver, and blood to suggest the compound will be a suitable cardiac imaging agent. If initial biodistribution studies are positive, further studies are generally aimed at demonstrating high specificity of cardiac retention of the tracer for presynaptic sympathetic nerve terminals. For example, administration of DMI (10 mg/kg i.p.) to block NET transporters prior to tracer administration is one way to assess specificity for sympathetic neurons (Rosenspire et al. 1990). Another approach has been administration of the neurotoxin 6-hydroxydopamine (6-OHDA; 100 mg/kg i.p.) to cause a chemical destruction of cardiac sympathetic nerve terminal axons (Raffel and Chen 2004; Schwaiger et al. 1992). Mechanistic studies of the importance of vesicular uptake on a tracer's neuronal retention have typically used administration of reserpine (1 mg/kg i.p., 3 h prior to tracer administration) to block VMAT2 function (Schwaiger et al. 1992). The influence of MAO metabolism has been assessed by administration of MAO inhibitors, including the MAO-A inhibitor clorgyline (10 mg/kg i.p., 60 min before tracer administration) (Del Rosario et al. 1996). Biodistribution studies in rodents are also frequently performed for generating initial estimates of human radiation absorbed doses. For these studies, comprehensive biodistribution data at several time points are needed to provide sufficient kinetic data for the dosimetry software package, such as OLINDA/EXM 1.0 (Stabin et al. 2005), to calculate radiation absorbed doses. For example, human radiation absorbed dose estimates for 4-[^{18}F]-fluoro-*meta*-hydroxyphenethylguanidine ([^{18}F]-4F-MHPG) have recently been reported based on biodistribution studies in rats (Jang et al. 2013).

Additional studies in rodent models have been aimed at better defining the ability of sympathetic nerve radiotracers to track changes in nerve density and neuronal function. One interesting study looked at the influence of modulating sympathetic outflow pharmacologically on the efflux of [^{125}I]-MIBG and [^{3}H]-labeled norepinephrine ([^{3}H]-NE) in rat hearts (Sisson et al. 1991). After injecting [^{125}I]-MIBG or [^{3}H]-NE intravenously into four groups of animals, their concentrations in the heart at $t=2$ h were measured in one group to establish baseline levels of each compound. The remaining three groups received intraperitoneal injection at $t=2$ h of one of the following: (a) the α_2-adrenergic receptor antagonist yohimbine (10 mg/kg) to stimulate neuronal activity; (b) the centrally acting α_2-adrenergic receptor agonist clonidine (0.2 mg/kg), which decreases norepinephrine release; or (c) the injection vehicle, physiologic saline. Cardiac concentrations of [^{3}H]-NE and [^{125}I]-MIBG were determined 4 h later to determine the effect of modulating cardiac sympathetic nerve activity. Yohimbine-induced stimulation of sympathetic nerve activity increased the fractional loss rates of [^{3}H]-NE and [^{125}I]-MIBG by 220 and 210 %, respectively, relative to the rate seen in vehicle-treated animals. Clonidine decreased the fractional loss rates of [^{3}H]-NE and [^{125}I]-MIBG to 51 and 32 % of control rates, respectively. These findings suggest that observed changes in MIBG clearance rates observed in diseased human hearts are at least to some degree modulated by sympathetic nerve activity. For example, this is widely thought to be true in patients with heart failure, where enhanced sympathetic outflow is a hallmark symptom (Leimbach et al. 1986). However, it is also possible that disease-induced changes to vesicular uptake and storage of radiotracers like MIBG may also contribute to enhanced efflux in heart diseases.

To better define the relationship between cardiac retention of [^{11}C]-mHED and regional nerve density, [^{11}C]-mHED retention levels were correlated to in vitro assays of NET density in rats injected with different amounts of the neurotoxin 6-hydroxydopamine (6-OHDA) (Raffel et al. 2006). Six groups of rats were used ($n=5$ each), with each group receiving a different dose of 6-OHDA: 0 (controls), 7, 11, 15, 22, and 100 mg/kg, (i.p.). The next day [^{11}C]-mHED was injected i.v. into each animal and the [^{11}C]-mHED concentrations in heart at $t=30$ min (HU; % injected dose/g) were measured. Hearts were then homogenized and processed with differential centrifugation techniques to generate a tissue preparation for saturation binding assays with [^{3}H]-mazindol to measure NET density (B_{max}; fmol/mg protein). The injected doses of 6-OHDA induced a wide range of cardiac NET densities, from control levels down to only 8 % of controls at the highest 6-OHDA dose of 100 mg/kg. Cardiac [^{11}C]-mHED retention (HU) had a strong linear correlation with NET density (B_{max}): $\text{HU}=(0.0077)B_{max} - 0.028$, $r=0.97$. Thus, [^{11}C]-mHED retention was found to be linearly dependent on NET density in rat hearts that have been partially denervated by 6-OHDA. This suggests that [^{11}C]-mHED retention is a good surrogate measure of NET density, at least for this particular animal model.

However, in similar studies in a dog model of cardiac denervation, a nonlinear relationship between [^{11}C]-mHED retention and regional nerve density was found (Raffel 2012). In this study, varying degrees of regional cardiac denervation were induced by painting the epicardial wall with varying concentrations of the neurotoxin phenol, which penetrates a few mm into the myocardium and causes sympathetic nerve destruction. A few weeks after recovery from surgery, animals were killed immediately following PET imaging with [^{11}C]-mHED. Each heart was carefully sectioned into 20 left ventricular samples, to provide 40 independent tissue samples. The concentration of norepinephrine was measured for each tissue section as a direct measure of regional nerve density. Correlation of the PET measure of regional [^{11}C]-mHED retention levels and tissue norepinephrine concentrations showed a nonlinear relationship between [^{11}C]-mHED retention and nerve density. Thus, the functional dependence of a tracer's retention on regional nerve density may vary between different animal models. One factor that may contribute to these differences is that NET densities may vary between different species. In our studies of saturation binding assays with [^{3}H]-mazindol (Raffel and Chen 2004), we found that NET density in male Sprague–Dawley rat hearts averaged 461 ± 58 fmol/mg protein ($n=6$). NET densities measured under identical assays conditions ranged from 624 to 1,120 fmol/mg in dog hearts ($n=6$ mongrel dogs) and ranged from 196 to 287 fmol/mg protein in New Zealand white rabbits ($n=3$). Binding assays done in normal human hearts under similar binding assay conditions with [^{3}H]-mazindol found cardiac NET densities of $1{,}102 \pm 37$ fmol/mg protein (Böhm et al. 1995). These data suggest that cardiac NET densities in different species follow the rank order: human > dog > rat > rabbit. Again, these interspecies differences should be kept in mind when interpreting results from different animal models.

Rodent models of heart disease have also been used to assess alterations in the uptake and retention of sympathetic nerve radiotracers in different disease conditions. For example, a rat model of diabetes mellitus induced chemically with streptozotocin (STZ) has been used for studies of MIBG (Dubois et al. 1996; Kurata et al. 1997; Kiyono et al. 2001, 2005) and [^{11}C]-mHED (Schmid et al. 1999; Thackeray et al. 2011). One of these studies showed that cardiac retention of [^{125}I]-MIBG was significantly lower in the inferior wall than in the anterior wall in STZ diabetic rats, while [^{125}I]-MIBG retention was uniform in control rats (Kiyono et al. 2001). Also, the lower [^{125}I]-MIBG retention in the inferior wall of STZ diabetic rats was correlated with a lower NET density in the inferior wall relative to the anterior wall. Another disease model that has been used to study sympathetic nerve radiotracers is the spontaneously hypertensive rat as a model of hypertension (Dubois et al. 1996; Schwebel et al. 1999; Pissarek et al. 2002). Studies in these disease models allow for more detailed comparisons in changes of components of presynaptic nerve terminals (e.g., tissue norepinephrine levels, NET densities) and their relationship to corresponding changes in key postsynaptic elements, such as β-adrenergic receptor densities.

Studies in canine models of heart disease have provided important insights into the clinical information provided by sympathetic nerve radiotracers. Studies with [^{123}I]-MIBG in globally denervated dog hearts, induced chemically using 6-OHDA, showed that early retention of MIBG ($t=5$ min) was not altered while delayed images at 3 h showed no MIBG retention (Dae et al. 1992). Cardiac norepinephrine concentrations were reduced to only 6 % of control levels by 6-OHDA treatment, indicating almost complete denervation. The preserved retention early in the study was attributed to extraneuronal uptake (uptake-2) in the dog hearts. In the same study, [^{123}I]-MIBG imaging in human subjects that were recent heart transplant recipients showed no early retention of MIBG, consistent with uptake-2 being insignificant in human hearts.

Rabinovitch and coworkers performed detailed studies of cardiac [^{131}I]-MIBG retention in normal dogs ($n=13$) and in dogs with mechanical overload ($n=10$) following surgical infrarenal aortocaval arteriovenous shunt formation (Rabinovitch et al. 1987). Of the 10 mechanical overload dogs, 5 developed overt heart failure while the remaining 5 had compensated left ventricular hypertrophy. In the dogs with overt heart failure, the rate of [^{131}I]-MIBG efflux from 0.5 to 2.0 h was accelerated relative to controls (0.260 h^{-1} vs. 0.137 h^{-1} for controls, $p<0.001$). However, in the mechanical overload dogs with compensated hypertrophy, the [^{131}I]-MIBG efflux rate was not significantly different from controls. These data suggest that enhanced clearance of MIBG in overt heart failure is due to enhanced sympathetic outflow or effects of heart failure that would enhance MIBG efflux, such as diminished vesicular retention of MIBG.

Sisson and coworkers studied the effects of yohimbine and clonidine on [^{123}I]-MIBG efflux rates from dog hearts ($n=4$) using scintigraphic imaging (Sisson et al. 1991). Similar to their findings in rats described above, yohimbine treatment accelerated the [^{123}I]-MIBG efflux rate (0.277±0.013 h^{-1} vs. 0.137±0.036 h^{-1} for controls, $p<0.05$), while clonidine treatment almost completely inhibited

[^{123}I]-MIBG efflux (rate = 0.012 ± 0.024 h^{-1}, $p < 0.007$ relative to controls). These data strongly support the view that enhanced sympathetic outflow at cardiac sympathetic nerve terminals can directly cause enhanced efflux of MIBG, while central inhibition of sympathetic outflow can slow MIBG efflux.

The retention of [^{11}C]-mHED in a canine model of ischemically injured myocardium and its dependence on blood flow in reperfused myocardium has been reported (Wolpers et al. 1991). In this study, a balloon catheter was used to induce occlusion of the left anterior descending artery for 90 min. Upon reperfusion, [^{11}C]-mHED and radiolabeled microspheres were injected to assess regional [^{11}C]-mHED uptake into sympathetic nerve terminals and regional blood flow. Histochemical staining was used to assess different regions for evidence of infarction or reversible tissue injury. In left ventricular regions with demonstrated infarction, [^{11}C]-mHED retention was significantly reduced by 68 ± 9 %. In areas with reversible tissue injury, [^{11}C]-mHED retention was less severely affected, but still was reduced by 22 ± 8 % from control levels. Retention of [^{11}C]-mHED was found to be highly dependent on blood flow, which points out the importance of having corresponding measures of perfusion to properly interpret observed defects in [^{11}C]-mHED retention. These studies demonstrated that ischemic injury causes damage to presynaptic sympathetic nerve terminals and can reduce tracer retention even in areas of reversibly injured myocardium.

In a more recent study, a chronic occlusion model of hibernating myocardium in pigs was used to assess the influence of therapeutic interventions designed to improve cardiac function on regional sympathetic innervation as demonstrated by [^{11}C]-mHED retention (Fallavollita et al. 2010). Pigs ($n = 11$) were instrumented with a 1.5 mm stenosis of the left anterior descending (LAD) artery. Initial PET imaging studies with [^{11}C]-mHED were performed 3 months later to get baseline assessments of regional damage to sympathetic nerve terminals. One pig died from sudden cardiac death before imaging. The first therapeutic intervention was administration of the 3-hydroxy-3-methylglutaryl-coenzyme A (HMG-CoA) reductase inhibitor pravastatin (160 mg/day, orally) to improve regional function in hibernating myocardium ($n = 7$ pigs). One of the pigs receiving pravastatin and the remaining 3 pigs underwent percutaneous revascularization as the second therapeutic intervention. [^{11}C]-mHED imaging was repeated at 4 weeks after starting the therapeutic interventions. Baseline scans showed significant [^{11}C]-mHED defects in the LAD region, with 48 ± 4 % of the left ventricle demonstrating abnormally low [^{11}C]-mHED retention. After the therapeutic interventions, there was no improvement in the extent of abnormal [^{11}C]-mHED retention (58 ± 9 % of the left ventricle, $p = 0.39$), despite demonstrated improvement in left ventricular function parameters in response to the therapies. Thus, in spite of functional improvements in the hibernating myocardium, the ischemic damage to presynaptic sympathetic nerve function persisted, suggesting the damage to the neurons was structural rather than functional in nature.

This brief review of studies performed in animal models, especially in experimental models of heart disease, illustrates their importance in defining changes in a tracer's retention and kinetics in response to disease conditions. The results of these studies greatly aid in the interpretation of the results of clinical studies of cardiac sympathetic innervation in different heart disease populations.

10.7 Imaging Studies

The increasing availability of single photon emission computed tomography (SPECT) and PET systems designed for small animal imaging has made it possible to do more elegant preclinical evaluations of sympathetic innervation radiotracers than were previously possible through biodistribution studies alone. Much more detailed analyses of neuronal retention mechanisms and tracer kinetics in response to various pharmacological challenges can be more accurately characterized. Many excellent examples of imaging studies in small animals can be found throughout the chapters in this book.

Most of our recent preclinical PET imaging studies have been performed in rhesus macaque monkeys. In our experience, studies in this species provide the most accurate predictions of the myocardial kinetics of sympathetic nerve radiotracers in human hearts. The absence of significant uptake-2 activity in the hearts of monkeys and humans undoubtedly contributes to this finding. However, the trade-off in performing imaging studies in monkeys is that it is not possible to induce various models of heart diseases or to correlate imaging or kinetic parameters with direct measures of tissue components, such as NET density measures.

Our studies of radiolabeled phenethylguanidines in isolated rat hearts identified at least two compounds that exhibited favorable kinetic properties for tracer kinetic analyses, *N*-[^{11}C]-guanyl-(−)-*meta*-octopamine ([^{11}C]-GMO) and [^{11}C]-4-fluoro-meta-hydroxyphenethylguanidine ([^{11}C]-4F-MHPG) (Fig. 10.5). Recently, we have [^{18}F] labeled the latter compound to prepare [^{18}F]-4F-MHPG (Jang et al. 2013). PET imaging studies with [^{11}C]-GMO and [^{18}F]-4F-MHPG in rhesus macaque monkeys have so far supported the hypotheses that led to their development. Specifically, the myocardial kinetics of [^{11}C]-GMO and [^{18}F]-4F-MHPG have each been successfully analyzed using compartmental modeling techniques and Patlak graphical analysis to yield quantitative measures of nerve density (Raffel et al. 2013b; Jang et al. 2013).

Transaxial cardiac PET images of [^{11}C]-GMO and [^{18}F]-4F-MHPG in rhesus macaque monkeys, acquired using a microPET P4 primate scanner (Siemens/CTI Concorde Microsystems, Knoxville, TN), are shown in Fig. 10.8. In addition to control studies, a series of studies with the NET inhibitor DMI were performed to evaluate the ability of quantitative parameters from tracer kinetic analyses to track declines in available NET density. For these studies, a DMI dose was dissolved in 2 mL of physiological saline and infused intravenously over 20 min using an infusion pump, and 10 min after DMI infusion, [^{11}C]-GMO or [^{18}F]-4F-MHPG (18–40 MBq/kg) was injected as PET acquisition was started. Increasingly higher doses of infused DMI caused progressive declines in the final myocardial retention of each radiotracer (Fig. 10.8).

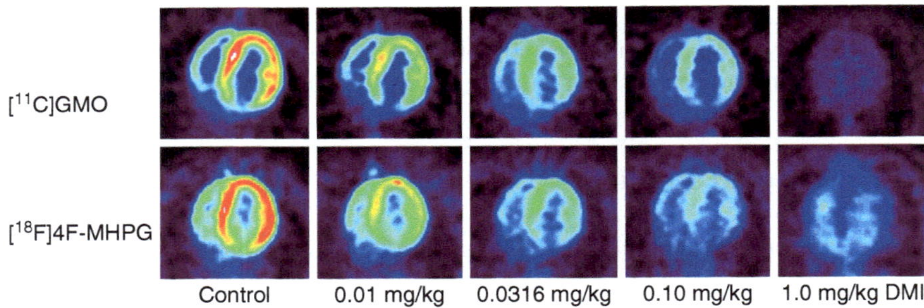

Fig. 10.8 Transaxial microPET images of [^{11}C]-GMO (top row) and [^{18}F]-4F-MHPG (*bottom row*) in rhesus macaque monkeys under control conditions and for progressively higher doses of the NET inhibitor DMI. The extremely low myocardial retention of each tracer at the highest DMI dose demonstrates their high selectivity for presynaptic sympathetic nerve terminals

Venous blood samples (n=4–6) were collected during PET imaging to assess radiotracer metabolism and partitioning of radioactivity between plasma and red blood cells (RBCs). Deproteinized plasma samples were adjusted to pH 6.5–7.0, filtered, and analyzed with reverse-phase high-performance liquid chromatography (HPLC) and radiodetection to determine the fraction of plasma radioactivity associated with parent radiotracer and metabolites. [^{11}C]-GMO in plasma was metabolized with a mean half-time $T_{1/2}=16.0\pm3.0$ min, while [^{18}F]-4F-MHPG was metabolized more quickly, with $T_{1/2}=2.5\pm0.8$ min. In both cases, a single major radiometabolite that was more polar than the parent compound was observed in the radio-HPLC data. Performing in vitro incubations of [^{18}F]-4F-MHPG with commercially available monkey or human liver cytosol fractions and the sulfotransferase cofactor adenosine-3′-phosphate-5′-phosphosulfate (PAPS) for 20 min at 37 °C, we were able to generate the major radiometabolite of [^{18}F]-4F-MHPG seen in monkey plasma. Thus, sulfur conjugation appears to be the major metabolism pathway for [^{18}F]-4F-MHPG in rhesus macaque monkeys. Similar in vitro metabolism studies with [^{11}C]-GMO, including sulfoconjugation studies, as well as glucuronidation studies with monkey liver microsomes and the glucuronidation cofactor uridine 5′-diphosphoglucuronic acid (UDPGA) were negative. Further studies are needed to identify the major radiometabolite of [^{11}C]-GMO. In terms of blood partitioning, [^{11}C]-GMO tended to stay in plasma with very little uptake into RBCs. The mean concentration ratio between plasma and whole blood was $C_p(t)/C_{wb}(t)=1.47\pm0.08$ (total of 48 blood samples). For [^{18}F]-4F-MHPG, this ratio typically averaged 1.24 ± 0.10. For each PET study, the data describing the metabolic breakdown of parent radiotracer and the blood partitioning data were used to convert an image-derived time–activity curve for radioactivity in whole blood, $C_{wb}(t)$, into an estimated plasma time–activity curve, $C_p(t)$, for tracer kinetic analyses.

Region-of-interest (ROI) analysis was used to extract time–activity curves for [^{18}F]-4F-MHPG and [^{11}C]-GMO in left ventricular tissue, $C_t(t)$, from the dynamic PET scans. A simplified compartmental model (Fig. 10.9) was used for compartmental modeling. This model assumes that all tracer molecules transported into

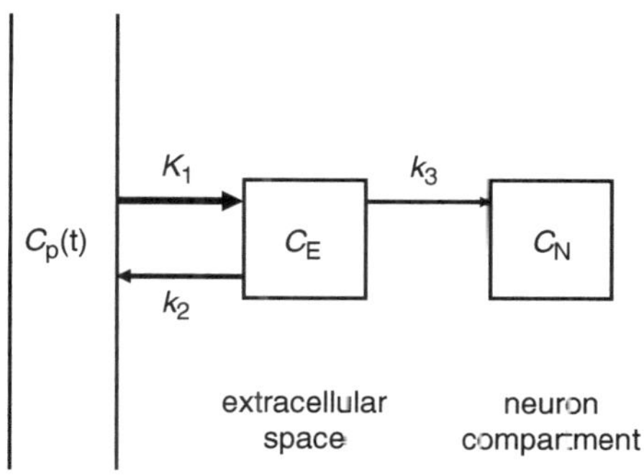

Fig. 10.9 Compartmental model structure used for compartmental modeling of the myocardial kinetics of [^{18}F]-4F-MHPG and [^{11}C]-GMO in rhesus macaque monkeys

sympathetic nerve terminals by NET are irreversibly trapped inside the neurons by rapid vesicular storage. This assumption is supported by the kinetics of these tracers in isolated rat hearts (Fig. 10.5). Compartmental modeling provided estimates of the rate constants K_1 (mL/min/g), k_2 (min^{-1}) and k_3 (min^{-1}) and a blood volume fraction *BV* (dimensionless). The estimated rate constants for each study were used to calculate the net uptake rate constant $K_i = (K_1 k_3)/(k_2 + k_3)$, with units mL/min/g, which reflects the rate of [^{18}F]-4F-MHPG or [^{11}C]-GMO accumulation into sympathetic nerve terminals. The kinetics of each radiotracer was also analyzed using Patlak graphical analysis (Patlak and Blasberg 1985). Patlak plots constructed from the kinetic data $C_p(t)$ and $C_t(t)$ were linear for points on the plot corresponding to PET image frames acquired from ~3 min after tracer injection until the end of the study. The linear portion of the Patlak plot was analyzed with linear regression to determine the Patlak slope, K_p (mL/min/g). Under ideal conditions, the Patlak slope K_p is a direct measure of the net uptake rate constant K_i and thus for the compartmental model structure used is also approximately equal to $(K_1 k_3)/(k_2 - k_3)$.

For both [^{11}C]-GMO and [^{18}F]-4F-MHPG, compartmental modeling of their kinetics was robust, converging quickly to a single global minimum for all studies. Representative examples of the myocardial kinetics of [^{18}F]-4F-MHPG and corresponding compartmental model fits are shown in Fig. 10.10. Similarly, Patlak analysis of [^{18}F]-4F-MHPG and [^{11}C]-GMO kinetics was successful, yielding highly linear Patlak plots, with linear correlation coefficients $r > 0.99$ in all cases. Patlak plots for PET studies with [^{11}C]-GMO in rhesus macaque monkeys are presented in Fig. 10.11, which show that the Patlak slopes K_p (mL/min/g) declined progressively with increases in the infused DMI dose. For control studies ($n = 4$), Patlak slopes $K_p = 0.103 \pm 0.005$ mL/min/g. Declines in measured K_p values for [^{11}C]-GMO versus increasing DMI doses were well described by a one-site sigmoidal dose–response function with variable slope (Fig. 10.12). For the Patlak slope data, a half maximal inhibitory concentration (IC_{50}) of 0.068 ± 0.010 mg/kg DMI was estimated, with a Hill slope $n_H = -0.54 \pm 0.05$. For compartmental modeling results, the net uptake rate constants calculated from parameter estimates as $K_i = (K_1 k_3)/(k_2 + k_3)$ also were found to provide good quantitative measures of sympathetic nerve density. A similar sigmoidal dose–response curve was seen for the K_i vs. DMI dose data (Fig. 10.12). In this case, $IC_{50} = 0.087 \pm 0.012$ mg/kg DMI, with a Hill slope $n_H = -0.70 \pm 0.07$.

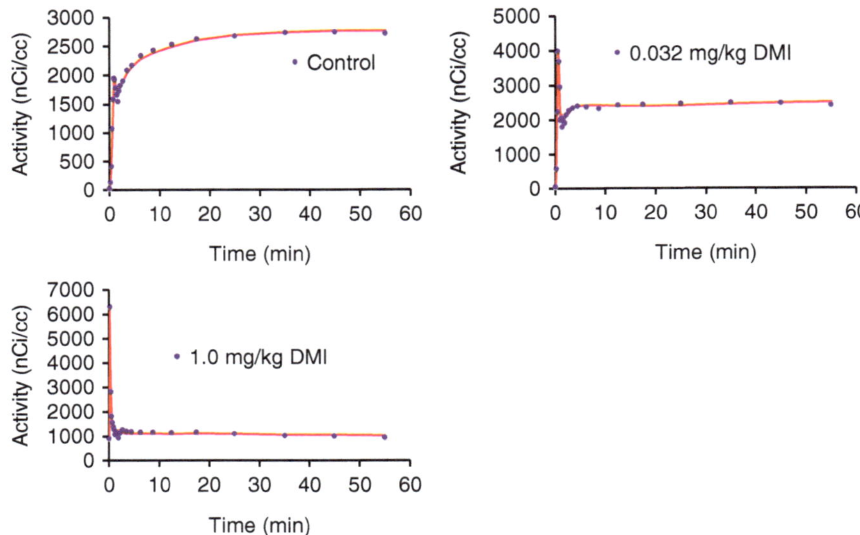

Fig. 10.10 Compartmental modeling of myocardial [^{18}F]-4F-MHPG kinetics in monkeys for a control study (*left top*), a moderate desipramine (DMI) dose study (*right*), and a high DMI dose study (*left bottom*). Compartmental modeling was successful under all experimental conditions tested

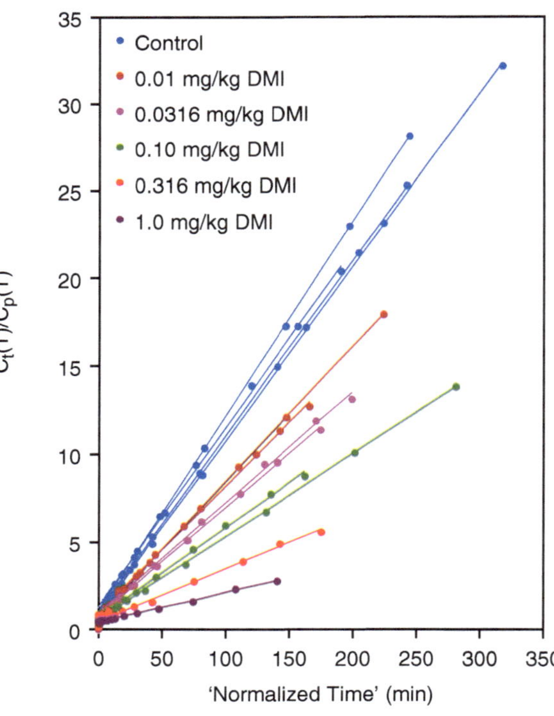

Fig. 10.11 Patlak graphical analysis of [^{11}C]-GMO kinetics in rhesus macaque monkeys under control conditions ($n = 4$) and following pharmacological blockade of cardiac NET at five different doses of DMI. Plots were highly linear in all cases ($r > 0.99$) and Patlak slopes declined in a dose-dependent manner with increasing DMI doses

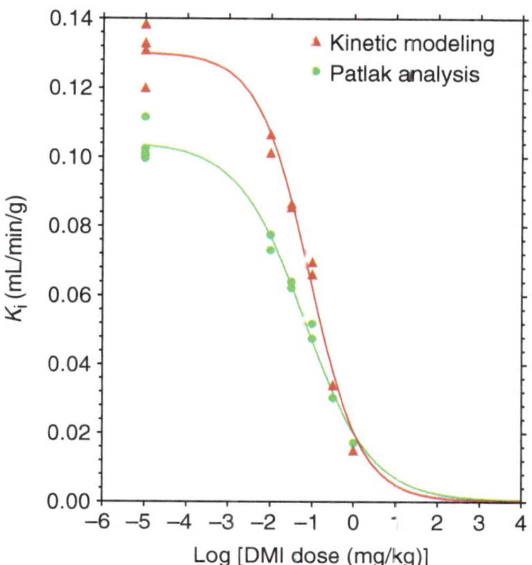

Fig. 10.12 Dose–response curves of "net uptake constants" K_i (mL/min/g) derived from either compartmental modeling (*red triangles*) or Patlak graphical analysis (*green circles*) of [^{11}C]-GMO kinetics in rhesus macaque monkeys. Each of the K_i parameters appears to serve as robust and reproducible quantitative measures of cardiac sympathetic nerve density

Comparable results were seen for compartmental modeling and Patlak graphical analysis of [^{18}F]-4F-MHPG kinetics in rhesus macaque monkeys (Jang et al. 2013).

The main difference between K_i values estimated from compartmental modeling versus Patlak analysis is that the latter method does not provide a means of accounting for blood volume and spillover effects in the tissue time–activity curve. This is managed by the blood volume term *BV* in compartmental modeling analysis. The result is that the Patlak slopes have a modest downward bias relative to corresponding K_i values calculated from compartmental modeling. For [^{11}C]-GMO, a strong linear correlation was seen between K_p and K_i, with $K_p=(0.758)K_i+0.001$ ($r=0.99$). K_p and K_i were similarly correlated for control and DMI-blocking studies with [^{18}F]-4F-MHPG, with $K_p=(0.829)K_i+0.010$ ($r=0.97$). Thus, kinetic analysis results with [^{11}C]-GMO and [^{18}F]-4F-MHPG demonstrate that either method of acquiring estimates of the net uptake rate constant K_i yields robust and reproducible estimates of cardiac sympathetic nerve density.

In clinical studies with [^{11}C]-mHED, the regional cardiac retention of the radiotracer is usually expressed as a "retention index" (RI, mL blood/min/mL tissue), which is the regional tissue concentration of [^{11}C]-mHED (kBq/mL tissue) in the final dynamic PET image divided by the integral of the whole-blood time–activity curve (kBq·min/mL blood) (Allman et al. 1993). For [^{11}C]-GMO, we calculated RI values using not only the integrated whole-blood time–activity curve (RI_{wb}) but also the integrated plasma time–activity curve corrected for metabolites that was used for compartmental modeling and Patlak analysis (RI_p). When RI_{wb} and RI_p values were plotted against the corresponding net uptake rate constants K_i from compartmental modeling or Patlak slopes from Patlak analysis K_p, highly linear correlations were seen in each case:

$$RI_{wb} = (0.340)K_i + 0.008 \quad (r = 0.96)$$

$$RI_{\mathrm{p}} = (0.765)K_{\mathrm{i}} + 0.002 \ (r = 0.99)$$

$$RI_{\mathrm{wb}} = (0.434)K_{\mathrm{p}} + 0.009 \ (r = 0.94)$$

$$RI_{\mathrm{p}} = (1.009)K_{\mathrm{p}} + 0.001 \ (r = 1.00)$$

Correlations were higher for the $\mathrm{RI_p}$ values versus K_i and K_p because the whole-blood time–activity data are not corrected for metabolites; thus, variations in the rate of tracer metabolism in different studies are not accounted for, leading to a larger spread in the calculated $\mathrm{RI_{wb}}$ values. The highest correlation was between the $\mathrm{RI_p}$ values and the Patlak slopes K_p. This is not completely surprising since in this case, the value of $\mathrm{RI_p}$ is equal to the slope of a line connecting the origin of the Patlak plot to the final time point in the Patlak plot, which would have a value slightly larger than the Patlak slope but highly correlated with it.

These results suggest that a retention index approach to analyzing the kinetics of [^{11}C]-GMO or [^{18}F]-4F-MHPG could potentially be used instead of compartmental modeling or Patlak analysis. However, if tracer metabolism in plasma is not corrected for, there will be higher variability in the RI values. Since these tracers have been designed specifically to minimize flow limitation effects, it is likely that retention index measurements made with these tracers will detect regional denervation earlier in its progression than is currently possible using [^{11}C]-mHED retention indices.

10.8 Case Study: Development of Radiolabeled Phenethylguanidines

The sequence of preclinical studies of a new radiopharmaceutical will likely vary on a case-by-case basis, depending on how much is already known about the class of compounds being studied. In the case of our recent work with radiolabeled phenethylguanidines, we knew from the literature that many of these compounds were potent depletors of cardiac norepinephrine stores at pharmacological doses due to their prolonged retention inside storage vesicles. Since we were specifically looking for a tracer with a slower NET transport rate than [^{11}C]-mHED and [^{123}I]-MIBG and long neuronal retention times, we initially screened a series of [^{11}C]-labeled phenethylguanidines in our isolated working rat heart system to identify compounds with these two kinetic properties (Raffel et al. 2007). One of the advantages of this system is that a new radiotracer's neuronal uptake rate constant (K_up, mL/min/g wet) and clearance kinetics from neuronal spaces can be measured in a single isolated rat heart study. During the structure–activity relation studies in isolated rat hearts, when a compound was identified to have the desired kinetic properties, then a biodistribution study in rats at $t=30$ min was performed. Some laboratories might choose instead to do small animal imaging studies at this point, but in our case, biodistribution studies allowed for quantitative comparisons with a wealth of biodistribution data archived for all of the sympathetic nerve radiotracers previously developed at our institution.

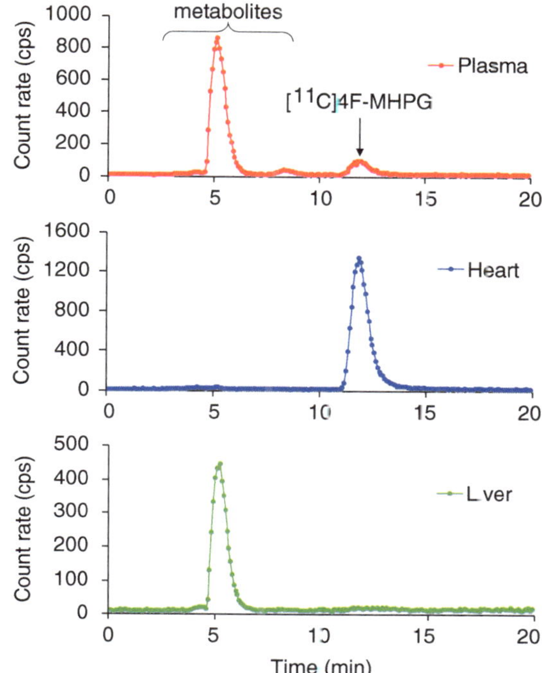

Fig. 10.13 Studies of the metabolic fate of [^{11}C]-4F-MHPG in a rat at $t=30$ min after tracer administration. Reverse-phase HPLC analysis with radiodetection of extracts from plasma, heart, and liver shows that the radiometabolites in plasma are not found in the heart, demonstrating that all heart activity is associated with the parent radiotracer

If the results of the biodistribution study showed sufficiently high heart-to-blood ratios and low lung uptake, we then performed a few studies of the metabolic fate of the tracer in rats to verify that radiometabolites were inactive at NET and did not accumulate in the heart. This is important because if any major radiometabolite is a NET substrate, it would complicate tracer kinetic analysis. For one of these studies, a single rat was injected with ~185 MBq of a [^{11}C]-labeled phenethylguanidine. At $t=30$ min, the animal was killed and a blood sample, the heart, and the liver were harvested. Theses samples were analyzed by radiodetection and reverse-phase HPLC. An example of a study performed for [^{11}C]-4F-MHPG is shown in Fig. 10.13. The data show that at 30 min after tracer administration, most of the [^{11}C]-4F-MHPG in plasma has been metabolized to one major and one minor radiometabolite. Activity in the liver is >99 % the major radiometabolite, while activity in the heart is >99 % authentic [^{11}C]-4F-MHPG. Thus, at least for the rat model, the radiometabolites are not active at NET and all heart retention of this tracer is associated with the parent compound.

Unfortunately, direct assessments of radiometabolite activity at NET are not feasible in nonhuman primates or human subjects. For example, in the case of [^{18}F]-4F-MHPG, the radiometabolite formed in rhesus macaque monkeys is different from that observed in the rat. As discussed in Sect. 10.8, our data strongly suggests that sulfur conjugation is the major metabolic pathway for [^{18}F]-4F-MHPG in the monkey. However, we can indirectly infer that the sulfur conjugate of [^{18}F]-4F-MHPG is inactive at NET based on the results of kinetic analyses. If the radiometabolite was active, Patlak plots constructed from plasma input functions that exclude activity associated with the radiometabolite would not be linear. Another approach to verifying the inactivity of the [^{18}F]-4F-MPHG metabolite would be to synthesize the [^{11}C]-labeled sulfur conjugate and test its activity in the isolated rat heart or a cellular-based in vitro transport assay.

The radiolabeled phenethylguanidines that successfully passed all of these initial screenings were evaluated in microPET imaging studies of their imaging properties and kinetics and metabolism in nonhuman primates as described in Sect. 10.8. Out of ~40 structures tested in the isolated rat heart, around 10 were ultimately evaluated in PET studies in nonhuman primates. Most PET studies to date have focused on [^{11}C]-GMO and [^{18}F]-4F-MHPG, but a few other fluorine-bearing structures deserve further bio-evaluations.

The steps taken in the radiotracer development process are not always linear. As information is gathered with compounds in different models, the information gleaned is fed back into improved tracer designs. For example, our microPET studies in monkeys tended to show that structures with a β-hydroxyl group in the side chain of a phenethylguanidine tended to have much higher liver uptake than those without this feature (Raffel et al. 2007). Thus, one drawback with [^{11}C]-GMO, which has a β-hydroxyl group, is its relatively high liver uptake. However, a strength of [^{11}C]-GMO is its low lipophilicity, which tends to keep the tracer in plasma and out of RBCs during an imaging study. This simplifies tracer kinetic analyses because conversion of an image-derived whole-blood time–activity curve into a plasma input function is more straightforward due to the consistent partition ratio between plasma and RBCs.

These previous compounds also tend to have very low binding to plasma proteins. We measured plasma free fractions of [^{11}C]-GMO and [^{18}F]-4F-MHPG in human plasma samples incubated with each tracer for 30 min at 37 °C using published ultrafiltration techniques (Gandelman et al. 1994). The plasma free fraction for [^{11}C]-GMO and [^{18}F]-4F-MHPG were 82.0 ± 1.1 % ($n = 6$) and 73.7 ± 1.9 % ($n = 6$), respectively. Thus, most of the radiotracer in the plasma fraction is free for extraction into heart tissue during passage through cardiac capillary beds.

Our current views on desirable properties for a radiotracer designed to measure regional cardiac sympathetic nerve density are as follows: (a) neuronal uptake rates of 0.20–0.80 mL/min/g in the isolated rat heart model; (b) very long neuronal retention times due to retention in vesicles or other irreversible mechanisms; (c) low lipophilicity, with a negative Log*P*, preferably <−1.0; (d) stable against intraneuronal metabolism by enzymes such as MAO; (e) metabolic breakdown rates in plasma that are not too fast (e.g., $T_{1/2} = 10$–30 min); (f) radiometabolites that are inactive at NET; and (g) high plasma free fractions. We are also currently avoiding structures with a β-hydroxyl group to minimize liver uptake. However, studies in human subjects might show that this structural element does not cause high liver uptake as it does in monkeys. Like any working model, these current views are subject to new data that show that one or more of these criteria need to be revised.

Conclusion

In conclusion, the studies presented in this chapter highlight some of the preclinical evaluations that have been performed in the development of cardiac sympathetic innervation tracers. The results of these studies provide fundamental insights into the mechanisms of action of these imaging agents. Clearly, the better our understanding of the interaction of these radiotracers with various physiological components of sympathetic nerve terminals, the better our ability to properly assess observed changes in their cardiac retention observed clinically in heart diseases.

References

Allman KC, Stevens MJ, Wieland DM et al (1993) Noninvasive assessment of cardiac diabetic neuropathy by C-11 hydroxyephedrine and positron emission tomography. J Am Coll Cardiol 22:1425–1432

Böhm M, La Rosée K, Schwinger RHG et al (1995) Evidence for reduction of norepinephrine uptake sites in the failing human heart. J Am Coll Cardiol 25:145–153

Burgen ASV, Iversen LL (1965) The inhibition of noradrenaline uptake by sympathomimetic amines in the rat isolated heart. Br J Pharmacol 25:34–49

Carr EA, Carroll M, Counsell RE et al (1979) Studies of uptake of the bretylium analogue, iodobenzyltrimethylammonum iodide, by non-primate, monkey and human heart. Br J Clin Pharmacol 8:425–432

Chakraborty PK, Gildersleeve DL, Jewett DM et al (1993) High yield synthesis of high specific activity R-(−)-[11C]epinephrine for routine PET studies in humans. Nucl Med Biol 20:939–944

Cohn JN, Levine TB, Olivari MT et al (1984) Plasma norepinephrine as a guide to prognosis in patients with chronic congestive heart failure. N Engl J Med 311:819–823

Costa E, Kunstman R, Gessa GL et al (1962) Structural requirements for bretylium and guanethidine-like activity in a series of guanidine derivatives. Life Sci 3:75–80

Dae MW, De Marco T, Botvinick EH et al (1992) Scintigraphic assessment of MIBG uptake in globally denervated human and canine hearts – implications for clinical studies. J Nucl Med 33:1444–1450

DeGrado TR, Hutchins GD, Toorongian SA et al (1993) Myocardial kinetics of carbon-11-meta-hydroxyephedrine: retention mechanisms and effects of norepinephrine. J Nucl Med 34:1287–1293

DeGrado TR, Zalutsky MR, Vaidyanathan G (1995) Uptake mechanisms of meta-[123I]iodobenzylguanidine in isolated rat heart. Nucl Med Biol 22(1):1–12

DeGrado TR, Zalutsky MR, Coleman RE et al (1998) Effects of specific activity on meta-[131I] iodobenzylguanidine kinetics in isolated rat heart. Nucl Med Biol 25:59–64

Del Rosario RB, Jung Y-W, Chakraborty PK et al (1996) Synthesis and preliminary evaluation of [11C]-(−)-phenylephrine as a functional heart neuronal PET agent. Nucl Med Biol 23: 611–616

Dubois EA, Kam KL, Somsen GA et al (1996) Cardiac iodine-123 metaiodobenzylguanidine uptake in animals with diabetes mellitus and/or hypertension. Eur J Nucl Med 23:901–908

Eisenhofer G, Smolich JJ, Esler MD (1992) Disposition of endogenous adrenaline compared to noradrenaline released by cardiac sympathetic nerves in the anaesthetized dog. Naunyn Schmiedebergs Arch Pharmacol 345:160–171

Fallavollita JA, Banas MD, Suzuki G et al (2010) 11C-meta-Hydroxyephedrine defects persist despite functional improvement in hibernating myocardium. J Nucl Cardiol 17:85–96

Fielden R, Green AL (1965) The effects of some aralkylguanidines in mice. Br J Pharmacol 24:408–417

Gandelman M, Baldwin RM, Zoghbi SS et al (1994) Evaluation of ultrafiltration for the free fraction determination of SPECT radiotracers: b-CIT, IBF and iomazenil. J Pharm Sci 83: 1014–1019

Glowniak J, Turner F, Gray L et al (1989) Iodine-123 metaiodobenzylguanidine imaging of the heart in idiopathic congestive cardiomyopathy and cardiac transplants. J Nucl Med 30:1182–1191

Graefe K-H (1981) The disposition of 3H-(−)-noradrenaline in the perfused cat and rabbit heart. Naunyn Schmiedebergs Arch Pharmacol 318:71–82
Graefe K-H, Bönisch H, Keller B (1978) Saturation kinetics of the adrenergic neurone uptake system in the perfused rabbit heart: a new method for determination of initial rates of amine uptake. Naunyn Schmiedebergs Arch Pharmacol 302:263–273
Green AL, Fielden R, Bartlett DC et al (1967) New norepinephrine-depleting agents. b-hydroxyphenethylguanidine and related compounds. J Med Chem 10:1006–1008
Hansch C, Leo A, Hoekman D (1995) Exploring QSAR: hydrophobic, electronic and steric constants. In: Computer applications in chemistry books, vol 2. ACS, Washington, DC
Hayer-Zillgen M, Brüss M, Bönisch H (2002) Expression and pharmacological profile of the human organic cation transporters hOCT1, hOCT2 and hOCT3. Br J Pharmacol 156:829–836
Hellmann G, Hertting G, Peskar B (1971) Uptake kinetics and metabolism of 7-3H-dopamine in the isolated perfused rat heart. Br J Pharmacol 41:256–269
Iversen LL (1963) The uptake of noradrenaline by the isolated perfused rat heart. Br J Pharmacol 21:523–537
Iversen LL (1965) The uptake of catechol amines at high perfusion concentrations in the rat isolated heart: a novel catechol amine uptake process. Br J Pharmacol 25:18–33
Iversen LL (1967) The uptake and storage of noradrenaline in sympathetic nerves. Cambridge University Press, Cambridge
Iversen LL (1971) Role of transmitter uptake mechanisms in synaptic neurotransmission. Br J Pharmacol 41:571–591
Jang KS, Jung YW, Gu G et al (2013) 4-[18 F]fluoro-m-hydroxyphenethylguanidine: a radiopharmaceutical for quantifying regional cardiac sympathetic nerve density with positron emission tomography. J Med Chem 56:7312–7323
Kiyono Y, Iida Y, Kawashima H et al (2001) Regional alterations of myocardial norepinephrine transporter density in streptozotocin-induced diabetic rats: implications for heterogeneous cardiac accumulation of MIBG in diabetes. Eur J Nucl Med 38:894–899
Kiyono Y, Kajiyama S, Fujiwara H et al (2005) Influence of the polyol pathway on norepinephrine transporter reduction in diabetic cardiac sympathetic nerves: implications for heterogeneous accumulation of MIBG. Eur J Nucl Med Mol Imaging 32:993–997
Kuntzman R, Jacobson MM (1963) Monoamine oxidase inhibition by a series of compounds structurally related to bretylium and guanethidine. J Pharmacol Exp Ther 141:166–172
Kurata C, Okayama K, Wakabayashi Y et al (1997) Cardiac sympathetic neuropathy and effects of aldose reductase inhibitor in streptozotocin-induced diabetic rats. J Nucl Med 38:1677–1680
Kvetnansky R, Sabban EL, Palkovits M (2009) Catecholaminergic systems in stress: structural and molecular genetic approaches. Physiol Rev 89:535–606
Lameris TW, van den Meiracker AH, Boomsma F et al (1999) Catecholamine handling in the porcine heart: a microdialysis approach. Am J Physiol 277:H1562–H1569
Leimbach WN, Wallin BG, Victor RG et al (1986) Direct evidence from intraneuronal recordings for increased central sympathetic outflow in patients with heart failure. Circulation 73: 913–919
Lightman SJ, Iversen LL (1969) The role of uptake-2 in the extraneuronal metabolism of catecholamines in the isolated rat heart. Br J Pharmacol 33:638–649
Ng CK, Holden JE, DeGrado TR et al (1991) Sensitivity of myocardial fluorodeoxyglucose lumped constant to glucose and insulin. Am J Physiol 260:H593–H603
Nguyen NTB, DeGrado TR, Chakraborty P et al (1997) Myocardial kinetics of C-11 epinephrine in the isolated working rat heart. J Nucl Med 38:780–785
Patlak CS, Blasberg RG (1985) Graphical evaluation of blood-to-brain transfer constants from multiple-time uptake data. Generalizations. J Cereb Blood Flow Metab 5:584–590
Pissarek M, Ermert J, Oesterreich G et al (2002) Relative uptake, metabolism, and b-receptor binding of (1R,2S)-4-18 F-fluorometaraminol and 123I-MIBG in normotensive and spontaneously hypertensive rats. J Nucl Med 43:366–373
Rabinovitch MA, Rose CP, Rouleau JL et al (1987) Metaiodobenzylguanidine [131I] scintigraphy detects impaired myocardial sympathetic neuronal transport function of canine mechanical-overload heart failure. Circ Res 61:797–804

Raffel DM (2012) Targeting norepinephrine transporters in cardiac sympathetic nerve terminals. In: Welch MJ, Eckelman WC (eds) Targeted molecular imaging. Imaging in medical diagnosis and therapy. CRC Press, Boca Raton, pp 305–320
Raffel DM, Chen W (2004) Binding of [3H]mazindol to cardiac norepinephrine transporters: kinetic and equilibrium studies. Naunyn Schmiedebergs Arch Pharmacol 370:9–16
Raffel DM, Wieland DM (1999) Influence of vesicular storage and monoamine oxidase activity on [11C]phenylephrine kinetics: studies in isolated rat heart. J Nucl Med 40(2):323–330
Raffel DM, Wieland DM (2001) Assessment of cardiac sympathetic nerve integrity with positron emission tomography. Nucl Med Biol 28:541–559
Raffel D, Loc'h C, Mardon K et al (1998) Kinetics of the norepinephrine analog [Br-76]-meta-bromobenzylguanidine in isolated working rat heart. Nucl Med Biol 25:1–16
Raffel DM, Corbett JR, del Rosario RB et al (1999) Sensitivity of [11C]phenylephrine kinetics to monoamine oxidase activity in normal human heart. J Nucl Med 40(2):232–238
Raffel DM, Chen W, Sherman PS et al (2006) Dependence of cardiac 11C-meta-hydroxyephedrine retention on norepinephrine transporter density. J Nucl Med 47:1490–1496
Raffel DM, Jung YW, Gildersleeve DL et al (2007) Radiolabeled phenethylguanidines: novel imaging agents for cardiac sympathetic neurons and adrenergic tumors. J Med Chem 50: 2078–2088
Raffel DM, Chen W, Jung YW et al (2013a) Radiotracers for cardiac sympathetic innervation: transport kinetics and binding affinities for the human norepinephrine transporter. Nucl Med Biol 40:331–337
Raffel DM, Koeppe RA, Jung YW et al (2013b) Quantification of cardiac sympathetic nerve density of N-11C-guanyl-meta-octopamine and tracer kinetic analysis. J Nucl Med 54: 1645–1652
Raisman R, Sette M, Pimoule C et al (1982) High-affinity [3H]desipramine binding in the peripheral and central nervous system: a specific site associated with the neuronal uptake of noradrenaline. Eur J Pharmacol 78:345–351
Rosenspire KC, Haka MS, Van Dort ME et al (1990) Synthesis and preliminary evaluation of carbon-11-meta-hydroxyephedrine: a false transmitter agent for heart neuronal imaging. J Nucl Med 31:1328–1334
Salt PJ (1972) Inhibition of noradrenaline uptake$_2$ in the isolated rat heart by steroids, clonidine and methoxylated phenylethylamines. Eur J Pharmacol 20:329–340
Schmid H, Forman LA, Cao X et al (1999) Heterogeneous cardiac sympathetic denervation and decreased myocardial nerve growth factor in streptozotocin-induced diabetic rats. Diabetes 48:603–608
Schwaiger M, Hutchins GD, Wieland DM (1992) Noninvasive evaluation of the cardiac sympathetic nervous system with positron emission tomography. In: Bergmann SR, Sobel BE (eds) Positron emission tomography of the heart. Futura Publishing, Mount Kisco, pp 231–254
Schwebel C, Durand A, Godin-Ribuot D et al (1999) Myocardial meta-[125I]iodobenzylguanidine uptake in awake genetically hypertensive rats at different ages: an autoradiographic study. Can J Physiol Pharmacol 77:398–406
Sisson JC, Bolgos G, Johnson J (1991) Measuring acute changes in adrenergic nerve activity of the heart in the living animal. Am Heart J 121:1119–1123
Stabin MG, Sparks RB, Crowe E (2005) OLINDA/EXM: the second-generation personal computer software for internal dose assessment in nuclear medicine. J Nucl Med 46:1023–1027
Taegtmeyer H, Hems R, Krebs HA (1980) Utilization of energy providing substrates in the isolated working rat heart. Biochem J 186:701–711
Thackeray JT, Radziuk J, Harper ME et al (2011) Sympathetic nervous dysregulation in the absence of systolic left ventricular dysfunction in a rat model of insulin resistance with hyperglycemia. Cardiovasc Diabetol 10:75. doi:10.1186/1475-2840-1110-1175
Ungerer M, Hartmann F, Karoglan M et al (1998) Regional in vivo and in vitro characterization of autonomic innervation in cardiomyopathic human heart. Circulation 97:174–180
Van Dort ME, Kim JH, Tluczek L et al (1997) Synthesis of carbon-11 labeled desipramine and its metabolite 2-hydroxydesipramine: potential radiotracers for PET studies of the norepinephrine transporter. Nucl Med Biol 24:707–711

Wieland DM, Brown LE, Rogers WL et al (1981) Myocardial imaging with a radioiodinated norepinephrine storage analog. J Nucl Med 22:22–31

Wolpers HG, Nguyen N, Rosenspire KC et al (1991) 11C-hydroxyephedrine as marker for neuronal catecholamine retention in reperfused canine myocardium. Coron Artery Dis 2:923–929

Wu X, Kekuda R, Huang W et al (1998) Identity of the organic cation transporter OCT3 as the extraneuronal monoamine transporter (uptake2) and evidence for the expression of the transporter in the brain. J Biol Chem 273:32776–32786

Zwart R, Verhaagh S, Buitelaar M et al (2001) Impaired activity of the extraneuronal monoamine transporter system known as uptake-2 in Orct3/Slc22a3-deficient mice. Mol Cell Biol 21:4188–4196

PET Imaging of Myocardial β-Adrenoceptors

11

Riemer H.J.A. Slart, Peter van der Meer, René A. Tio, Dirk J. van Veldhuisen, and Philip H. Elsinga

Contents

Abstract

β-adrenoceptors are important in the regulation of heart function and have been studied extensively in recent decades. In vitro studies have shown downregulation of β-adrenoceptor density in heart failure and cardiac conditions that may lead to heart failure.

R.H.J.A. Slart, MD, PhD (✉) • P.H. Elsinga, PhD
Department of Nuclear Medicine and Molecular Imaging, University Medical Center Groningen, University of Groningen,
Hanzeplein 1, 30001, Groningen 9700 RB, The Netherlands
e-mail: r.h.j.a.slart@umcg.nl

P. van der Meer, MD, PhD • R.A. Tio, MD, PhD • D.J. van Veldhuisen, MD, PhD
Division Cardiology, Thorax Center, University Medical Center Groningen, University of Groningen, Groningen, The Netherlands

R.H.J.A. Slart et al. (eds.), *Autonomic Innervation of the Heart: Role of Molecular Imaging*, DOI 10.1007/978-3-662-45074-1_11

Novel methods have been developed to measure β-adrenoceptors in vivo with the use of positron emission tomography (PET). A PET study with the radioligand [^{11}C]-CGP-12177 has shown promising results and measurements of β-adrenoceptor density with [^{11}C]-CGP-12177 were shown to be reproducible and in agreement with in vitro studies. [^{11}C]-CGP-12388 using a simpler method of radiochemical synthesis has been presented as an alternative. Also, transportable [^{18}F]-labeled PET ligands are in development and applicable for more general use in PET centers lacking a cyclotron. Most PET studies with CGP radioligands were performed in the 1990s. The main limitation of [^{11}C]-CGP-12177 and [^{11}C]-CGP-12388, besides the troublesome production of the former, is the lack of subtype selectivity. Future perspectives may include the development of subtype-selective β-adrenergic receptor ligands to obtain more information about the pathophysiological role of the different subpopulations in vivo.

Using the full potential of PET, performance of regional measurements and longitudinal studies might add further knowledge to the pathophysiological role of the β-adrenoceptor in cardiac disease and the effect of interventions. This chapter will give an overview of the background of different β-adrenergic receptor types, their role in cardiac diseases, current PET imaging possibilities of the β-adrenergic receptor, and new developments in this field.

Abbreviations

CRT	Cardiac synchronization therapy
DCM	Dilated cardiomyopathy
eNOS	Endothelial isoform of NO synthase
ICD	Implantable cardioverter defibrillator
IDC	Idiopathic dilated cardiomyopathy
LV	Left ventricle
LVEF	Left ventricular ejection fraction
NO	Nitric oxide
PET	Positron emission tomography

11.1 Introduction

Heart failure and arrhythmia are a major cause of mortality and morbidity (Bui et al. 2011; Heidenreich et al. 2011; Jhund et al. 2009; Rathi and Deedwania 2012). Cardiac sympathetic nervous system dysfunction is associated with heart failure and sudden cardiac death (Brunner-La Rocca et al. 2001). A common finding in heart failure and sudden cardiac death is a disturbed cardiac β-adrenergic receptor expression (Bristow 1984). Current status in the clinic is that patients are suboptimally selected for treatment, leading to over- and underdiagnosis of heart failure patients. Better selection of patients with high risk of fatal arrhythmias and risk of heart failure is needed for optimal targeted therapy. Also, patient selection for costly implantable cardioverter defibrillator (ICD) to prevent fatal arrhythmias should be improved. Finally, the prediction of the success rate of the costly cardiac synchronization therapy (CRT) in heart failure patients can be optimized by non-invasive imaging of the β-adrenoceptor density of the heart as the effect of CRT is related to the β-adrenoceptor density of the heart (Chakir et al. 2009).

PET is an accurate technique for non-invasive imaging of cardiac β-adrenergic receptor expression (Doze et al. 2002; Elsinga et al. 1998). The β-adrenoceptor plays an important role in the relation with heart failure development and arrhythmias and is therefore a potential therapeutic target for these pathologies (de Jong et al. 2005; Lefroy et al. 1993; Schafers et al. 1998; Wichter et al. 2000). A general feature of the failing human heart is a decrease in cardiac β-adrenoceptors that in most (but not all) cases is due to a selective decrease in β_1-adrenoceptors leading to a shift in the β_1-:β_2-adrenoceptor ratio towards β_2-adrenoceptors (Brodde et al. 2001). The PET tracers [^{11}C]-CGP-12177 and [^{11}C]-CGP-12388 are developed to image and quantify the cardiac β-adrenergic receptor density (Delforge et al. 1991; Doze et al. 2002; Elsinga et al. 1997). Due to the short half-life of carbon-11 (~20 min), these radiopharmaceuticals can only be used in PET centers with an on-site cyclotron. Another disadvantage is the nonselective binding of these PET tracers to different types of β-adrenergic receptors.

11.2 β-Adrenergic Receptors of the Heart

11.2.1 Background of β-Adrenergic Receptors in the Normal Heart

Four different β-adrenoceptor subtypes have been cloned so far and identified pharmacologically; they are designated β_1-, β_2-, β_3-, and β_4-adrenoceptors (Bylund et al. 1994, 1998; Kaumann and Molenaar 1997). It is generally accepted that, in the human heart, functional β_1- and β_2-adrenoceptors coexist. The expression of both receptors has been first demonstrated by radionuclide ligand binding studies and was subsequently confirmed by functional experiments (Bristow et al. 1990; Brodde et al. 1992a). The number of β-adrenoceptors is more or less evenly distributed in the right and left atrial and ventricular tissue; however, the proportion of β_2-adrenoceptors is slightly higher in the atria (approximately 1/3 of the total β-adrenoceptors expression) than in the ventricles (about 20 % of the total β-adrenoceptors expression) (Brodde 1991; Steinfath et al. 1992a) and may be even higher (~50 %) in the atrioventricular conducting system (Elnatan et al. 1994). In the healthy human heart, the β_1-adrenoceptor is the dominant subtype (β_1 to β_2 ratio = 3:1).

Both β_1- and β_2-adrenoceptors bind to adenylyl cyclase and cause increase of the intracellular amount of cAMP (Bristow et al. 1989; Brodde et al. 1984). In the human heart, adenylyl cyclase is preferentially activated by β_2-adrenoceptor stimulation although β_1-adrenoceptors predominate. This has been demonstrated in human right atrium (Brodde et al. 1984; Bruckner et al. 1984) and in human ventricular myocardium (Bristow et al. 1989; Kaumann et al. 1989). The mechanism underlying these different coupling efficiencies of human cardiac β_1- and β_2-adrenoceptors to adenylyl cyclase is not known. It can be explained by a general phenomenon that β_2-adrenoceptors couple more efficiently to adenylyl cyclase than β_1-adrenoceptors. In vitro experiments have convincingly shown that both β_1- and β_2-adrenoceptors can mediate positive inotropic effects of β-adrenoceptor agonists in isolated electrically driven atrial and ventricular preparations (Brodde et al. 2001). In right and left atria, β_1- and β_2-adrenoceptor stimulation can evoke maximum positive inotropic effects, while in right and left ventricles, only β_1-adrenoceptor stimulation can evoke maximum positive inotropic effects and β_2-adrenoceptor stimulation only submaximal positive inotropic effects (Kaumann et al. 1989; Motomura et al. 1990). High proportions of the β_2 adrenoceptor are also found in the pacemaker and conduction regions, where they may be important in controlling heart rate and rhythm (Dzimiri 1999).

During the last few years, evidence has accumulated that, in addition to β_1- and β_2-adrenoceptors, a third or fourth (or both) β-adrenoceptor might exist in the human heart.

β_3-adrenoceptor transcripts have been detected in the human heart (Pott et al. 2006). Stimulation of the β_3-adrenoceptor produces a negative inotropic effect. The inhibition of contractility includes the inhibitory G protein, $G_{i/O,}$ and results from the production of nitric oxide (NO) by the endothelial isoform of NO synthase (eNOS) and an increase in intracellular cGMP level (Gauthier et al. 1996, 1998). Compared to β_1- and β_2-adrenoceptor, the β_3-adrenoceptor presents a relative in vitro and in vivo lack of desensitization following activation with agonists (Nantel et al. 1993). These features suggest that the expression of β_3-adrenoceptor in heart may have pathophysiological significance.

Opposite regulation has been described for β_1-adrenoceptor and β_3-adrenoceptor in the failing human heart (Moniotte et al. 2001). In addition to the classically observed β_1-adrenoceptor downregulation (Bristow et al. 1982), an upregulation of β_3-adrenoceptor was described (Moniotte et al. 2001). Despite increased β_3-adrenoceptor expression, the negative inotropic effect was slightly reduced in failing heart tissue compared with responses observed in non-failing samples because of concurrent alterations in post-receptor coupling mechanisms, especially decreased eNOS expression. Nevertheless, the reduction in β_3-adrenoceptor response is less than that obtained with β_1-adrenoceptor stimulation.

In addition to the possible existence of cardiodepressant β_3-adrenoceptors, Kaumann and colleagues had postulated the existence of a putative β_4-adrenoceptor in the human heart that upon stimulation causes positive inotropic effects (Brodde and Michel 1999; Gauthier et al. 2000; Kaumann and Molenaar 1997). This receptor type, which had never been cloned and was primarily stimulated by CGP-12177, had properties clearly different from the β_3-adrenoceptor. The β_4-adrenoceptor interacts with nonconventional partial agonists, e.g., CGP-12177, that cause cardiostimulant effects at concentrations considerably higher than those that block β_1- and β_2,-adrenoceptors.

11.2.2 β-Adrenergic Receptor Expression in the Failing Heart

Chronic excessive sympathetic activation leads to substantial and pathologic downregulation of postsynaptic β-adrenergic receptors. The distribution of β_1- and β_2-adrenoceptors in the human heart can be inhomogeously altered in pathological situations such as heart failure or by pharmacological interventions. A general feature of the failing human heart is a decrease in cardiac β-adrenoceptors that in most cases is due to a selective decrease in β_1-adrenoceptors leading to a shift in the β_1-:β_2-adrenoceptor ratio towards β_2-adrenoceptors (Brodde et al. 2001). In patients with biventricular failure, β-adrenoceptors are downregulated in both right and the left ventricle (Pitschner et al. 1993). Interestingly, it appears that the decrease in β-adrenoceptors is more pronounced in ventricular tissue than in atrial tissue (Brodde et al. 1998). On the other hand, in patients with primary pulmonary hypertension who exhibit isolated right ventricular failure, β-adrenoceptors are chamber specifically downregulated only in right ventricles (Bristow et al. 1991). β_3-adrenoceptors are overexpressed in heart failure and hypertension and could constitute a new therapeutic target (Moniotte et al. 2001).

Myocardial ischemia will result in upregulation of membrane-bound β-adrenoceptors (Maisel et al. 1985; Majmudar and Nahrendorf 2012). However, some studies also find downregulation of β-adrenoceptors in ischemic hearts (Rhee and Tyler 1985). Conflicting results may be explained by the fact that ongoing ischemia or hypertension proceeding to heart failure may cause downregulation of β-adrenoceptors, whereas short-term ischemia may cause upregulation. Diabetes may also be related to altered adrenergic receptor properties and density (Heyliger et al. 1982; Williams et al. 1983). Altered adrenergic receptor properties may underlie, at least in part, the chronotropic and inotropic abnormalities of cardiac performance that are associated with the diabetic state.

Also, the use of chemotherapy may influence the β-adrenoceptor density. Kenk and colleagues found that adriamycin-induced toxicity did not change presynaptic noradrenaline uptake but decreased β-adrenergic receptors in cardiac tissues (Kenk et al. 2010).

The transplanted human heart is a denervated organ; animal studies have shown that denervation can induce β-adrenoceptor sensitization (Brodde 1993). Whether this also occurs in the transplanted human heart is not completely understood at present. Assessment of β-adrenoceptor density over a long period after heart transplantation did not result in any upregulation (Brodde et al. 1991).

There was, however, a redistribution of β_1- and β_2-adrenoceptors with time after heart transplantation: β_1-adrenoceptors decreased whereas β_2-adrenoceptors increased (Brodde et al. 1991; Farrukh et al. 1993; Steinfath et al. 1992b). Finally, treatment of patients with β-adrenoceptor blockers can affect distribution of cardiac β_1- and β_2-adrenoceptors. Thus, chronic treatment of patients with coronary artery disease with β_1-adrenoceptor blockers such as metoprolol, atenolol, or bisoprolol leads to a selective increase of cardiac β_1-adrenoceptors (Brodde 1990). This indicates that chronic treatment with β_1-adrenoceptors blockers sensitizes cardiac β_2-adrenoceptors. A similar cardiac β_2-adrenoceptor sensitizing effect of chronic

β_1-adrenoceptor blocker treatment has also been found in vivo, in patients with coronary artery disease (Hall et al. 1991) as well as in healthy volunteers (Hall et al. 1993). The mechanism of this cardiac β_1-/β_2-adrenoceptor crossover interaction is, however, not known. A previous study has demonstrated that carvedilol rather than metoprolol is the drug of choice for improving the hemodynamics and ventricular remodeling in the failing heart (Zhao et al. 2007). The blockade of β_3-adrenoceptors may play a part in these beneficial effects on both left and right ventricles. In patients with heart failure, carvedilol is associated with a larger increase in left ventricular ejection fraction (LVEF) at rest, left ventricular stroke volume, and stroke work during exercise than metoprolol (Metra et al. 2000). Metoprolol diminishes left ventricular remodeling, but unlike carvedilol, it has no significant impact on right ventricular remodeling during chronic heart failure.

11.3 In Vitro Measurement of β-Adrenoceptor Density

The role of the β-adrenoceptor in the regulation of myocardial contraction has been extensively investigated, both in animal models and in human tissue. Assessment of β-adrenoceptor density in a membrane preparation became possible with the introduction of high-affinity, radiolabeled β-adrenergic antagonists, $[^3H]$-DHA (Lefkowitz et al. 1974) and $[^{125}I]$-IHYP (Aurbach et al. 1974). A disadvantage of these assays is the use of lipophilic radionuclide ligands, which leads to high non-specific binding and binding to internalized receptors. With the introduction of $[^3H]$-CGP-12177, a hydrophilic β-adrenergic receptor ligand, and the development of methods to measure cardiac β-adrenoceptors in isolated cells (Buxton and Brunton 1985) and tissue (Watson-Wright et al. 1989), it was a breakthrough to measure β-adrenoceptors at the surface of intact cells (Staehelin et al. 1983) in a physiological state. In vitro measurements in human cardiac tissue in the non-failing human heart have shown that β-adrenoceptor density varies between 70 and 100 fmol/mg protein (Brodde 1991). This variation may be due to the different circumstances in which tissues are obtained, different methods of transportation of tissues to the laboratory, different radionuclide ligands, and/or differences in the methodology of the measurements.

One of the first papers in the early 1980s reported a decreased β-adrenoceptor density in the failing human heart using in vitro ligand binding to homogenized myocardial samples of hearts excised from cardiac transplant recipients (Bristow et al. 1982) (Table 11.1). They found reductions in β-adrenoceptor density of approximately 50 %. In the late 1980s, it was found that the severity of heart failure is related to the reduction of the β-adrenoceptor density and the responsiveness to agonists (Bohm et al. 1988). This downregulation of β-adrenoceptors has been explained by an enhanced sympathetic drive to the heart and hence endogenous downregulation by an elevated release of cardiac-derived noradrenaline (Ruffolo and Kopia 1986), leading to a loss of cardiac contractility (Brodde et al. 1992b). The reduction in receptor density in idiopathic dilated cardiomyopathy is selective for the β_1-adrenoceptor subtype (Bristow et al. 1986; Brodde 1991) and is accompanied

Table 11.1 Experimental in vitro B_{max} studies

Disease	B_{max} alternation
Heart failure	→ ↓
Myocardial ischemia	→ ↑↓
Hypertension	→ ↑↓
Diabetes	↓
Cardiotoxicity	↓

→ no change in B_{max}, ↓ decrease of B_{max}, ↑ increase in B_{max}, B_{max} β-adrenoceptor density

by a similar decrease in β_1-adrenoceptor mRNA levels (Ihl-Vahl et al. 1996). This results in a physiological loss of receptors (Pitschner et al. 1993) and is correlated with the severity of heart failure (Engelhardt et al. 1996).

The levels of β_2-adrenoceptor and β_2-adrenoceptor mRNA remain unaffected but it is believed that these receptors become uncoupled (Brodde 1991). Patients with severe left ventricular dysfunction showed fewer β-adrenergic receptors in lymphocytes, as measured in radioligand binding assays (Colucci et al. 1981). However, although changes in lymphocyte β_2-adrenoceptors are significantly correlated with changes in cardiac β_2-adrenoceptors, they are not related to changes in cardiac β_1-adrenoceptors, which predominate in all parts of the human heart. Furthermore, circulating lymphocytes are not exposed to the local environment of neuronally released catecholamines in the myocardial interstitium. The use of lymphocyte β_2-adrenoceptors as a tool for predicting the status of cardiac β-adrenoceptors is therefore quite limited (Brodde et al. 1989), and thus cardiac tissue will be needed to evaluate cardiac β-adrenoceptor function. Abnormal sympathetic nervous system and β-adrenoceptor signaling is also associated with diabetes. Thackeray and colleagues used [^{3}H]-CGP-12177 to examine altered β-adrenoceptor expression in diabetic rat hearts (Thackeray et al. 2011). Reduced cardiac [^{3}H]-CGP-12177 binding in the presence of sustained hyperglycemia corresponded to a decrease in relative β-adrenoceptor expression. Their study indirectly supports the use of [^{11}C]-CGP-12177 for assessment of cardiac dysfunction in diabetes, by evaluating the cardiac β-adrenoceptor density.

11.4 Non-invasive Imaging of Cardiac β-Adrenergic Receptors

11.4.1 PET Imaging and Density Measurement of Cardiac β-Adrenergic Receptors

Several postsynaptic receptor ligands have been labeled and proposed as PET tracers for cardiac quantification and imaging (Elsinga et al. 1998; Law et al. 2010; Tseng et al. 2001). However, the clinical use of receptor-targeted tracers has been limited to a few studies and still faces significant challenge. High specific binding, high affinity, and hydrophilicity, which avoids binding to internalized inactive receptors, lack of pharmacologic effects, and, finally, a simple and reliable tracer synthesis, are requirements that must be met for a widespread application of receptor ligands for cardiac PET. [^{11}C]-CGP-12177, a hydrophilic nonselective β-adrenoreceptor antagonist, is still the most widely used tracer for adrenergic receptor imaging (Caldwell et al. 2008; Elsinga et al. 1998; Link et al. 2003; Naya et al. 2009) Synthesis of this tracer is not simple and requires [^{11}C]-phosgene as a precursor, which has prevented a broader clinical application until now. CGP-12177 has high receptor affinity and fast plasma clearance, suggesting feasibility for clinical imaging. A graphical method, which adjusts for kinetics related to metabolites, has been established for quantification in humans (Delforge et al. 2002). This approach requires a dual-injection protocol with tracer doses of high and low specific activity (Fig. 11.1). β-Adrenergic receptor density (B_{max}) measured by [^{11}C]-CGP-12177 PET correlated well with in vitro measurements of myocardial samples in both healthy volunteers and patients with congestive cardiomyopathy (Delforge et al. 2002). [^{11}C]-CGP-12388 is a non-subtype-selective β-adrenergic receptor antagonist and an isopropyl analog of CGP-12177. CGP-12388 can be labeled easier than CGP-12177 via a one-step procedure using 2-[^{11}C]-acetone (Elsinga et al. 1994). It is equally hydrophilic compared to [^{11}C]-CGP-12177 and the biodistribution and retention of CGP-12388 is reported to be similar to CGP-12177 (Doze et al. 2002). Both CGP ligands have been applied in the biologically active S-enantiomer and can be blocked by pindolol (Fig. 11.1).

[^{18}F]-fluorocarazolol and [^{11}C]-carazolol are non-subtype-selective, lipophilic radioligands with high affinity for β_1- and β_2-adrenoceptors. The use of fluorine-18 instead of carbon-11 has the advantages of higher specific activity and a longer half-life, which enables prolonged PET studies.

[^{11}C]-carazolol has been evaluated by Berridge and coworkers in mice and pigs (Berridge et al. 1994). The pig heart was clearly visualized. Specific

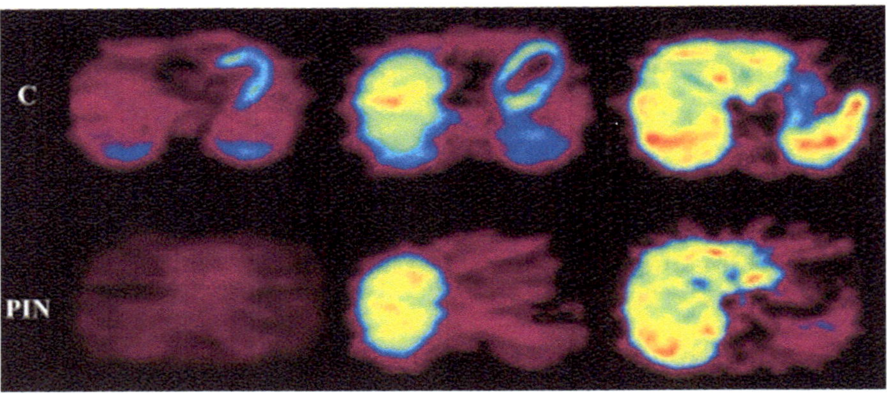

Fig. 11.1 PET images of a human volunteer acquired with [^{11}C]-CGP-12388. Transaxial cross sections in the time frame 14–60 min postinjection are displayed. The *upper row* is the control study; the *bottom row* is the pindolol-blocked study (Elsinga et al. 2001)

binding to β-adrenoceptors was demonstrated by injection of the bioactive [^{11}C]-isomer (specific and nonspecific binding), followed by a second injection of the (R)-isomer (only nonspecific binding). [^{18}F]-fluorocarazolol has been evaluated in several animal models and in humans. Specific binding to β-adrenoceptors of [^{18}F]-fluorocarazolol was demonstrated: (1) by injection of the (S)-isomer and subsequent injection of the (R)-isomer, (2) by blocking experiments with various β-adrenoceptor agonists and antagonists (van Waarde et al. 1995), and (3) by saturation experiments (Doze et al. 1998). The in vivo binding of fluorocarazolol was found to be stereospecific (activity residing in the (S)-isomer). It could be blocked by drugs that bind to β_1- and β_2-adrenoceptors, and specific binding was in good agreement with β-adrenoceptor densities determined by in vitro assays. Metabolite analyses of [^{18}F]-fluorocarazolol showed a rapid (<5 min) appearance of polar metabolites in plasma, while at 60 min postinjection, 92 and 82 % of the total radioactivity in lung and heart remained native [^{18}F]-fluorocarazolol (van Waarde et al. 1995). In PET images of male Wistar rats, the lungs were clearly visible and pulmonary uptake of radioactivity was strongly decreased (>90 %) after pretreatment of the animals with propranolol. The heart could not be visualized. However, PET scans after i.v. injection of [^{18}F]-fluorocarazolol in human volunteers clearly showed β-adrenoceptors in both lung and heart (Visser et al. 1997). Cardiac uptake of radioactivity was strongly inhibited after ingestion of pindolol (to 39 % of the control value at 60 min postinjection). These pilot studies in humans were performed with noncarrier-added [^{18}F]-fluorocarazolol (~1 nmol), after it had been shown that fluorocarazolol is not acutely toxic in rodents at doses >10,000-fold higher than were administered to volunteers. For quantification of receptor densities with compartment models, a dual-injection protocol is required involving the administration of a pharmacological dose of the radioligand (~100 nmol). Such protocols can only be carried out after extensive toxicological screening of the experimental drug. Unfortunately, fluorocarazolol showed a positive Ames test (mutagenicity in bacterial strains) during such examination. Therefore, it was decided to terminate all human studies with [^{18}F]-fluorocarazolol. In contrast to fluorocarazolol, the available toxicological data of carazolol show that the compound is nontoxic even at very high doses. Evaluation in humans should indicate the suitability of [^{11}C]-carazolol as a radiopharmaceutical for clinical PET, although this PET ligand is lipophilic.

11.4.2 PET Imaging of β-Adrenergic Receptors in the Failing Heart

Several factors may induce changes of membrane-bound β-adrenergic receptor density. Major causes are (1) heart failure, (2) myocardial ischemia with or without diabetes, (3) hypertension, and (4) toxic damage. The first study measuring β-adrenoceptor density with [^{11}C]-CGP-12177 PET in patients showed a decreased β-adrenoceptor density in vivo in a group of patients with heart failure due to

Table 11.2 Human (clinical) in vitro B_{max} studies

Disease	B_{max} alternation
Dilated cardiomyopathy	↓
Myocardial ischemia	↓
Valvular disease	↓
Exercise	↑

↓ decrease of B_{max}, ↑ increase in B_{max}, B_{max} β-adrenoceptor density

idiopathic dilated cardiomyopathy (Merlet et al. 1993) (Table 11.2). The [11C]-CGP-12177 PET measurements correlated with β-adrenoceptor density in endomyocardial biopsy. Moreover, these in vivo measurements correlated with functional measurements of β-contractile responsiveness to intracoronary dobutamine infusion. These studies were followed by reports of the group of Camici concerning patients with hypertrophic cardiomyopathy in different phases of disease. Their first report using [11C]-CGP-12177 PET showed a slightly reduced β-adrenoceptor density in patients with primary hypertrophic cardiomyopathy with preserved left ventricular function (Lefroy et al. 1993). These results were in agreement with the hypothesis of an increased sympathetic activity in the heart, which is supported by an elevated myocardial noradrenaline content (Kawai et al. 1983; Tsukamoto et al. 2007) and cardiac spillover of noradrenaline (Brush et al. 1989) in patients with hypertrophic cardiomyopathy. A group with secondary hypertrophic cardiomyopathy due to hypertension and aortic stenosis without heart failure showed a comparable reduction in β-adrenoceptor with [11C]-CGP-12177 PET (Choudhury et al. 1996b). A study in a mixed group of patients with hypertrophic cardiomyopathy with and without signs of heart failure showed a lower β-adrenoceptor density in patients with signs of heart failure and a correlation between β-adrenoceptor density and ventricular function using [11C]-CGP-12177 PET (Choudhury et al. 1996a). From these studies it might be concluded that β-adrenoceptor downregulation precedes clinical heart failure and may be an early clinical marker of left ventricular dysfunction. A study of de Jong and colleagues investigated whether decreased myocardial β-adrenoceptor density in patients with idiopathic dilated cardiomyopathy (IDC) can be estimated using [11C]-CGP-12388 PET (de Jong et al. 2005). They concluded that [11C]-CGP-12388 PET is applicable for the measurement of myocardial β-adrenoceptor density in patients. A highly significant reduction in β-adrenoceptor density was found with a significant difference in β-adrenoceptor density ($p<0.005$) between patients with IDC (B_{max} 5.4 ± 1.3 pmol/g) and healthy controls (B_{max} 8.4 ± 1.5 pmol/g). A prospective longitudinal study may yield further evidence to support this finding (de Jong et al. 2005).

Link and colleagues used [11C]-meta-hydroxyephedrine ([11C]-mHED) to image norepinephrine transporter function as an indicator of presynaptic function and [11C]-CGP-12177 to measure global and regional cell surface β-adrenoceptor density as an indicator of postsynaptic function in 19 normal subjects and 9 congestive heart failure patients (Link et al. 2003). Presynaptic, but not postsynaptic, function was significantly different between normals and congestive heart failure patients.

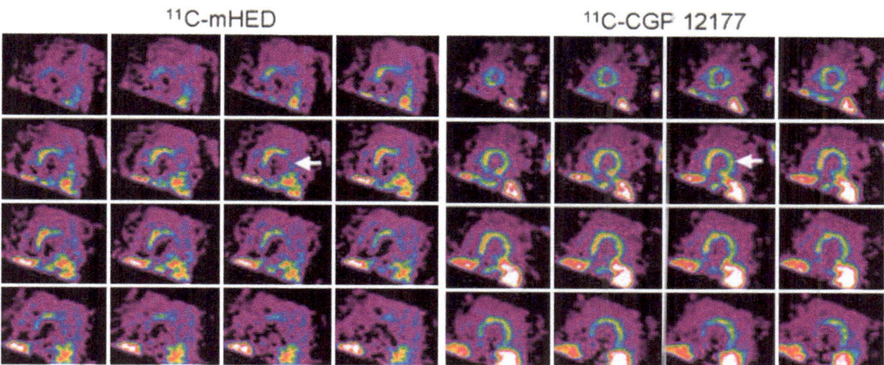

Fig. 11.2 Short-axis PET images of [^{11}C]-mHED (35- to 45 min sum) and [^{11}C]-CGP-12177 (10- to 20 min sum from injection 1) showing left ventricular activity in a chronic congestive heart failure patient. Apical slices are at *upper left* and basal slices are at *lower right* of each panel. *Arrows indicate* extensive mismatch between [^{11}C]-mHED and [^{11}C]-CGP (Caldwell et al. 2008)

Presynaptic function was well matched to postsynaptic function in the normal hearts but significantly different and poorly matched in the congestive heart failure patients studied.

Caldwell and colleagues evaluated in 13 patients with ischemic congestive heart failure and 25 aged-matched healthy volunteers the presynaptic function with [^{11}C]-mHED and the postsynaptic function with [^{11}C]-CGP-12177 (Caldwell et al. 2008) (Fig. 11.2).

Myocardial blood flow was assessed with [^{15}O]-water PET, but global and regional mean blood flow was not different between congestive heart failure and healthy subjects. They found reduced [^{11}C]-mHED and [^{11}C]-CGP-12177 activity in congestive heart failure patients compared with the healthy volunteers and also a mismatch (ratio B_{max} of [^{11}C]-CGP-12177 to [^{11}C]-mHED uptake) between pre- and postsynaptic left ventricular sympathetic function in patients with severe congestive heart failure. After 1.5 year of follow-up, four individuals had an adverse outcome (congestive heart failure death, new or recurrent cardiac arrest or progressive congestive heart failure leading to transplantation). Three of the four patients had mismatch scores >3 times that of the healthy subjects or the congestive heart failure patients without an adverse outcome. Sympathetic signaling in such regions would be more dependent on circulating catecholamines, which are probably lower than those in a normally functioning myoneural junction (Bristow et al. 1992). This decrease could lead to β-adrenoceptor upregulation. However, in patients with dilated cardiomyopathy, [^{11}C]-mHED PET is significantly correlated with the density but not the affinity of uptake-1 sites in the human heart, suggesting either loss of neurons or downregulation of uptake-1 in dilated cardiomyopathy (Ungerer et al. 1998).

After myocardial infarction, LV (left ventricle) remodeling is observed in noninfarcted LV myocardium. LV remodeling is closely associated with systolic heart failure. Myocardial dysfunction is related to the downregulation of cardiac postsynaptic β-adrenoceptors. A recent [^{11}C]-CGP-12177 PET study found out that in the remote non-infarcted region in patients, β-adrenoceptor downregulation was observed, which was related to deterioration of local myocardial systolic function (Ohte et al. 2012).

Furthermore, noradrenaline uptake-1 mechanism and β-adrenoceptor density are reduced in the myocardium of patients with chronic LV dysfunction and evidence of hibernating myocardium (John et al. 2007). The increased sympathetic activity to the heart in these patients is a generalized rather than regional phenomenon which is likely to contributing to the remodeling process of the whole left ventricle rather than playing a causative role in hibernating myocardium.

In patients with syndrome X (Rosen et al. 1996) and asthma (Qing et al. 1997b), i.e., patients with normal left ventricular function, myocardial β-adrenoceptor density was found to be equal to that in normal volunteers, which is in agreement with the general hypothesis that β-adrenoceptor downregulation is only associated with heart failure. Interestingly, myocardial β-adrenoceptor downregulation was also observed in patients with arrhythmogenic right ventricular cardiomyopathy (Schafers et al. 1998). Although these patients have no heart failure, some evidence suggests that their local synaptic catecholamine levels are increased, which apparently causes downregulation of β-adrenoceptor similar to that in patients with heart failure (Wichter et al. 2000). A pharmacological intervention study has been performed in healthy volunteers. This study showed downregulation of pulmonary (Hayes et al. 1996) as well as myocardial β-adrenoceptors (Qing et al. 1997a) after 2 weeks of treatment with a β_2-adrenoceptor agonist (albuterol). Naya and colleagues examined if [^{11}C]-CGP-12177 PET could predict improvement of cardiac function by beta-blocker carvedilol treatment in patients with IDC (Naya et al. 2009). They found that myocardial β-adrenoceptor density is more tightly related to improvement of LVEF due to carvedilol than is cardiac contractile reserve as assessed by dobutamine stress echocardiography in patients with IDC. Patients with decreased myocardial β-adrenoceptor have higher resting adrenergic drive, as reflected by plasma norepinephrine, and may receive greater benefit from being treated by anti-adrenergic drugs.

11.5 New Developments

So far, production methods of β-receptor PET ligands were very complex, hampering their widespread use. Because of the potential clinical importance of cardiac β-adrenergic receptor imaging with PET, radiopharmaceuticals should be developed for PET sites without proper production facilities. To this end new radiopharmaceuticals need to be developed which are labeled with [^{18}F] instead of [^{11}C], as [^{18}F] has a longer half-life (110 min) and can be transported to sites within a range of 4 h transport time, which is routinely done on a commercial basis for [^{18}F]-FDG. Beside the disadvantage of the short half-life of carbon-11, CGP-derivatives are non-subtype-selective β-adrenergic receptor ligands. A more selective β-adrenergic receptor ligand characterized with fast plasma clearance and with a high affinity is needed, and β-adrenergic receptor 1 subtype will be the optimal choice in heart studies.

A [^{18}F]-labeled β_1-adrenoceptor PET ligand with these optimal properties as mentioned before is needed. Law and colleagues developed and applied a fluoroethoxy derivative of the β_1-adrenoceptor antagonist ICI 89406, labeled with fluorine-18 [(S)-[^{18}F]-FICI] (Law et al. 2010) in an animal study. Although in vitro membrane studies showed that (S)-FICI had high affinity and selectivity for β_1- adrenoceptors, this study in mice and rats failed to demonstrate high specific binding of (S)-[^{18}F]-F-ICI to myocardial β_1-adrenoceptor.

Novel [^{18}F]-fluorination techniques, such as click chemistry, new lead molecules can be synthesized that showed high affinity for β-adrenoceptors. In this click reaction, the bio-orthogonal functional groups alkyne and azide react to form triazoles.

The "click reaction" catalyzed by Cu(I) is a well-established method for rapid and highly efficient synthesis of 1,4-disubstituted triazoles from a wide variety of substrates. Using this method to prepare a β-adrenoceptor ligand, the hydroxyl propylamine moiety (crucial for binding to β-adrenoceptors) can partially be maintained and [^{18}F] is introduced as a novel moiety, hopefully not causing mutagenicity of the carazolol derivatives. A lead compound being a [^{18}F]-fluorinated analog of carazolol, [^{18}F]-FPTC, was produced by a click reaction between a PEGylated [^{18}F]-alkyne and an azidoalcohol derivative of 4-hydroxycarbazol.

A number of studies, either in animals or in human patients, have demonstrated that functionally active autoantibodies targeting the human β_1-adrenergic receptor (anti-b1AR-abs) may play an important role in the development and clinical course of progressive cardiac dilatation and failure and increase the risk of developing malignant arrhythmia (Iwata et al. 2001a, b; Magnusson et al. 1994). The presence of these autoantibodies is associated with a markedly worse prognosis in patients with dilated cardiomyopathy (DCM) and ischemic heart disease.

The disadvantage of these anti-b1AR-antibodies is the interaction with the [^{18}F]-labeled β_1-adrenoceptor PET ligands which may cause interference with the PET tracer binding to β_1-adrenergic receptors.

Future perspectives may include the development of [^{18}F]-labeled subtype-selective β-adrenoceptor ligands to obtain more information about the pathophysiological role of the different subpopulations in vivo. Subtype-selective ligands are being developed for the β_1-adrenoceptor as well as the β_2-adrenoceptor, but thus far no suitable ligands have been produced and evaluated in clinical studies.

PET has been shown to be a promising technique for the investigation of the role of β-adrenoceptors in cardiac diseases. So far most studies have focused on their role in patients with systolic heart failure (i.e., with a reduced LVEF). However, it is currently unknown whether β-receptor density plays also a role in the development of heart failure and specifically in the development of heart failure with a preserved ejection fraction. The lifetime risk for developing heart failure is 20 % (Lloyd-Jones et al. 2002). Due to the ageing population, the incidence and prevalence of heart failure will increase, not only systolic heart failure but even more heart failure with a preserved ejection fraction (Brouwers et al. 2013). Several studies have identified risk factors for new onset of heart failure, including age, the presence of hypertension, and a history of ischemic heart disease. However, so far the role of β-adrenoreceptor in this is unknown and warrants further investigation.

Conclusions

The development of new methods to measure β-adrenoceptor in vivo might help us to further understand β-adrenoceptor function and provide additional prognostic information and assist in clinical decisions about therapeutic interventions. New perspectives will lie in the development and application of [^{18}F]-labeled subtype-selective ligands and in using the full potential of PET to perform regional and longitudinal studies.

References

Aurbach GD, Fedak SA, Woodard CJ et al (1974) Beta-adrenergic receptor: stereospecific interaction of iodinated beta-blocking agent with high affinity site. Science 186:1223–1224

Berridge MS, Nelson AD, Zheng L et al (1994) Specific beta-adrenergic receptor binding of carazolol measured with PET. J Nucl Med 35:1665–1676

Bohm M, Beuckelmann D, Brown L et al (1988) Reduction of beta-adrenoceptor density and evaluation of positive inotropic responses in isolated, diseased human myocardium. Eur Heart J 9:844–852

Bristow MR (1984) Myocardial beta-adrenergic receptor downregulation in heart failure. Int J Cardiol 5:648–652

Bristow MR, Ginsburg R, Minobe W et al (1982) Decreased catecholamine sensitivity and beta-adrenergic-receptor density in failing human hearts. N Engl J Med 307:205–211

Bristow MR, Ginsburg R, Umans V et al (1986) Beta 1- and beta 2-adrenergic-receptor subpopulations in nonfailing and failing human ventricular myocardium: coupling of both receptor subtypes to muscle contraction and selective beta 1-receptor down-regulation in heart failure. Circ Res 59:297–309

Bristow MR, Hershberger RE, Port JD et al (1989) Beta 1- and beta 2-adrenergic receptor-mediated adenylate cyclase stimulation in nonfailing and failing human ventricular myocardium. Mol Pharmacol 35:295–303

Bristow MR, Hershberger RE, Port JD et al (1990) Beta-adrenergic pathways in nonfailing and failing human ventricular myocardium. Circulation 82:I12–I25

Bristow MR, Anderson FL, Port JD et al (1991) Differences in beta-adrenergic neuroeffector mechanisms in ischemic versus idiopathic dilated cardiomyopathy. Circulation 84:1024–1039

Bristow MR, Minobe W, Rasmussen R et al (1992) Beta-adrenergic neuroeffector abnormalities in the failing human heart are produced by local rather than systemic mechanisms. J Clin Invest 89:803–815

Brodde OE (1990) Beta- and alpha-adrenoceptor-agonists and -antagonists in chronic heart failure. Basic Res Cardiol 85(Suppl 1):57–66

Brodde OE (1991) Beta 1- and beta 2-adrenoceptors in the human heart: properties, function, and alterations in chronic heart failure. Pharmacol Rev 43:203–242

Brodde OE (1993) Beta-adrenoceptors in cardiac disease. Pharmacol Ther 60:405–430

Brodde OE, Michel MC (1999) Adrenergic and muscarinic receptors in the human heart. Pharmacol Rev 51:651–690

Brodde OE, O'Hara N, Zerkowski HR et al (1984) Human cardiac beta-adrenoceptors: both beta 1- and beta 2-adrenoceptors are functionally coupled to the adenylate cyclase in right atrium. J Cardiovasc Pharmacol 6:1184–1191

Brodde OE, Michel MC, Gordon EP et al (1989) Beta-adrenoceptor regulation in the human heart: can it be monitored in circulating lymphocytes? Eur Heart J 10(Suppl B):2–10

Brodde OE, Khamssi M, Zerkowski HR (1991) Beta-adrenoceptors in the transplanted human heart: unaltered beta-adrenoceptor density, but increased proportion of beta 2-adrenoceptors with increasing posttransplant time. Naunyn Schmiedebergs Arch Pharmacol 344:430–436

Brodde OE, Broede A, Daul A et al (1992a) Receptor systems in the non-failing human heart. Basic Res Cardiol 87(Suppl 1):1–14

Brodde OE, Hillemann S, Kunde K et al (1992b) Receptor systems affecting force of contraction in the human heart and their alterations in chronic heart failure. J Heart Lung Transplant 11:S164–S174

Brodde OE, Vogelsang M, Broede A et al (1998) Diminished responsiveness of Gs-coupled receptors in severely failing human hearts: no difference in dilated versus ischemic cardiomyopathy. J Cardiovasc Pharmacol 31:585–594

Brodde OE, Bruck H, Leineweber K et al (2001) Presence, distribution and physiological function of adrenergic and muscarinic receptor subtypes in the human heart. Basic Res Cardiol 96:528–538

Brouwers FP, de Boer RA, van der Harst P et al (2013) Incidence and epidemiology of new onset heart failure with preserved vs. reduced ejection fraction in a community-based cohort: 11-year follow-up of PREVEND. Eur Heart J 34:1424–1431

Bruckner R, Meyer W, Mugge A et al (1984) Alpha-adrenoceptor-mediated positive inotropic effect of phenylephrine in isolated human ventricular myocardium. Eur J Pharmacol 99:345–347

Brunner-La Rocca HP, Esler MD, Jennings GL et al (2001) Effect of cardiac sympathetic nervous activity on mode of death in congestive heart failure. Eur Heart J 22:1136–1143

Brush JE Jr, Eisenhofer G, Garty M et al (1989) Cardiac norepinephrine kinetics in hypertrophic cardiomyopathy. Circulation 79:836–844

Bui AL, Horwich TB, Fonarow GC (2011) Epidemiology and risk profile of heart failure. Nat Rev Cardiol 8:30–41

Buxton IL, Brunton LL (1985) Direct analysis of beta-adrenergic receptor subtypes on intact adult ventricular myocytes of the rat. Circ Res 56:126–132

Bylund DB, Eikenberg DC, Hieble JP et al (1994) International Union of Pharmacology nomenclature of adrenoceptors. Pharmacol Rev 46:121–136

Bylund DB, Bond RA, Clarke DE, Eikenburg DC, Hieble JP, Langer SZ, Lefkowitz RJ, Minneman PB, Milinoff PB, Ruffolo RR, Strosberg AD, Trendelenburg UG (1998) Adrenoceptors. In: Bylund DB, Bond RA, Clarke DE, Eikenburg DC, Hieble JP, Langer SZ, Lefkowitz RJ, Minneman PB, Milinoff PB, Ruffolo RR, Strosberg AD, Trendelenburg UG (eds) The IUPHAR compendium of receptor characterization and classification. IUPHAR Media, London, pp 58–74

Caldwell JH, Link JM, Levy WC et al (2008) Evidence for pre- to postsynaptic mismatch of the cardiac sympathetic nervous system in ischemic congestive heart failure. J Nucl Med 49:234–241

Chakir K, Daya SK, Aiba T et al (2009) Mechanisms of enhanced beta-adrenergic reserve from cardiac resynchronization therapy. Circulation 119:1231–1240

Choudhury L, Guzzetti S, Lefroy DC et al (1996a) Myocardial beta adrenoceptors and left ventricular function in hypertrophic cardiomyopathy. Heart 75:50–54

Choudhury L, Rosen SD, Lefroy DC et al (1996b) Myocardial beta adrenoceptor density in primary and secondary left ventricular hypertrophy. Eur Heart J 17:1703–1709

Colucci WS, Alexander RW, Williams GH et al (1981) Decreased lymphocyte beta-adrenergic-receptor density in patients with heart failure and tolerance to the beta-adrenergic agonist pirbuterol. N Engl J Med 305:185–190

de Jong RM, Willemsen AT, Slart RH et al (2005) Myocardial beta-adrenoceptor downregulation in idiopathic dilated cardiomyopathy measured in vivo with PET using the new radioligand (S)-[11C]CGP12388. Eur J Nucl Med Mol Imaging 32:443–447

Delforge J, Syrota A, Lancon JP et al (1991) Cardiac beta-adrenergic receptor density measured in vivo using PET, CGP 12177, and a new graphical method. J Nucl Med 32:739–748

Delforge J, Mesangeau D, Dolle F et al (2002) In vivo quantification and parametric images of the cardiac beta-adrenergic receptor density. J Nucl Med 43:215–226

Doze P, van Waarde A, Elsinga PH et al (1998) Validation of S-1′-[18F]fluorocarazolol for in vivo imaging and quantification of cerebral beta-adrenoceptors. Eur J Pharmacol 353:215–226

Doze P, Elsinga PH, van Waarde A et al (2002) Quantification of beta-adrenoceptor density in the human heart with (S)-[11C]CGP 12388 and a tracer kinetic model. Eur J Nucl Med Mol Imaging 29:295–304

Dzimiri N (1999) Regulation of beta-adrenoceptor signaling in cardiac function and disease. Pharmacol Rev 51:465–501

Elnatan J, Molenaar P, Rosenfeldt FL et al (1994) Autoradiographic localization and quantitation of beta 1- and beta 2-adrenoceptors in the human atrioventricular conducting system: a comparison of patients with idiopathic dilated cardiomyopathy and ischemic heart disease. J Mol Cell Cardiol 26:313–323

Elsinga PH, van Waarde A, Visser GM et al (1994) Synthesis and preliminary evaluation of (R, S)-1-[2-((carbamoyl-4-hydroxy)phenoxy)-ethylamino]-3-[4-(1-[11C]-met hyl-4-trifluoromethyl-2-imidazolyl)phenoxy]-2-propanol ([11C]CGP 20712A) as a selective beta 1-adrenoceptor ligand for PET. Nucl Med Biol 21:211–217

Elsinga PH, van Waarde A, Jaeggi KA et al (1997) Synthesis and evaluation of (S)-4-(3-(2′-[11C] isopropylamino)-2-hydroxypropoxy) -2H-benzimidazol -2-one ((S)-[11C]CGP 12388) and (S)-4-(3-((1′-[18F]-fluoroisopropyl)amino)-2-hydroxypropoxy) -2H- benzimidazol-2-one ((S)-[18F]fluoro-CGP 12388) for visualization of beta-adrenoceptors with positron emission tomography. J Med Chem 40:3829–3835

Elsinga PH, van Waarde A, Visser TJ et al (1998) Visualization of beta-adrenoceptors using PET. Clin Positron Imaging 1:81–94

Elsinga PH, Doze P, van Waarde A et al (2001) Imaging of beta-adrenoceptors in the human thorax using (S)-[(11)C]CGP12388 and positron emission tomography. Eur J Pharmacol 433:173–176

Engelhardt S, Bohm M, Erdmann E et al (1996) Analysis of beta-adrenergic receptor mRNA levels in human ventricular biopsy specimens by quantitative polymerase chain reactions: progressive reduction of beta 1-adrenergic receptor mRNA in heart failure. J Am Coll Cardiol 27:146–154

Farrukh HM, White M, Port JD et al (1993) Up-regulation of beta 2-adrenergic receptors in previously transplanted, denervated nonfailing human hearts. J Am Coll Cardiol 22:1902–1908

Gauthier C, Tavernier G, Charpentier F et al (1996) Functional beta3-adrenoceptor in the human heart. J Clin Invest 98:556–562

Gauthier C, Leblais V, Kobzik L et al (1998) The negative inotropic effect of beta3-adrenoceptor stimulation is mediated by activation of a nitric oxide synthase pathway in human ventricle. J Clin Invest 102:1377–1384

Gauthier C, Langin D, Balligand JL (2000) Beta3-adrenoceptors in the cardiovascular system. Trends Pharmacol Sci 21:426–431

Hall JA, Petch MC, Brown MJ (1991) In vivo demonstration of cardiac beta 2-adrenoreceptor sensitization by beta 1-antagonist treatment. Circ Res 69:959–964

Hall JA, Ferro A, Dickerson JE et al (1993) Beta adrenoreceptor subtype cross regulation in the human heart. Br Heart J 69:332–337

Hayes MJ, Qing F, Rhodes CG et al (1996) In vivo quantification of human pulmonary beta-adrenoceptors: effect of beta-agonist therapy. Am J Respir Crit Care Med 154:1277–1283

Heidenreich PA, Trogdon JG, Khavjou OA et al (2011) Forecasting the future of cardiovascular disease in the United States: a policy statement from the American Heart Association. Circulation 123:933–944

Heyliger CE, Pierce GN, Singal PK et al (1982) Cardiac alpha- and beta-adrenergic receptor alterations in diabetic cardiomyopathy. Basic Res Cardiol 77:610–618

Ihl-Vahl R, Eschenhagen T, Kubler W et al (1996) Differential regulation of mRNA specific for beta 1- and beta 2-adrenergic receptors in human failing hearts. Evaluation of the absolute cardiac mRNA levels by two independent methods. J Mol Cell Cardiol 28:1–10

Iwata M, Yoshikawa T, Baba A et al (2001a) Autoantibodies against the second extracellular loop of beta1-adrenergic receptors predict ventricular tachycardia and sudden death in patients with idiopathic dilated cardiomyopathy. J Am Coll Cardiol 37:418–424

Iwata M, Yoshikawa T, Baba A et al (2001b) Autoimmunity against the second extracellular loop of beta(1)-adrenergic receptors induces beta-adrenergic receptor desensitization and myocardial hypertrophy in vivo. Circ Res 88:578–586

Jhund PS, Macintyre K, Simpson CR et al (2009) Long-term trends in first hospitalization for heart failure and subsequent survival between 1986 and 2003: a population study of 5.1 million people. Circulation 119:515–523

John AS, Mongillo M, Depre C et al (2007) Pre- and post-synaptic sympathetic function in human hibernating myocardium. Eur J Nucl Med Mol Imaging 34:1973–1980

Kaumann AJ, Molenaar P (1997) Modulation of human cardiac function through 4 beta-adrenoceptor populations. Naunyn Schmiedebergs Arch Pharmacol 355:667–681

Kaumann AJ, Hall JA, Murray KJ et al (1989) A comparison of the effects of adrenaline and noradrenaline on human heart: the role of beta 1- and beta 2-adrenoceptors in the stimulation of adenylate cyclase and contractile force. Eur Heart J 10(Suppl B):29–37

Kawai C, Yui Y, Hoshino T et al (1983) Myocardial catecholamines in hypertrophic and dilated (congestive) cardiomyopathy: a biopsy study. J Am Coll Cardiol 2:834–840

Kenk M, Thackeray JT, Thorn SL et al (2010) Alterations of pre- and postsynaptic noradrenergic signaling in a rat model of adriamycin-induced cardiotoxicity. J Nucl Cardiol 17:254–263

Law MP, Wagner S, Kopka K et al (2010) Preclinical evaluation of an 18F-labelled beta1-adrenoceptor selective radioligand based on ICI 89,406. Nucl Med Biol 37:517–526

Lefkowitz RJ, Mukherjee C, Coverstone M et al (1974) Stereospecific (3H)(minus)-alprenolol binding sites, beta-adrenergic receptors and adenylate cyclase. Biochem Biophys Res Commun 60:703–709

Lefroy DC, De Silva R, Choudhury L et al (1993) Diffuse reduction of myocardial beta-adrenoceptors in hypertrophic cardiomyopathy: a study with positron emission tomography. J Am Coll Cardiol 22:1653–1660

Link JM, Stratton JR, Levy W et al (2003) PET measures of pre- and post-synaptic cardiac beta adrenergic function. Nucl Med Biol 30:795–803

Lloyd-Jones DM, Larson MG, Leip EP et al (2002) Lifetime risk for developing congestive heart failure: the Framingham Heart Study. Circulation 106:3068–3072

Magnusson Y, Wallukat G, Waagstein F et al (1994) Autoimmunity in idiopathic dilated cardiomyopathy. Characterization of antibodies against the beta 1-adrenoceptor with positive chronotropic effect. Circulation 89:2760–2767

Maisel AS, Motulsky HJ, Insel PA (1985) Externalization of beta-adrenergic receptors promoted by myocardial ischemia. Science 230:183–186

Majmudar MD, Nahrendorf M (2012) Cardiovascular molecular imaging: the road ahead. J Nucl Med 53:673–676

Merlet P, Delforge J, Syrota A et al (1993) Positron emission tomography with 11C CGP-12177 to assess beta-adrenergic receptor concentration in idiopathic dilated cardiomyopathy. Circulation 87:1169–1178

Metra M, Giubbini R, Nodari S et al (2000) Differential effects of beta-blockers in patients with heart failure: a prospective, randomized, double-blind comparison of the long-term effects of metoprolol versus carvedilol. Circulation 102:546–551

Moniotte S, Kobzik L, Feron O et al (2001) Upregulation of beta(3)-adrenoceptors and altered contractile response to inotropic amines in human failing myocardium. Circulation 103:1649–1655

Motomura S, Deighton NM, Zerkowski HR et al (1990) Chronic beta 1-adrenoceptor antagonist treatment sensitizes beta 2-adrenoceptors, but desensitizes M2-muscarinic receptors in the human right atrium. Br J Pharmacol 101:363–369

Nantel F, Bonin H, Emorine LJ et al (1993) The human beta 3-adrenergic receptor is resistant to short term agonist-promoted desensitization. Mol Pharmacol 43:548–555

Naya M, Tsukamoto T, Morita K et al (2009) Myocardial beta-adrenergic receptor density assessed by 11C-CGP12177 PET predicts improvement of cardiac function after carvedilol treatment in patients with idiopathic dilated cardiomyopathy. J Nucl Med 50:220–225

Ohte N, Narita H, Iida A et al (2012) Cardiac beta-adrenergic receptor density and myocardial systolic function in the remote noninfarcted region after prior myocardial infarction with left ventricular remodeling. Eur J Nucl Med Mol Imaging 39:1246–1253

Pitschner HF, Droege A, Mitze M et al (1993) Down-regulated beta-adrenoceptors in severely failing human ventricles: uniform regional distribution, but no increased internalization. Basic Res Cardiol 88:179–191

Pott C, Brixius K, Bloch W et al (2006) Beta3-adrenergic stimulation in the human heart: signal transduction, functional implications and therapeutic perspectives. Pharmazie 61:255–260

Qing F, Rahman SU, Hayes MJ et al (1997a) Effect of long-term beta2-agonist dosing on human cardiac beta-adrenoceptor expression in vivo: comparison with changes in lung and mononuclear leukocyte beta-receptors. J Nucl Cardiol 4:532–538

Qing F, Rahman SU, Rhodes CG et al (1997b) Pulmonary and cardiac beta-adrenoceptor density in vivo in asthmatic subjects. Am J Respir Crit Care Med 155:1130–1134

Rathi S, Deedwania PC (2012) The epidemiology and pathophysiology of heart failure. Med Clin North Am 96:881–890

Rhee HM, Tyler L (1985) Myocardial ischemic injury and beta-adrenergic receptors in perfused working rabbit hearts. Adv Exp Med Biol 191:281–288

Rosen SD, Boyd H, Rhodes CG et al (1996) Myocardial beta-adrenoceptor density and plasma catecholamines in syndrome X. Am J Cardiol 78:37–42

Ruffolo RR Jr, Kopia GA (1986) Importance of receptor regulation in the pathophysiology and therapy of congestive heart failure. Am J Med 80:67–72

Schafers M, Lerch H, Wichter T et al (1998) Cardiac sympathetic innervation in patients with idiopathic right ventricular outflow tract tachycardia. J Am Coll Cardiol 32:181–186

Staehelin M, Simons P, Jaeggi K et al (1983) CGP-12177. A hydrophilic beta-adrenergic receptor radioligand reveals high affinity binding of agonists to intact cells. J Biol Chem 258:3496–3502

Steinfath M, Lavicky J, Schmitz W et al (1992a) Regional distribution of beta 1- and beta 2-adrenoceptors in the failing and nonfailing human heart. Eur J Clin Pharmacol 42:607–611

Steinfath M, von der Leyen H, Hecht A et al (1992b) Decrease in beta 1- and increase in beta 2-adrenoceptors in long-term follow-up after orthotopic cardiac transplantation. J Mol Cell Cardiol 24:1189–1198

Thackeray JT, Parsa-Nezhad M, Kenk M et al (2011) Reduced CGP12177 binding to cardiac beta-adrenoceptors in hyperglycemic high-fat-diet-fed, streptozotocin-induced diabetic rats. Nucl Med Biol 38:1059–1066

Tseng H, Link JM, Stratton JR et al (2001) Cardiac receptor physiology and its application to clinical imaging: present and future. J Nucl Cardiol 8:390–409

Tsukamoto T, Morita K, Naya M et al (2007) Decreased myocardial beta-adrenergic receptor density in relation to increased sympathetic tone in patients with nonischemic cardiomyopathy. J Nucl Med 48:1777–1782

Ungerer M, Hartmann F, Karoglan M et al (1998) Regional in vivo and in vitro characterization of autonomic innervation in cardiomyopathic human heart. Circulation 97:174–180

van Waarde A, Elsinga PH, Brodde OE et al (1995) Myocardial and pulmonary uptake of S-1′-[18F]fluorocarazolol in intact rats reflects radioligand binding to beta-adrenoceptors. Eur J Pharmacol 272:159–168

Visser TJ, van Waarde A, van der Mark TW et al (1997) Characterization of pulmonary and myocardial beta-adrenoceptors with S-1′-[fluorine-18]fluorocarazolol. J Nucl Med 38:169–174
Watson-Wright WM, Armour JA, Johnstone DE et al (1989) Myocardial slice: a physiological approach to beta-adrenergic ([3H] CGP-12177) receptor binding in hamster and guinea pig heart. J Pharmacol Methods 22:37–47
Wichter T, Schafers M, Rhodes CG et al (2000) Abnormalities of cardiac sympathetic innervation in arrhythmogenic right ventricular cardiomyopathy: quantitative assessment of presynaptic norepinephrine reuptake and postsynaptic beta-adrenergic receptor density with positron emission tomography. Circulation 101:1552–1558
Williams RS, Schaible TF, Scheuer J et al (1983) Effects of experimental diabetes on adrenergic and cholinergic receptors of rat myocardium. Diabetes 32:881–886
Zhao Q, Wu TG, Jiang ZF et al (2007) Effect of beta-blockers on beta3-adrenoceptor expression in chronic heart failure. Cardiovasc Drugs Ther 21:85–90

Autonomic PET-CT Imaging in Heart Failure

12

Juhani Knuuti

Contents

Abstract

The studies suggest a potential role for sympathetic and parasympathetic neuronal and receptor positron emission tomography (PET) imaging in patients with heart failure. This information could be valuable in predicting the progression of ventricular remodeling and outcome in heart failure. Although innervation imaging with PET in heart failure holds great promise, the method has not received wider clinical acceptance. Larger randomized studies are required to confirm the incremental value of innervation imaging in various specific indications.

J. Knuuti, MD, PhD
Turku PET Centre, University of Turku and Turku University Hospital, Turku, Finland
e-mail: juhani.knuuti@utu.fi

R.H.J.A. Slart et al. (eds.), *Autonomic Innervation of the Heart: Role of Molecular Imaging*, DOI 10.1007/978-3-662-45074-1_12

Abbreviations

DCM Dilated cardiomyopathy
NE Norepinephrine
NYHA New York Heart Association
PET Positron emission tomography
SPECT Single photon emission computed tomography

12.1 Introduction

Derangements in autonomic function have been detected in heart failure. These have been regarded as hallmarks of cardiac remodeling during the development of heart failure (Thackeray and Bengel 2013). Abnormalities both in presynaptic and postsynaptic neural functions have been detected in cardiomyopathy and heart failure, and these changes also appear also to have a significant prognostic value. Positron emission tomography (PET) imaging is powerful technique to investigate the autonomic functions of the heart. In patients with heart failure, both presynaptic and postsynaptic abnormalities have been detected (Backs et al. 2001).

12.2 Autonomic Imaging in the Dilated Cardiomyopathy

12.2.1 Presynaptic Function

Similarly to [^{123}I]-MIBG, impaired uptake of [^{11}C]-mHED has been detected on patients with dilated cardiomyopathy (DCM) (Hartmann et al. 1999; Vesalainen et al. 1999) (Fig. 12.1). Furthermore, the degree of abnormality is associated with the severity of heart failure (Hartmann et al. 1999) (Fig. 12.2). In one study, the results of in vivo [^{11}C]-mHED PET were compared to changes in tissue of explanted human hearts (Ungerer et al. 1998). The authors found that uptake-1 density and tissue norepinephrine content varied significantly in left ventricles of patients with cardiomyopathy and that [^{11}C]-mHED PET correlated significantly to the density of the uptake-1 sites in the human heart.

It has been shown that reduced myocardial [^{11}C]-mHED uptake correlates with blunted vascular sympathetic effector responses, as measured by baroreflex testing (Vesalainen et al. 1999). Furthermore, the tracer uptake has been also found to be correlated with metabolic changes, reduced contractile function, and myocardial efficiency (Bengel et al. 2001, 2002). It has been suggested that reduced amount of presynaptic catecholamine uptake sites increases myocardial overexposure to catecholamines and may facilitate progress and further deterioration of congestive heart failure (Henneman et al. 2008).

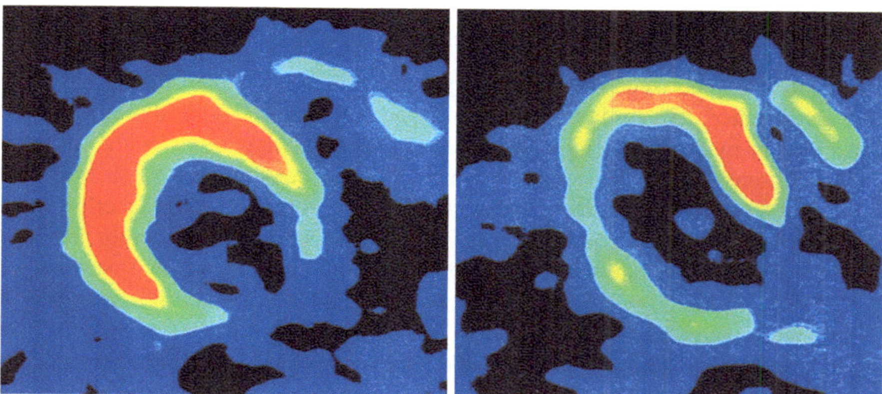

Fig. 12.1 Representative transaxial plane of the left ventricle demonstrating the myocardial [^{11}C]-mHED retention in a healthy control (*left*) and in a heart failure patient with previous lateral myocardial infarction (*right*). Notice the reduced [^{11}C]-mHED retention not only at the site of myocardial infarction but also at the remote myocardial regions (With permission from Vesalainen et al. (1999))

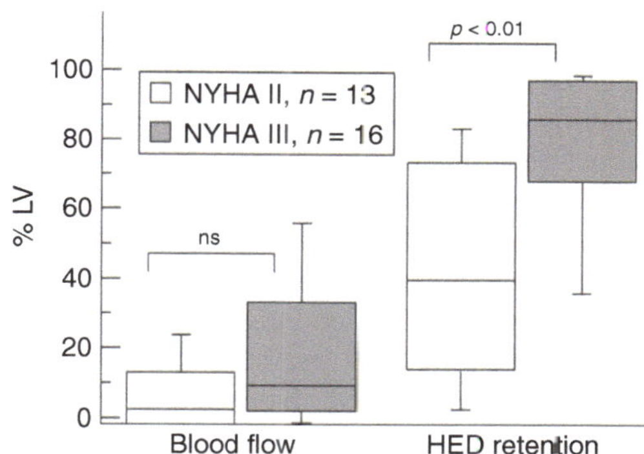

Fig. 12.2 Extent of neuronal and blood flow inhomogeneities in dilated cardiomyopathy, expressed as percentage of polar map area <2.5 SD below control values (% left ventricular). [^{11}C]-mHED retention was significantly different in NYHA II v NYHA III patients ($p<0.01$) (With permission from Hartmann et al. (1999)). *ns* non significant

Whether these abnormalities can be reversed in patients with heart failure has been sparsely studied. The effects of a 6-month exercise training program on [^{11}C]-mHED uptake and several other cardiovascular parameters were investigated in small group of 13 patients with NYHA class II–III heart failure (Pietila et al. 1997). The myocardial [^{11}C]-mHED uptake was enhanced from 0.228 ± 0.099 to 0.263 ± 0.066 1/s ($p<0.05$) by training, and the changes correlated with changes in R-R interval variability. The systolic blood pressure variability reduced from 4.89 ± 1.03 to 3.18 ± 0.48 ($p<0.05$), and these changes correlated inversely with the enhancement of [^{11}C]-mHED retention ($r=-0.66$; $p<0.05$). These parallel changes allowed the authors to conclude that exercise training induces a shift toward normalization of the compensatory autonomic nervous imbalance in heart failure although they did not give any mechanistic explanations.

12.2.2 Postsynaptic Sympathetic Function

The relationship between pre- and postsynaptic functions in heart failure has been also investigated. In a study by Tsukamoto and colleagues (2007), β-adrenoceptor density was measured using [^{11}C]-CGP-12177 PET in patients with nonischemic cardiomyopathy. They demonstrated that the density was 50 % lower as compared to healthy volunteers and it significantly correlated with ejection fraction (Tsukamoto et al. 2007). Interestingly, parallel to β-adrenoceptor density, [^{123}I]-MIBG washout rate was enhanced. This can be understood that washout of [^{123}I]-MIBG is linked with increased sympathetic firing rate and norepinephrine (NE) release, and this will then create a downregulation of β-adrenoceptors. This hypothesis is also in agreement with the results of a study by Caldwell and colleagues (2008) who demonstrated reduced NE transport and lower β-adrenoceptor density in ischemic congestive heart failure patients, by using [^{11}C]-mHED and [^{11}C]-CGP-12177 PET. In addition, the mismatch between [^{11}C]-CGP-12177 and [^{11}C]-mHED uptake was clearly higher in patients with heart failure as compared to healthy controls.

Naya and colleagues (2009) investigated ten patients with idiopathic dilated cardiomyopathy using a β-adrenoceptor tracer [^{11}C]-CGP-12177. The left ventricle contractile reserve was evaluated using dobutamine echocardiography prior and after the carvedilol (beta-blocker) therapy. Patients with the lowest [^{11}C]-CGP-12177 binding showed the greatest improvement of left ventricular ejection fraction and reduction of plasma NE levels after carvedilol. Baseline myocardial β-adrenergic density correlated with the change of ejection fraction by carvedilol therapy ($r = -0.88$, $p < 0.001$). Myocardial β-adrenergic density was independent predictor of the change in ejection fraction by carvedilol ($r = -0.88$, $p < 0.001$), and, in addition, myocardial β-adrenergic density was significantly correlated with plasma norepinephrine ($r = -0.79$, $p < 0.01$) and ejection fraction ($r = 0.70$, $p < 0.05$). Thus, the patients with decreased myocardial β-adrenergic receptor density can be suggested to have higher resting adrenergic drive and this seems to be able to predict the response to beta-blocker therapy.

In contrast to these findings, in patients with more advanced congestive heart failure, [^{11}C]-mHED uptake was markedly reduced but β-adrenoceptor density as measured using [^{11}C]-CGP-12177 was not significantly different as compared to healthy volunteers (Link et al. 2003) but levels of βARK-1, a marker of postsynaptic adrenergic signal transduction, were inversely related to ($r = -0.61$, $p = 0.04$) presynaptic changes (Ungerer et al. 2000). Also in other studies in patients with terminal heart failure, no correlations between [^{11}C]-mHED retention and β-adrenoceptor density studied using [^{3}H]-CGP-12177 were detected, but β-adrenoceptor kinase expression, an intracellular protein involved in the desensitization and internalization of receptors, was found to be changed (Ungerer et al. 1998, 2000).

Taken together, increased sympathetic tone with or without reduced nerve density is associated with eventual downregulation of β-adrenoceptors in cardiomyopathy, but in more advanced stage of the disease, this receptor downregulation seems not to exist. Since these changes seem to be linked with the severity of the heart failure, they could be potentially used as biomarkers of ventricular remodeling and in the assessment of the progression of heart failure. However, prospective studies are needed to prove such an approach.

12.2.3 Postsynaptic Parasympathetic Function

The parasympathetic signaling in patients with heart failure is less well studied. [^{11}C]-MQNB, a muscarinic receptor antagonist, was used in 20 patients with congestive heart failure due to idiopathic dilated cardiomyopathy and compared with 12 normal subjects (Le Guludec et al. 1997). The mean receptor concentration was significantly higher in patients than in control subjects suggesting that congestive heart failure is associated with an upregulation of myocardial muscarinic receptors. This was considered to be an adaptive mechanism to beta-agonist stimulation (Le Guludec et al. 1997). The authors suggested that the enhanced parasympathetic postsynaptic signaling counteracts to increased sympathetic tone observed in heart failure. Moreover, regional mismatch of pre- and postsynaptic function may have detrimental consequences on electrical conduction and contribute to ventricular arrhythmias observed in cardiomyopathy heart failure (Thackeray and Bengel 2013).

12.3 Autonomic Imaging in the Hypertrophic Cardiomyopathy

In hypertrophic cardiomyopathy patients, β-adrenoceptor density was found to be reduced by using [^{11}C]-CGP-12177 PET (Lefroy et al. 1993) and the severity of reduction correlated with disease progression (Choudhury et al. 1996). In the subsequent studies, a decrease in [^{11}C]-mHED uptake paralleling with the decrease of β-adrenoceptor density was identified. These findings are consistent with reduced local NE reuptake and increased catecholamine levels and consequent downregulation of postsynaptic receptors (Schafers et al. 1998).

Studies also with [^{18}F]-fluorodopamine have been performed in patients with hypertrophic cardiomyopathy (Li et al. 2000). [^{18}F]-fluorodopamine accumulation was decreased despite preserved myocardial perfusion measured using [^{13}N]NH3. The changes were limited to the hypertrophied myocardial regions. Decreased neuronal uptake could reflect local relative hypoinnervation, decreased numbers of neuronal uptake sites, or metabolic limitations on cell membrane transport (Li et al. 2000). The decreased uptake-1 activity can be expected to augment delivery of locally released and circulating catecholamines to adrenoceptors during sympathetic or adrenomedullary activation, and this, in turn, could induce hypercontractility, vulnerability to ventricular arrhythmias, and reduced coronary perfusion reserve in patients with hypertrophic cardiomyopathy (Li et al. 2000).

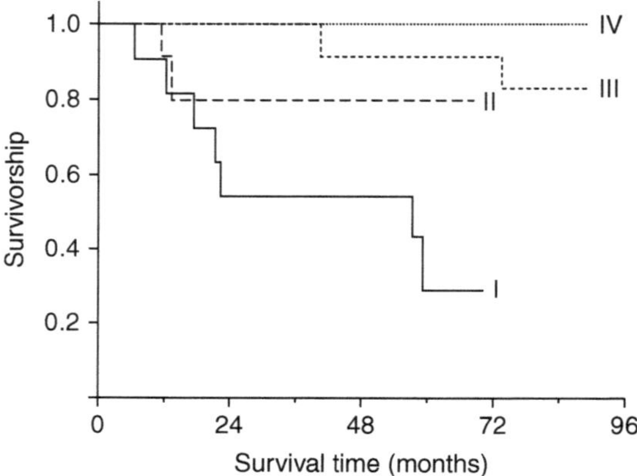

Fig. 12.3 Survival for the cardiac end points in patient groups divided into quartiles based on myocardial [^{11}C]-mHED retention. The survival (freedom from cardiac death or transplantation) was poorest in the group with the lowest [^{11}C]-mHED retention values ($p<0.05$ between the two quartiles with lowest [^{11}C]-mHED retention). The Roman numerals refer to quartiles of [^{11}C]-mHED retention (*I* quartile with the lowest [^{11}C]-mHED retention, *IV* quartile with the highest [^{11}C]-mHED retention) (With permission from Pietilä et al. (2001))

12.4 Prognosis

Abnormalities of the autonomic nervous system are known to be of prognostic significance in chronic heart failure. Consistent with the studies using single photon emission computed tomography (SPECT) with [^{123}I]-MIBG, prognostic value of quantitative [^{11}C]-mHED PET findings in patients with heart failure can be expected.

Unfortunately, limited number of studies have investigated this aspect with PET and [^{11}C]-mHED or other tracers. In a study by Pietilä and colleagues (2001), 46 NYHA class II–III patients with dilated cardiomyopathy were investigated with quantitative [^{11}C]-mHED and PET. During the follow-up period of about 4.5 years, [^{11}C]-mHED retention together with peak oxygen uptake and left ventricular end-diastolic volume was statistically significantly linked with the cardiac events. The lower was the [^{11}C]-mHED uptake, the poorer was the prognosis (Fig. 12.3). There are no studies demonstrating the prognostic value of the mismatch between pre- and postsynaptic functions.

12.5 Innervation Imaging in the Future

Innervation imaging with PET can be expected to hold great promise for the clinical use. However, the method has not yet received wider clinical acceptance mainly due to limited access to PET tracers. In addition, the clinical studies for prognostic value are very limited. To ascertain the clinical value of innervation PET imaging in various specific indications such as heart failure, randomized studies are required. New expensive therapies for heart failure (e.g., biventricular pacemakers) are being introduced, and innervation imaging could be one of the methods to identify those patients who would benefit the most from these expensive therapies.

12.6 Summary

The studies suggest a potential role for sympathetic and parasympathetic neuronal and receptor PET imaging in patients with heart failure. This information could be valuable in predicting the progression of ventricular remodeling and outcome in heart failure. Although innervation imaging with PET in heart failure holds great promise, the method has not received wider clinical acceptance. Larger randomized studies are required to confirm the incremental value of innervation imaging in various specific indications.

Acknowledgments The author has been supported by the Finnish Foundation of Cardiovascular Research, and work was conducted within the Finnish Centre of Excellence in Cardiovascular and Metabolic Diseases supported by the Academy of Finland, University of Turku, Turku University Hospital, and Åbo Akademi University.

References

Backs J, Haunstetter A, Gerber SH, Metz J, Borst MM, Strasser RH, Kubler W, Haass M (2001) The neuronal norepinephrine transporter in experimental heart failure: evidence for a posttranscriptional downregulation. J Mol Cell Cardiol 33:461–472

Bengel FM, Permanetter B, Ungerer M, Nekolla SG, Schwaiger M (2001) Relationship between altered sympathetic innervation, oxidative metabolism and contractile function in the cardiomyopathic human heart; a non-invasive study using positron emission tomography. Eur Heart J 22:1594–1600

Bengel FM, Permanetter B, Ungerer M, Nekolla SG, Schwaiger M (2002) Alterations of the sympathetic nervous system and metabolic performance of the cardiomyopathic heart. Eur J Nucl Med Mol Imaging 29:198–202

Caldwell JH, Link JM, Levy WC, Poole JE, Stratton JR (2008) Evidence for pre- to postsynaptic mismatch of the cardiac sympathetic nervous system in ischemic congestive heart failure. J Nucl Med 49:234–241

Choudhury L, Guzzetti S, Lefroy DC, Nihoyannopoulos P, McKenna WJ, Oakley CM, Camici PG (1996) Myocardial beta adrenoceptors and left ventricular function in hypertrophic cardiomyopathy. Heart 75:50–54

Hartmann F, Ziegler S, Nekolla S, Hadamitzky M, Seyfarth M, Richardt G, Schwaiger M (1999) Regional patterns of myocardial sympathetic denervation in dilated cardiomyopathy: an analysis using carbon-11 hydroxyephedrine and positron emission tomography. Heart 81:262–270

Henneman MM, Bengel FM, van der Wall EE, Knuuti J, Bax JJ (2008) Cardiac neuronal imaging: application in the evaluation of cardiac disease. J Nucl Cardiol 15:442–455

Le Guludec D, Cohen-Solal A, Delforge J, Delahaye N, Syrota A, Merlet P (1997) Increased myocardial muscarinic receptor density in idiopathic dilated cardiomyopathy: an in vivo PET study. Circulation 96:3416–3422

Lefroy DC, de Silva R, Choudhury L, Uren NG, Crake T, Rhodes CG, Lammertsma AA, Boyd H, Patsalos PN, Nihoyannopoulos P et al (1993) Diffuse reduction of myocardial beta-adrenoceptors in hypertrophic cardiomyopathy: a study with positron emission tomography. J Am Coll Cardiol 22:1653–1660

Li ST, Tack CJ, Fananapazir L, Goldstein DS (2000) Myocardial perfusion and sympathetic innervation in patients with hypertrophic cardiomyopathy. J Am Coll Cardiol 35:1867–1873

Link JM, Stratton JR, Levy W, Poole JE, Shoner SC, Stuetzle W, Caldwell JH (2003) PET measures of pre- and post-synaptic cardiac beta adrenergic function. Nucl Med Biol 30:795–803

Naya M, Tsukamoto T, Morita K, Katoh C, Nishijima K, Komatsu H, Yamada S, Kuge Y, Tamaki N, Tsutsui H (2009) Myocardial beta-adrenergic receptor density assessed by 11C-CGP12177 PET predicts improvement of cardiac function after carvedilol treatment in patients with idiopathic dilated cardiomyopathy. J Nucl Med 50:220–225

Pietila MJ, Ukkonen H, Saraste M, Nagren K, Lehikoinen P, Knuuti J, VoipioPulkki LM (1997) Exercise training improves myocardial sympathetic innervation and may improve reduced myocardial blood flaw in patients with congestive heart failure: a PET study. Circulation 96:459

Pietilä M, Malminiemi K, Ukkonen H, Saraste M, Nagren K, Lehikoinen P, Voipio-Pulkki LM (2001) Reduced myocardial carbon-11 hydroxyephedrine retention is associated with poor prognosis in chronic heart failure. Eur J Nucl Med 28:373–376

Schafers M, Dutka D, Rhodes CG, Lammertsma AA, Hermansen F, Schober O, Camici PG (1998) Myocardial presynaptic and postsynaptic autonomic dysfunction in hypertrophic cardiomyopathy. Circ Res 82:57–62

Thackeray JT, Bengel FM (2013) Assessment of cardiac autonomic neuronal function using PET imaging. J Nucl Cardiol 20:150–165

Tsukamoto T, Morita K, Naya M, Inubushi M, Katoh C, Nishijima K, Kuge Y, Okamoto H, Tsutsui H, Tamaki N (2007) Decreased myocardial beta-adrenergic receptor density in relation to increased sympathetic tone in patients with nonischemic cardiomyopathy. J Nucl Med 48: 1777–1782

Ungerer M, Hartmann F, Karoglan M, Chlistalla A, Ziegler S, Richardt G, Overbeck M, Meisner H, Schomig A, Schwaiger M (1998) Regional in vivo and in vitro characterization of autonomic innervation in cardiomyopathic human heart. Circulation 97:174–180

Ungerer M, Weig HJ, Kubert S, Overbeck M, Bengel F, Schomig A, Schwaiger M (2000) Regional pre- and postsynaptic sympathetic system in the failing human heart–regulation of beta ARK-1. Eur J Heart Fail 2:23–31

Vesalainen RK, Pietila M, Tahvanainen KU, Jartti T, Teras M, Nagren K, Lehikoinen P, Huupponen R, Ukkonen H, Saraste M, Knuuti J, Voipio-Pulkki LM (1999) Cardiac positron emission tomography imaging with [11C]hydroxyephedrine, a specific tracer for sympathetic nerve endings, and its functional correlates in congestive heart failure. Am J Cardiol 84:568–574

Conventional Radionuclide Imaging of Autonomic Function in Heart Failure

13

Arnold F. Jacobson and Jagat Narula

Contents

A.F. Jacobson, MD, PhD
Diagram Consulting, 10 Lio Poele Place, Kihei, HI 96753, USA
e-mail: afjacobsonmd@gmail.com

J. Narula, MD, PhD, FACC, FAHA, FRCP [Edin] (✉)
Cardiovascular Imaging Program, Zena and Michael A. Wiener Cardiovascular Institute and Marie-Josée and Henry R. Kravis Center for Cardiovascular Health of Mount Sinai School of Medicine, Mount Sinai Medical Center,
One Gustave L. Levy Place, New York, NY 10029, USA
e-mail: jagat.narula@mountsinai.org

R.H.J.A. Slart et al. (eds.), *Autonomic Innervation of the Heart: Role of Molecular Imaging*, DOI 10.1007/978-3-662-45074-1_13

Abstract
Conventional nuclear imaging with single-photon emitting radionuclides can be used for qualitative and quantitative assessment of cardiac autonomic function in patients with heart failure. Status of sympathetic innervation can be assessed using [^{123}I]-metaiodobenzylguanidine ([^{123}I]-MIBG), an analogue of norepinephrine. Reduced myocardial [^{123}I]-MIBG uptake is common in heart failure patients, and the severity of global and regional abnormalities is indicative of the level of risk for mortality and occurrence of ventricular arrhythmias. [^{123}I]-MIBG imaging can identify early damage from cardiotoxic chemotherapy and early evidence of reinnervation in transplanted hearts. The extent of [^{123}I]-MIBG tomographic defects provides an indicator of the likelihood of appropriate implantable cardioverter-defibrillator (ICD) activation and may be useful in assessment of patients being considered for these devices. In the future, [^{123}I]-MIBG imaging may provide a non-invasive means to evaluate the effectiveness of heart failure treatments that reduce autonomic nervous system imbalances common in heart failure patients.

Abbreviations

ACE	Angiotensin-converting enzyme
AHA	American Heart Association
ARB	Angiotensin receptor blocker
AUC	Area under the curve
BNP	B-type natriuretic peptide
CRT	Cardiac resynchronization therapy
CT	Computed tomography
FDG	Fluorodeoxyglucose
H/M	Heart-to-mediastinum ratio
HF	Heart failure
HRV	Heart rate variability
ICD	Implantable cardioverter-defibrillator
[123I]	Iodine-123
LV	Left ventricular
LVAD	Left ventricular Assist Device
LVEF	Left ventricular ejection fraction
MCE	Major cardiac event
MIBG	Metaiodobenzylguanidine
MPI	Myocardial perfusion imaging
NE	Norepinephrine
NET	Norepinephrine transporter
NYHA	New York Heart Association
PET	Positron emission tomography
ROC	Receiver Operating Characteristic
ROI	Region of interest

SCD	Sudden cardiac death
SHFM	Seattle Heart Failure Model
SPECT	Single-photon emission computed tomography
[99mTc]	Technetium-99m
VMAT	Vesicular monoamine transporter

13.1 Underlying Physiological Principles of Scintigraphic Imaging for Assessing Autonomic Function

The principles that underlie the use of radiolabeled compounds for nuclear imaging of physiological processes have been described in earlier chapters. With particular reference to radiopharmaceuticals used for single-photon emission computed tomography (SPECT) imaging, most such compounds are labeled with either technetium-99m ([^{99m}Tc]) or iodine-123 ([^{123}I]). While compounds labeled with [^{99m}Tc] tend to be easier to produce because the precursor can be formulated as a lyophilized kit to which generator-produced pertechnetate solution is added, compounds labeled with radioiodine often have greater physiological activity because the radionuclide can be incorporated into the molecule without the need for additional chelators or other linking compounds. Creation of SPECT imaging compounds that bind to cell surface receptors and other proteins is thus more often accomplished using iodine as the radiolabel.

For the past 30 years, the dominant conventional nuclear imaging pharmaceutical for examining a component of the autonomic nervous system has been metaiodobenzylguanidine (MIBG) (Wieland et al. 1981). MIBG is a structural and functional analogue of norepinephrine (NE), but it possesses only weak sympathomimetic effects and is a poor ligand for adrenergic receptors (Shapiro et al. 1984; Smets et al. 1988; Ekelund et al. 2001). MIBG is taken up by the norepinephrine transporter (NET) with a higher affinity than NE (K_m=0.31 and 1.8 μM, respectively), but with a similar capacity. MIBG uptake is also sensitive to the vesicular monoamine transporter (VMAT) inhibitor reserpine (Smets et al. 1989), and radiolabeled MIBG has been observed in vesicles using electron spectroscopic imaging (Gaze et al. 1991), indicating vesicular uptake. MIBG is not metabolized by either monoamine oxidase (MAO) or catechol-*O*-methyltransferase (COMT) (Mangner et al. 1986; Tobes et al. 1989); therefore, the majority of MIBG taken up by the NET is available for VMAT uptake into vesicles. MIBG is also known to enter cells via non-NET-dependent uptake$_2$ activity (Dae et al. 1992; DeGrado et al. 1995). MIBG is therefore subject to the same uptake and accumulation pathways as NE, but does not share the same catabolic pathways or pharmacodynamic effects. After every cycle of vesicular exocytosis and reuptake, NE is subject to MAO catabolism in the cytoplasm, prior to VMAT uptake into the vesicles, whereas MIBG is not. This favors MIBG vesicular storage over that of NE, particularly over repeated cycles of uptake and release (Sisson and Wieland 1986).

Based upon whole-body images acquired as part of biodistribution studies, it is estimated that in a normal individual, slightly less than 1 % of an intravenously injected dose of MIBG localizes to the myocardium (Kline et al. 1981). In patients with congestive heart failure, a close correlation is observed between elevated levels of plasma and urinary NE and the severity of left ventricular dysfunction (Cohn et al. 1984; Leimbach et al. 1986). This was reported to be due to decreased cardiac NE uptake (Bohm et al. 1995; Liang et al. 1989; Ungerer et al. 1998) and a reduced expression of cardiac NET by posttranscriptional downregulation (Backs et al. 2001). The NET therefore has profound effects on the pharmacology of NE and consequently also on that of MIBG.

The loss of adrenergic innervation and inhibition of NET or VMAT activity reduce the uptake and retention of MIBG. High levels of circulating NE may also reduce accumulation by competing for NET uptake. Chronically high levels of NE and certain drugs of abuse may also reduce the expression of NET and thus reduce neuronal accumulation. A loss of MIBG uptake is commonly observed in heart failure patients, most likely as a result of a decrease in the number of adrenergic neurons in combination with an overall increase in sympathetic activity, leading to increased vesicular exocytosis and efflux of MIBG from the synapse.

The functional attributes of MIBG as a NE analogue establish the utility of the compound as a diagnostic product. Analogous to the use of F-18 FDG, functionally a marker of glucose metabolism, for PET imaging demonstration of epileptogenic foci, viable myocardium, and active tumor, MIBG scintigraphy identifies tissues capable of concentrating neuroadrenergic amines, thereby providing a means to document the loss of autoregulatory sympathetic neuronal function. In the heart, MIBG imaging is a sensitive marker for sympathetic neuronal injury, often showing changes prior to other imaging or clinical evidence of damage. Cardiac [^{123}I]-MIBG imaging has been shown to be useful for investigating the severity of heart failure (Merlet et al. 1992a, b) and for assessing response to standard therapies such as ACE inhibitors and beta-blockers (Kasama et al. 2005a, b; Agostini et al. 2000). In recent years, reduced myocardial [^{123}I]-MIBG uptake has been demonstrated to be a powerful prognostic indicator in HF patients, with those with the greatest myocardial denervation having the poorest outcomes (Merlet et al. 1999a, b; Wakabayashi et al. 2001). These observations apply to morbidity and mortality resulting from pump failure as well as to unstable arrhythmias that often precede occurrence of sudden cardiac death (SCD) (Nishisato et al. 2010).

The following sections summarize published results examining the use of [^{123}I]-MIBG as a diagnostic and prognostic imaging agent in patients with HF of various etiologies.

13.2 [^{123}I]-MIBG Imaging Principles and Procedures

13.2.1 Semiquantitative and Quantitative Analyses

For more than 20 years, the most common approach to examination of [^{123}I]-MIBG myocardial images in HF patients has been to obtain quantitative measures of uptake for comparison with reference data from individuals without heart disease. The most

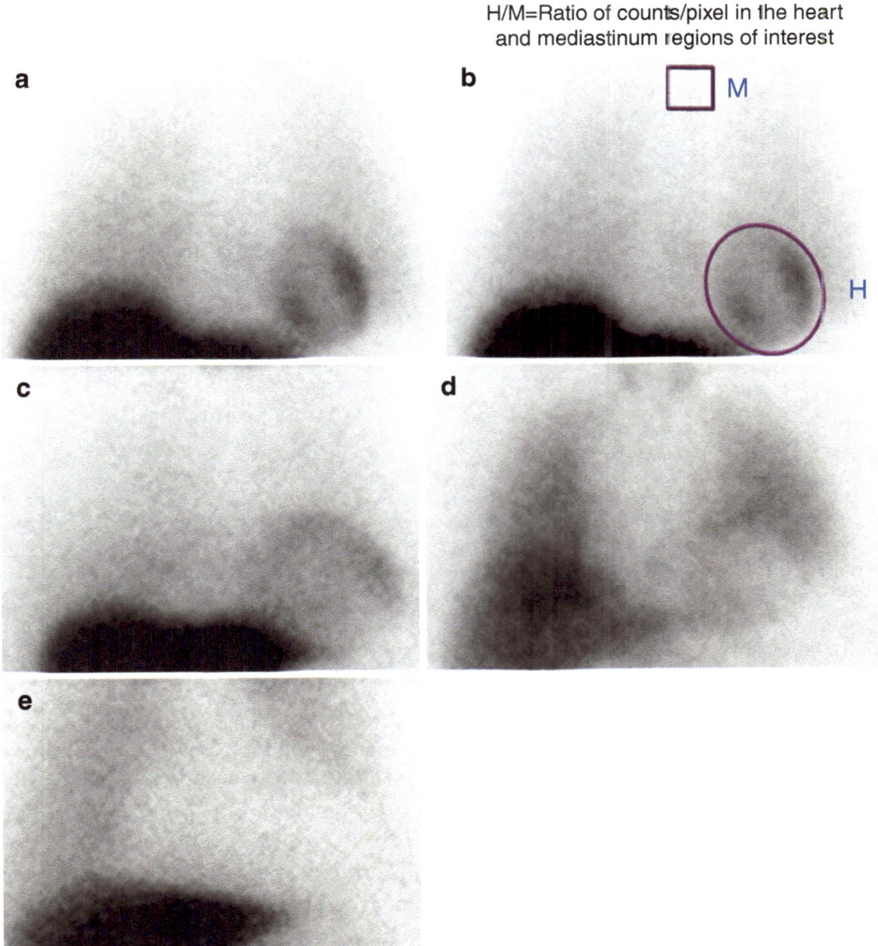

Fig. 13.1 Anterior planar [^{123}I]-MIBG images of the chest in a healthy control without heart disease (**a**) and 3 heart failure patients (**c**–**e**). Image (**b**) reproduces the image of the healthy control with regions of interest (ROIs) drawn around the visible myocardium (*H*) and the upper mediastinum (*M*), from which the H/M ratio is calculated by dividing the mean counts per pixel in the former and latter ROIs. H/M is 2.40 in the healthy patient (**a**), 1.83 in the HF patient with preserved sympathetic innervation (**c**), 1.34 in the HF patient with moderately reduced uptake (**d**), and 0.96 in the HF patient with no visible cardiac uptake (**e**). The finding in image (**e**) represents the worst prognosis; this patient died from HF progression 8 months after being studied

widely used technique involves a comparison of global uptake in the heart to another region within the same image (Fig. 13.1). As the mediastinum is usually included in images of the thorax and this area lacks specific NET-associated uptake, it has become the standard reference region for the so-called heart-to-mediastinum ratio (H/M). The H/M was first employed in analysis of planar images and more recently

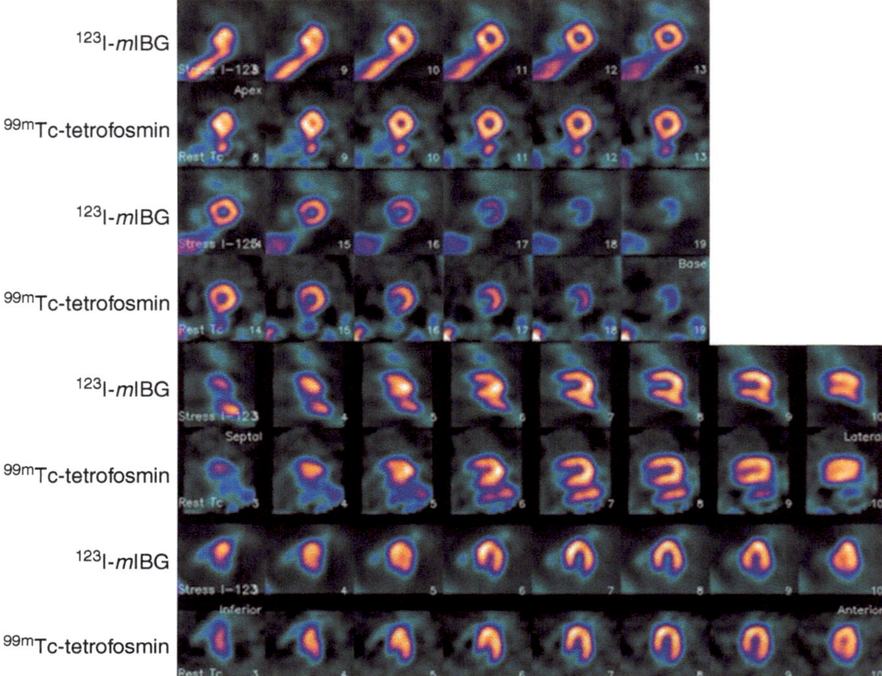

Fig. 13.2 Aligned [^{123}I]-MIBG and ^{99m}Tc-tetrofosmin MPI SPECT images from an 82-year-old female with no history of heart disease show normal innervation and perfusion. *Top* four rows represent reoriented short-axis images, followed by vertical and horizontal long-axis views

has been adapted for similar analyses using SPECT (Fig. 13.2) (Chen et al. 2012). In general, [^{123}I]-MIBG results are presented in terms of the relationship between a quantitative value of myocardial uptake (on planar or SPECT imaging) and a specific outcome event (such as worsening of HF, occurrence of a cardiac event, or death) or another quantitative parameter (such as change in left ventricular ejection fraction (LVEF) or MPI defect score). While differences in methodologies and study objectives limit the degree to which data from various studies can be combined, there is near unanimity of opinion concerning the direct relationship between quantitative [^{123}I]-MIBG uptake values and clinical outcome (whether representing the natural history of the disease or its likelihood of responding to a particular therapy). The overwhelmingly consistent finding has been that the greater the reduction in [^{123}I]-MIBG uptake, the poorer is the outcome (Verberne et al. 2008).

13.2.2 Proof of Principle of [^{123}I]-MIBG Imaging: Heart Transplantation

In end-stage HF, the final remaining therapeutic option is often heart transplantation. In several earlier studies (Merlet et al. 1992a, 1999a, b), many native hearts prior to removal demonstrated virtually no visible MIBG uptake (H/M ratio approximately 1.0). However, in an interesting irony, [^{123}I]-MIBG imaging of the transplanted heart has in some instances provided compelling validation of the method as a measure of sympathetic innervation, in that initially the transplanted heart is totally denervated and demonstrates no specific uptake of MIBG, essentially the same finding as for the organ that was removed. However, over time the transplanted heart serves as a model of the potential for recovery of this innervation. This has been best demonstrated in a study by Estorch et al. (1999), in which 31 subjects from 6 months to 12 years posttransplant underwent planar and SPECT [^{123}I]-MIBG imaging. Considering an H/M ratio <1.3 as no significant uptake, 4 of 9 subjects within 2 years of transplant and 18 of 22 at 2–12 years posttransplant showed visible myocardial activity. For all subjects in these groups, mean H/M ratio was significantly higher in the latter (1.62 (0.2) vs. 1.34 (0.2)). Regional MIBG uptake on SPECT imaging was seen almost exclusively in the anterior and lateral walls. However, in a more recent study by Yap et al. (2006), none of the eight patients studied 1.1–6.3 years post-heterotopic transplantation showed detectable uptake on either planar or SPECT [^{123}I]-MIBG imaging. While these results indicate that reinnervation does occur in some transplanted hearts, the clinical significance of whether it occurs in specific patients is still uncertain.

13.3 [^{123}I]-MIBG Imaging Findings in HF Patients

The following section contains a brief review of a representative selection of the several hundred [^{123}I]-MIBG imaging studies in HF patients published in the past 20 years. This literature has provided a clear picture of the importance of cardiac sympathetic innervation as a prognostic factor in patients with HF.

A large number of investigators have demonstrated that HF patients with lower cardiac uptake of [^{123}I]-MIBG, typically quantified using the H/M ratio, have poorer prognosis in terms of all-cause and cardiac mortality. The mean planar H/M ratio in patients who died was typically 0.2–0.3 less than in the surviving patients (Wakabayashi et al. 2001; Momose et al. 1999; Yamada et al. 2003; Merlet et al. 1999a, b; Nakata et al. 2005). Several recent meta-analyses confirmed these individual observations in aggregations of over 2,000 HF patients (Verberne et al. 2008; Kuwabara et al. 2011).

It has long been appreciated that derangements of the sympathetic nervous system play a role in the loss of myocardial contractile function. The increased circulating NE levels commonly seen in patients with HF and the poor prognosis of individuals with particularly high NE levels are associated with a decreased responsiveness of the heart to adrenergic stimulation and downregulation of cardiac β-receptors (Cohn et al. 1984; Bohm et al. 1995; Backs et al. 2001; Tsukamoto et al. 2007). The success of beta-blocker therapy as a treatment for HF is associated with recovery of at least some of the sympathetic neuronal function in the myocardium, particularly among those with sufficient myocardial viability to sustain a reasonable level of pump function. Imaging of myocardial sympathetic innervation provides a means to judge the recovery of this regulatory system in HF patients receiving standard of care medical therapy (Agostini et al. 2000). More recent research suggests that such imaging may also be of value in assessing effectiveness of therapy using devices such as biventricular pacemakers and left ventricular assist devices (Cha et al. 2008).

Most studies of [^{123}I]-MIBG imaging in patients with HF have examined the prognostic value of the method for prediction of specific clinical outcomes. Some have been longitudinal studies to determine the relationship between imaging and clinical variables and long-term survival, while others have examined the potential role of [^{123}I]-MIBG imaging in managing or optimizing medical therapy for HF. Most earlier studies relied upon planar imaging and H/M ratios, while many more recent trials have incorporated SPECT imaging as a significant component of the investigational plan.

13.3.1 Overall Prognosis

Numerous investigators have examined the utility of [^{123}I]-MIBG imaging as a predictor of clinical outcome in HF patients being treated with standard therapeutic regimens (digoxin, diuretics, beta-blockers, ACE inhibitors, etc.). The following table summarizes a representative selection of such studies, with outcome events generally being cardiac death or heart transplantation. In all studies, the mean H/M for subjects with events was significantly lower than for subjects without events (Table 13.1).

In the studies of Merlet et al. (1992a, 1999a, b), multivariate discriminant analysis showed quantitation of [^{123}I]-MIBG uptake as the most powerful independent predictor of mortality. Many other studies, including those of Momose et al. (1999), Nakata et al. (1998), Wakabayashi et al. (2001), Ebina et al. (2002), Kyuma et al. (2004), Agostini et al. (2008), and Tamaki et al. (2009) showed similar results in multivariate models for cardiac death and other adverse cardiac outcomes.

The objective of the study of Matsui et al. (2002) was somewhat different than those cited above, in that [^{123}I]-MIBG imaging was performed twice, before and after 6 months of intensive therapy, to determine the prognostic significance of the change in quantitative uptake. Although 85 subjects were studied at entry, only 74 had the second imaging study and then were followed clinically. During follow-up, there were 12 deaths and 11 other adverse outcomes. Although there was no difference in the mean H/M ratios at baseline between subjects who did and did not survive, 11 of those who died showed decrease in H/M ratio between the two [^{123}I]-MIBG studies, a finding not seen among survivors. Overall, the change in [^{123}I]-MIBG uptake was a better predictor of adverse long-term outcome than either NE or b-type natriuretic peptide (BNP) levels, which were also measured at baseline and after the first 6 months of treatment.

In the study published by Agostini et al. (2008), [^{123}I]-MIBG scans obtained on 290 HF patients (262 with LVEF <50 %) from six European centers were reanalyzed using a standardized methodology to determine the H/M ratio on delayed planar images. Major cardiac events (MCE) (cardiac death; cardiac transplant; potentially fatal arrhythmia, including ICD discharge) during a 24-month follow-up were confirmed by an adjudication committee of cardiologists. Such events occurred

Table 13.1 Outcome data for cardiomyopathy patients – selected studies with group comparisons based upon mean H/M ratios

Reference	No. HF patients	Mean follow-up (mo)	Outcome event	No. outcome events	Mean H/M ratio (SD) outcome events	Mean H/M ratio (SD) no outcome events
Momose et al. (1999)	59	25	Cardiac death	16	1.48 (0.29)	1.76 (0.24)
Merlet et al. (1999a, b)	112	27	Cardiac death	25	1.10 (0.09)	1.34 (0.14)
			Heart transplant	19	1.05 (0.15)	
Wakabayashi et al. (2001)	132	54	Cardiac death	48	Ischemic: 1.67 (0.34)	Ischemic: 1.84 (0.37)
					Nonischemic: 1.56 (0.35)	Nonischemic: 1.79 (0.40)
Ebina et al. (2002)	62	16	Cardiac death	12	1.71 (0.37)	2.21 (0.44)
Kioka et al. (2007)	97	65	Sudden death	14	1.54 (0.27)	1.77 (0.30)
Kuramoto et al. (2011)	106	82	Cardiac death	32	1.57 (0.24)	1.79 (0.32)

No number, *HF* heart failure, *SD* standard deviation, *H/M* heart-to-mediastinum ratio, *mo* months

in 67 subjects (26 %), and mean H/M ratios were significantly lower in this group than in those who did not have events (1.51 ± 0.30 for MCE group, 1.97 ± 0.54 for non-MCE group ($p < 0.001$)). Two-year event-free survival using an "optimum" H/M ratio threshold of 1.75 was 62 % for H/M ratio <1.75, 95 % for H/M ratio ≥1.75 ($p < 0.0001$). Logistic regression showed H/M ratio and LVEF as the only significant predictors of MCE. For the lower and upper H/M quartiles of ≤1.45 and >2.17, 2-year event-free survival was 52 and 98 %, respectively.

The results of the largest prospective trial examining the prognostic significance of [^{123}I]-MIBG imaging in HF were published in 2010 (Jacobson et al. 2010). In the ADMIRE-HF study, 961 NYHA class II and III HF patients with LVEF ≤35 % underwent [^{123}I]-MIBG imaging and clinical follow-up for a mean of 17 months. Time to first occurrence of NYHA functional class progression, potentially life-threatening arrhythmic event, or cardiac death was compared with H/M in relation to an estimated lower limit of normal of 1.60. A total of 237 subjects (25 %) experienced events, of which only 25 occurred in the 201 subjects with H/M ≥1.60. Two-year event rate was 15 % for H/M ≥1.60 and 37 % for H/M <1.60; hazard ratios for individual event categories were HF progression, 0.49 ($p = 0.002$); arrhythmic events, 0.37 ($p = 0.02$); and cardiac death, 0.14 ($p = 0.006$). In a multivariate Cox proportional hazards model, significant variables were H/M, LVEF, BNP, and NYHA functional class. The predictive value of the H/M was subsequently reconfirmed in analyses of all-cause mortality following additional follow-up to a median of 24 months (Narula et al. 2010) (Fig. 13.3).

There is overwhelming evidence from the cited studies and numerous others performed in the past 20 years that significant myocardial denervation is associated with a substantial increase in the occurrence of severe adverse outcomes in HF patients. With the increasing methodological standardization of planar and SPECT [^{123}I]-MIBG imaging (Flotats et al. 2010), broader use of this technique as part of risk stratification of HF patients appears justified. During the past decade, it has become increasingly evident that this method provides information that should be of substantial value to the clinicians responsible for managing these patients.

13.3.2 Monitoring Therapeutic Response

One of the major challenges in the management of HF is the optimization of the medical regimen, with drugs such as beta-blockers and ACE inhibitors requiring careful titration to achieve the maximum therapeutic benefit with the fewest side effects. Patients with significantly impaired cardiac function often have a relatively narrow window for therapeutic efficacy, with adverse reactions acting as a potentially significant disincentive for adherence to often complex multidrug regimens. While imaging studies are widely used to monitor parameters of cardiac function such as LVEF and end-diastolic volume, there remains a need for more sophisticated means to judge the likely success of proposed therapeutic strategies, in order to improve the selection of drugs and dosages in clinical practice.

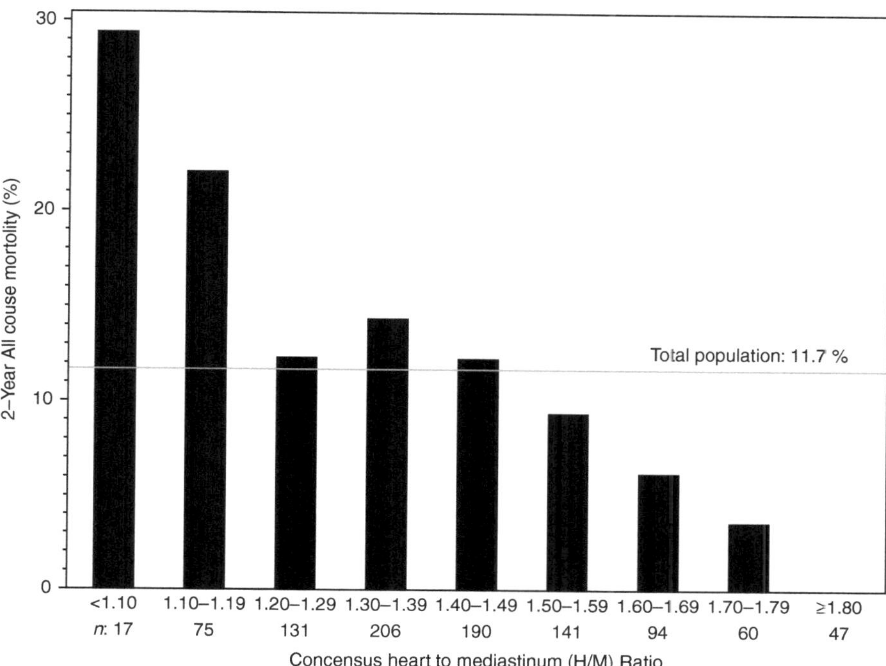

Fig. 13.3 Two-year all-cause mortality rates from the prospective multicenter international ADMIRE-HF extension trial of 961 NYHA class II/III HF patients with LVEF ≤35 %. There was a progressive decrease of all-cause and cardiac mortality (latter not shown) with increasing planar H/M ratio. No deaths occurred in the 47 subjects (5 %) with H/M ≥1.8

[^{123}I]-MIBG imaging has been employed as a method for quantitative assessment of therapeutic response in a number of small prospective studies. As a marker of cardiac sympathetic innervation, it is not surprising that [^{123}I]-MIBG has been used most often in studies examining the effectiveness of beta-blockers. Two such studies were reported by Merlet et al. (1999a) and Suwa et al. (1997). In the former, 18 subjects underwent planar [^{123}I]-MIBG imaging at baseline and after 6 months of treatment with metoprolol titrated to a maximum daily dosage of 150 mg. Effectiveness of the treatment was documented in terms of increased mean H/M ratio (1.29 (0.1) to 1.38 (0.17)), increased mean LVEF (20 % to 27 %), and decreased mean plasma NE (0.93 to 0.72 ng/ml), and all changes were statistically significant. In the study of Suwa et al. (1997), 45 subjects with nonischemic dilated cardiomyopathy had [^{123}I]-MIBG scans prior to initiation of bisoprolol therapy, and the response was assessed after 6 months. Overall, 30 subjects responded to treatment (as reflected by >20 % increase in LV fractional shortening on echocardiography); mean H/M ratio of responders was 2.1 (0.4) versus 1.5 (0.2) for non-responders ($p<0.001$). Using an H/M ratio threshold of 1.7 allowed prediction of response with sensitivity of 91 % and specificity of 92 %. Kasama et al. (2002) reported data from a study of 30 HF patients, 15 of whom were randomized to receive spironolactone in addition to their standard therapeutic regimen. [^{123}I]-MIBG planar imaging performed at baseline and 6 months showed improvement in the mean H/M ratio only in the spironolactone group (1.62 (0.2)–1.83 (0.2) vs. 1.7 (0.2)–1.67 (0.2)). Corresponding to this imaging improvement, only this group was judged clinically improved (based upon NYHA classifications). These data were published only a few years following completion of the first large clinical trial documenting the survival benefit of aldosterone inhibition in patients with severe HF (Pitt et al. 1999).

Studies have shown beneficial effects on cardiac sympathetic innervation (assessed by [^{123}I]-MIBG imaging) for almost all contemporary HF therapies. These include angiotensin receptor blockers (Kasama et al. 2003, 2005a), cardiac resynchronization therapy (Nishioka et al. 2007; Cha et al. 2008), and ventricular assist devices (Drakos et al. 2010). In total, more than 40 studies comparing cardiac uptake of [^{123}I]-MIBG before and after initiation of various HF therapies have been published in the past 15 years. A recent review of the medication dosages at entry into the ADMIRE-HF trial demonstrated that the H/M retained its prognostic validity regardless of the intensity of treatment (based upon range of dosage) using beta-blockers, ACE inhibitors, ARBs, and aldosterone inhibitors (Pina et al. 2012).

In aggregate, the above-cited studies demonstrate the potential benefit of neurocardiac imaging as an aid for rationalizing selection of drug therapy in HF. [^{123}I]-MIBG imaging might be used initially to judge the likelihood of success of a category of drugs (such as beta-blockers) based upon the severity of the adrenergic deficiency and later might provide insight regarding optimal drug dosage through quantitative measures of changes in myocardial uptake parameters. Analogous to the use of this modality for prognostic assessment of HF patients, [^{123}I]-MIBG imaging is a tool that could be particularly valuable for the HF specialist in managing more difficult cases such as individuals with multiple comorbidities.

13.3.3 [^{123}I]-MIBG Imaging in Pre-heart Failure: Patients with Malignancy Receiving Cardiotoxic Chemotherapeutic Agents

Analogous to the documented reduction in cardiac uptake of [^{123}I]-MIBG in patients with HF, similar observations have been made in cancer patients who experienced cardiac toxicity as a result of chemotherapeutic agents. Particularly for known cardiotoxic drugs such as the anthracyclines, studies have shown decreased myocardial [^{123}I]-MIBG uptake as a result of such treatment. In one study of 21 patients treated with either doxorubicin or epirubicin (Valdes Olmos et al. 1995), the most significant reduction in cardiac [^{123}I]-MIBG uptake was seen in the patients who received the highest doses. In 8 patients who developed persistently reduced LVEF at high doxorubicin cumulative dose levels, [^{123}I]-MIBG imaging performed after discontinuation of chemotherapy remained abnormal. In another study of 59 patients who received Adriamycin (Niitsu et al. 1995), increase in washout rate (WR) was related to the total dose of Adriamycin, and as the WR increased, the frequency of ventricular arrhythmias also increased. The WR usually normalized 3–6 months after the discontinuation of Adriamycin. Finally, Carrio et al. (1995) reported on 36 patients who received doxorubicin and had normal [^{123}I]-MIBG uptake (H/M 1.85 ± 0.29) and LVEF (61 % ± 8 %) before chemotherapy. At a cumulative dose of 240–300 mg/m^2 doxorubicin, [^{123}I]-MIBG uptake was unchanged (mean H/M 1.80 ± 0.2), but after 420–600 mg/m^2, both [^{123}I]-MIBG uptake (mean H/M 1.76 ± 0.2, $p < 0.05$) and LVEF (mean 52 % ± 8 % ($p < 0.05$)) were decreased. These results are all consistent with the larger HF literature, reflecting that HF induced by cardiotoxic drugs produces the same reduction in cardiac [^{123}I]-MIBG neuronal uptake as occurs in association with ischemic and nonischemic cardiomyopathy.

13.3.4 [^{123}I]-MIBG Imaging and Risk of Life-Threatening Arrhythmia

Heterogeneity of sympathetic innervation has been associated with increased arrhythmogenicity (Inoue and Zipes 1987; Stanton and Zipes 1991; Mitrani et al. 1993). The coexistence of denervated and hyperinnervated areas in the diseased myocardium produces increased electrophysiological heterogeneity during sympathetic activation, leading to ventricular arrhythmia and SCD (Chen et al. 2007). Adrenergic denervation of viable myocardium may also result in denervation supersensitivity, with exaggerated response of myocardium to sympathetic stimulation and increased vulnerability to ventricular arrhythmias (Dae et al. 1995; Minardo et al. 1988). Therefore, [^{123}I]-MIBG imaging provides the capability to identify presence of denervated but viable myocardium as a means to judge risk for ventricular arrhythmic events.

Although patients with both ischemic and nonischemic HF have abnormal cardiac uptake of [^{123}I]-MIBG, the pattern of such abnormalities tends to differ between the two types of HF. In patients with previous myocardial infarction (MI), there is usually a discrete focal defect on [^{123}I]-MIBG SPECT images, corresponding to the location of the MI but typically larger in size than the defect seen on MPI SPECT (McGhie et al. 1991; Yukinaka et al. 1998; Simoes et al. 2004) (Fig. 13.4). In patients with nonischemic cardiomyopathy, the pattern of uptake on [^{123}I]-MIBG SPECT is usually heterogeneous, and focal defects are usually smaller than in patients with prior MI (Maeno et al. 1993; Parthenakis et al. 2002). Total [^{123}I]-MIBG SPECT defect scores are usually smaller in nonischemic than ischemic HF patients; in some of the former patients, MPI SPECT is qualitatively normal (Clements et al. 2012). While there is a growing body of evidence that larger [^{123}I]-MIBG SPECT defect is associated with increased risk for SCD and ICD activations (Boogers et al. 2010), it remains to be determined if different thresholds for interpretation of [^{123}I]-MIBG SPECT findings in ischemic and nonischemic patients are needed.

Current available methods for precise identification of individuals at risk for SCD and therefore at the greatest need for ICDs have definite limitations. For example, non-invasive tests reflecting autonomic function, such as heart rate variability

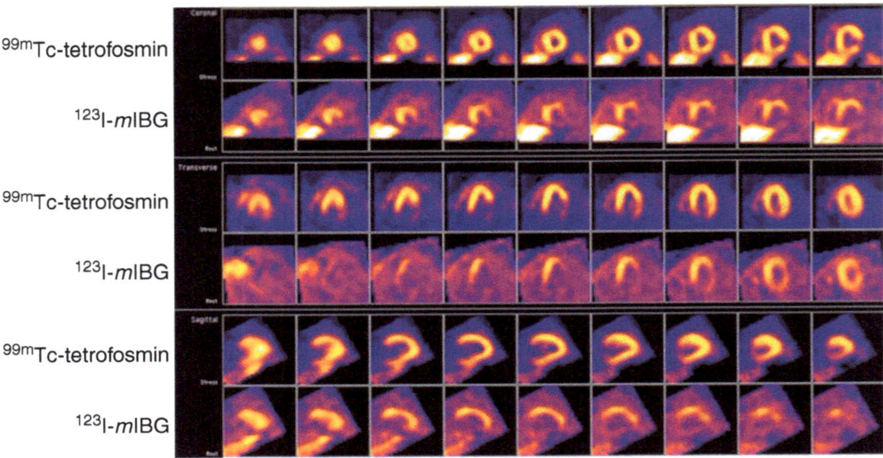

Fig. 13.4 Aligned ^{99m}Tc-tetrofosmin MPI and [^{123}I]-MIBG SPECT images from a 42-year-old male with history of lateral wall myocardial infarction. *Top* two rows represent reoriented short-axis images, followed by vertical and horizontal long-axis views. There is a small perfusion defect at the base of the lateral wall, corresponding to the known infarct. There is a much larger innervation defect, including both the region of the lateral infarct and almost the entire inferior wall. This pattern of innervation-perfusion mismatch is associated with an increased risk for ventricular arrhythmias

(HRV), signal-averaged ECG (SAECG), and microvolt t-wave alternans (MTA), have limited sensitivity and positive predictive value (Bailey et al. 2001; Gehl et al. 2005). This has led to increased interest in the potential of [^{123}I]-MIBG imaging for such assessments. One of the earliest examinations of this use of the [^{123}I]-MIBG imaging method was published by Arora et al. (2003), who evaluated 17 patients with ICDs using [^{123}I]-MIBG cardiac imaging (as means of assessing myocardial sympathetic innervation) and spectral analysis of HRV (as means of assessing central autonomic tone). Patients with previous ICD discharges had lower early H/M, more extensive [^{123}I]-MIBG SPECT defects, and more [^{123}I]-MIBG/^{99m}Tc-sestamibi MPI mismatch segments (denervation in areas of myocardial viability) as compared with patients without previous ICD discharges. The combined non-invasive evaluation of local cardiac autonomic innervation and systemic autonomic function by means of [^{123}I]-MIBG and HRV allowed correct identification of patients at high and low risk for potentially fatal arrhythmias.

Another study which examined several indicators of autonomic function in relation to arrhythmic events was reported by Koutelou et al. (2009). Twenty-five patients with NYHA class I or II HF and recent ICD implants were studied for baroreflex sensitivity, 24-h heart rate variability, and [^{123}I]-MIBG imaging. During mean 32 months follow-up, the frequency of fast ventricular arrhythmic episodes correlated with measures from all three tests, and among the tests there was limited interdependence. These results suggest that various measures of autonomic dysfunction can provide complementary information for assessing degree of risk for fast ventricular arrhythmias in HF patients.

There has been considerable recent interest in determining if defect size on [^{123}I]-MIBG SPECT imaging can identify HF patients most and least likely to need ICDs as protection from occurrence of SCD. Studies examining this question have generally involved a mixture of patients receiving devices for primary and secondary prevention. Results for several such studies are summarized below.

A prospective pilot study was performed to determine whether alterations in cardiac sympathetic innervation as measured by [^{123}I]-MIBG scintigraphy were related to inducibility of ventricular tachyarrhythmias during electrophysiology (EP) testing in patients with previous myocardial infarction (Bax et al. 2008). Of 50 subjects with complete data, including ^{99m}Tc-tetrofosmin MPI SPECT, 30 had positive and 20 negative EP tests. Of all the imaging and clinical variables, only the [^{123}I]-MIBG SPECT defect size discriminated between subjects with positive and negative EP tests (42.7 ± 8.8 vs. 34.9 ± 9.8; $p = 0.005$). A 4-h [^{123}I]-MIBG SPECT defect score of ≥37 yielded a sensitivity of 77 % and specificity of 75 % for predicting EP results.

A study of 116 HF subjects referred for ICD therapy included both [^{123}I]-MIBG and MPI SPECT procedures at baseline (Boogers et al. 2010). During a mean follow-up of 23 ± 15 months, appropriate ICD therapy occurred in 24 (21 %) patients and cardiac death occurred in 8 (28 %) patients. Late [^{123}I]-MIBG SPECT defect score was an independent predictor for both end points. Patients with a late [^{123}I]-MIBG SPECT defect score >26 showed significantly more appropriate ICD therapy (52 % vs. 5 %, $p < 0.01$) and appropriate ICD therapy or cardiac death (57 % vs. 10 %, $p < 0.01$) than patients with smaller defects.

In the study of Nishisato et al. (2010), 60 ICD patients underwent [^{123}I]-MIBG planar and SPECT imaging and rest ^{99m}Tc-tetrofosmin MPI and then were followed for a mean 29 months. During this time, 30 patients (50 %) experienced at least one appropriate ICD discharge. Patients with impaired [^{123}I]–MIBG uptake (H/M <1.9) and tetrofosmin defect score >12 had a significantly greater event rate (94 %) than did the group with impaired uptake of [^{123}I]-MIBG and preserved uptake of tetrofosmin [45 %; $p < 0.05$] and the group with preserved uptake of both agents (18 %). These results suggest that [^{123}I]-MIBG and MPI provide complementary information for identifying patients most in need of ICD protection against SCD.

In the recent study by Kasama et al. (2012), the relationship between [^{123}I]-MIBG results and late ventricular potentials (LP) was examined in 56 patients with dilated cardiomyopathy. [^{123}I]-MIBG SPECT defect score was significantly higher (35 ± 8 vs. 28 ± 6, $p < 0.005$), and the H/M ratio was significantly lower (1.57 ± 0.23 vs. 1.78 ± 0.20, $p < 0.005$) in patients who were LP positive. During a mean follow-up time of 4.5 years, there were nine sudden deaths, and occurrence of these events was significantly higher in LP-positive patients with washout rate ≥50 %. This study provided further evidence of the increased risk for SCD associated with large innervation abnormalities on [^{123}I]-MIBG imaging.

13.3.5 Combination of [^{123}I]-MIBG Imaging and Clinical Risk Models

Many clinical models of prognosis from HF have been developed in the past 20 years. These models generally incorporate patient demographics, medical history, medication usage, and selected laboratory and imaging measurements to provide estimates of all-cause and cardiac mortality rates and risk for nonfatal events such as HF hospitalization or need for heart transplantation. Although providing greater rigor for categorizing relative risk in the HF population, clinical models have not gained wide acceptance as a tool to assist in the management of patient care. Especially for cardiologists who employ cardiology society guidelines as the basis for HF management decisions, the additional value of model calculations of future morbidity and mortality risk may not be obvious.

The subjectivity associated with definition of risk contributes to the reticence of clinicians to employ such calculations in patient-care decisions. Nevertheless, concern about overutilization of ICDs has raised awareness of the potential value of accurate identification of low-risk patients as a means to reduce the number of implanted devices that never fire. The basic logic is that if a clinical model or diagnostic test can identify patients with a very low risk of dying from any cause, those individuals do not require interventions to protect them from possible SCD. There is a growing body of evidence that addition of results of [^{123}I]-MIBG imaging to clinical prediction models produces improved accuracy for identifying both high- and low-risk HF patients.

One of the most widely used and well-validated HF prediction models, developed by Levy and associates, is known as the Seattle HF Model (SHFM) (Levy et al. 2006). SHFM includes a variety of demographic and clinical markers to predict 1–5-year mortality in HF patients. It also shows changes in life expectancy with alterations in heart failure medications and by placement of ICDs, biventricular CRT, and left ventricular assist devices (LVADs).

None of the variables included in the SHFM provide a direct measure of cardiac sympathetic neuronal status. An indication that addition of [^{123}I]-MIBG imaging results could improve performance of the SHFM was provided by a recent analysis of data from a small HF trial in the pre-beta-blocker era (Kuramoto et al. 2011). A larger analysis of SHFM in conjunction with the ADMIRE-HF dataset demonstrated improvement in multiple indices of predictive accuracy for all-cause mortality, including receiver operating characteristic (ROC) curve area under the curve (AUC) and net reclassification improvement (NRI) (Ketchum et al. 2012). The observed 2-year mortality in the highest-risk SHFM subjects (rounded SHFM score of 1) was 24 %, but varied from 46 % with H/M <1.2 to 0 % with H/M ≥ 1.80. NRI was 22.7 % ($p<0.001$), with 14.9 % of subjects who died reclassified into a higher-risk category than suggested by SHFM score alone ($p=0.01$) and 7.9 % of subjects who survived reclassified into a lower-risk category ($p<0.0001$). The 1-year ROC curve AUC showed significant improvement for the combined model with H/M compared to the SHFM alone (+0.04, $p=0.026$).

13.4 Limitations of [^{123}I]-MIBG SPECT for Cardiac Neuronal Evaluation

As noted earlier, an important element of the evaluation of cardiac sympathetic neuronal function with [^{123}I]-MIBG is quantitation of uptake of the radiopharmaceutical. However, the known limitations associated with quantitative analyses of imaging with SPECT agents must be acknowledged. Unlike PET imaging, whose characteristics tend to be suitable for quantitative analysis, imaging with conventional single-photon tracers requires a number of corrections, such as for scatter and attenuation, in order to produce numerical values that approximate the in vitro distribution of these agents. Such corrections have not been routinely used in most studies involving [^{123}I]-MIBG. In addition, the complexity of the photon emissions from [^{123}I], including both high-energy (>500 kev) gamma photons and low-energy (<30 keV) characteristic x-rays, requires use of additional corrections to account for image degradation due to collimator septal penetration and errors in measurements of administered activity in nuclear medicine dose calibrators. Several of these issues are discussed further in this section.

While the most common quantitative measurement used in [^{123}I]-MIBG imaging is the H/M, the values of this parameter, whether determined from planar or SPECT images, represent relative rather than absolute estimators. Whereas the normal value of the H/M on planar images acquired using a low-energy high-resolution (LEHR) collimator is in the range of 2–2.5, phantom experiments have demonstrated that the absolute concentration ratio which yields this range is on the order of eight to ten times higher (Chen et al. 2006). Uncorrected SPECT images provide H/M values somewhat closer to reality (normal range 3.5–5), but only with scatter, attenuation, and septal penetration corrections do SPECT H/M ratios approach the actual values associated with the measurements (Chen et al. 2006). While medium-energy collimators result in H/M values about 10–20 % higher than LEHR collimators, the magnitude of this difference is small compared to the effect achieved by the various SPECT correction techniques (Inoue et al. 2003; Fletcher et al. 2010). In this regard, reasonable quantitation of [^{123}I]-MIBG SPECT images requires similarly sophisticated correction techniques as are routinely employed in analysis of PET images.

Accurate determination of the amount of [^{123}I]-MIBG activity administered to a patient is required both to insure adequate image counts and limit radiation dose to the minimum required to produce diagnostic images. Nuclear medicine dose calibrators are typically adjusted for a single conversion factor (ionization current to activity) for [^{123}I], and this factor can be as much as 20–30 % low or high depending upon the container in which the radiopharmaceutical is measured (Jacobson et al. 2011). This range reflects the effect of variable penetration of low-energy characteristic x-rays on the photon flux detected by the dose calibrator ionization chamber. While determining the appropriate correction factor for a syringe or vial is not difficult, it is nevertheless important as a routine quality control activity for a nuclear medicine laboratory that performs [^{123}I]-MIBG imaging.

On the most basic level, the greatest challenge for performing [^{123}I]-MIBG SPECT imaging in HF patients is the low level of specific myocardial uptake present in significant numbers of such patients. Nuclear imaging is much better for detecting physiological processes with increased rather than decreased uptake, which is one reason techniques such as FDG PET and radionuclide bone imaging are highly effective. MPI SPECT and PET have been successful because there is usually high contrast between normally perfused myocardial regions and adjacent areas of ischemia and infarction. In contrast, the normal myocardium demonstrates a lower level of [^{123}I]-MIBG than MPI tracer uptake, and uptake of the former tends to be reduced more in non-infarcted regions, regardless of whether the patient has HF of ischemic or nonischemic etiology. These phenomena produce images with relatively low target-to-background ratios which can be difficult to interpret. Additional complexity in interpretation results from persistent high liver activity (particularly problematic for the inferior wall) and frequent presence of significant lung activity (affecting visualization of anterior and lateral walls). These various SPECT challenges have contributed to the use of global [^{123}I]-MIBG uptake determinations in most studies, as these are less affected by the various confounding factors. Nevertheless, there remains potential for significant improvement in SPECT imaging through the use of iterative reconstruction techniques and the various correction procedures described earlier (Chen et al. 2012). Image fusion with MPI SPECT also holds promise as a means to provide more accurate quantitation of regional [^{123}I]-MIBG defects. As all aspects of SPECT imaging (equipment and software) continue to improve, the clinical value of [^{123}I]-MIBG SPECT imaging will also become greater.

13.5 Future Directions

In the USA, HF is one of the most common reasons for medical care visits, responsible for more than one million hospitalizations and more than 3.4 million doctors' office visits (Rosamond et al. 2008). The annual cost ($39 billion) and human consequences of HF (mentioned on >277,000 death certificates and as the underlying cause of >56,000 of those deaths (Lloyd-Jones et al. 2010; Roger et al. 2012)) are substantial. In spite of many recent advances in treatments for HF and resultant improvements in clinical outcome, many patients still do not respond adequately to medical therapy as recommended in professional society guidelines (Hunt et al. 2009). Such patients now often receive implanted devices for additional therapy, despite the fact that the majority of patients who receive ICDs for primary prevention of SCD never experience an appropriate device discharge (Ezekowitz et al. 2003) and a significant minority who receive biventricular pacemakers for CRT do not improve (Birnie and Tang 2006).

Effectiveness of treatments, procedures, and devices in HF patients has been established among groups participating in prospective clinical trials (Hunt et al. 2009). However, determining whether an individual patient will benefit from a particular therapeutic strategy requires an understanding of his/her prognosis, particularly with regard to risk of near-term mortality. Although physicians employ both professional society guidelines and their own clinical judgment in providing treatment for their HF patients, they often do not obtain quantitative estimates of mortality risk as a further guide to management decisions. Individualized assessment of risk (e.g., estimated 1- and 2-year mortality), and in some instances specific subcategorization of that risk (e.g., relative risk for death from pump failure vs. ventricular arrhythmias), would be important in assuring that patients receive the best and most appropriate therapies for their specific circumstances.

In current clinical practice, HF patients who require reevaluation of their condition typically undergo a battery of laboratory and imaging tests. However, none of these provide an indication of the status of cardiac sympathetic neurons. Important decisions on use of potentially lifesaving treatments, such as ICDs or biventricular pacemakers for CRT, are often based on measurements such as left ventricular ejection fraction (LVEF) from echocardiography and QRS duration from 12-lead electrocardiogram (ECG), which define populations that may benefit from such treatments but not specific characteristics of individual patients (Tung et al. 2008; Buxton 2009). For example, if clinical trials of patients with LVEF of 30–35 % showed that treatment A had a 40 % response rate that was significantly better than the 20 % response rate for treatment B, treatment A might be recommended for all such patients even though 60 % would not benefit from receiving it. There is a need to introduce more specific individualized quantitative risk assessment procedures for HF patient evaluation, particularly for patients judged to be at intermediate risk by the physicians who must make decisions that could involve significant risk and/or high costs. [^{123}I]-MIBG imaging for quantitation of sympathetic neuronal integrity can be used alone or in combination with a validated clinical risk model to provide physicians with valuable new information on mortality risk.

The combination of [^{123}I]-MIBG imaging and clinical risk models can provide a reliable estimate of a patient's mortality risk, which would be of particular importance for determining whether an apparently intermediate-risk patient (such as a patient with NYHA class II or III HF and moderate LV dysfunction (LVEF 30–35 %)) actually has a low (e.g., 2 %) or high (e.g., 20 %) annual risk of dying. For example, a patient with average mortality risk per SHFM-D could have a three times higher or lower event likelihood with inclusion of [^{123}I]-MIBG H/M results (Ketchum et al. 2012). In clinical circumstances, availability of a reliable means to estimate where the patient falls on the continuum of risk for all-cause mortality (the most robust and unbiased end point) and cardiac mortality (the most relevant end point for etiology-specific therapies) will empower clinicians to make better quantitative assessments of benefit versus risk relative to available treatment options for HF patients.

How will assessing the functional status of myocardial sympathetic innervation provide benefit to the clinical cardiologist and his/her HF patients? By quantifying myocardial uptake of [^{123}I]-MIBG, the cardiologist will be able to determine the likelihood of patient death in the following years and take appropriate steps to incorporate this insight into a management strategy. If [^{123}I]-MIBG uptake is poor, the physician will know that the patient is at above-average risk for a fatal outcome and can consider therapeutic options accordingly. On the other hand, if cardiac uptake is preserved, the physician will be able to inform the patient of this positive outcome and maintain a stable therapeutic approach. Finally, if cardiac uptake is heterogeneous and discordant with regional myocardial perfusion, the cardiologist will be alerted to the increased risk of arrhythmic events and SCD. [^{123}I]-MIBG imaging provides clinicians with a robust quantitative tool for further stratifying intermediate-risk HF patients, thereby improving their ability to individualize their approach to such patients.

13.6 Summary

[^{123}I]-MIBG imaging provides unique information on the status of sympathetic innervation of the myocardium, a key target of most modern HF therapies, that cannot be replicated by any of the anatomical imaging procedures or biomarker assays in common use for evaluating these patients. While the anatomical information provided by echocardiography, coronary angiography, CT, and MRI can be useful in the initial diagnostic assessment and subsequent follow-up of HF patients, results of [^{123}I]-MIBG imaging provide insight into functional impairment at the cellular level which previously could not be quantified. Similarly, blood levels of BNP and NE provide indirect evidence of cardiac pathology and sympathetic nervous system hyperactivity, but neither offers an assessment of the status of sympathetic nerves in the heart.

Given that derangements of cardiac sympathetic innervation are common in HF patients and most guidelines-based HF therapies have been shown to improve the function of this system, quantitative measures of the condition of the cardiac sympathetic nervous system can provide useful supplementary information for the clinician. In the same way that assessment of myocardial perfusion supplements the information about coronary artery disease provided by angiographic procedures, assessment of myocardial sympathetic innervation adds to the information on LV function provided by echocardiography and gated SPECT myocardial perfusion imaging to provide the clinician with improved understanding of the status of symptomatic, intermediate-risk HF patients.

The results of [^{123}I]-MIBG imaging can provide benefits to both the HF patient and the cardiologist responsible for managing his/her care. Estimates of prognosis for death and morbidity such as HF hospitalization can help the cardiologist better identify his/her truly high- and low-risk patients and facilitate development of strategies best suited to meeting the individual needs of each patient. In addition, [^{123}I]-MIBG imaging provides new information about a fundamental physiologic attribute of the heart, thereby supplementing other methods (LVEF, NYHA classification, BNP, etc.) currently used by clinicians as part of routine clinical care. The ultimate beneficiary of [^{123}I]-MIBG imaging is the patient, who has a better understanding of the severity of his/her condition and is better able to judge whether the potential benefits of proposed therapeutic options are sufficient to justify any associated risks.

References

Agostini D, Belin A, Amar MH, Darlas Y, Hamon M, Grollier G, Potier JC, Bouvard G (2000) Improvement of cardiac neuronal function after carvedilol treatment in dilated cardiomyopathy: a [^{123}I]-MIBG scintigraphic study. J Nucl Med 41:845–851

Agostini D, Verberne HJ, Burchert W, Knuuti J, Povinec P, Sambuceti G, Unlu M, Estorch M, Banerjee G, Jacobson AF (2008) I-^{123}-MIBG myocardial imaging for assessment of risk for a major cardiac event in heart failure patients: insights from a retrospective European multicenter study. Eur J Nucl Med Mol Imaging 35:535–546

Arora R, Ferrick KJ, Nakata T, Kaplan RC, Rozengarten M, Latif F, Ng K, Marcano V, Heller S, Fisher JD, Travin MI (2003) I-^{123} MIBG imaging and heart rate variability analysis to predict the need for an implantable cardioverter defibrillator. J Nucl Cardiol 10:121–131

Backs J, Haunstetter A, Gerber SH, Metz J, Borst MM, Strasser RH et al (2001) The neuronal norepinephrine transporter in experimental heart failure: evidence for a posttranscriptional downregulation. J Mol Cell Cardiol 33:461–472

Bailey JJ, Berson AS, Handelsman H, Hodges M (2001) Utility of current risk stratification tests for predicting major arrhythmic events after myocardial infarction. J Am Coll Cardiol 38:1902–1911

Bax JJ, Kraft O, Buxton AE, Fjeld JG, Parizek P, Agostini D et al (2008) ^{123}I-MIBG scintigraphy to predict inducibility of ventricular arrhythmias on cardiac electrophysiology testing: a prospective multicenter pilot study. Circ Cardiovasc Imaging 1:131–140

Birnie DH, Tang AS (2006) The problem of non-response to cardiac resynchronization therapy. Curr Opin Cardiol 21:20–26

Bohm M, La Rosee K, Schwinger RH, Erdmann E (1995) Evidence for reduction of norepinephrine uptake sites in the failing human heart. J Am Coll Cardiol 25:146–153

Boogers MJ, Borleffs CJ, Henneman MM, van Bommel RJ, van Ramshorst J, Boersma E, Dibbets-Schneider P, Stokkel MP, van der Wall EE, Schalij MJ, Bax JJ (2010) Cardiac sympathetic denervation assessed with ^{123}-iodine metaiodobenzylguanidine imaging predicts ventricular arrhythmias in implantable cardioverter-defibrillator patients. J Am Coll Cardiol 55:2769–2777

Buxton AE (2009) Risk stratification for sudden death in patients with coronary artery disease. Heart Rhythm 6:836–847

Carrio I, Estorch M, Berna L, Lopez-Pousa J, Tabernero J, Torres G (1995) Indium-111-antimyosin and iodine-^{123}-MIBG studies in early assessment of doxorubicin cardiotoxicity. J Nucl Med 36:2044–2049

Cha YM, Oh J, Miyazaki C, Hayes DL, Rea RF, Shen WK, Asirvatham SJ, Kemp BJ, Hodge DO, Chen PS, Chareonthaitawee P (2008) Cardiac resynchronization therapy upregulates cardiac autonomic control. J Cardiovasc Electrophysiol 19:1045–1052

Chen J, Garcia EV, Galt JR, Folks RD, Carrio I (2006) Optimized acquisition and processing protocols for I-^{123} cardiac SPECT imaging. J Nucl Cardiol 13:251–260

Chen LS, Zhou S, Fishbein MC, Chen PS (2007) New perspectives on the role of autonomic nervous system in the genesis of arrhythmias. J Cardiovasc Electrophysiol 18:123–127

Chen J, Folks RD, Verdes L, Manatunga DN, Jacobson AF, Garcia EV (2012) Quantitative I^{123} MIBG SPECT in differentiating abnormal and normal MIBG myocardial uptake. J Nucl Cardiol 19:92–99

Clements IP, Wiseman GA, Hodge DO (2012) Differences in myocardial [^{123}I]-MIBG uptake in ischemic and non-ischemic cardiomyopathy (abstr). Eur J Nucl Med Mol Imaging 39:S192

Cohn JN, Levine TB, Olivari MT, Garberg V, Lura D, Francis GS et al (1984) Plasma norepinephrine as a guide to prognosis in patients with chronic congestive heart failure. N Engl J Med 311:819–823

Dae MW, De Marco T, Botvinick EH, O'Connell JW, Hattner RS, Huberty JP, Yuen-Green MS (1992) Scintigraphic assessment of MIBG uptake in globally denervated human and canine hearts–implications for clinical studies. J Nucl Med 33:1444–1450

Dae MW, O'Connell JW, Botvinick EH, Chin MC (1995) Acute and chronic effects of transient myocardial ischemia on sympathetic nerve activity, density, and norepinephrine content. Cardiovasc Res 30:270–280

DeGrado TR, Zalutsky MR, Vaidyanathan G (1995) Uptake mechanisms of meta-[^{123}I]iodobenzylguanidine in isolated rat heart. Nucl Med Biol 22:1–12

Drakos SG, Athanasoulis T, Malliaras KG, Terrovitis JV, Diakos N, Koudoumas D, Ntalianis AS, Theodoropoulos SP, Yacoub MH, Nanas JN (2010) Myocardial sympathetic innervation and long-term left ventricular mechanical unloading. JACC Cardiovasc Imaging 3:64–70

Ebina T, Takahashi N, Mitani I, Sumita S, Ishigami T, Ashino K, Minamisawa K, Kuji N, Ochiai H, Ishikawa Y, Oka T, Inoue T, Matsubara S, Umemura S (2002) Clinical implications of cardiac (^{123})I-meta-iodobenzylguanidine scintigraphy and cardiac natriuretic peptides in patients with heart disease. Nucl Med Commun 23:795–801

Ekelund S, Nygren P, Larsson R (2001) Guanidino-containing drugs in cancer chemotherapy: biochemical and clinical pharmacology. Biochem Pharmacol 61:1183–1193

Estorch M, Camprecios M, Flotats A, Mari C, Berna L, Catafau AM, Ballester M, Narula J, Carrio I (1999) Sympathetic reinnervation of cardiac allografts evaluated by [^{123}I]-MIBG imaging. J Nucl Med 40:911–916

Ezekowitz JA, Armstrong PW, McAlister FA (2003) Implantable cardioverter defibrillators in primary and secondary prevention: a systematic review of randomized, control trials. Ann Intern Med 138:445–452

Fletcher AM, Motherwell DW, Small AD, McCurrach GM, Goodfield NE, Petrie MC, Martin W, Cobbe SM (2010) I-^{123} MIBG cardiac uptake measurements: limitations of collimator choice and scatter correction in the clinical context. Nucl Med Commun 31:629–636

Flotats A, Carrio I, Agostini D, Le Guludec D, Marcassa C, Schaffers M, Somsen GA, Unlu M, Verberne HJ (2010) Proposal for standardization of (^{123})I-metaiodobenzylguanidine (MIBG) cardiac sympathetic imaging by the EANM Cardiovascular Committee and the European Council of Nuclear Cardiology. Eur J Nucl Med Mol Imaging 37:1802–1812

Gaze MN, Huxham IM, Mairs RJ, Barrett A (1991) Intracellular localisation of metaiodobenzyl guanidine in human neuroblastoma cells by electron spectroscopic imaging. Int J Cancer 47:875–880

Gehl AK, Stein RH, Metz LD, Gomes A (2005) Microvolt t-wave alternans for the risk stratification of ventricular tachyarrhythmic events. J Am Coll Cardiol 46:75–82

Hunt SA, Abraham WT, Chin MH et al (2009) Focused update incorporated into the ACC/AHA 2005 guidelines for the diagnosis and management of heart failure in adults. Circulation 119:e391–e479

Inoue H, Zipes DP (1987) Results of sympathetic denervation in the canine heart: supersensitivity that may be arrhythmogenic. Circulation 75:877–887

Inoue Y, Suzuki A, Shirouzu I, Machida T, Yoshizawa Y, Akita F, Ohnishi S, Yoshikawa K, Ohtomo K (2003) Effect of collimator choice on quantitative assessment of cardiac iodine ^{123}MIBG uptake. J Nucl Cardiol 10:623–632

Jacobson AF, Senior R, Cerqueira MD, Wong ND, Thomas GS, Lopez VA et al (2010) Myocardial iodine-^{123} meta-iodobenzylguanidine imaging and cardiac events in heart failure results of the prospective ADMIRE-HF (AdreView Myocardial Imaging for Risk Evaluation in Heart Failure) study. J Am Coll Cardiol 55:2212–2221

Jacobson AF, Centofanti R, Babalola OI, Dean B (2011) Survey of commercial dose calibrator performance for measurement of [^{123}I] activity. J Nucl Med Technol 39:302–306

Kasama S, Toyama T, Kumakura H, Takayama Y, Ichikawa S, Suzuki T, Kurabayashi M (2002) Spironolactone improves cardiac sympathetic nerve activity and symptoms in patients with congestive heart failure. J Nucl Med 43:1279–1285

Kasama S, Toyama T, Kumakura H, Takayama Y, Ichikawa S, Suzuki T, Kurabayashi M (2003) Addition of valsartan to an angiotensin-converting enzyme inhibitor improves cardiac sympathetic nerve activity and left ventricular function in patients with congestive heart failure. J Nucl Med 44:884–890

Kasama S, Toyama T, Kumakura H, Takayama Y, Ichikawa S, Suzuki T, Kurabayashi M (2005a) Effects of perindopril on cardiac sympathetic nerve activity in patients with congestive heart failure: comparison with enalapril. Eur J Nucl Med Mol Imaging 32:964–971

Kasama S, Toyama T, Kumakura H, Takayama Y, Ichikawa S, Suzuki T, Kurabayashi M (2005b) Effects of candesartan on cardiac sympathetic nerve activity in patients with congestive heart failure and preserved left ventricular ejection fraction. J Am Coll Cardiol 45:661–667

Kasama S, Toyama T, Kaneko Y, Iwasaki T, Sumino H, Kumakura H, Minami K, Ichikawa S, Matsumoto N, Sato Y, Kurabayashi M (2012) Relationship between late ventricular potentials and myocardial [123I]-metaiodobenzylguanidine scintigraphy in patients with dilated cardiomyopathy with mild to moderate heart failure: results of a prospective study of sudden death events. Eur J Nucl Med Mol Imaging 39:1056–1064

Ketchum ES, Jacobson AF, Caldwell JH, Senior R, Cerqueira MD, Thomas GS, Agostini D, Narula J, Levy WC (2012) Selective improvement in Seattle heart failure model risk stratification using iodine-123 meta-iodobenzylguanidine imaging. J Nucl Cardiol 19:1007–1016

Kioka H, Yamada T, Mine T, Morita T, Tsukamoto Y, Tamaki S, Masuda M, Okuda K, Hori M, Fukunami M (2007) Prediction of sudden death by using cardiac Iodine-123 Metaiodobenzylguanidine imaging in patients with mild to moderate chronic heart failure. Heart 93:1213–1218

Kline RC, Swanson DP, Wieland DM, Thrall JH, Gross MD, Pitt B, Beierwaltes WH (1981) Myocardial imaging in man with I-123 meta-iodobenzylguanidine. J Nucl Med 22:129–132

Koutelou M, Katsikis A, Flevari P, Theodorakis G, Livanis E, Georgiadis M, Voudris V, Kremastinos D (2009) Predictive value of cardiac autonomic indexes and MIBG washout in ICD recipients with mild to moderate heart failure. Ann Nucl Med 23:677–684

Kuramoto Y, Yamada T, Tamaki S, Okuyama Y, Morita T, Furukawa Y (2011) Usefulness of cardiac iodine-123 meta-iodobenzylguanidine imaging to improve prognostic power of Seattle heart failure model in patients with chronic heart failure. Am J Cardiol 107:1185–1190

Kuwabara Y, Tamaki N, Nakata T, Yamashina S, Yamazaki J (2011) Determination of the survival rate in patients with congestive heart failure stratified by [123I]-MIBG imaging: a meta-analysis from the studies performed in Japan. Ann Nucl Med 25:101–107

Kyuma M, Nakata T, Hashimoto A, Nagao K, Sasao H, Takahashi T, Tsuchihashi K, Shimamoto K (2004) Incremental prognostic implications of brain natriuretic peptide, cardiac sympathetic nerve innervation, and noncardiac disorders in patients with heart failure. J Nucl Med 45:155–163

Leimbach WN Jr, Wallin BG, Victor RG, Aylward PE, Sundlof G, Mark AL (1986) Direct evidence from intraneural recordings for increased central sympathetic outflow in patients with heart failure. Circulation 73:913–919

Levy WC, Mozaffarian D, Linker DT, Sutradhar SC, Anker SD, Cropp AB et al (2006) The Seattle heart failure model: prediction of survival in heart failure. Circulation 113:1424–1433

Liang CS, Fan TH, Sullebarger JT, Sakamoto S (1989) Decreased adrenergic neuronal uptake activity in experimental right heart failure. A chamber-specific contributor to beta-adrenoceptor downregulation. J Clin Invest 84:1267–1275

Lloyd-Jones D, Adams RJ, Brown TM et al (2010) Heart disease and stroke statistics – 2010 update. A report from the American Heart Association Statistics Committee and Stroke Statistics Subcommittee. Circulation 121:e1–e170

Maeno M, Ishida Y, Shimonagata T, Hayashida K, Toyama T, Hirose Y, Nagata M, Miyatake K, Uehara T, Nishimura T (1993) The significance of 201Tl/[123I] MIBG (metaiodobenzylguanidine) mismatched myocardial regions for predicting ventricular tachycardia in patients with idiopathic dilated cardiomyopathy. Kaku Igaku 30:1221–1229

Mangner TJ, Tobes MC, Wieland DW, Sisson JC, Shapiro B (1986) Metabolism of iodine-131 metaiodobenzylguanidine in patients with metastatic phaeochromocytoma. J Nucl Med 27:37–44

Matsui T, Tsutamoto T, Maeda K, Kusukawa J, Kinoshita M (2002) Prognostic value of repeated [123I]-metaiodobenzylguanidine imaging in patients with dilated cardiomyopathy with congestive heart failure before and after optimized treatments–comparison with neurohumoral factors. Circ J 66:537–543

Mcghie AI, Corbett JR, Akers MS, Kulkarni P, Sills MN, Kremers M, Buja LM, Durant-Reville M, Parkey RW, Willerson JT (1991) Regional cardiac adrenergic function using I-[123] meta-iodobenzylguanidine tomographic imaging after acute myocardial infarction. Am J Cardiol 67:236–242

Merlet P, Dubois-Rande JL, Adnot S, Bourguignon MH, Benvenuti C, Loisance D, Valette H, Castaigne A, Syrota A (1992a) Myocardial beta-adrenergic desensitization and neuronal norepinephrine uptake function in idiopathic dilated cardiomyopathy. J Cardiovasc Pharmacol 19:10–16

Merlet P, Valette H, Dubois-Rande JL, Moyse D, Duboc D, Dove P, Bourguignon MH, Benvenuti C, Duval AM, Agostini D (1992b) Prognostic value of cardiac metaiodobenzylguanidine imaging in patients with heart failure. J Nucl Med 33:471–477

Merlet P, Benvenuti C, Moyse D, Pouillart F, Dubois-Rande JL, Duval AM, Loisance D, Castaigne A, Syrota A (1999a) Prognostic value of MIBG imaging in idiopathic dilated cardiomyopathy. J Nucl Med 40:917–923

Merlet P, Pouillart F, Dubois-Rande JL, Delahaye N, Fumey R, Castaigne A, Syrota A (1999b) Sympathetic nerve alterations assessed with [^{123}I]-MIBG in the failing human heart. J Nucl Med 40:224–231

Minardo JD, Tuli MM, Mock BH, Weiner RE, Pride HP, Wellman HN, Zipes DP (1988) Scintigraphic and electrophysiological evidence of canine myocardial sympathetic denervation and reinnervation produced by myocardial infarction or phenol application. Circulation 78:1008–1019

Mitrani RD, Klein LS, Miles WM, Hackett FK, Burt RW, Wellman HN, Zipes DP (1993) Regional cardiac sympathetic denervation in patients with ventricular tachycardia in the absence of coronary artery disease. J Am Coll Cardiol 22:1344–1353

Momose M, Kobayashi H, Iguchi N, Matsuda N, Sakomura Y, Kasanuki H, Kusakabe K, Okawa T (1999) Comparison of parameters of [^{123}I]-MIBG scintigraphy for predicting prognosis in patients with dilated cardiomyopathy. Nucl Med Commun 20:529–535

Nakata T, Miyamoto K, Doi A, Sasao H, Wakabayashi T, Kobayashi H, Tsuchihashi K, Shimamoto K (1998) Cardiac death prediction and impaired cardiac sympathetic innervation assessed by MIBG in patients with failing and nonfailing hearts. J Nucl Cardiol 5:579–590

Nakata T, Wakabayashi T, Kyuma M, Takahashi T, Tsuchihashi K, Shimamoto K (2005) Cardiac metaiodobenzylguanidine activity can predict the long-term efficacy of angiotensin-converting enzyme inhibitors and/or beta-adrenoceptor blockers in patients with heart failure. Eur J Nucl Med Mol Imaging 32:186–194

Narula J, Cerqueira MD, Senior R, Travin M, Thomas GS, Clements IP, Jacobson AF (2010) [^{123}I]-MIBG myocardial scintigraphy and left ventricular ejection fraction for defining risk for ventricular arrhythmic events and death in heart failure patients: results from the ADMIRE-HF Extension (X) Trial (abstr). Presented at the American Heart Association annual meeting, Chicago

Niitsu N, Yamazaki J, Nakayama M, Umeda M, Morishita T (1995) Usefulness of [^{123}I]-MIBG myocardial SPECT in patients with hematologic malignancies with chemotherapeutic agent-induced cardiomyopathy. Gan To Kagaku Ryoho 22:1941–1945

Nishioka SA, Martinelli FM, Brandao SC, Giorgi MC, Vieira ML, Costa R, Mathias W, Meneghetti JC (2007) Cardiac sympathetic activity pre and post resynchronization therapy evaluated by [^{123}I]-MIBG myocardial scintigraphy. J Nucl Cardiol 14:852–859

Nishisato K, Hashimoto A, Nakata T, Doi T, Yamamoto H, Nagahara D, Shimoshige S, Yuda S, Tsuchihashi K, Shimamoto K (2010) Impaired cardiac sympathetic innervation and myocardial perfusion are related to lethal arrhythmia: quantification of cardiac tracers in patients with ICDs. J Nucl Med 51:1241–1249

Parthenakis FI, Prassopoulos VK, Koukouraki SI, Zacharis EA, Diakakis GF, Karkavitsas NK, Vardas PE (2002) Segmental pattern of myocardial sympathetic denervation in idiopathic dilated cardiomyopathy: relationship to regional wall motion and myocardial perfusion abnormalities. J Nucl Cardiol 9:15–22

Pina IL, Carson P, Lindenfeld J, Archambault T, Jacobson AF (2012) Is there a relationship between adequacy of medical therapy for heart failure and results of imaging of sympathetic neuronal status using I-[123] meta iodobenzylguanidine (MIBG)? (abstr). Presented at European Society of Cardiology annual meeting, Munich, Germany

Pitt B, Zannad F, Remme WJ et al (1999) The effect of spironolactone on morbidity and mortality in patients with severe heart failure. Randomized Aldactone Evaluation Study Investigators. N Engl J Med 341:709–717

Roger VL, Go AS, Lloyd-Jones DM et al (2012) American Heart Association heart disease and stroke statistics–2012 update: a report from the American Heart Association. Circulation 125:e2–e220

Rosamond W, Flegal K, Furie K et al (2008) Heart disease and stroke statistics – 2008 Update. A report from the American Heart Association Statistics Committee and Stroke Statistics Subcommittee. Circulation 117:e25–e146

Shapiro B, Wieland D, Brown LE, Nakajo M, Sisson JC, Beierwaltes WH (1984) 131-meta-iodobenzylguanidine (MIBG) adrenal medullary scintigraphy. In: Interventional nuclear medicine. Grune and Stratton, Inc, New York, pp 451–481

Simoes MV, Barthel P, Matsunari I, Nekolla SG, Schomig A, Schwaiger M, Schmidt G, Bengel FM (2004) Presence of sympathetically denervated but viable myocardium and its electrophysiologic correlates after early revascularised, acute myocardial infarction. Eur Heart J 25:551–557

Sisson JC, Wieland DM (1986) Radiolabelled meta-iodobenzylguanidine: pharmacology and clinical studies. Am J Physiol Imaging 1:96–103

Smets LA, Bout B, Wisse J (1988) Cytotoxic and antitumor effects of the norepinephrine analogue meta-iodo-benzylguanidine (MIBG). Cancer Chemother Pharmacol 21:9–13

Smets LA, Loesberg C, Janssen M, Metwally EA, Huiskamp R (1989) Active uptake and extravesicular storage of m-iodobenzylguanidine in human neuroblastoma SK-N-SH cells. Cancer Res 49:2941–2944

Stanton MS, Zipes DP (1991) Modulation of drug effects by regional sympathetic denervation and supersensitivity. Circulation 84:1709–1714

Suwa M, Otake Y, Moriguchi A, Ito T, Hirota Y, Kawamura K, Adachi I, Narabayashi I (1997) Iodine-[123] metaiodobenzylguanidine myocardial scintigraphy for prediction of response to beta-blocker therapy in patients with dilated cardiomyopathy. Am Heart J 133:353–358

Tamaki S, Yamada T, Okuyama Y, Morita T, Sanada S, Tsukamoto Y, Masuda M, Okuda K, Iwasaki Y, Yasui T, Hori M, Fukunami M (2009) Cardiac iodine-[123] metaiodobenzylguanidine imaging predicts sudden cardiac death independently of left ventricular ejection fraction in patients with chronic heart failure and left ventricular systolic dysfunction: results from a comparative study with signal-averaged electrocardiogram, heart rate variability, and QT dispersion. J Am Coll Cardiol 53:426–435

Tobes MC, Fig LM, Carey J, Geatti O, Sisson JC, Shapiro B (1989) Alterations of iodine-131 MIBG biodistribution in an anephric patient: comparison to normal and impaired renal function. J Nucl Med 30:1476–1482

Tsukamoto T, Morita K, Naya M, Inubushi M, Katoh C, Nishijima K, Kuge Y, Okamoto H, Tsutsui H, Tamaki N (2007) Decreased myocardial beta-adrenergic receptor density in relation to increased sympathetic tone in patients with nonischemic cardiomyopathy. J Nucl Med 48:1777–1782

Tung R, Zimetbaum P, Josephson MB (2008) A critical appraisal of implantable cardioverter-defibrillator therapy for the prevention of sudden cardiac death. J Am Coll Cardiol 52:1111–1121

Ungerer M, Hartmann F, Karoglan M, Chlistalla A, Ziegler S, Richardt G, Overbeck M, Meisner H, Schomig A, Schwaiger M (1998) Regional in vivo and in vitro characterisation of autonomic innervation in cardiomyopathic human heart. Circulation 97:174–180

Valdes Olmos RA, Bokkel Huinink WW, ten Hoeve RF, van Tinteren H, Bruning PF, van Vlies B, Hoefnagel CA (1995) Assessment of anthracycline-related myocardial adrenergic derangement by [^{123}I]-metaiodobenzylguanidine scintigraphy. Eur J Cancer 31:26–31

Verberne HJ, Brewster LM, Somsen GA, Eck-Smit BL (2008) Prognostic value of myocardial [^{123}I]-metaiodobenzylguanidine (MIBG) parameters in patients with heart failure: a systematic review. Eur Heart J 29:1147–1159

Wakabayashi T, Nakata T, Hashimoto A, Yuda S, Tsuchihashi K, Travin MI, Shimamoto K (2001) Assessment of underlying etiology and cardiac sympathetic innervation to identify patients at high risk of cardiac death. J Nucl Med 42:1757–1767

Wieland DM, Brown LE, Rogers WL et al (1981) Myocardial imaging with a radioiodinated norepinephrine storage analog. J Nucl Med 22:22–31

Yamada T, Shimonagata T, Fukunami M et al (2003) Comparison of the prognostic value of cardiac iodine-^{123} MIBG imaging and heart rate variability in patients with chronic heart failure: a prospective study. J Am Coll Cardiol 41:231–238

Yap KS, Gould P, Kalff V, Kaye DM, Esmore D, Kelly MJ (2006) Evaluation of sympathetic reinnervation in heterotopic cardiac transplants by iodine-^{123}-metaiodobenzylguanidine (I-1^{23}-MIBG) imaging. J Heart Lung Transplant 25:977–980

Yukinaka M, Nomura M, Ito S, Nakaya Y (1998) Mismatch between myocardial accumulation of [^{123}I]-MIBG and 99mTc-MIBI and late ventricular potentials in patients after myocardial infarction: association with the development of ventricular arrhythmias. Am Heart J 136:859–867

Autonomic Imaging in Myocardial Ischemia

14

Ichiro Matsunari and Junichi Taki

Contents

Abstract

Autonomic nerve function plays an important role in the pathogenesis of ischemically compromised myocardium. Autonomic imaging using pre- or postsynaptic sympathetic tracers such as [^{123}I]-metaiodobenzylguanidine ([^{123}I]-MIBG) has been applied successfully to characterize ischemia-related alterations in view of cardiac autonomic function. A number of studies using [^{123}I]-MIBG and flow tracers have consistently demonstrated a larger [^{123}I]-MIBG defect than

I. Matsunari, MD, PhD (✉)
Clinical Research Department, The Medical and Pharmacological Research Center Foundation, Foundation. Wo 32, Inoyama, Hakui, Ishikawa 925-0613, Japan
e-mail: matsunari@mprcf.or.jp

J. Taki, MD, PhD
Department of Nuclear Medicine, Kanazawa University Hospital, Kanazawa, Japan

R.H.J.A. Slart et al. (eds.), *Autonomic Innervation of the Heart: Role of Molecular Imaging*, DOI 10.1007/978-3-662-45074-1_14

perfusion defect, indicating that sympathetic nerve terminals are more susceptible to ischemia than myocardial tissue. Furthermore, there is an increasing body of evidence that autonomic imaging provides important clinical information such as prognosis and therapy response in patients with coronary heart disease (CHD). Autonomic positron emission tomography (PET) imaging using pre- or postsynaptic sympathetic tracers such as [^{11}C]-metahydroxyephedrine (mHED) is particularly useful when regional assessment of sympathetic nerve function is of concern such as those encountered in CHD. However, inconsistent autonomic imaging results have been published in vasospastic angina, silent myocardial ischemia, and reinnervation after myocardial infarction. Therefore, more work needs to be done to establish its clinical role in these circumstances.

Abbreviations

CHD	Coronary heart disease
CHF	Chronic heart failure
CRT	Cardiac resynchronization therapy
EPI	Epinephrine
H/M	Heart to mediastinum
ICD	Implantable cardioverter defibrillator
LV	Left ventricle
LVEF	Left ventricular ejection fraction
mHED	Metahydroxyephedrine
MIBG	Metaiodobenzylguanidine
PET	Positron emission tomography
SCD	Sudden cardiac death
SPECT	Single photon emission computed tomography
SROC	Summary receiver operating characteristic
TMR	Transmyocardial laser revascularization

14.1 Introduction

Despite recent advances in diagnostic and therapeutic options, myocardial ischemia/infarction continues to be a major cause of mortality and morbidity in many countries (Go et al. 2013). Autonomic nerve function is known to play an important role in the pathogenesis of ischemically compromised myocardium (Zipes 1992). Therefore, efforts have been made to characterize myocardial ischemia/infarction in view of autonomic neuronal function using invasive (Eisenhofer et al. 1996) or non-invasive techniques (Lautamaki et al. 2007). Autonomic imaging using norepinephrine analogues such as [^{123}I]-metaiodobenzylguanidine ([^{123}I]-MIBG) (Wieland et al. 1981) or [^{11}C]-metahydroxyephedrine (mHED) (Schwaiger et al. 1990)/epinephrine (EPI) (Munch et al. 2000) is suitable for non-invasive assessment of presynaptic sympathetic neuronal integrity of the heart. Postsynaptic receptor function can also be measured non-invasively using positron emission tomography (PET) and postsynaptic tracers such as [^{11}C]-CGP-12177 (Delforge et al. 1991). In this chapter, we describe the state-of-the-art knowledge of autonomic imaging and its future perspectives in ischemic heart disease.

14.2 Autonomic Imaging in Myocardial Infarction

It has been well documented, both experimentally (Dae et al. 1991; Minardo et al. 1988; Nishimura et al. 1992; Sisson et al. 1990) and clinically (Fagret et al. 1989; McGhie et al. 1991), that myocardial ischemia causes sympathetic neuronal damage exceeding the area of necrosis/scar. A number of studies (Dae et al. 1995; Fagret et al. 1989; Hartikainen et al. 1994; Lekakis et al. 1994; Mantysaari et al. 1995; McGhie et al. 1991; Nakajima et al. 1995; Spinnler et al. 1993; Tomoda et al. 1994) using [^{123}I]-MIBG and flow tracers have consistently demonstrated a larger [^{123}I]-MIBG defect than perfusion defect since the introduction of this tracer. A representative case example showing a larger [^{123}I]-MIBG defect than perfusion is illustrated in Fig. 14.1. By contrast, none of the published studies have shown a smaller [^{123}I]-MIBG defect than perfusion defect. Figure 14.2 displays polar maps of myocardial area at risk, infarct size, and [^{123}I]-MIBG images

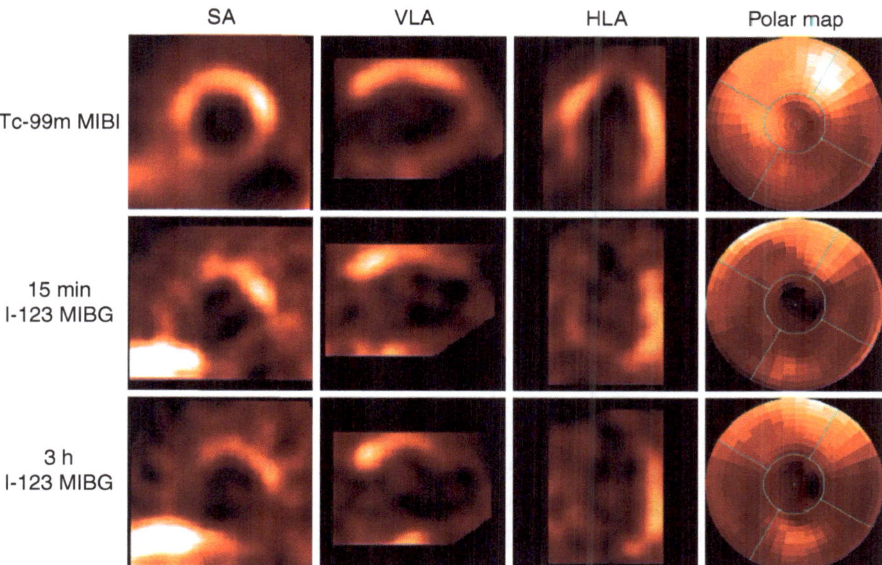

Fig. 14.1 [^{99m}Tc]-MIBI (upper) and 15 min (*middle*) and 3 h (*lower*) [^{123}I]-MIBG SPECT images and polar maps from a patient with inferior myocardial infarction. Both 15 min and 3 h [^{123}I]-MIBG images show a larger inferior defect than [^{99m}Tc]-MIBI perfusion images. *SA* indicates short axis, *VLA* vertical long axis, *HLA* horizontal long axis

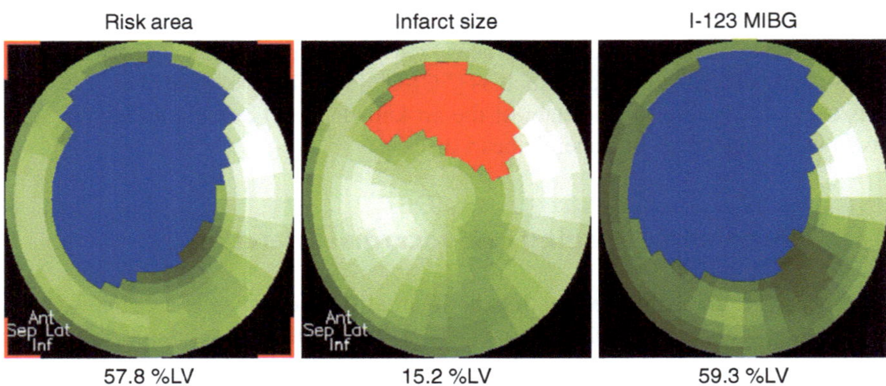

Fig. 14.2 Polar maps of myocardium at risk (*left*) and infarct size (*center*) and [^{123}I]-MIBG (*right*) images from a patient with anterior myocardial infarction. Quantified defect areas on each polar map are filled with *blue* or *red color*, and measured defect sizes are expressed as the percentage of left ventricular myocardium (%LV)

from a patient with anterior myocardial infarction. The area at risk image shows a large defect that involves the anterior to septal wall. After reperfusion, defect size remarkably decreased, from 57.8 to 15.2 % of left ventricular myocardium. The [^{123}I]-MIBG defect, on the other hand, was similar to the area at risk in both size and location. As such, the extent of sympathetic neuronal damage is determined by the area of ischemia in patients with acute coronary syndromes (Matsunari et al. 2000). These observations indicate that sympathetic nerve terminals are more susceptible to ischemia than myocardial tissue. Such dysinnervated but viable myocardium may be linked to the pathogenesis of lethal ventricular arrhythmias (Zipes 1992).

Using PET and [^{11}C]-mHED as a tracer for cardiac sympathetic presynaptic function, Allman et al. have demonstrated a more extensive area of [^{11}C]-mHED abnormalities than that of blood flow, which is essentially similar to the observations reported using [^{123}I]-MIBG single photon emission computed tomography (SPECT) (Allman et al. 1993). Although [^{11}C]-mHED PET is technically more demanding, including the necessity for on-site cyclotron, it consistently yields better quality images and appears to be more suitable for assessing regional abnormalities than [^{123}I]-MIBG SPECT as typically illustrated in Fig. 14.3 (Matsunari et al. 2010). Furthermore, although there is a close correlation between [^{123}I]-MIBG heart-to-mediastinum (H/M) uptake ratio and [^{11}C]-mHED retention (Matsunari et al. 2010), PET imaging using presynaptic sympathetic tracers such as [^{11}C]-mHED or [^{11}C]-epinephrine provides the possibility of absolute quantification of cardiac sympathetic innervation on regional basis by routine use of attenuation/scatter correction. This feature may become important when regional, rather than global, cardiac sympathetic innervation is of concern (Sasano et al. 2008). However, clinical experience with PET autonomic imaging is still limited, and therefore more work needs to be done to determine its clinical role in assessing myocardial infarction.

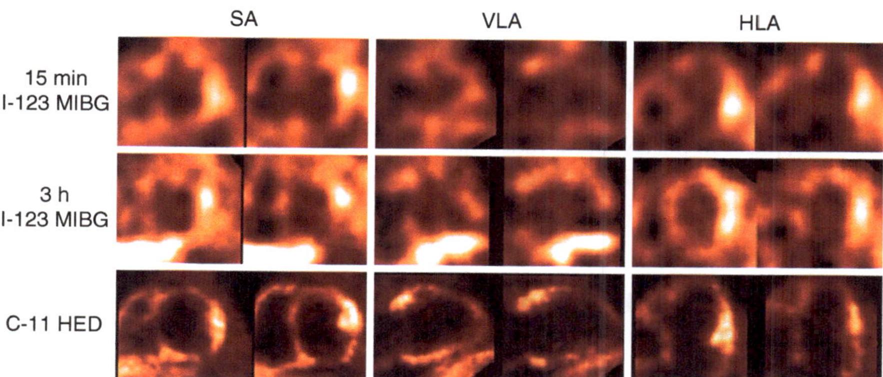

Fig. 14.3 [^{123}I]-MIBG SPECT (*upper and middle*) and [^{11}C]-mHED PET (*lower*) images from a male patient with anterior and inferior myocardial infarction. The quality of 15 min and 3 h [^{123}I]-MIBG SPECT and [^{11}C]-mHED PET images was judged as fair, poor, and good, respectively. In particular, the low myocardial tracer uptake and intense adjacent liver activity on the late [^{123}I]-MIBG SPECT degrade the image quality. *SA* indicates short axis, *VLA* vertical long axis, *HLA* horizontal long axis

14.3 Autonomic Imaging in Remote Myocardium in Patients After Myocardial Infarction

After myocardial infarction, the left ventricular remodeling involves not only the infarcted but also non-infarcted myocardium. From a therapeutic viewpoint, attenuation of remodeling process is expected to result in reduced morbidity and better prognosis (Pfeffer and Braunwald 1991). Therefore, characterization of such non-infarcted myocardium is important as a target of medical treatments. To date, however, there is only limited data available in literature that focused on remote myocardium after myocardial infarction. A planar [^{123}I]-MIBG imaging study in patients after acute myocardial infarction has demonstrated a faster myocardial [^{123}I]-MIBG washout involving remote myocardium as compared with normal subjects, indicating increased sympathetic nerve tone (Bengel et al. 1999). Spyrou et al. performed PET imaging using [^{11}C]-CGP-12177, a β-adrenergic receptor ligand, in patients soon after myocardial infarction and found that β-adrenergic receptor density was decreased in both infarcted and remote myocardia (Spyrou et al. 2002). They also found that the degree of β-adrenergic receptor density reduction was correlated with later left ventricular dilation. The downregulation of postsynaptic β-adrenergic density in remote myocardium was also confirmed in a PET study by Ohte et al. (2012). In a study using [^{123}I]-MIBG SPECT by Sakata et al., patients with left ventricle (LV) dilatation had more severe [^{123}I]-MIBG abnormality than those without left ventricular dilatation, suggesting the contribution of cardiac sympathetic neuronal function in left ventricular remodeling (Sakata et al. 2000). However, sympathetic innervation in non-infarcted myocardium could not be assessed in that study, because absolute quantification of tracer uptake was not possible with [^{123}I]-MIBG imaging due to non-quantitative nature of SPECT, which usually relies on relative rather than absolute uptake values. Caldwell et al. performed PET imaging using [^{11}C]-mHED and [^{11}C]-CGP-12177 in patients with ischemic heart failure and found decreased presynaptic function combined with a small decrease in postsynaptic function (mismatch) in non-infarcted myocardium (Caldwell et al. 2008). Thus, autonomic dysfunction in non-infarcted myocardium may play a role in the pathogenesis of left ventricular remodeling.

14.4 Autonomic Imaging in Myocardial Ischemia Without Infarction

14.4.1 Stable Coronary Artery Disease

Although many of the studies on autonomic imaging in CHD mainly focused on patients after myocardial infarction, cardiac sympathetic nerve terminals are more sensitive to ischemia than myocardial cells as described earlier (Matsunari et al. 2000). Therefore, it is conceivable that ischemic sympathetic neuronal damage would occur even in the absence of infarction. This was confirmed by clinical studies demonstrating [^{123}I]-MIBG defects exceeding perfusion defects in patients without a history of myocardial infarction (Guertner et al. 1993; Hartikainen et al. 1997). Similar results were observed using [^{11}C]-mHED PET (Bulow et al. 2003). This concept was also supported by an experimental study by Luisi et al. using a pig model of chronic hibernation without infarction showing extensive defects in [^{11}C]-mHED uptake in the area of hibernating but viable myocardium (Luisi et al. 2005).

14.4.2 Vasospastic Angina

Vasospastic angina is a form of angina characterized by a sudden spasm of one of the coronary arteries without significant stenosis. It is known that vasospastic angina is often associated with altered autonomic nervous activity (Ricci et al. 1979). Because coronary vasospasm causes a transient ischemia in that vascular territory, such an ischemic episode may cause reduction in [^{123}I]-MIBG uptake despite preserved perfusion. The results of meta-analysis using Meta-DiSc software (Zamora et al. 2006) from seven published studies (Ha et al. 1998; Hirano et al. 2002; Inobe et al. 1997; Sakata et al. 1997; Takano et al. 1995; Taki et al. 1998; Watanabe et al. 2002a) that reported the diagnostic value of [^{123}I]-MIBG imaging are summarized in Fig. 14.4. The pooled estimates of sensitivity and specificity were 77 % (95 % confident intervals: 70–82 %) and 77 % (95 % confident intervals: 70–83 %), respectively. The area under the summary receiver operating characteristic analysis (SROC) curve and its Q*-point were 89 ± 5% and 82 ± 5 %, respectively. However, both sensitivities and specificities had significant heterogeneity ($P < 0.0001$ for both), as is evident from the wide range (42–100 % for sensitivity and 40–100 % for

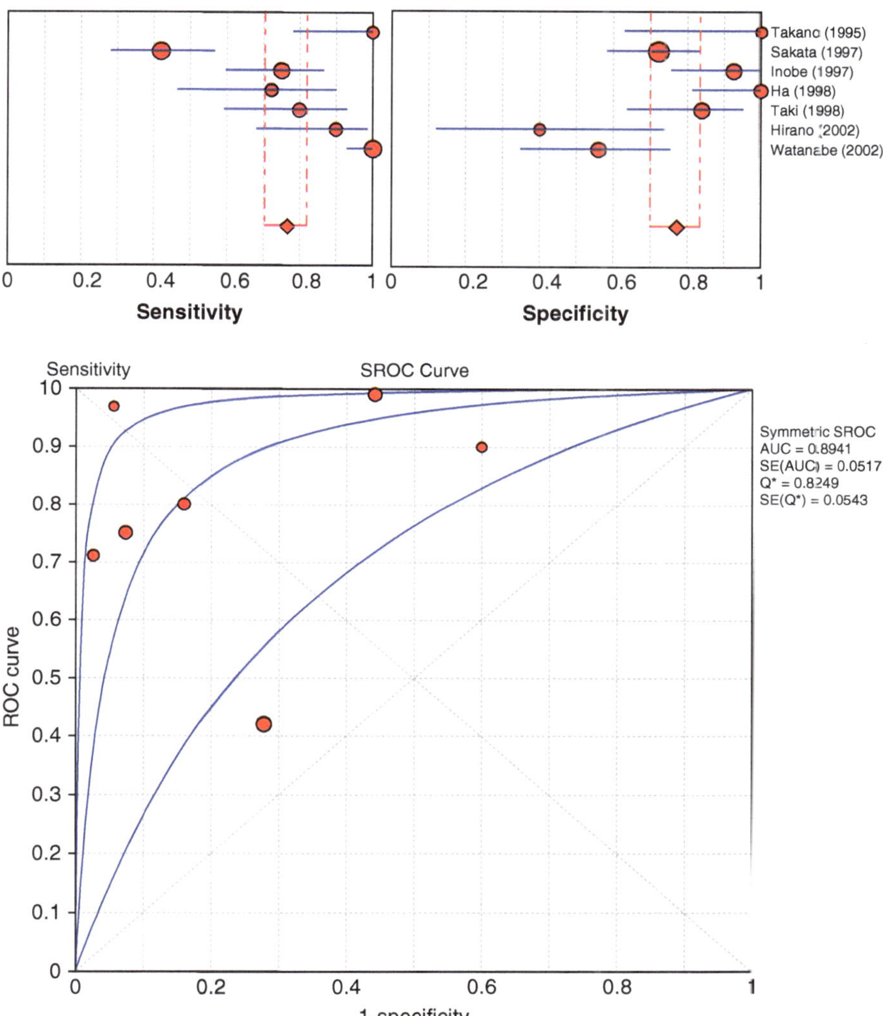

Fig. 14.4 Forrest plot of sensitivities (*upper left*) and specificities (*upper right*) from published [^{123}I]-MIBG studies in the diagnostic performance of vasospastic angina on patient basis and summary receiver operating characteristic (*SROC*) curve (*lower*). Each *red circle* represents individual study in meta-analysis, with size of circle proportional to sample size of study. *Red diamond denotes* an estimate of pooled values with 95 % confidence intervals (CI) in *red line*. *Blue lines* in the forest plots represent 95 % CI of each study. Best-fit curve (*middle curve*) in the SROC curve lies between two curves that demarcate its 95 % CI

specificity) and the high inconsistency index (90.8 % for sensitivity and 80.8 % for specificity). The heterogeneity in diagnostic performance is also evident from the wide 95 % confidence intervals in SROC curves. In a study by Sakata et al., the use of lower [^{123}I]-MIBG washout rate rather than reduced [^{123}I]-MIBG uptake as a marker of vasospastic angina significantly improved sensitivity and specificity from 42 to 76 % and 72 to 87 %, respectively, indicating that cardiac sympathetic nerve activity in vasospastic angina is suppressed probably because of the enhanced parasympathetic nerve activity (Sakata et al. 1997). Furthermore, a subsequent study from the same authors has demonstrated that high H/M ratio or lower washout rate was a marker of future cardiac events (Sakata et al. 2005). By contrast, Inobe et al. have demonstrated that the patients with higher disease activity were frequently associated with either the uptake reduction or the abnormally high washout of [^{123}I]-MIBG (Inobe et al. 1997). Although these inconsistent published results could be explained in part by different patient characteristics such as disease severity and duration and by different methodologies among the studies (Ha et al. 1998; Hirano et al. 2002; Inobe et al. 1997; Sakata et al. 1997; Takano et al. 1995; Taki et al. 1998; Watanabe et al. 2002a), the exact underlying mechanisms are still unclear. Thus, the clinical use of autonomic imaging in vasospastic angina remains to be established by further work.

14.4.3 Silent Myocardial Ischemia

Silent myocardial ischemia is defined as evidence for ischemia without symptoms such as chest pain (Gutterman 2009). It is important to note that patients with silent myocardial ischemia often have a poor prognosis as compared with those with painful ischemia. Therefore, early detection and monitoring of patients with silent myocardial ischemia before hard cardiac events is clinically relevant. Although the exact mechanism is yet to be determined, impairment in cardiac sympathetic innervation is likely to be linked with the occurrence of silent myocardial ischemia. In this regard, autonomic imaging may play a role for characterization of silent ischemia. However, published results focusing on this topic using [^{123}I]-MIBG imaging are inconclusive so far. In a study by Shakespeare et al. using delayed (4 h) [^{123}I]-MIBG SPECT, no evidence of denervation was observed in silent ischemia (Shakespeare et al. 1993). Hartikainen et al. found that the patients with silent ischemia revealed smaller areas of viable but denervated myocardium than those with chest pain (Hartikainen et al. 1994). Studies by other groups (Langer et al. 1995; Matsuo et al. 1996; Shimonagata et al. 1995), however, have suggested a link between silent ischemia and abnormalities on [^{123}I]-MIBG SPECT. A study by Langer et al. have demonstrated that diabetic patients with silent myocardial ischemia had evidence of a diffuse abnormality in [^{123}I]-MIBG uptake (Langer et al. 1995). A subsequent study by Matsuo et al. showed decreased [^{123}I]-MIBG uptake particularly in the inferior wall in patients with silent ischemia (Matsuo et al. 1996). All these studies were based on relatively small patient sample size, which may have contributed to the inconclusive results among the studies. It should also be noted that all these studies mainly relied on interpretation of [^{123}I]-MIBG SPECT images, where accurate assessment of regional abnormalities may sometimes be difficult due to poor image quality (Matsunari et al. 2010). Thus, much work still needs to be done to determine the value of autonomic imaging to characterize silent myocardial ischemia.

14.5 Reinnervation After Myocardial Infarction or Ischemia

Restoration of cardiac catecholamine uptake and storage site (i.e., reinnervation) is known to occur after heart transplantation (Schwaiger et al. 1991), where postganglionic sympathetic nerve fibers of the donor heart are interrupted, resulting in complete denervation. It is also known that reinnervation following heart transplantation is partial and not consistently observed (Bengel et al. 2001). In an experimental dog study by Minardo et al., [^{123}I]-MIBG scintigraphic images returned to normal at 14 weeks after myocardial infarction, which is consistent with the presence of reinnervation (Minardo et al. 1988). However, in a pig model of myocardial hibernation (Fallavollita et al. 2010), [^{11}C]-mHED defects persisted despite functional improvement at 4 weeks after successful percutaneous coronary intervention or pravastatin therapy, indicating the lack of plasticity of sympathetic neurons within a short term. Likewise, conflicting results have been published as to whether and when reinnervation occurs after myocardial infarction as summarized in Table 14.1. Allman et al. performed [^{11}C]-mHED PET in patients after myocardial infarction and did not observe changes in [^{11}C]-mHED defect size between 1 week and 8 months (Allman et al. 1993). By contrast, Hartikainen et al. found partial reinnervation using [^{123}I]-MIBG SPECT in peri-infarcted area during the follow-up period of 12 months (Hartikainen et al. 1996). In patients with stable coronary heart disease undergoing percutaneous coronary intervention, Guetner et al. performed [^{123}I]-MIBG SPECT before and 3–4 months after the intervention and observed partial reinnervation in 5 of 16 (31 %) patients (Guertner et al. 1993). All of these studies were based on relatively small sample sizes and were performed more than a decade ago using older-generation cameras. It is also important to note that sympathetic dysinnervation after ischemic insult can be either functional (stunning), structural (anatomical denervation), or both (Fallavollita and Canty 2010), which may affect the likelihood and time course of reinnervation. Thus, whether and how reinnervation occurs as well as its clinical implications after myocardial infarction or ischemia remain to be determined by further studies.

14.6 Clinical Applications

14.6.1 Prognostic Value

There is an increasing body of evidence that autonomic imaging using [^{123}I]-MIBG provides important prognostic information in patients with heart failure (Agostini et al. 2008; Jacobson et al. 2010; Kuwabara et al. 2011; Merlet et al. 1992; Nakata et al. 1998; Verberne et al. 2008). Patients with a reduced late H/M ratio or increased washout rate are likely to be associated with poor prognosis. Although there are only a few data available that have specifically looked at patients with coronary heart disease (Kasama et al. 2011; Wakabayashi et al. 2001), many published studies regarding prognostic value of [^{123}I]-MIBG imaging included a considerable number of ischemic heart failure patients. In a large prospective study (ADMIRE-HF) by

Table 14.1 Summary of studies on reinnervation after acute myocardial infarction

Author	Publication year	Tracer	Number of patients	Imaging time points	Reinnervation	Remarks
Allman et al.	1993	$[^{11}C]$-HED	8	1 week to 8 months	No	
Podio et al.	1995	$[^{123}I]$-MIBG	10	1 week to 30 months	No	
Hartikainen et al.	1996	$[^{123}I]$-MIBG	13	3–12 months	Yes?	Only in peri-infarcted area
Abe et al.	1997	$[^{123}I]$-MIBG	1	2 weeks to 12 months	Yes	A case report
Fallen et al.	1999	$[^{18}F]$-fluorodopamine	10	2 weeks to 6 months	Yes	
Simula et al.	2000	$[^{123}I]$-MIBG	15	1 week to 3 months	No	

Jacobson et al. involving 961 patients, for example, 61 % of total study population had ischemic heart failure (Jacobson et al. 2010). Additionally, it is known that myocardial adrenergic nerve activity measured by [^{123}I]-MIBG imaging is accelerated in proportion to severity of heart failure, independent of the underlying cause (Imamura et al. 1995). Furthermore, in a study by Kasama et al. that focused on patients with ST-segment elevation myocardial infarction, increased [^{123}I]-MIBG washout rate was a significant predictor of cardiac events, independent of left ventricular ejection fraction (LVEF) (Kasama et al. 2011). Thus, it is possible that [^{123}I]-MIBG imaging predicts prognosis in patients with ischemic heart disease as does in general heart failure population. However, it should be noted that the cutoff thresholds of H/M ratio to identify high-risk patients may not be identical between ischemic and non-ischemic heart failure, as demonstrated in a study by Wakabayashi et al. (2001).

At present, data on the prognostic value of autonomic PET imaging in CHD is still limited. Pietila et al. performed [^{11}C]-mHED PET imaging in 46 chronic heart failure (CHF) patients (72 % of total population were CHD) and found that a low [^{11}C]-mHED retention was a predictor of poor prognosis (Pietila et al. 2001). Gaemperli et al. have found that reduced myocardial β-adrenergic receptor density measured by [^{11}C]-CGP-12177 PET was associated with development of CHF during a median follow-up period of 12.7 years (Gaemperli et al. 2010). Thus, autonomic PET imaging also seems to be promising for risk stratification in CHD patients.

14.6.2 Therapy Monitoring and Prediction of Therapy Response

14.6.2.1 Medical

[^{123}I]-MIBG imaging has been used for monitoring of medical therapies such as beta-blockers in heart failure patients (Agostini et al. 2000; Gerson et al. 2002; Kasama et al. 2003; Kramer et al. 1999; Lotze et al. 2001; Nakata et al. 2005; Toyama et al. 2003, 2008; Watanabe et al. 2002b; Yamazaki et al. 2001). Likewise, it should be possible that autonomic imaging can be used to monitor medical therapies in ischemic heart failure. In patients with acute myocardial infarction, Kasama et al. (2005, 2007) have demonstrated improved [^{123}I]-MIBG defect score, H/M ratio, and washout rate after short- or long-term nicorandil therapy. [^{123}I]-MIBG imaging has also been used to predict therapy response in heart failure patients (Choi et al. 2001; Fujimoto et al. 2004; Fukuoka et al. 1997; Kakuchi et al. 1999; Suwa et al. 1997), where those with higher H/M ratio and/or lower washout rate are likely to improve after treatment. However, there is only limited data available that specifically focused on the predictive power of [^{123}I]-MIBG imaging in patients with coronary heart disease.

14.6.2.2 Cardiac Resynchronization Therapy

Cardiac resynchronization therapy (CRT) has emerged as an effective option to treat patients with drug-refractory heart failure and left ventricular desynchrony (Abraham et al. 2002; St John Sutton et al. 2003). In general heart failure population, [^{123}I]-MIBG imaging is known to be useful in monitoring CRT response (Burri et al. 2008;

Cha et al. 2008; Erol-Yilmaz et al. 2005; Higuchi et al. 2006; Shinohara et al. 2011) and in selecting patients who are likely to improve in response to CRT (Cha et al. 2011; Nishioka et al. 2007; Tanaka et al. 2012). Patients with significant response to CRT are likely to be associated with improved H/M ratio and slowed washout on [^{123}I]-MIBG imaging after therapy, whereas those with no response are with no improvement in these imaging parameters. Furthermore, patients with preserved [^{123}I]-MIBG H/M ratio and slower washout rate are likely to be associated with significant improvement in function after CRT. These concepts may also apply to the patients with ischemic heart failure. However, there are no studies that specifically looked at patients with ischemic heart failure, and therefore more work needs to be done to clarify the value of [^{123}I]-MIBG imaging in this clinical setting.

14.6.2.3 Implantable Cardioverter Defibrillators (ICDs)

Sudden cardiac death (SCD) due to lethal arrhythmia represents an important cause of mortality in patients with CHD (Deo and Albert 2012). Implantable cardioverter defibrillators (ICDs) have emerged as novel devices to prevent SCD (Mirowski et al. 1980). Generally accepted criteria for ICD therapy include severely depressed LVEF (30–40 %) in patients with coronary heart disease, history of cardiac arrest due to ventricular arrhythmias, sustained ventricular tachycardias, positive electrophysiologic testing, and the like. However, many patients who die from SCD actually have a low-risk profile and are missed for diagnosis by the current LVEF-based criteria. Thus, we still need a better strategy to identify high-risk CHD patients for SCD who are most likely to benefit from ICD therapy. In an animal model of post-infarct ventricular tachycardia, Sasano et al. have demonstrated that the degree of perfusion/innervation mismatch was significantly correlated with the earliest site of ventricular activation during ventricular tachycardia (Sasano et al. 2008). In patients after acute myocardial infarction, Simoes et al. have demonstrated a significant correlation between the extent of sympathetically denervated but viable myocardium and electrophysiological parameters characterizing repolarization and depolarization (Simoes et al. 2004). Bax et al. performed [^{123}I]-MIBG imaging and electrophysiologic testing in patients with a history of myocardial infarction and depressed LV function and found a significant relationship between late [^{123}I]-MIBG defect score and inducibility of sustained ventricular arrhythmias (Bax et al. 2008). These observations suggest that autonomic imaging may have a role to identify high-risk CHD patients for SCD. This concept was further supported by subsequent [^{123}I]-MIBG imaging studies involving patients with ICD placement, in whom detailed information on arrhythmic events is easily available (Boogers et al. 2010; Nishisato et al. 2010). Thus, although further prospective large studies are required, autonomic imaging seems to be useful to identify candidates for ICD placement in CHD.

14.6.2.4 Effects of Revascularization on Cardiac Sympathetic Innervation in Stable CHD

Although coronary revascularization is a powerful therapeutic option to treat patients with stable CHD, there are only limited data available that have focused on the effect of revascularization on cardiac sympathetic innervation. As described in earlier Sect. 14.5, inconsistent results have been published as to whether reinnervation occurs after coronary revascularization (Fallavollita et al. 2010; Guertner et al. 1993).

Transmyocardial laser revascularization (TMR) is another therapeutic option particularly for patients with severe CHD with refractory angina (Frazier et al. 1999). Although TMR alone may not necessarily improve survival rate, a combination of TMR and coronary revascularization is reportedly useful in relieving angina as compared to traditional revascularization therapy (Fihn et al. 2012). There have been several studies that investigated the effects of TMR on cardiac sympathetic innervation. Al-Sheikh et al. performed [^{11}C]-mHED PET imaging before and after TMR and found that TMR causes LV cardiac sympathetic denervation without affecting myocardial blood flow at rest or during stress, suggesting that the improvement in angina may be due to sympathetic denervation (Al-Sheikh et al. 1999). Subsequent experimental (Le et al. 2007) and clinical (Beek et al. 2004; Muxi et al. 2003; Teresinska et al. 2004) studies using [^{123}I]-MIBG have confirmed TMR-induced denervation, although one experimental study using swine model and autoradiography did not show significant reduction in [^{125}I]-MIBG uptake 3 days after the treatment (Johnson et al. 2002). Furthermore, similar to those reported for coronary revascularization, whether reinnervation occurs after TMR is still a matter of discussion (Beek et al. 2004; Muxi et al. 2003; Teresinska et al. 2004). Thus, although regional denervation after TMR is likely to be related to angina relief, clinical value of autonomic imaging in this area remains to be determined.

14.7 Conclusion and Future Perspectives

There is a general consensus that sympathetic nerve terminals are more sensitive to ischemia than myocardial tissue, as confirmed by a number of studies using [^{123}I]-MIBG. Autonomic imaging has also been applied to characterize various ischemia-related alterations in sympathetic nerves such as those encountered in non-infarcted remote myocardium, stable CHD, and vasospastic angina. Furthermore, there is an increasing body of evidence that autonomic imaging provides important clinical information such as prognosis and therapy response in CHD patients. In addition, autonomic imaging may play a role for selecting patients who are likely to benefit from CRT/ICD therapy. However, inconsistent [^{123}I]-MIBG imaging results have been published in vasospastic angina, silent myocardial ischemia, and reinnervation after myocardial infarction. Thus, there are several areas where the role of autonomic imaging in CHD remains to be established by further studies.

Autonomic PET imaging using pre- or postsynaptic sympathetic tracers such as [^{11}C]-mHED or [^{11}C]-CGP-12177 has also been applied to characterize ischemia-related alterations, which is particularly useful when regional assessment of sympathetic nerve function is of concern such as those encountered in CHD. However, its availability is still limited, resulting in limited clinical experience. New [^{18}F]-labeled tracers such as [^{18}F]-LMI1195 (Yu et al. 2011) may facilitate its wider clinical use in future.

References

Abraham WT, Fisher WG, Smith AL et al (2002) Cardiac resynchronization in chronic heart failure. N Engl J Med 346:1845–1853

Agostini D, Belin A, Amar MH et al (2000) Improvement of cardiac neuronal function after carvedilol treatment in dilated cardiomyopathy: a ^{123}I-MIBG scintigraphic study. J Nucl Med 41:845–851

Agostini D, Verberne HJ, Burchert W et al (2008) I-123-mIBG myocardial imaging for assessment of risk for a major cardiac event in heart failure patients: insights from a retrospective European multicenter study. Eur J Nucl Med Mol Imaging 35:535–546

Allman KC, Wieland DM, Muzik O et al (1993) Carbon-11 hydroxyephedrine with positron emission tomography for serial assessment of cardiac adrenergic neuronal function after acute myocardial infarction in humans. J Am Coll Cardiol 22:368–375

Al-Sheikh T, Allen KB, Straka SP et al (1999) Cardiac sympathetic denervation after transmyocardial laser revascularization. Circulation 100:135–140

Bax JJ, Kraft O, Buxton AE et al (2008) ^{123}I-mIBG scintigraphy to predict inducibility of ventricular arrhythmias on cardiac electrophysiology testing: a prospective multicenter pilot study. Circ Cardiovasc Imaging 1:131–140

Beek JF, van der Sloot JA, Huikeshoven M et al (2004) Cardiac denervation after clinical transmyocardial laser revascularization: short-term and long-term iodine 123-labeled metaiodobenzylguanide scintigraphic evidence. J Thorac Cardiovasc Surg 127:517–524

Bengel FM, Barthel P, Matsunari I et al (1999) Kinetics of ^{123}I-MIBG after acute myocardial infarction and reperfusion therapy. J Nucl Med 40:904–910

Bengel FM, Ueberfuhr P, Schiepel N et al (2001) Effect of sympathetic reinnervation on cardiac performance after heart transplantation. N Engl J Med 345:731–738

Boogers MJ, Borleffs CJ, Henneman MM et al (2010) Cardiac sympathetic denervation assessed with 123-iodine metaiodobenzylguanidine imaging predicts ventricular arrhythmias in implantable cardioverter-defibrillator patients. J Am Coll Cardiol 55:2769–2777

Bulow HP, Stahl F, Lauer B et al (2003) Alterations of myocardial presynaptic sympathetic innervation in patients with multi-vessel coronary artery disease but without history of myocardial infarction. Nucl Med Commun 24:233–239

Burri H, Sunthorn H, Somsen A et al (2008) Improvement in cardiac sympathetic nerve activity in responders to resynchronization therapy. Europace 10:374–378

Caldwell JH, Link JM, Levy WC et al (2008) Evidence for pre- to postsynaptic mismatch of the cardiac sympathetic nervous system in ischemic congestive heart failure. J Nucl Med 49:234–241

Cha YM, Oh J, Miyazaki C et al (2008) Cardiac resynchronization therapy upregulates cardiac autonomic control. J Cardiovasc Electrophysiol 19:1045–1052

Cha YM, Chareonthaitawee P, Dong YX et al (2011) Cardiac sympathetic reserve and response to cardiac resynchronization therapy. Circ Heart Fail 4:339–344

Choi JY, Lee KH, Hong KP et al (2001) Iodine-123 MIBG imaging before treatment of heart failure with carvedilol to predict improvement of left ventricular function and exercise capacity. J Nucl Cardiol 8:4–9

Dae MW, Herre JM, O'Connell JW et al (1991) Scintigraphic assessment of sympathetic innervation after transmural versus nontransmural myocardial infarction. J Am Coll Cardiol 17:1416–1423

Dae MW, O'Connell JW, Botvinick EH et al (1995) Acute and chronic effects of transient myocardial ischemia on sympathetic nerve activity, density, and norepinephrine content. Cardiovasc Res 30:270–280

Delforge J, Syrota A, Lancon JP et al (1991) Cardiac beta-adrenergic receptor density measured in vivo using PET, CGP 12177, and a new graphical method. J Nucl Med 32:739–748

Deo R, Albert CM (2012) Epidemiology and genetics of sudden cardiac death. Circulation 125:620–637

Eisenhofer G, Friberg P, Rundqvist B et al (1996) Cardiac sympathetic nerve function in congestive heart failure. Circulation 93:1667–1676

Erol-Yilmaz A, Verberne HJ, Schrama TA et al (2005) Cardiac resynchronization induces favorable neurohumoral changes. Pacing Clin Electrophysiol 28:304–310

Fagret D, Wolf JE, Comet M (1989) Myocardial uptake of meta-[123I]-iodobenzylguanidine [(123I]-MIBG) in patients with myocardial infarct. Eur J Nucl Med 15:624–628

Fallavollita JA, Canty JM Jr (2010) Dysinnervated but viable myocardium in ischemic heart disease. J Nucl Cardiol 17:1107–1115

Fallavollita JA, Banas MD, Suzuki G et al (2010) ^{11}C-meta-hydroxyephedrine defects persist despite functional improvement in hibernating myocardium. J Nucl Cardiol 17:85–96

Fihn SD, Gardin JM, Abrams J et al (2012) 2012 ACCF/AHA/ACP/AATS/PCNA/SCAI/STS guideline for the diagnosis and management of patients with stable ischemic heart disease: a report of the American College of Cardiology Foundation/American Heart Association task force on practice guidelines, and the American College of Physicians, American Association for Thoracic Surgery, Preventive Cardiovascular Nurses Association, Society for Cardiovascular Angiography and Interventions, and Society of Thoracic Surgeons. Circulation 126:e354–e471

Frazier OH, March RJ, Horvath KA (1999) Transmyocardial revascularization with a carbon dioxide laser in patients with end-stage coronary artery disease. N Engl J Med 341:1021–1028

Fujimoto S, Inoue A, Hisatake S et al (2004) Usefulness of ^{123}I-metaiodobenzylguanidine myocardial scintigraphy for predicting the effectiveness of beta-blockers in patients with dilated cardiomyopathy from the standpoint of long-term prognosis. Eur J Nucl Med Mol Imaging 31:1356–1361

Fukuoka S, Hayashida K, Hirose Y et al (1997) Use of iodine-123 metaiodobenzylguanidine myocardial imaging to predict the effectiveness of beta-blocker therapy in patients with dilated cardiomyopathy. Eur J Nucl Med 24:523–529

Gaemperli O, Liga R, Spyrou N et al (2010) Myocardial beta-adrenoceptor down-regulation early after infarction is associated with long-term incidence of congestive heart failure. Eur Heart J 31:1722–1729

Gerson MC, Craft LL, McGuire N et al (2002) Carvedilol improves left ventricular function in heart failure patients with idiopathic dilated cardiomyopathy and a wide range of sympathetic nervous system function as measured by iodine 123 metaiodobenzylguanidine. J Nucl Cardiol 9:608–615

Go AS, Mozaffarian D, Roger VL et al (2013) Heart disease and stroke statistics–2013 update: a report from the American Heart Association. Circulation 127:e6–e245

Guertner C, Klepzig H Jr, Maul FD et al (1993) Noradrenaline depletion in patients with coronary artery disease before and after percutaneous transluminal coronary angioplasty with iodine-123 metaiodobenzylguanidine and single-photon emission tomography. Eur J Nucl Med 20:776–782

Gutterman DD (2009) Silent myocardial ischemia. Circ J 73:785–797

Ha JW, Lee JD, Jang Y et al (1998) ^{123}I-MIBG myocardial scintigraphy as a noninvasive screen for the diagnosis of coronary artery spasm. J Nucl Cardiol 5:591–597

Hartikainen J, Mantysaari M, Kuikka J et al (1994) Extent of cardiac autonomic denervation in relation to angina on exercise test in patients with recent acute myocardial infarction. Am J Cardiol 74:760–763

Hartikainen J, Kuikka J, Mantysaari M et al (1996) Sympathetic reinnervation after acute myocardial infarction. Am J Cardiol 77:5–9

Hartikainen J, Mustonen J, Kuikka J et al (1997) Cardiac sympathetic denervation in patients with coronary artery disease without previous myocardial infarction. Am J Cardiol 80:273–277

Higuchi K, Toyama T, Tada H et al (2006) Usefulness of biventricular pacing to improve cardiac symptoms, exercise capacity and sympathetic nerve activity in patients with moderate to severe chronic heart failure. Circ J 70:703–709

Hirano Y, Ozasa Y, Yamamoto T et al (2002) Diagnosis of vasospastic angina by hyperventilation and cold-pressor stress echocardiography: comparison to I-MIBG myocardial scintigraphy. J Am Soc Echocardiogr 15:617–623

Imamura Y, Ando H, Mitsuoka W et al (1995) Iodine-123 metaiodobenzylguanidine images reflect intense myocardial adrenergic nervous activity in congestive heart failure independent of underlying cause. J Am Coll Cardiol 26:1594–1599
Inobe Y, Kugiyama K, Miyagi H et al (1997) Long-lasting abnormalities in cardiac sympathetic nervous system in patients with coronary spastic angina: quantitative analysis with iodine 123 metaiodobenzylguanidine myocardial scintigraphy. Am Heart J 134:112–118
Jacobson AF, Senior R, Cerqueira MD et al (2010) Myocardial iodine-123 meta-iodobenzylguanidine imaging and cardiac events in heart failure. Results of the prospective ADMIRE-HF (AdreView Myocardial Imaging for Risk Evaluation in Heart Failure) study. J Am Coll Cardiol 55:2212–2221
Johnson LL, Thambar S, Donahay T et al (2002) Effect of endomyocardial laser channels on regional innervation shown with (125)I-MIBG and autoradiography. J Nucl Med 43:551–555
Kakuchi H, Sasaki T, Ishida Y et al (1999) Clinical usefulness of ^{123}I meta-iodobenzylguanidine imaging in predicting the effectiveness of beta blockers for patients with idiopathic dilated cardiomyopathy before and soon after treatment. Heart 81:148–152
Kasama S, Toyama T, Kumakura H et al (2003) Effect of spironolactone on cardiac sympathetic nerve activity and left ventricular remodeling in patients with dilated cardiomyopathy. J Am Coll Cardiol 41:574–581
Kasama S, Toyama T, Kumakura H et al (2005) Effects of nicorandil on cardiac sympathetic nerve activity after reperfusion therapy in patients with first anterior acute myocardial infarction. Eur J Nucl Med Mol Imaging 32:322–328
Kasama S, Toyama T, Sumino H et al (2007) Long-term nicorandil therapy improves cardiac sympathetic nerve activity after reperfusion therapy in patients with first acute myocardial infarction. J Nucl Med 48:1676–1682
Kasama S, Toyama T, Sumino H et al (2011) Prognostic value of cardiac sympathetic nerve activity evaluated by [123I]m-iodobenzylguanidine imaging in patients with ST-segment elevation myocardial infarction. Heart 97:20–26
Kramer CM, Nicol PD, Rogers WJ et al (1999) Beta-blockade improves adjacent regional sympathetic innervation during postinfarction remodeling. Am J Physiol 277:H1429–H1434
Kuwabara Y, Tamaki N, Nakata T et al (2011) Determination of the survival rate in patients with congestive heart failure stratified by $^{(1)(2)(3)}$I-MIBG imaging: a meta-analysis from the studies performed in Japan. Ann Nucl Med 25:101–107
Langer A, Freeman MR, Josse RG et al (1995) Metaiodobenzylguanidine imaging in diabetes mellitus: assessment of cardiac sympathetic denervation and its relation to autonomic dysfunction and silent myocardial ischemia. J Am Coll Cardiol 25:610–618
Lautamaki R, Tipre D, Bengel FM (2007) Cardiac sympathetic neuronal imaging using PET. Eur J Nucl Med Mol Imaging 34(Suppl 1):S74–S85
Le DE, Powers ER, Bin JP et al (2007) Transmyocardial revascularization ameliorates ischemia by attenuating paradoxical catecholamine-induced vasoconstriction. J Nucl Cardiol 14:207–214
Lekakis J, Antoniou A, Vassilopoulos N et al (1994) I-123 metaiodobenzylguanidine–thallium-201 mismatch following myocardial infarction. Clin Cardiol 17:21–25
Lotze U, Kaepplinger S, Kober A et al (2001) Recovery of the cardiac adrenergic nervous system after long-term beta-blocker therapy in idiopathic dilated cardiomyopathy: assessment by increase in myocardial ^{123}I-metaiodobenzylguanidine uptake. J Nucl Med 42:49–54
Luisi AJ Jr, Suzuki G, Dekemp R et al (2005) Regional ^{11}C-hydroxyephedrine retention in hibernating myocardium: chronic inhomogeneity of sympathetic innervation in the absence of infarction. J Nucl Med 46:1368–1374
Mantysaari M, Kuikka J, Hartikainen J et al (1995) Myocardial sympathetic nervous dysfunction detected with iodine-123-MIBG is associated with low heart rate variability after myocardial infarction. J Nucl Med 36:956–961
Matsunari I, Schricke U, Bengel FM et al (2000) Extent of cardiac sympathetic neuronal damage is determined by the area of ischemia in patients with acute coronary syndromes. Circulation 101:2579–2585

Matsunari I, Aoki H, Nomura Y et al (2010) Iodine-123 metaiodobenzylguanidine imaging and carbon-11 hydroxyephedrine positron emission tomography compared in patients with left ventricular dysfunction. Circ Cardiovasc Imaging 3:595–603

Matsuo S, Takahashi M, Nakamura Y et al (1996) Evaluation of cardiac sympathetic innervation with iodine-123-metaiodobenzylguanidine imaging in silent myocardial ischemia. J Nucl Med 37:712–717

McGhie AI, Corbett JR, Akers MS et al (1991) Regional cardiac adrenergic function using I-123 meta-iodobenzylguanidine tomographic imaging after acute myocardial infarction. Am J Cardiol 67:236–242

Merlet P, Valette H, Dubois-Rande JL et al (1992) Prognostic value of cardiac metaiodobenzylguanidine imaging in patients with heart failure. J Nucl Med 33:471–477

Minardo JD, Tuli MM, Mock BH et al (1988) Scintigraphic and electrophysiological evidence of canine myocardial sympathetic denervation and reinnervation produced by myocardial infarction or phenol application. Circulation 78:1008–1019

Mirowski M, Reid PR, Mower MM et al (1980) Termination of malignant ventricular arrhythmias with an implanted automatic defibrillator in human beings. N Engl J Med 303:322–324

Munch G, Nguyen NT, Nekolla S et al (2000) Evaluation of sympathetic nerve terminals with [(11)C]epinephrine and [(11)C]hydroxyephedrine and positron emission tomography. Circulation 101:516–523

Muxi A, Magrina J, Martin F et al (2003) Technetium 99m-labeled tetrofosmin and iodine 123-labeled metaiodobenzylguanidine scintigraphy in the assessment of transmyocardial laser revascularization. J Thorac Cardiovasc Surg 125:1493–1498

Nakajima K, Shuke N, Nitta Y et al (1995) Comparison of 99Tcm-pyrophosphate, ^{201}T1 perfusion, ^{123}I-labelled methyl-branched fatty acid and sympathetic imaging in acute coronary syndrome. Nucl Med Commun 16:494–503

Nakata T, Miyamoto K, Doi A et al (1998) Cardiac death prediction and impaired cardiac sympathetic innervation assessed by MIBG in patients with failing and nonfailing hearts. J Nucl Cardiol 5:579–590

Nakata T, Wakabayashi T, Kyuma M et al (2005) Cardiac metaiodobenzylguanidine activity can predict the long-term efficacy of angiotensin-converting enzyme inhibitors and/or beta-adrenoceptor blockers in patients with heart failure. Eur J Nucl Med Mol Imaging 32:186–194

Nishimura T, Oka H, Sago M et al (1992) Serial assessment of denervated but viable myocardium following acute myocardial infarction in dogs using iodine-123 metaiodobenzylguanidine and thallium-201 chloride myocardial single photon emission tomography. Eur J Nucl Med 19:25–29

Nishioka SA, Martinelli Filho M, Brandao SC et al (2007) Cardiac sympathetic activity pre and post resynchronization therapy evaluated by ^{123}I-MIBG myocardial scintigraphy. J Nucl Cardiol 14:852–859

Nishisato K, Hashimoto A, Nakata T et al (2010) Impaired cardiac sympathetic innervation and myocardial perfusion are related to lethal arrhythmia: quantification of cardiac tracers in patients with ICDs. J Nucl Med 51:1241–1249

Ohte N, Narita H, Iida A et al (2012) Cardiac beta-adrenergic receptor density and myocardial systolic function in the remote noninfarcted region after prior myocardial infarction with left ventricular remodelling. Eur J Nucl Med Mol Imaging 39(8):1246–1253

Pfeffer MA, Braunwald E (1991) Ventricular enlargement following infarction is a modifiable process. Am J Cardiol 68:127D–131D

Pietila M, Malminiemi K, Ukkonen H et al (2001) Reduced myocardial carbon-11 hydroxyephedrine retention is associated with poor prognosis in chronic heart failure. Eur J Nucl Med 28:373–376

Ricci DR, Orlick AE, Cipriano PR et al (1979) Altered adrenergic activity in coronary arterial spasm: insight into mechanism based on study of coronary hemodynamics and the electrocardiogram. Am J Cardiol 43:1073–1079

Sakata K, Shirotani M, Yoshida H et al (1997) Iodine-123 metaiodobenzylguanidine cardiac imaging to identify and localize vasospastic angina without significant coronary artery narrowing. J Am Coll Cardiol 30:370–376

Sakata K, Yoshida H, Nawada R et al (2000) Scintigraphic assessment of regional cardiac sympathetic nervous system in patients with single-vessel coronary artery disease. Ann Nucl Med 14:151–158

Sakata K, Iida K, Kudo M et al (2005) Prognostic value of I-123 metaiodobenzylguanidine imaging in vasospastic angina without significant coronary stenosis. Circ J 69:171–176

Sasano T, Abraham MR, Chang KC et al (2008) Abnormal sympathetic innervation of viable myocardium and the substrate of ventricular tachycardia after myocardial infarction. J Am Coll Cardiol 51:2266–2275

Schwaiger M, Kalff V, Rosenspire K et al (1990) Noninvasive evaluation of sympathetic nervous system in human heart by positron emission tomography. Circulation 82:457–464

Schwaiger M, Hutchins GD, Kalff V et al (1991) Evidence for regional catecholamine uptake and storage sites in the transplanted human heart by positron emission tomography. J Clin Invest 87:1681–1690

Shakespeare CF, Page CJ, O'Doherty MJ et al (1993) Regional sympathetic innervation of the heart by means of metaiodobenzylguanidine imaging in silent ischemia. Am Heart J 125:1614–1622

Shimonagata T, Ishida Y, Hayashida K et al (1995) Scintigraphic assessment of silent myocardial ischaemia after early infarction using myocardial SPET imaging with ^{201}Tl and ^{123}I-MIBG. Nucl Med Commun 16:893–900

Shinohara T, Takahashi N, Saito S et al (2011) Effect of cardiac resynchronization therapy on cardiac sympathetic nervous dysfunction and serum C-reactive protein level. Pacing Clin Electrophysiol 34:1225–1230

Simoes MV, Barthel P, Matsunari I et al (2004) Presence of sympathetically denervated but viable myocardium and its electrophysiologic correlates after early revascularised, acute myocardial infarction. Eur Heart J 25:551–557

Sisson JC, Johnson J, Bolgos G et al (1990) Portrayal of adrenergic denervation in the presence of myocardial infarction: a feasibility study. Am J Physiol Imaging 5:151–166

Spinnler MT, Lombardi F, Moretti C et al (1993) Evidence of functional alterations in sympathetic activity after myocardial infarction. Eur Heart J 14:1334–1343

Spyrou N, Rosen SD, Fath-Ordoubadi F et al (2002) Myocardial beta-adrenoceptor density one month after acute myocardial infarction predicts left ventricular volumes at six months. J Am Coll Cardiol 40:1216–1224

St John Sutton MG, Plappert T, Abraham WT et al (2003) Effect of cardiac resynchronization therapy on left ventricular size and function in chronic heart failure. Circulation 107:1985–1990

Suwa M, Otake Y, Moriguchi A et al (1997) Iodine-123 metaiodobenzylguanidine myocardial scintigraphy for prediction of response to beta-blocker therapy in patients with dilated cardiomyopathy. Am Heart J 133:353–358

Takano H, Nakamura T, Satou T et al (1995) Regional myocardial sympathetic dysinnervation in patients with coronary vasospasm. Am J Cardiol 75:324–329

Taki J, Yasuhara S, Takamatsu T et al (1998) Value of iodine-123 metaiodobenzylguanidine scintigraphy in patients with vasospastic angina. Eur J Nucl Med 25:229–234

Tanaka H, Tatsumi K, Fujiwara S et al (2012) Effect of left ventricular dyssynchrony on cardiac sympathetic activity in heart failure patients with wide QRS duration. Circ J 76:382–389

Teresinska A, Sliwinski M, Konieczna S et al (2004) Changes in cardiac adrenergic nervous system after transmyocardial laser revascularisation assessed by I-123-MIBG SPECT. A preliminary report. Kardiol Pol 60:15–26

Tomoda H, Yoshioka K, Shiina Y et al (1994) Regional sympathetic denervation detected by iodine 123 metaiodobenzylguanidine in non-Q-wave myocardial infarction and unstable angina. Am Heart J 128:452–458

Toyama T, Hoshizaki H, Seki R et al (2003) Efficacy of carvedilol treatment on cardiac function and cardiac sympathetic nerve activity in patients with dilated cardiomyopathy: comparison with metoprolol therapy. J Nucl Med 44:1604–1611

Toyama T, Hoshizaki H, Yoshimura Y et al (2008) Combined therapy with carvedilol and amiodarone is more effective in improving cardiac symptoms, function, and sympathetic nerve activity in patients with dilated cardiomyopathy: comparison with carvedilol therapy alone. J Nucl Cardiol 15:57–64

Verberne HJ, Brewster LM, Somsen GA et al (2008) Prognostic value of myocardial ^{123}I-metaiodobenzylguanidine (MIBG) parameters in patients with heart failure: a systematic review. Eur Heart J 29:1147–1159

Wakabayashi T, Nakata T, Hashimoto A et al (2001) Assessment of underlying etiology and cardiac sympathetic innervation to identify patients at high risk of cardiac death. J Nucl Med 42:1757–1767

Watanabe K, Takahashi T, Miyajima S et al (2002a) Myocardial sympathetic denervation, fatty acid metabolism, and left ventricular wall motion in vasospastic angina. J Nucl Med 43:1476–1481

Watanabe K, Takahashi T, Nakazawa M et al (2002b) Effects of carvedilol on cardiac function and cardiac adrenergic neuronal damage in rats with dilated cardiomyopathy. J Nucl Med 43:531–535

Wieland DM, Brown LE, Rogers WL et al (1981) Myocardial imaging with a radioiodinated norepinephrine storage analog. J Nucl Med 22:22–31

Yamazaki J, Muto H, Kabano T et al (2001) Evaluation of beta-blocker therapy in patients with dilated cardiomyopathy–clinical meaning of iodine 123-metaiodobenzylguanidine myocardial single-photon emission computed tomography. Am Heart J 141:645–652

Yu M, Bozek J, Lamoy M et al (2011) Evaluation of LMI1195, a novel 18F-labeled cardiac neuronal PET imaging agent, in cells and animal models. Circ Cardiovasc Imaging 4:435–443

Zamora J, Abraira V, Muriel A et al (2006) Meta-DiSc: a software for meta-analysis of test accuracy data. BMC Med Res Methodol 6:31

Zipes DP (1992) Ischemic modulation of myocardial innervation. G Ital Cardiol 22:615–621

Imaging the Cardiac Automatic Nervous System in Diabetes Mellitus

15

Arthur J.H.A. Scholte and Hein J. Verberne

Contents

Abstract

Patients with diabetes mellitus are at an increased risk of silent myocardial infarction and are associated with poor outcome related to ventricular arrhythmias and sudden cardiac death. Although the cardiac sympathetic nervous system can be evaluated via the relatively simple and non-invasive assessment of heart rate variability, the evaluation with cardiac nuclear imaging using [^{123}I]-metaiodobenzylguanidine ([^{123}I]-MIBG) scintigraphy seems to be more sensitive. In addition, cardiac [^{123}I]-MIBG-derived semiquantitative parameters are important predictors of outcome in patients with diabetes mellitus and heart failure.

A.J.H.A. Scholte, MD, PhD (✉)
Department of Cardiology, Leiden University Medical Center, University of Leiden, Leiden, The Netherlands
e-mail: a.j.h.a.scholte@lumc.nl

H.J. Verberne, MD, PhD
Department of Nuclear Medicine, Academic Medical Center, University of Amsterdam, Amsterdam, The Netherlands

R.H.J.A. Slart et al. (eds.), *Autonomic Innervation of the Heart: Role of Molecular Imaging*, DOI 10.1007/978-3-662-45074-1_15

Abbreviations

CAD	Coronary artery disease
CAN	Cardiac autonomic neuropathy
DM	Diabetes mellitus
ECG	Electrocardiogram
H/M	Heart/mediastinum
HF	Heart failure
HRV	Heart rate variability
LV	Left ventricle
LVEF	Left ventricular ejection fraction
NYHA	New York Heart Association
PET	Positron emission tomography
RR	R-wave to R-wave interval
SPECT	Single-photon emission computer tomography

15.1 Diabetes Mellitus

Diabetes mellitus (DM) is the most common endocrine disease and is primarily defined by the level of hyperglycemia. Criteria of the American Diabetes Association for the diagnosis of DM (American Diabetes Association 2008) are:

- Fasting (no caloric intake for at least 8 h) venous plasma glucose concentration ≥7.0 mmol/l (126 mg/dl)
- Symptoms of hyperglycemia and a casual plasma glucose ≥11.1 mmol/l (200 mg/ dl)
- Two-hour plasma glucose ≥11.1 mmol/l during an oral glucose tolerance test

Recent estimates indicate that there were 171 million people in the world with DM in the year 2000 and this is projected to increase to 366 million by 2030 (Wild et al. 2004).

In 2005, an estimated 1.1 million people died from the complications of DM and almost half of deaths by DM occurred in people under the age of 70 years. Moreover, 55 % of DM deaths occurred in women (www.diabetes.org 2009).

DM can be classified in type 1 and type 2. DM type 1 (also called type 1 diabetes, T1D, T1DM, insulin-dependent DM, juvenile diabetes) is an autoimmune disease, which results in destruction of insulin-producing β-cells of the pancreas. The consequential lack of insulin causes an increase of fasting blood glucose, and eventually glucose begins to appear in the urine when the urine glucose level is above the renal reabsorption threshold. The subsequent glycosuria or glucose in the urine causes the patient to urinate more frequently and drink more than normal (polydipsia). These characteristic symptoms often prompted the diagnosis DM.

DM type 2 (formerly called non-insulin-dependent or adult-onset DM) results from the body's ineffective use of insulin that is characterized by high blood glucose in the context of insulin resistance and relative insulin deficiency. DM type 2 comprises 90 % of people with diabetes around the world and is largely the result of excess body weight and physical inactivity. While DM type 2 is initially often managed by increasing exercise and dietary modification, medications are typically needed as the disease progresses. Furthermore, DM type 2 is not only associated with obesity but also with hypertension and elevated cholesterol (combined hyperlipidemia). The combination of these conditions is often referred to as the metabolic syndrome. The symptoms of DM type 2 may be similar to those of DM type 1, but are often less pronounced.

The long-term complications of DM include microvascular damage of the eyes, kidneys, and nerves, and macrovascular complications including ischemic heart disease, stroke, and peripheral vascular disease. Coronary artery disease (CAD) is the leading cause of morbidity and death in individuals with DM type 2 (American Diabetes Association 1998). The 10-year mortality rate in patients with known CAD and diabetes exceeds 70 %. Some studies suggest that the risk for future cardiac death in patients with diabetes without known CAD is similar to that in nondiabetic patients with overt clinical CAD (Haffner et al. 1998). In addition, early and late outcomes of diabetic patients with acute coronary syndromes are worse than those of their nondiabetic counterparts. To compound the problem, myocardial ischemia is often asymptomatic in patients with DM, and CAD is frequently in an advanced state, when it becomes clinically manifest (The Bari Investigators 1997, 2000).

The adverse clinical outcomes in patients with DM underscore the need to develop practical approaches to detect CAD in an early stage before clinical symptoms occur. Thus, early detection of CAD and myocardial ischemia seems to be important to reduce cardiovascular disease, morbidity, and mortality in asymptomatic patients with DM type 2. From a management perspective, patients with high-risk characteristics on testing for myocardial ischemia may benefit from coronary revascularization. With regard to pharmacological therapy, the knowledge that a patient with diabetes has CAD may indicate the need to initiate or intensify pharmacological therapy with aspirins, statins, and angiotensin-converting enzymes inhibitors.

Another important complication of DM is diabetic neuropathy. Diabetic neuropathies are a heterogeneous group of diabetic complications that affect different parts of the peripheral nervous system. Its pathophysiology is likely to be multifactorial, involving alterations in metabolism, micro- and macrovascular dysfunction, deficiency of neurohormonal growth factor, and autoimmune nerve damage (Vinik and Ziegler 2007). Cardiac autonomic neuropathy (CAN) is one of the most important neuropathies for patients with DM, because it is related with poor cardiac outcome.

15.2 Cardiac Autonomic Neuropathy

CAN due to structural and functional changes has been described in many disease states. The classical case of cardiac denervation exists after cardiac transplantation, but autonomic dysfunction is also common in heart failure, chronic kidney disease, myocardial ischemia, hibernating myocardium, and DM (Ji and Travin 2010; Fallavollita and Canty 2010).

The prevalence of CAN in type 2 diabetic patients is estimated to be around 20–30 % of patients. Although diabetic autonomic neuropathy can affect every system in the body, CAN is particularly associated with an increased risk of silent myocardial infarction and associated with poor outcome related to ventricular arrhythmias and sudden cardiac death (Gerritsen et al. 2001; Zipes and Wellens 1998) thus contributing to significant cardiovascular morbidity and mortality (Boulton et al. 2005).

CAN results from damage to the autonomic nerve fibers innervating the heart and blood vessels, which causes abnormalities in heart rate control and impairs vascular dynamics. Clinical manifestations of CAN include resting tachycardia (heart rate >100 beats/min), exercise intolerance due to blunting of cardiac output in response to exercise, orthostatic hypotension (fall in systolic blood pressure >20 mmHg or diastolic blood pressure >10 mmHg on standing) without an appropriate reflex increase in heart rate, asymptomatic (silent) ischemia or painless myocardial infarction, and intraoperative cardiovascular instability (Vinik et al. 2003).

15.3 Heart Rate Variability

In clinical practice, it is possible to assess CAN by measuring heart rate variability (HRV). HRV is the physiological phenomenon of variation in the time between heart beats. It can be measured by the variation in the beat-to-beat interval. Measuring the HRV has shown to be a simple, non-invasive method to evaluate both the parasympathetic and sympathetic nervous systems using a range of different tests. These tests can be recorded, for instance, with the aid of a Holter electrocardiogram (ECG).

Drugs influencing HRV, such as β-adrenergic blockers, angiotensin-converting enzyme inhibitors, angiotensin receptor blocker, and neuroleptic drugs or clozapine, have to be stopped 1 week before HRV measurement.

Assessment of the parasympathetic nervous system includes:

1. HRV at rest over 150 consecutive beats.
2. Beat-to-beat variation (the mean longest RR interval) with deep breathing at 6 cycles per minute over 120 consecutive beats, the so-called E(xpiration):I(nspiration) ratio.
3. Immediate heart rate response in reaction to change in position from recumbent to standing. This can be calculated as the "30–15 ratio," defined as the longest RR interval of beats 20–40 divided by the shortest RR interval of beat 5–25 with beat one being the first one during the process of getting up.
4. HRV during Valsalva maneuver (i.e., moderately forceful attempted exhalation against a closed airway, usually done by closing one's mouth, pinching one's nose shut while pressing out as if blowing up a balloon): calculated as the ratio of the longest RR interval following the pressure release to the shortest RR interval during the maneuver.

Assessment of the sympathetic nervous system includes the resting heart rate, spectral analysis of heart rate variation, postural blood pressure, handgrip blood pressure, cold pressor response, sympathetic skin galvanic response, sudorometry (i.e., assessment of perspiration), and cutaneous blood flow (Vinik and Ziegler 2007).

A decrease in systolic blood pressure equal to or greater than 30 mmHg within 2 min after standing can also be defined as an abnormal heart rate response (Clarke et al. 1979). Finally, two or more abnormal cardiovascular reflex tests can be defined as CAN positive (ECG-based CAN) and one or less as CAN negative (Rose and Blackburn 1968; Turpeinen et al. 1996; Schnell et al. 2002).

15.4 Prognosis of CAN Measured with HRV

The presence of CAN conveys a poor clinical outcome. In 1976 already, Ewing et al. published the results of 37 diabetic patients with symptoms and clinical features suggestive of autonomic neuropathy who were followed for 33 months (Ewing et al. 1976). The authors concluded that simple autonomic function tests provided significant prognostic information, with abnormal tests being associated with a high mortality. These results were confirmed in a larger population ($n = 605$) of the Hoorn study with a follow-up period of 9 years (Gerritsen et al. 2001). Mortality during the follow-up was 17 % ($n = 101$ patients), and patients with diabetes and impaired autonomic function had a twofold mortality risk. Meta-analysis by Vinik and coworkers assessed also the prognostic value of CAN in diabetic patients (Vinik et al. 2003). Using the pooled analyses from 12 studies involving 1,486 study subjects, they estimated that the pooled prevalence rate risk for silent myocardial infarction in diabetic patients was 1.96 (95 % confidence interval 1.53–2.51, $P < 0.001$) (Vinik et al. 2003). In the same review, the pooled estimate of the relative risk for mortality, based on 15 studies with 2,900 patients, was 2.14 (95 % confidence interval 1.83–2.51, $P < 0.0001$) for diabetic patients with CAN. The role of CAN in asymptomatic diabetic patients has been described by Valensi and colleagues (Valensi et al. 2001). In this study, 75 patients with at least two cardiovascular risk factors were evaluated for silent myocardial ischemia and CAN with a 3–7 years follow-up period. Eleven (15 %) patients had a major cardiovascular event, and multivariate analysis demonstrated that CAN was a better predictor of major cardiac events than silent myocardial ischemia.

Thus, it was estimated that the 5-year mortality rate is five times higher in diabetic patients with CAN compared with patients without evidence of CAN (Vinik et al. 2003; Vinik and Ziegler 2007). Therefore, early diagnosis and recognition of CAN are crucial as it may impact on the clinical decision-making of these patients.

However, all these tests are indirect assessments of the autonomic nervous system and are less sensitive than direct assessments by cardiac radionuclide imaging with single-photon emission computer tomography (SPECT) or positron emission tomography (PET) (Ziegler et al. 1998; Stevens et al. 1998).

15.5 Radionuclide Imaging of CAN in DM

SPECT and PET imaging are nowadays available for the assessment of cardiac sympathetic adrenergic innervation and activation. Both techniques can evaluate abnormalities in cardiac sympathetic innervation by visualizing the uptake and storage of radiolabeled neurotransmitters transported into the presynaptic nerve terminals.

15.5.1 [^{123}I]-MIBG SPECT

At present, several studies using [^{123}I]-MIBG imaging have demonstrated the presence of global and regional abnormalities in sympathetic innervation in diabetic patients (Turpeinen et al. 1996; Nagamachi et al. 2002, 2006; Kreiner et al. 1995; Scognamiglo et al. 1998). Turpeinen and colleagues performed [^{123}I]-MIBG scintigraphy to evaluate regional abnormalities in sympathetic innervation pattern in 7 type 1 and 13 type 2 diabetic patients (Turpeinen et al. 1996). Type 2 diabetic patients showed reduced [^{123}I]-MIBG uptake in the inferoposterior segments compared with type 1 diabetic patients. However, conventional indirect measures of autonomic function by power spectral analysis of HRV failed to detect any differences between the two groups. Nagamachi and colleagues subsequently evaluated the prognostic value of cardiac [^{123}I]-MIBG imaging by retrospectively evaluating 144 type 2 diabetic patients for the occurrence of cardiac events (arrhythmia, heart failure, or acute myocardial infarction) and all-cause mortality (Nagamachi et al. 2006). After a mean follow-up period of 7.2 ± 3.2 years, 17 (11.8 %), patients experienced a cardiac event, of which seven died. An additional 9 patients died due to noncardiac causes. On multivariate analysis, the presence of CAN, defined as a combination of the delayed heart/mediastinum (H/M) ratio and coefficient of R-wave to R-wave (RR) interval, was an independent predictor of cardiac events on follow-up (relative risk 6.75, 95 % confidence interval 1.16–39.3, $P = 0.03$). Similarly, the presence of CAN (relative risk 17.1, 95 % confidence interval 1.07–27.9, $P = 0.04$) and a reduced H/M ratio on delayed [^{123}I]-MIBG imaging (relative risk 6.0, 95 % confidence interval 1.18–30.6, $P = 0.04$) were independent predictors of all-cause mortality.

Previous data have suggested that [^{123}I]-MIBG scintigraphy may be more sensitive than HRV for detection of CAN in diabetic subjects (Schnell et al. 2002; Ziegler et al. 1998). Langer and colleagues investigated CAN according to HRV and [^{123}I]-MIBG scintigraphy in 23 normal subjects and 65 asymptomatic patients with diabetes type 2 and silent myocardial ischemia (Langer et al. 1995). The authors showed that [^{123}I]-MIBG uptake was largely diminished in diabetic patients, especially in those with clinically detectable CAN; moreover, diffuse abnormalities in [^{123}I]-MIBG uptake were observed in patients with silent myocardial ischemia. Scholte and coworkers performed a systematic, head-to-head comparison between HRV and [^{123}I]-MIBG scintigraphy in 88 patients with type 2 diabetes asymptomatic for CAD to evaluate the presence of CAN (Scholte et al. 2010). The study included much more patients than the previous studies, but although the inclusion

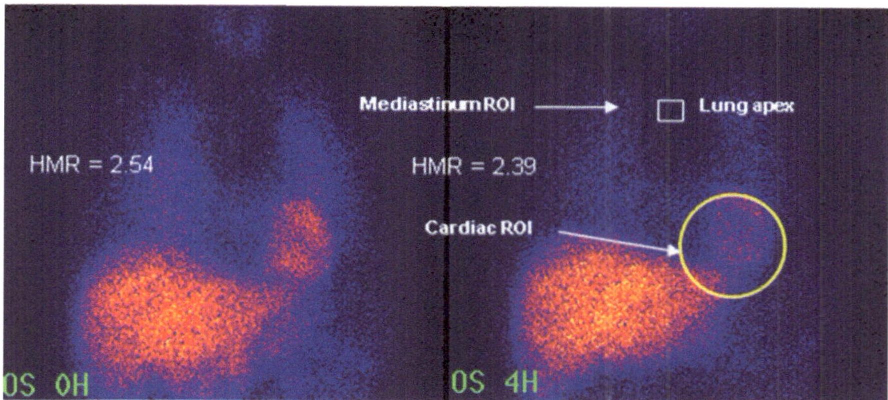

Fig. 15.1 A 61-year-old female with DM-2 and no cardiac complaints. Myocardial perfusion scintigraphy showed normal perfusion at rest and during exercise. Planar cardiac [^{123}I]-MIBG scintigraphy at 15 min (i.e., early) and 4 h (i.e., late) postinjection (*left and right panels*). The early and late [^{123}I]-MIBG H/M ratios are to be considered as normal. The calculated myocardial washout of [^{123}I]-MIBG was approximately 6 % (also within the normal range). However, the reconstructed cardiac [^{123}I]-MIBG SPECT images clearly showed reduced [^{123}I]-MIBG uptake in the inferior myocardial wall

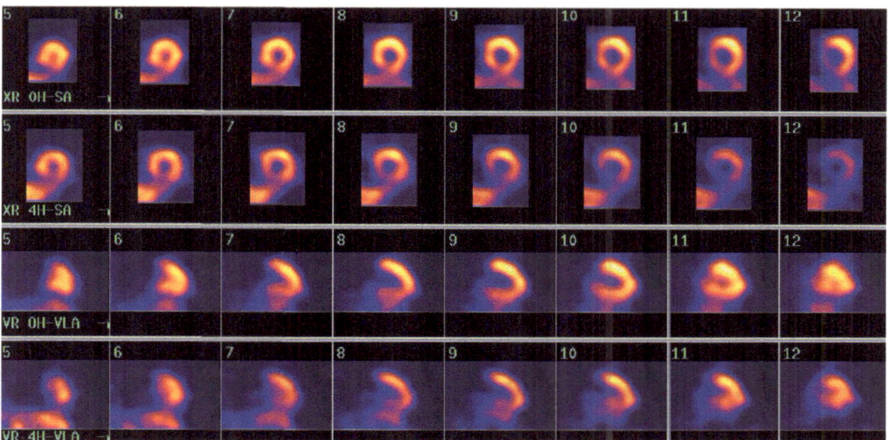

Fig. 15.2 Early and delayed short-axis (*SA*) and vertical long-axis (*VLA*) views

criteria were different, the results were in line with previous reports observing a significantly higher proportion of CAN with [^{123}I]-MIBG scintigraphy compared to HRV (Schnell et al. 1995, 1996, 2002). The fact that more patients exhibit abnormalities on cardiac [^{123}I]-MIBG imaging as compared to HRV, as illustrated in a patient in Figs. 15.1, 15.2, and 15.3, underscores the suggestion that abnormalities in cardiac sympathetic innervation occur prior to ECG-based (HRV) cardiac autonomic dysfunction (Schnell et al. 2002). An alternative explanation is that

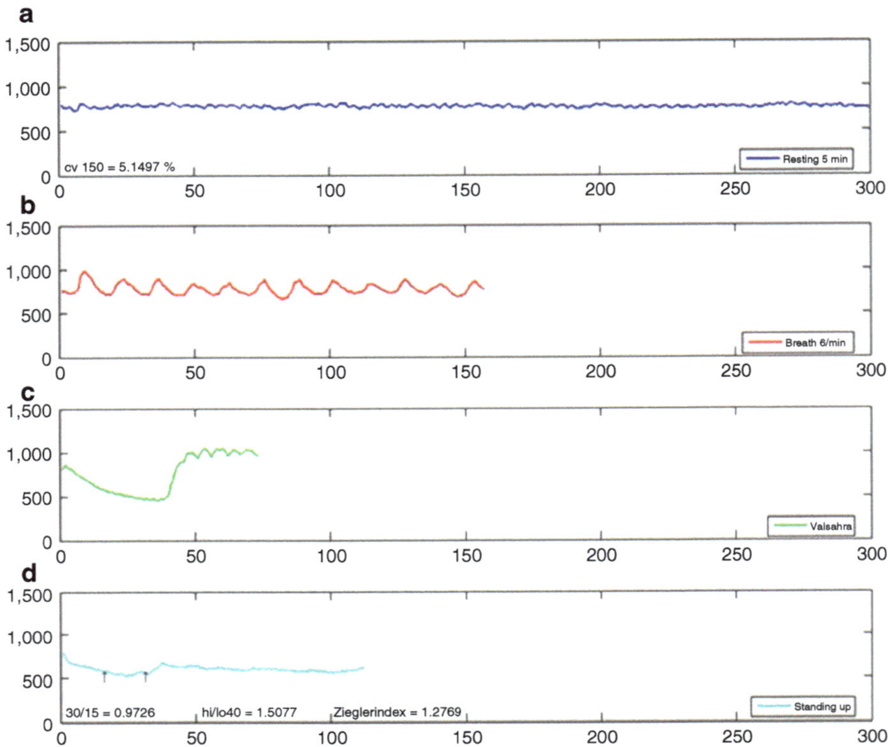

Fig. 15.3 Normal HRV registration measurement of the same patient as depicted in Fig. 15.2. This nicely illustrates that cardiac [^{123}I]-MIBG seems to be more sensitive for detecting possible cardiac autonomic neuropathy. (**a**) Beat-to-beat variation during 5 min at rest. (**b**) RR interval during 2 min of deep inspiration and expiration. (**c**) RR interval during Valsalva maneuver of 15 s. (**d**) RR interval during laying to standing test

[^{123}I]-MIBG scintigraphy mainly reflects sympathetic innervation, whereas HRV may be more related to parasympathetic function (Ewing and Clarke 1982). In addition, HRV is more a reflection of global/systemic autonomic innervation/function, whereas cardiac [^{123}I]-MIBG reflects organ-specific sympathetic innervation and function. Although it remains to be determined which of these two parameters may be more useful to predict long-term outcome, HRV and cardiac [^{123}I]-MIBG imaging may be complementary and add incremental value to each other.

While HRV and other traditional parameters provide an impression of global innervation abnormalities, [^{123}I]-MIBG scintigraphy with SPECT provides information on regional innervation. The findings in the study from Scholte indicated that regional abnormalities occur often in patients with asymptomatic diabetes. Other studies using [^{123}I]-MIBG scintigraphy, in populations with varying cardiovascular diseases, have also shown regional innervation abnormalities (Schnell et al. 1995, 1996, 2002; Scott and Kench 2004). For example, Langer and colleagues, evaluated

65 diabetic patients and noted significantly impaired [^{123}I]-MIBG uptake in the inferior wall and apex (Langer et al. 1995). Additional studies have shown that abnormalities in CAN tend to occur first in the inferior regions of the myocardium and then progressively spread to adjacent segments (Schnell et al. 1997; Hattori et al. 1996).

15.5.2 Positron Emission Tomography

Absolute quantification of myocardial sympathetic innervation is possible with PET imaging. Using carbon-11 metahydroxyephedrine ([^{11}C]-mHED) in PET imaging has the advantage of accurately detecting regional abnormalities in sympathetic innervation. Regional abnormalities in cardiac sympathetic innervation with [^{11}C]-mHED PET imaging in 29 diabetic patients compared with ten healthy subjects has been studied by Stevens and coworkers (Stevens et al. 1998). The diabetic patients were categorized into the presence of mild or severe diabetic autonomic neuropathy. Using the absolute difference in myocardial tracer uptake, the extent of regional sympathetic denervation was expressed as the percentage of the left ventricle (LV) in all subjects with diabetes. The study showed that the extent of regional sympathetic denervation was significantly larger in patients with severe autonomic neuropathy compared with patients with mild autonomic neuropathy (48 ± 19 % vs. 6 ± 5 %, $P < 0.01$). Furthermore, there was evidence of sympathetic dysinnervation with increased innervation in the basal myocardial segments but decreased innervation in the apical myocardial segments. This variation in regional myocardial variation in sympathetic innervation could contribute to myocardial electrical instability and potentially life-threatening arrhythmias.

15.6 DM CAN in Heart Failure Patients

The role of [^{123}I]-MIBG scintigraphy in predicting heart failure (HF) progression in patients with and without DM has been worked out in a substudy of the ADMIRE-HF study (Gerson et al. 2011; Jacobson et al. 2010). In this international multicenter study, the prognostic value of [^{123}I]-MIBG cardiac imaging in 961 subjects with NYHA class II-III heart failure and left ventricular ejection fraction (LVEF) < 35 % has been evaluated. Progression of HF, defined as an increase in NYHA class (from II to III/IV or from III to IV), was observed in 22 % of patients with DM compared to 14 % in those without DM ($P = 0.005$). In patients with DM, the late H/M ratio was lower than in those without DM, and only 21 % of patients with DM in the study had a late H/M ratio ≥ 1.6. This is consistent with cardiac autonomic neuropathy in patients with HF in general, regardless of the presence of DM. Moreover, in heart failure patients with H/M ratio < 1.6, DM was associated with an three times increased risk of HF progression over 2 years compared to those with DM with normal [^{123}I]-MIBG uptake (RR, 2.99; $P < 0.001$). The late H/M ratio was an independent, incremental predictor of HF progression in addition to B-type natriuretic peptide, LVEF, and NYHA class, supporting the association of DM with alterations in cardiac structure and function and highlighting the contribution of cardiac autonomic denervation to the development and progression of HF (Boudina and Abel 2007).

As discussed by Gerson and colleagues, different pathways may be responsible for this observation (Gerson et al. 2011). A defective angina warning system can interfere with identification of myocardial ischemia and infarction (i.e., silent) preventing application of effective therapies for ischemic heart disease. In addition, this defective warning system leads to an activation of the renin-angiotensin-aldosterone system, tachycardia by uninhibited sympathetic activity, orthostatic hypotension, and uncontrolled hypertension (Gerson et al. 2011). As a result, left ventricular systolic and diastolic dysfunction can progress. Also, autonomic dysfunction involving cardiac efferent sympathetic nerve transmission is an important determinant of coronary blood flow under conditions of increased sympathetic stimulation. In response to sympathetic activation by cold pressor stress, Di Carli and colleagues showed a 31 ± 12 % increase in myocardial blood flow with a 13 % fall in coronary vascular resistance in diabetics without sympathetic nerve dysfunction compared to only a 14 ± 10 % increase in myocardial blood flow and a 5 % increase in coronary resistance in diabetics with sympathetic nerve dysfunction (Di Carli et al. 1999).

15.7 Clinical Implications and Conclusions

Of all established diabetes mellitus-related and cardiac risk factors in patients with diabetes, poor glycemic control is of great importance in the development and progression of CAN (Ziegler et al. 1998; Schnell et al. 1997). Accordingly, early detection of CAN is of utmost importance, and cardiac [^{123}I]-MIBG scintigraphy appears more sensitive than HRV to detect CAN in diabetic patients. Identification of these patients may permit risk factor modification, and intensive medical treatment, aiming at better glycemic control, which in turn may favorably affect outcome (Anan et al. 2005, 2006, 2007a, b). Indeed, several studies have shown that improvement of CAN (as evidenced by HRV) can be achieved by weight loss as a result of regular exercise (Howorka et al. 1997; Kontopoulos et al. 1997). Furthermore, progression of CAN can also be delayed by intensive medical therapy, thereby reducing the risk of premature mortality and progression of heart failure (Ziegler 1994).

References

American Diabetes Association (1998) Consensus development conference on the diagnosis of coronary heart disease in people with diabetes: 10–11 February 1998, Miami, Florida. Diabetes Care 21:1551–1559

American Diabetes Association (2008) Diagnosis and classification of diabetes mellitus. Diabetes Care 31:S55–S60

Anan F, Takahashi N, Nakagawa M, Ooie T, Saikawa T, Yoshimatsu H (2005) High-sensitivity C-reactive protein is associated with insulin resistance and cardiovascular autonomic dysfunction in type 2 diabetic patients. Metabolism 54:552–558

Anan F, Takahashi N, Shinohara T et al (2006) Smoking is associated with insulin resistance and cardiovascular autonomic dysfunction in type 2 diabetic patients. Eur J Clin Invest 36: 459–465

Anan F, Masaki T, Yonemochi H et al (2007a) Abdominal visceral fat accumulation is associated with the results of (123)I-metaiodobenzylguanidine myocardial scintigraphy in type 2 diabetic patients. Eur J Nucl Med Mol Imaging 34:1189–1197

Anan F, Yonemochi H, Masaki T et al (2007b) Homocysteine levels are associated with the results of 123I-metaiodobenzylguanidine myocardial scintigraphy in type 2 diabetic patients. Eur J Nucl Med Mol Imaging 34:28–35

Boudina S, Abel ED (2007) Diabetic cardiomyopathy revisited. Circulation 115:3213–3223

Boulton AJ, Vinik AI, Arezzo JC et al (2005) Diabetic neuropathies: a statement by the American diabetes association. Diabetes Care 28:956–962

Clarke BF, Ewing DJ, Campbell IW (1979) Diabetic autonomic neuropathy. Diabetologia 17: 195–212

Di Carli MF, Bianco-Batlles D, Landa ME et al (1999) Effects of autonomic neuropathy on coronary blood flow in patients with diabetes mellitus. Circulation 100:813–819

Ewing DJ, Clarke BF (1982) Diagnosis and management of diabetic autonomic neuropathy. Br Med J 285:916–918

Ewing DJ, Campbell IW, Clarke BF (1976) Mortality in diabetic autonomic neuropathy. Lancet 1:601–603

Fallavollita JA, Canty JM Jr (2010) Dysinnervated but viable myocardium in ischemic heart disease. J Nucl Cardiol 17:1107–1115

Gerritsen J, Dekker JM, Ten Voorde BJ et al (2001) Impaired autonomic function is associated with increased mortality, especially in subjects with diabetes, hypertension, or a history of cardiovascular disease: the Hoorn study. Diabetes Care 24:1793–1798

Gerson MC, Caldwell JH, Ananthasubramaniam K et al (2011) Influence of diabetes mellitus on prognostic utility of imaging of myocardial sympathetic innervation in heart failure patients. Circ Cardiovasc Imaging 4:87–93

Haffner SM, Lehto S, Ronnemaa T, Pyorala K, Laakso M (1998) Mortality from coronary heart disease in subjects with type 2 diabetes and in nondiabetic subjects with and without prior myocardial infarction. N Engl J Med 339:229–234

Hattori N, Tamaki N, Hayashi T et al (1996) Regional abnormality of iodine-123-MIBG in diabetic hearts. J Nucl Med 37:1985–1990

Howorka K, Pumprla J, Haber P, Koller-Strametz J, Mondrzyk J, Schabmann A (1997) Effects of physical training on heart rate variability in diabetic patients with various degrees of cardiovascular autonomic neuropathy. Cardiovasc Res 34:206–214

Jacobson AF, Senior R, Cerqueira MD et al (2010) Myocardial iodine-123 meta-iodobenzylguanidine imaging and cardiac events in heart failure. Results of the prospective ADMIRE-HF (AdreView myocardial imaging for risk evaluation in heart failure) study. J Am Coll Cardiol 55: 2212–2221

Ji SY, Travin MI (2010) Radionuclide imaging of cardiac autonomic innervation. J Nucl Cardiol 17:655–666

Kontopoulos AG, Athyros VG, Didangelos TP et al (1997) Effect of chronic quinapril administration on heart rate variability in patients with diabetic autonomic neuropathy. Diabetes Care 20:355–361

Kreiner G, Wolzt M, Fasching P et al (1995) Myocardial m-[123I]iodobenzylguanidine scintigraphy for the assessment of adrenergic cardiac innervation in patients with IDDM. Comparison with cardiovascular reflex tests and relationship to left ventricular function. Diabetes 44: 543–549

Langer A, Freeman MR, Josse RG, Armstrong PW (1995) Metaiodobenzylguanidine imaging in diabetes mellitus: assessment of cardiac sympathetic denervation and its relation to autonomic dysfunction and silent myocardial ischemia. J Am Coll Cardiol 25:610–618

Nagamachi S, Jinnouchi S, Kurose T et al (2002) Serial change in 123I-MIBG myocardial scintigraphy in non-insulin-dependent diabetes mellitus. Ann Nucl Med 16:33–38

Nagamachi S, Fujita S, Nishii R et al (2006) Prognostic value of cardiac I-123 metaiodobenzylguanidine imaging in patients with non-insulin-dependent diabetes mellitus. J Nucl Cardiol 13:34–42

Rose GA, Blackburn H (1968) Cardiovascular survey methods. Monogr Ser World Health Organ 56:1–188

Schnell O, Kirsch CM, Stemplinger J, Haslbeck M, Standl E (1995) Scintigraphic evidence for cardiac sympathetic dysinnervation in long-term IDDM patients with and without ECG-based autonomic neuropathy. Diabetologia 38:1345–1352

Schnell O, Muhr D, Weiss M, Dresel S, Haslbeck M, Standl E (1996) Reduced myocardial 123I-metaiodobenzylguanidine uptake in newly diagnosed IDDM patients. Diabetes 45:801–805

Schnell O, Muhr D, Dresel S, Weiss M, Haslbeck M, Standl E (1997) Partial restoration of scintigraphically assessed cardiac sympathetic denervation in newly diagnosed patients with insulin-dependent (type 1) diabetes mellitus at one-year follow-up. Diabet Med 14:57–62

Schnell O, Hammer K, Muhr-Becker D et al (2002) Cardiac sympathetic dysinnervation in Type 2 diabetes mellitus with and without ECG-based cardiac autonomic neuropathy. J Diabetes Complications 16:220–227

Scholte AJ, Schuijf JD, Delgado V et al (2010) Cardiac autonomic neuropathy in patients with diabetes and no symptoms of coronary artery disease: comparison of 123I-metaiodobenzylguanidine myocardial scintigraphy and heart rate variability. Eur J Nucl Med Mol Imaging 37:1698–1705

Scognamiglio R, Avogaro A, Casara D et al (1998) Myocardial dysfunction and adrenergic cardiac innervation in patients with insulin-dependent diabetes mellitus. J Am Coll Cardiol 31: 404–412

Scott LA, Kench PL (2004) Cardiac autonomic neuropathy in the diabetic patient: does 123I-MIBG imaging have a role to play in early diagnosis? J Nucl Med Technol 32:66–71

Stevens MJ, Raffel DM, Allman KC et al (1998) Cardiac sympathetic dysinnervation in diabetes: implications for enhanced cardiovascular risk. Circulation 98:961–968

The BARI Investigators (1997) Influence of diabetes on 5-year mortality and morbidity in a randomized trial comparing CABG and PTCA in patients with multivessel disease: the Bypass Angioplasty Revascularization Investigation (BARI). Circulation 96:1761–1769

The BARI Investigators (2000) Seven-year outcome in the Bypass Angioplasty Revascularization Investigation (BARI) by treatment and diabetic status. J Am Coll Cardiol 35:1122–1129

Turpeinen AK, Vanninen E, Kuikka JT, Uusitupa MI (1996) Demonstration of regional sympathetic denervation of the heart in diabetes. Comparison between patients with NIDDM and IDDM. Diabetes Care 19:1083–1090

Valensi P, Sachs RN, Harfouche B et al (2001) Predictive value of cardiac autonomic neuropathy in diabetic patients with or without silent myocardial ischemia. Diabetes Care 24:339–343

Vinik AI, Ziegler D (2007) Diabetic cardiovascular autonomic neuropathy. Circulation 115: 387–397

Vinik AI, Maser RE, Mitchell BD, Freeman R (2003) Diabetic autonomic neuropathy. Diabetes Care 26:1553–1579

Website: http://www.diabetes.org/diabetes-statistics/prevalence.jsp. Consulted in 2009

Wild S, Roglic G, Green A, Sicree R, King H (2004) Global prevalence of diabetes: estimates for the year 2000 and projections for 2030. Diabetes Care 27:1047–1053

Ziegler D (1994) Diabetic cardiovascular autonomic neuropathy: prognosis, diagnosis and treatment. Diabetes Metab Rev 10:339–383

Ziegler D, Weise F, Langen KJ et al (1998) Effect of glycaemic control on myocardial sympathetic innervation assessed by [123I]metaiodobenzylguanidine scintigraphy: a 4-year prospective study in IDDM patients. Diabetologia 41:443–451

Zipes DP, Wellens HJ (1998) Sudden cardiac death. Circulation 98:2334–2351

Imaging of the Autonomic Nervous System in Cardiac Amyloidosis

16

Walter Noordzij, Andor W.J.M. Glaudemans, Riemer H.J.A. Slart, and Bouke P.C. Hazenberg

Contents

Abstract

Cardiac amyloidosis is a restrictive cardiomyopathy with potentially fatal consequences due to amyloid deposition in the myocardial tissue, but also to amyloid infiltration in the nerve conduction system. The prognosis is poor because of progressive cardiac disease. Early detection of cardiac involvement has become of major clinical interest, because its occurrence and severity limits the choice of treatment. The use of iodine-123 labelled metaiodobenzylguanidine

W. Noordzij, MD (✉) • A.W.J.M. Glaudemans, MD, PhD • R.H.J.A. Slart, MD, PhD
Department of Nuclear Medicine and Molecular Imaging, University of Groningen, University Medical Center Groningen, Hanzeplein 1, 9700 RB Groningen, The Netherlands
e-mail: w.noordzij@umcg.nl

B.P.C. Hazenberg, MD, PhD
Department of Rheumatology and Clinical Immunology, University of Groningen, University Medical Center Groningen, Hanzeplein 1, 9700 RB Groningen, The Netherlands

R.H.J.A. Slart et al. (eds.), *Autonomic Innervation of the Heart: Role of Molecular Imaging*, DOI 10.1007/978-3-662-45074-1_16

([^{123}I]-MIBG), a chemical modified analogue of norepinephrine, is well established in patients with heart failure and plays an important role in cardiac amyloidosis. [^{123}I]-MIBG is stored in vesicles in the sympathetic nerve terminals and is not catabolised like norepinephrine. Decreased heart-to-mediastinum ratios (HMR) on late planar images and increased wash-out rates indicate cardiac sympathetic denervation and are associated with poor prognosis. Single-photon emission computed tomography (SPECT) provides additional information and has advantages for evaluating abnormalities in regional distribution in the myocardium. However, inferior wall defects should be interpreted with caution.

Abbreviations

AA	Serum amyloid A protein type of amyloidosis
AF	Atrial fibrillation
AL	Immunoglobulin light chain type of amyloidosis
ANS	Autonomic nervous system
ATTR	Transthyretin type of amyloidosis
HMR	Heart-to-mediastinum ratio
HRV	Heart rate variability
LVEF	Left ventricular ejection fraction
MHED	Meta-hydroxy-ephedrine
MIBG	Meta-iodobenzylguanidine
MRI	Magnetic resonance imaging
SAP	Serum amyloid P component
SPECT	Single-photon emission computed tomography
TTE	Transthoracic echocardiography

16.1 Introduction

Cardiac amyloidosis is a rare disorder. Amyloidosis is caused by misfolded soluble serum proteins that are deposited extracellularly as insoluble amyloid fibrils throughout the body. All major types of systemic amyloidosis may display cardiac involvement. About 50 % of all amyloidosis patients experience some cardiac manifestations related to the disease. The prevalence of this cardiac involvement varies widely among the different types. It is frequent in AL type (immunoglobulin light chain derived) and ATTR type (transthyretin derived) but infrequent in AA type (serum amyloid A protein derived) amyloidosis (Falk et al. 1997; Sipe et al. 2012). Cardiac involvement eventually leads to a type of cardiomyopathy that does not present with ventricular hypertrophy or dilatation. Instead, it leads to restricted ventricular filling, resulting in symptoms and signs of heart failure. Heart failure occurs in at least 25 % of all patients (Dubrey et al. 1998). In ATTR amyloidosis, however, cardiac involvement initially leads less frequently to systolic dysfunction and heart failure. Furthermore, symptoms are milder and progression is slower, when compared to AL amyloidosis. Restrictions in ventricular filling result in persistently elevated venous pressures, liver enlargement, ascites and oedema, i.e. the clinical picture of right-sided heart failure. Consequently, patients usually suffer from dyspnoea and fatigue. Amyloidosis is the most common cause of this so-called restrictive cardiomyopathy.

The diagnosis is based on histological proof from endomyocardial biopsy, especially when amyloidosis is limited to the heart. Four samples provide a sensitivity of nearly 100 %, and a negative biopsy almost always rules out the disease. But this gold standard is not met in most patients, because the diagnosis is very likely when amyloid has been detected in extra-cardiac tissue (e.g. in subcutaneous abdominal fat tissue, see Fig. 16.1) in combination with the typical clinical picture of amyloid cardiomyopathy (Gertz et al. 2005). Since endomyocardial biopsy harbours a risk in these patients, a non-invasive diagnostic tool is clinically valuable. Different imaging modalities are used for haemodynamics and determination of prognosis. Correct and early recognition of cardiac amyloidosis and its various types remains a challenge.

The prognosis of cardiac amyloidosis is worse compared to other manifestations of the disease. Cardiac AL amyloidosis is often rapidly progressive, and, in patients with ventricular septum thickness >15 mm, left ventricular ejection fraction (LVEF) <40 % and symptoms of heart failure, the median survival is less than 6 months (Ronsyn et al. 2011). No specific treatment exists for cardiac amyloidosis or restrictive cardiomyopathy. However, heart failure should be treated with diuretics, and cardiac transplantation might be considered in selected cases. Early detection of cardiac involvement is essential as the presence and severity of cardiac amyloidosis clearly influence the treatment options to stop progression of the disease and, even more importantly, directly affect prognosis.

16.1.1 The Role of Non-scintigraphic Imaging Modalities

A detailed outline on the role of non-scintigraphic imaging modalities to assess potential cardiac amyloidosis is not in the scope of this book chapter. In short, transthoracic echocardiography and cardiac magnetic resonance imaging with gadolinium enhancement are discussed.

Transthoracic echocardiography plays an important role in the evaluation of cardiac manifestation of amyloidosis. Nowadays, it is the modality of choice for the evaluation of amyloid deposition in the heart (Falk et al. 1987). The most common finding is left ventricular wall thickening due to amyloid deposition in the myocardium. This is often associated with right ventricular wall thickening, diffuse valvular infiltration, dilated atria and pericardial effusion (Klein et al. 1990). Although echocardiography plays a major role, the diagnosis of cardiac amyloidosis is often only possible when the disease has reached an advanced stage, where irreversible functional and structural myocardial changes have occurred. There is an obvious need for methods that detect cardiac amyloidosis in an earlier and preferentially presymptomatic phase.

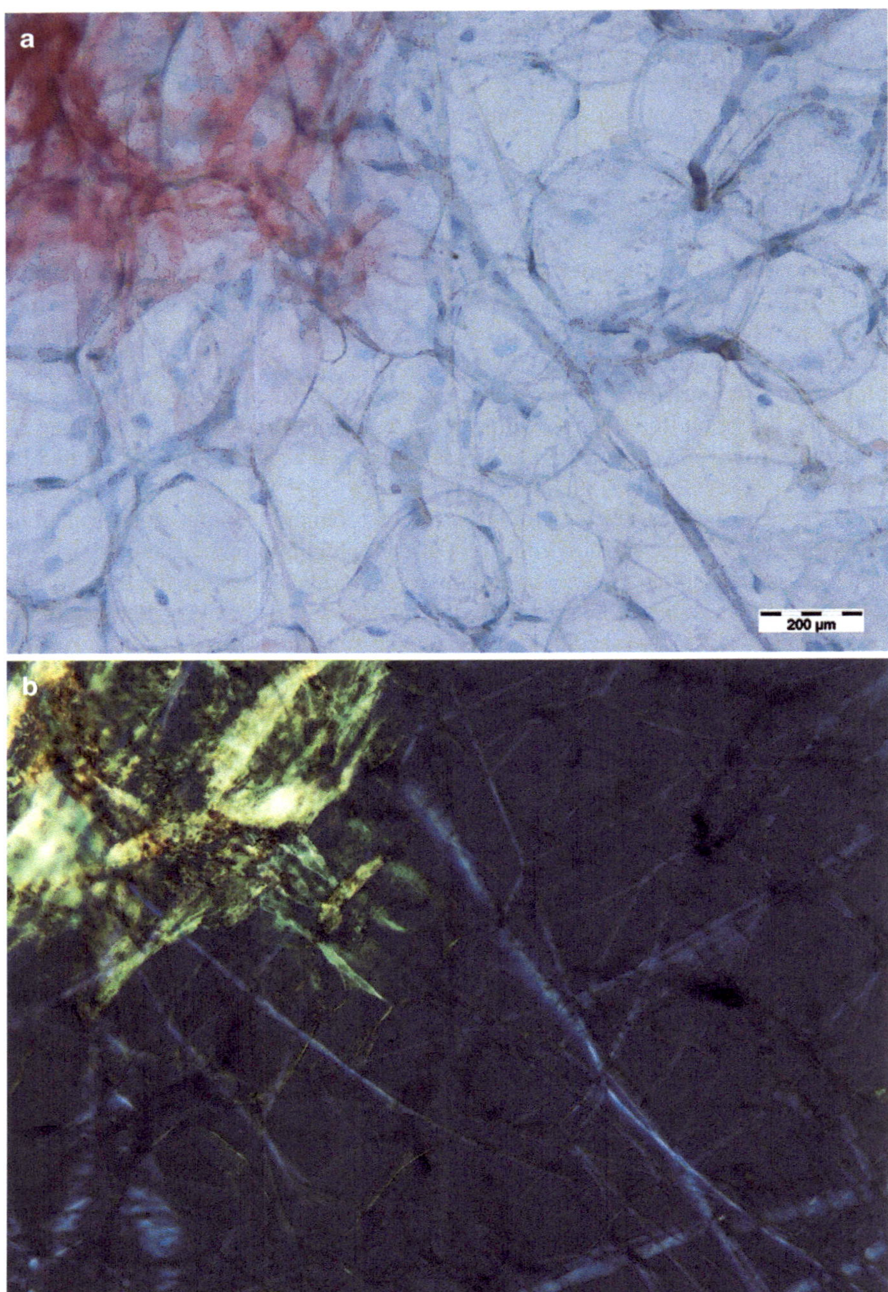

Fig. 16.1 An example of an abdominal subcutaneous fat aspirate exposing amyloid deposits, stained with Congo red. (**a**) Viewed in normal light: amyloid is stained red. Bar length is 200 µm. (**b**) Viewed in polarised light: amyloid shows apple-green birefringence (collagen is bluish white)

If echocardiography is inconclusive, cardiac magnetic resonance imaging with gadolinium enhancement might be useful. Gadolinium is an extracellular fluid tracer which accumulates in expanded interstitial place. Usually, in the intact myocardium, the distribution of gadolinium is very low, and therefore gadolinium enhancement is absent. However, in the case of myocardial interstitial space expansion, such as in amyloidosis due to extracellular amyloid infiltration, gadolinium concentration may increase within myocardial tissue. Global subendocardial late gadolinium enhancement can be found in approximately two-thirds of patients with systemic amyloidosis (Maceira et al. 2005). However, the value of MRI for the early detection of cardiac involvement is not clear.

16.1.2 The Role of Scintigraphic Imaging Modalities

Scintigraphy, using labelled serum amyloid P component (SAP), provides not only information on different organ distributions, but serial scans can provide evidence of progression and regression of the disease (Hawkins 2002). Unfortunately, these SAP scans are unsuitable for detecting amyloid deposition in the myocardium, due to size of the tracer, heart movement, blood-pool content and residual tracer uptake in the spleen.

Autonomic innervation abnormalities resulting in impaired gastric emptying is fairly common in patients with hereditary ATTR amyloidosis, in which disease a TTR mutation causes amyloid deposition (Wixner et al. 2012). Scintigraphic gastric emptying studies can play a role in identifying gastric retention due to ATTR amyloidosis. This same modality had been used to evaluate the effect of liver transplantation on gastric emptying. It showed that liver transplantation eventually had no effect on the gastric emptying time in these patients (Suhr et al. 2003).

Myocardial adrenergic denervation, using iodine-123 meta-iodobenzylguanidine ([^{123}I]-MIBG), has been shown present in patients with amyloidosis (Nakata et al. 1995; Tanaka et al. 1997; Delahaye et al. 1999). Indirectly, [^{123}I]-MIBG visualises the effect of amyloid deposition in the myocardium. This technique might be able to detect early cardiac denervation before ongoing deposition of amyloid leads to actual heart failure. Table 16.1 provides an overview of the diagnostic criteria for the assessment of cardiac amyloidosis, using the above-mentioned imaging modalities. The purpose of this book chapter is to discuss the role of [^{123}I]-MIBG in the assessment of cardiac amyloidosis.

16.2 Consequences of Impaired Sympathetic Innervation in Cardiac Amyloidosis

Cardiac amyloidosis is a form of restrictive cardiomyopathy, due to the progressive deposition of amyloid fibrils in myocardium and direct depression of diastolic function. Usually this occurs in both left and right ventricles, causing biventricular heart failure. But cardiac amyloidosis often presents itself as severe right-sided heart failure only. Eventually, systolic dysfunction leads to congestive heart failure. This

Table 16.1 Diagnostic criteria for cardiac amyloidosis

Imaging modality	Findings in cardiac amyloidosis	Remarks
Endomyocardial biopsy	Positive Congo red staining	Gold standard, however invasive method
Transthoracic echocardiography	Main findings:	Modality of choice, however often only positive in advanced stage of disease
	Left ventricular wall thickening	
	Highly refractile (sparkling cardiac echoes)	
	Associated findings:	
	Right ventricular wall thickening	
	Diffuse valvular infiltration	
	Dilated atria	
	Pericardial effusion	
Magnetic resonance imaging	Global subendocardial late gadolinium enhancement	Aspecific finding. No role in early stage of disease
[^{123}I]-MIBG scintigraphy	Planar views:	Restricted to AL and ATTR patients. Positive test results before abnormalities on echocardiography
	Low heart-to-mediastinum ratio (HMR, <1.6) at 4 h post injection	However, inferior wall defect on SPECT can be false positive
	High wash-out rate (>20 %) at 4 h post injection	
	SPECT:	
	Segmental defect on polar map view	

occurs only in late stages because the left ventricular ejection fraction (LVEF) remains (nearly) normal until late in disease. Symptoms caused by heart failure are dyspnoea, orthopnoea, peripheral oedema and sometimes, in late stages of the disease, ascites.

Amyloid deposition in the atria can cause atrial fibrillation (AF) that causes complaints of fast and irregular heart action. Also, AF is associated with the development of thromboembolism. A poor LVEF and amyloid infiltration can contribute to the complications of embolisms (e.g. cerebral infarction).

Furthermore, microvascular disease does not only cause complaints of angina due to myocardial ischemia (Mueller et al. 2000), it also often leads to syncope (Chamarthi et al. 1997). The development of syncope seems to be based on multiple factors. First, it may be a consequence of bradycardia due to amyloid infiltration in the conduction system. Secondly, a syncope can be a result of sustained ventricular tachycardia. Third, it may be caused by hypotension due to autonomic neuropathy or forward failure, sometimes aggravated by overuse of diuretic drugs. Finally, it may be the onset of sudden cardiac death due to electromechanical dissociation rather than ventricular dysrhythmias (Falk et al. 1984).

16.3 Use of Planar Images of [^{123}I]-MIBG in Amyloidosis

The use of [^{123}I]-MIBG is studied most intensively in patients with hereditary ATTR amyloidosis with polyneuropathy, formerly called familial amyloidotic polyneuropathy. The first reported case of severe peripheral neuropathy due to hereditary ATTR, in which 111 MBq [^{123}I]-MIBG was used, did not show any definite myocardial activity in all cardiac regions on either early (30 min post injection (pi)) or late images (4 h pi) (Nakata et al. 1995); see also an example of a normal and abnormal [^{123}I]-MIBG scan in Figs. 16.2 and 16.3. Although the cardiac walls were markedly thickened by amyloid, the left ventricular ejection fraction was normal on radionuclide ventriculography, as well as myocardial perfusion using thallium-201 ([^{201}Tl]). Analysis of heart rate variability (HRV) suggested highly damaged vagal and sympathetic activities. Thus, the defects on the [^{123}I]-MIBG scan were considered to represent impaired sympathetic nerve endings in the heart due to amyloid deposition.

The lack of [^{123}I]-MIBG uptake in myocardial tissue was also seen in a second case report (Arbab et al. 1997). In this patient with hereditary ATTR, a [^{123}I]-MIBG scan was performed, which showed no uptake in the heart, indicating severe impairment of cardiac sympathetic function. Also several other investigations were performed, including technetium-99m-labelled dimercaptosuccinic acid ([^{99m}Tc]-DMSA),

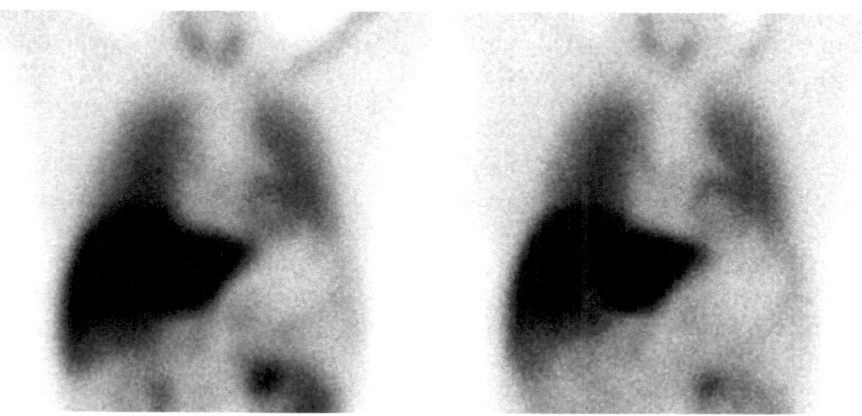

Fig. 16.2 An example of normal [^{123}I]-MIBG uptake. HMR on early (*left*) image 2.50, HMR on late (*right*) image 2.50, wash-out 0 %

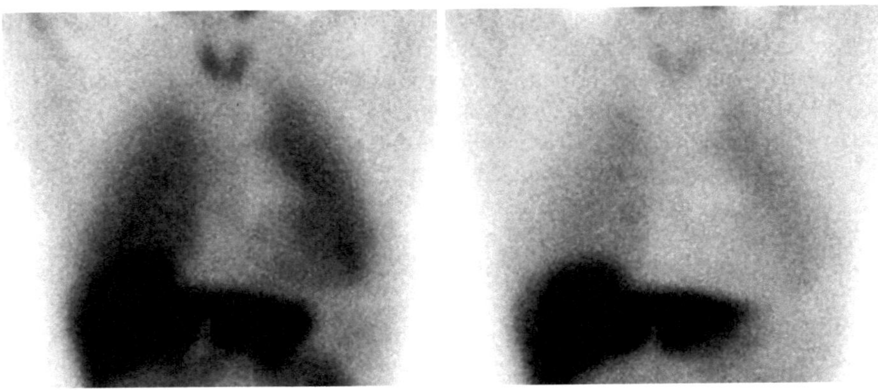

Fig. 16.3 An example of abnormal [^{123}I]-MIBG uptake in a patient with amyloid deposition. HMR on early (*left*) image 1.89, HMR on late (*right*) image 1.37, wash-out 27 %

[^{201}Tl] and iodine-123-labelled 15-(p-iodophenyl)-3-(R,S)-methyl-pentadecanoic acid ([^{123}I]-BMIPP) studies. These studies showed myocardial involvement of amyloidosis ([^{99m}Tc]-DMSA), normal myocardial perfusion ([^{201}Tl]) and normal fatty acid metabolism ([^{123}I]-BMIPP), respectively.

In the first clinical study, 12 patients with hereditary ATTR and polyneuropathy were prospectively followed, using [^{123}I]-MIBG and comparing it to echocardiography, and to [^{201}Tl] and [^{99m}Tc]-labelled pyrophosphate ([^{99m}Tc]-PYP) imaging studies (Tanaka et al. 1997). All 12 patients suffered from biopsy-proven cardiac amyloidosis. Four mCi (148 MBq) [^{123}I]-MIBG was administered and scans were performed 30 min and 3 h post injection (pi). In 8 out of these 12 patients no myocardial uptake of [^{123}I]-MIBG was found on either the early or the late images. The remaining four patients showed only limited uptake in the anterior wall on both early and late images. Four patients had left ventricle (LV) wall thickening on echocardiography, with otherwise normal results. There was no significant correlation found between the prevalence of decreased uptake of [^{123}I]-MIBG and LV wall thickness and results of [^{99m}Tc]-PYP scans. All 12 patients had normal myocardial perfusion on [^{201}Tl] scan. So, in conclusion, patients with hereditary ATTR amyloidosis and polyneuropathy were found to have a high incidence of myocardial adrenergic denervation with viable myocardium, which can be found early in cardiac amyloidosis in the absence of clinically apparent heart disease.

In the second clinical study, 17 patients with hereditary ATTR amyloidosis and polyneuropathy were analysed before liver transplantation (Delahaye et al. 1999). All patients had biopsy-proven ATTR amyloid by specimens from either rectal mucosa or peripheral nerves. These patients underwent [^{123}I]-MIBG (300 MBq) scanning at 20 min and 4 h pi, heart rate variability analysis, coronary angiography, radionuclide ventriculography, rest [^{201}Tl] scan, echocardiography and measurement of plasma catecholamine levels. [^{123}I]-MIBG scans were also performed in 12 age-matched control subjects. Planar [^{123}I]-MIBG images were analysed using

HMR and wash-out rate, defined as percent change in activity from early to late images within the LV. No patients showed evidence of coronary artery disease, perfusion defects or diminished LVEF. However, cardiac [^{123}I]-MIBG uptake was dramatically decreased in ATTR patients compared to the age-matched control population, on both early and late images (HMR at 4 h: 1.36±0.26 vs. 1.98±0.35, $p<0.001$). The wash-out rate was not significantly different. On the other hand, cardiac [^{123}I]-MIBG uptake at 4 h correlated with the severity of polyneuropathy. In concordance to the results of the former mentioned study, these patients with ATTR amyloidosis had sympathetic denervation as assessed by [^{123}I]-MIBG imaging, despite normal LV systolic function and myocardial perfusion.

In continuation of these findings a subsequent study in 31 patients with hereditary ATTR amyloidosis and polyneuropathy was performed after liver transplantation (Delahaye et al. 2006). The purpose of this study was to evaluate the outcomes of cardiac sympathetic innervation and amyloid infiltration after liver transplantation. Cardiac sympathetic innervation was assessed in the same manner as the study published in 1999 by the same authors: 300 MBq [^{123}I]-MIBG, scans at 20 min and 4 h pi and the use of HMR and wash-out rates. A similar age-matched control population was used for normal values of HMR and wash-out rate. All patients also underwent a [^{201}Tl] scan at rest, heart rate variability analysis, echocardiography, and right heart catheterisation. Sympathetic denervation was found in patients before liver transplantation compared to the control population (HMR 1.45±0.29 vs. 1.98±0.35, $p<0.001$) After liver transplantation, there was no significant change in global [^{123}I]-MIBG HMR (1.46±0.28). This may implicate that progression of cardiac sympathetic denervation stops after liver transplantation and that early re-innervation cannot be measured within 2 years after liver transplantation. There was no correlation found between age and echocardiographic findings. However, conduction disturbances, ventricular arrhythmias and LV wall thickening were associated with low [^{123}I]-MIBG uptake and progressed after liver transplantation. This may implicate progression of cardiac amyloid infiltration after liver transplantation (Haagsma et al. 2007). Low cardiac [^{123}I]-MIBG uptake was also in this study associated with severity of polyneuropathy, which worsened after liver transplantation. The authors conclude that [^{123}I]-MIBG imaging can provide an objective measurement of cardiac sympathetic innervation, which could help to guide the indications for liver transplantation in patients with early stage of hereditary ATTR amyloidosis and polyneuropathy.

Although symptoms and consequences of cardiac amyloid deposition in AL amyloidosis are often more frequent and severe than in ATTR amyloidosis (causing more frequently fatal dysfunction), the use of [^{123}I]-MIBG in this type of disease has hardly been studied. In fact only one major study has been performed in which the presence of impaired myocardial sympathetic innervation was related to clinical autonomic abnormalities and congestive heart failure in AL amyloidosis (Hongo et al. 2002). In this study 25 patients with biopsy-proven cardiac manifestation of AL amyloidosis underwent autonomic function tests, echocardiography, heart rate variability analysis and [^{123}I]-MIBG scanning. The [^{123}I]-MIBG scans were performed using 111 MBq [^{123}I]-MIBG with uptake at 30 min and 3 h pi. Myocardial uptake and wash-out rates were calculated using HMR. Furthermore, 20 of 25 patients underwent [^{201}Tl] scan at rest for myocardial perfusion. Of the 25 patients, 9 suffered from autonomic dysfunction and 16 did not. Five of 9 patients with autonomic dysfunction and 10 of 16 without had congestive heart failure. Between the two groups with and without autonomic dysfunction, no significant difference was found in amyloid deposition in the right and left ventricular wall based on echocardiographic thickness. None of the patients had myocardial perfusion defects. In patients with autonomic dysfunction, HMR (1.37 ± 0.05 vs. 1.66 ± 0.09 after 30 min, $p < 0.001$, and 1.29 ± 0.05 vs. 1.53 ± 0.06 after 3 h, $p < 0.001$) and wash-out rates (30.8 ± 4.0 % vs. 41.5 ± 4.8 %) were significantly decreased compared to the patients without autonomic dysfunction. In both groups, HMR was significantly decreased and wash-out rate increased in patients with heart failure (10 of 16 without autonomic dysfunction, 5 of 9 with autonomic symptoms) compared to the patients without heart failure. Therefore, myocardial uptake and turnover of [^{123}I]-MIBG in patients with AL amyloidosis are heterogeneous and seem to depend on the presence of both congestive heart failure and cardiac autonomic dysfunction.

In the most recent study, 61 patients with biopsy-proven amyloidosis (39 AL, 11 AA, 11 ATTR) underwent general clinical work-up, echocardiography and [^{123}I]-MIBG scintigraphy (Noordzij et al. 2012). Using echocardiography, left ventricular internal dimensions and wall thickness were measured, and highly refractile ('sparkling') cardiac echoes were assessed. These findings were compared with the early (15 min) and late (4 h) HMR and wash-out rates, determined after administration of [^{123}I]-MIBG. The echocardiographic parameters did not significantly differ among the three patient groups. Sparkling was present in 72 % of ATTR patients, in 54 % of AL patients and in 45 % of AA patients. Mean late HMR in all patients was 2.3 ± 0.75, and the mean wash-out rate was 8.6 ± 14 % (the latter did not significantly differ among the patient groups). Late HMR was significantly lower in patients with echocardiographic signs of amyloidosis than in patients without (2.0 ± 0.70 vs. 2.8 ± 0.58, $p < 0.001$). Also, wash-out rates were significantly higher in these patients (17 ± 10 % vs. −3.3 ± 9.9 %, $p < 0.001$). Furthermore, in ATTR patients with polyneuropathy but without echocardiographic signs of amyloidosis, HMR was lower than in patients with other types of amyloidosis (2.0 ± 0.59 vs. 2.9 ± 0.50, $p = 0.007$).

So, in conclusion, this study confirms that [^{123}I]-MIBG HMR is lower and wash-out rate is higher in patients with echocardiographic signs of amyloidosis. Also, [^{123}I]-MIBG scintigraphy is able to detect cardiac denervation in ATTR patients before signs of amyloidosis are evident on echocardiography.

16.4 Discussion

Amyloidoses are systemic diseases that affect multiple organs and tissues and carry a poor prognosis. The need to identify cardiac involvement is very urgent, because of high rates of arrhythmia, rapid deterioration and sudden cardiac death. Diagnostic imaging is important for risk assessment and decision making concerning drug treatment, liver transplantation, Implantable Cardioverter Defibrillator (ICD) implants and heart transplantation. This book chapter focuses on the use of [^{123}I]-MIBG, being the best literature-based imaging modality for cardiac sympathetic denervation. Myocardial defects in [^{123}I]-MIBG activity correlate with impaired cardiac sympathetic function due to amyloid deposition. This can be identified early in the disease. Furthermore, lower HMR and higher wash-out rates correspond to severity of the disease.

The use of HMR and wash-out rates have also been used in patients with other forms of heart failure. These studies have shown that decreased HMR on late images and increased wash-out rates are related to an increase in systolic dysfunction. Lower [^{123}I]-MIBG uptake was even reported to indicate poorer prognosis in patients with heart failure. In the recently published ADMIRE-HF (AdreView Myocardial for Risk Evaluation in Heart Failure, AdreView = [^{123}I]-MIBG) study, 961 patients with NYHA (New York Heart Association) functional class II/III and LVEF $\leq$ 35 % were followed for 2 years. All underwent [^{123}I]-MIBG (early and late) and myocardial perfusion imaging. The primary goal was to relate HMR <1.60 to a composite end point, including progression of NYHA functional class (worsening of heart failure), potentially life-threatening arrhythmic event or cardiac death. The cumulative 2-year event rate of the composite end point was significantly lower in patients with HMR $\geq$1.60 (15 % vs. 38 %, $p < 0.001$) (Jacobson et al. 2010). Imaging with [^{123}I]-MIBG seemed to be of independent prognostic value in patients with heart failure. In a subsequent multivariate analysis, HMR was reported to be an independent predictor of both cardiac and all-cause death (Travin et al. 2009). Surprisingly, this multivariate analysis showed that diabetes was no independent predictor. Patients with diabetes are considered to develop autonomic neuropathy during their life. However, another group did show that patients with diabetes, without clinical symptoms of myocardial ischemia, had low HMR and high wash-out (Scholte et al. 2010). [^{123}I]-MIBG scintigraphy even identified autonomic neuropathy in more patients than sequential performed heart rate variety analysis. Furthermore, in the past it was already shown that HMR of patients with diabetes was lower than healthy control subjects (Langer et al. 1995). This may indicate that in patients with amyloidosis, diabetes may play a confounding role.

As mentioned before, normal values for HMR and wash-out rates seem to vary, not only among different ages but also among different image acquisitions protocols. Concerning the image acquisition, the most important factor seems to be the collimator used for [^{123}I]-MIBG imaging. In addition to the 159 keV peak which is used for imaging, [^{123}I]-MIBG also has a 529 keV peak. Collimators exhibit different degree of scattering by gamma rays of 529 keV, so that these rays mix in with the data from 159 keV rays. The image quality is impaired by these scattered rays, when using low-energy collimators. A medium energy collimator seems to solve this problem, although not every institution will have access to such a collimator (Verberne et al. 2005; Dobbeleir et al. 1999; Inoue et al. 2003). Other factors causing differences in HMR and wash-out rates are the methods of setting regions of interest (ROIs) (especially concerning site, size and form), the moment of late images, the duration of an acquisition and the correction for decay (Yamashino and Yamazaki 2007; Verberne et al. 2008). On the other hand, according to blood activity, the slope of vascular clearance curves or estimated renal function (eGFR), variations in the quantity of vascular structures in the mediastinum and the rate of renal clearance of [^{123}I]-MIBG from the blood pool do not seem to contribute to increased inter individual variation in uptake on either early or late images (Verberne et al. 2011). In a recent proposal to standardise [^{123}I]-MIBG cardiac sympathetic imaging, evidence-based recommendations for, among others, image acquisition, collimator choice and data analysis are enlisted for routine clinical application. Standardisation of [^{123}I]-MIBG cardiac imaging should contribute to its clinical applicability and integration into current nuclear cardiology practice (Verberne et al. 2008; Flotats et al. 2010).

16.4.1 Single-Photon Emission Computed Tomography (SPECT)

The focus of this book chapter was the role of planar images of [^{123}I]-MIBG in cardiac amyloidosis and their place in the evaluation of cardiac sympathetic function. The acquisition of SPECT has also been reported and has advantages for evaluating abnormalities in regional distribution in the myocardium (Nakata et al. 1995; Tanaka et al. 1997; Delahaye et al. 1999, 2006; Arbab et al. 1997; Hongo et al. 2002). Usually, the reconstructed data are displayed in three planes (short axis, horizontal long axis and vertical long axis), which is similar to that used in myocardial perfusion SPECT. Various distribution patterns of myocardial [^{123}I]-MIBG accumulation have been reported. In 16 patients with AL amyloidosis who had no autonomic dysfunction, only two had a homogeneous distribution of [^{123}I]-MIBG (Hongo et al. 2002). The reduced uptake in the other patients was mainly localised in inferior and inferoposterior wall segments. Of the nine patients with autonomic dysfunction, five had only [^{123}I]-MIBG accumulation in the anterior wall. The reduced uptake and focal defects in the inferior wall were also reported in the ATTR patients studied before liver transplantation (Delahaye et al. 1999). These inferior wall defects should be interpreted carefully, hence substantial [^{123}I]-MIBG uptake in the liver may overlap the myocardial inferoposterior wall. In addition, even in normal cases, [^{123}I]-MIBG uptake is relatively low in the inferior wall, especially in the elderly (Gill et al. 1993; Estorch et al. 1995; Tsuchimochi et al. 1995).

Analogue to myocardial perfusion imaging, the use of polar maps can be used to calculate extent and severity scores for segmental defects. Comparing perfusion imaging to [^{123}I]-MIBG distribution provides extra information about the presence or absence of mismatch patterns. Myocardial ischemia or infarction disrupts sympathetic transmission, which may lead to denervation of a region larger than affected by ischemia only. Furthermore, sympathetic nervous tissue is more sensitive to ischemia than cardiomyocytes. The presence of innervation/perfusion imaging mismatches correlates with electrophysiological abnormalities and increasing inducibility of potential lethal dysrhythmia (Simoes et al. 2004; Sasano et al. 2008).

16.4.2 Future Perspectives

Various positron emission tomography (PET) analogues of norepinephrine are evaluated in heart diseases (Bengel and Schwaiger 2004). These PET tracers even show more similarities to norepinephrine than [^{123}I]-MIBG and bear several advantages for imaging. [^{11}C]-meta-hydroxy-ephedrine ([^{11}C]-mHED) is the most commonly used PET tracer. It has a higher sensitivity for the uptake-1 mechanism than [^{123}I]-MIBG and is not influenced by the uptake-2 mechanism, which might implicate a better differentiation between innervated and denervated myocardium. In a group of 21 patients with left ventricular dysfunction who underwent both [^{123}I]-MIBG and [^{11}C]-mHED imaging, the correlation between [^{123}I]-MIBG wash-out rate and mHED wash-out rate was poor ($r = 0.57$). But the defect size on both early ($r = 0.94$) and late images ($r = 0.88$) was more closely related between these two modalities. [^{11}C]-mHED seems to have advantages over [^{123}I]-MIBG in regional abnormalities (Matsunari et al. 2010). Other [^{11}C]-labelled tracers like [^{11}C]-phenethylguanidine are currently under investigation. Promising results from a study using rats show that [^{11}C]-phenethylguanidine and its analogues are transported slower than MIBG and mHED and therefore might provide a more accurate measurement of cardiac nerve activation (Raffel et al. 2007). Finally, a fluorine-18 ([^{18}F])-labelled PET tracer has been developed: N-[3-Bromo-4-(3-[^{18}F]fluoro-propoxy)-benzyl]-guanidine (LMI1195), which is a norepinephrine transporter substrate (Yu et al. 2011). In rats, the uptake of LM1195 in the heart appeared to be similar to [^{123}I]-MIBG, whereas the heart-to-lung ratios were significantly higher. Chemical cardiac sympathetic denervation resulted in a decrease in cardiac LM1195 uptake.

We are not aware that PET tracers already have been used to visualise cardiac denervation in patients with cardiac manifestation of amyloidosis.

Conclusions

The use of [^{123}I]-MIBG in cardiac sympathetic denervation is well established. Several studies point out the value of HMR and wash-out rate as parameters for sympathetic innervation abnormalities in cardiac amyloidosis. The method is highly reproducible and easily accessible, thereby making substitution by other modalities less attractive. However, there is an increasing urge to standardise quantitative values, such as HMR and wash-out rate.

References

Arbab AS, Koizumi K, Toyama K et al (1997) Scan findings of various myocardial SPECT agents in a case of amyloid polyneuropathy with suspected myocardial involvement. Ann Nucl Med 11:139–141

Bengel FM, Schwaiger M (2004) Assessment of cardiac sympathetic neuronal function using PET imaging. J Nucl Cardiol 11:603–616

Chamarthi B, Dubrey SW, Cha K et al (1997) Features and prognosis of exertional syncope in light-chain associated AL cardiac amyloidosis. Am J Cardiol 80:1242–1245
Delahaye N, Dinanian S, Slama MS et al (1999) Cardiac sympathetic denervation in familial amyloid polyneuropathy assessed by iodine-123 metaiodobenzylguanidine scintigraphy and heart rate variability. Eur J Nucl Med 26:416–424
Delahaye N, Rouzet F, Sarda L et al (2006) Impact of liver transplantation on cardiac autonomic denervation in familial amyloid polyneuropathy. Medicine 85:229–238
Dobbeleir AA, Hambye AS, Franken PR (1999) Influence of high energy photons on the spectrum of iodine-123 with low- and medium-energy collimators: consequences for imaging with 123I labelled compounds in clinical practice. Eur J Nucl Med 26:655–658
Dubrey SW, Cha K, Anderson J et al (1998) The clinical features of immunoglobulin light-chain (AL) amyloidosis with heart involvement. QJM 91:141–157
Estorch M, Carrio I, Berna L et al (1995) Myocardial iodine-labeled metaiodobenzylguanidine 123 uptake relates to age. J Nucl Cardiol 2:126–132
Falk RH, Rubinow A, Cohen AS (1984) Cardiac arrhythmias in systemic amyloidosis: correlation with echocardiographic abnormalities. J Am Coll Cardiol 3:107–113
Falk RH, Plehn J, Deering T et al (1987) Sensitivity and specificity of the echocardiographic features of cardiac amyloidosis. Am J Cardiol 59:418–422
Falk RH, Comenzo RL, Skinner M (1997) The systemic amyloidosis. N Engl J Med 337: 898–909
Flotats A, Carrió I, Agostini D et al (2010) Proposal for standardization of 123I-metaiodobenzylguanidine (MIBG) cardiac sympathetic imaging by the EANM Cardiovascular Committee and the European Council of Nuclear Cardiology. Eur J Nucl Med Mol Imaging 37:1802–1812
Gertz MA, Comenzo R, Falk RH et al (2005) Definition of organ involvement and treatment response in immunoglobulin light chain amyloidosis (AL): a consensus opinion from the 10th International Symposium on Amyloid and Amyloidosis. Am J Hematol 79:319–328
Gill JS, Hunter GJ, Gane G et al (1993) Heterogeneity of the human myocardial sympathetic innervation: in vivo demonstration by iodine 123-labeled meta-iodobenzylguanidine scintigraphy. Am Heart J 126:390–398
Haagsma EB, van Gameren II, Bijzet J et al (2007) Familial amyloidotic polyneuropathy: long-term follow-up of abdominal fat tissue aspirate in patients with and without liver transplantation. Amyloid 14:221–226
Hawkins PN (2002) Serum amyloid P component scintigraphy for diagnosis and monitoring amyloidosis. Curr Opin Nephrol Hypertens 11:649–655
Hongo M, Urushibata K, Kai R et al (2002) Iodine-123 metaiodobenzylguanidine scintigraphic analysis of myocardial sympathetic innervation in patients with AL (primary) amyloidosis. Am Heart J 144:122–129
Inoue Y, Suzuki A, Shirouzu I et al (2003) Effect of collimator choice on quantitative assessment of cardiac iodine 123 MIBG uptake. J Nucl Cardiol 10:623–632
Jacobson AF, Senior R, Cerqueira MD et al (2010) Myocardial iodine-123 meta-iodobenzylguanidine imaging and cardiac events in heart failure: Results of the prospective ADMIRE-HF (AdreView myocardial imaging for risk evaluation in heart failure) study. J Am Coll Cardiol 55: 2212–2221
Klein AL, Hatle LK, Taliercio CP et al (1990) Serial Doppler echocardiographic follow-up of left ventricular diastolic function in cardiac amyloidosis. J Am Coll Cardiol 16:1135–1141
Langer A, Freeman MR, Josse RG et al (1995) Metaiodobenzylguanidine imaging in diabetes mellitus: assessment of cardiac sympathetic denervation and its relation to autonomic dysfunction and silent myocardial ischemia. J Am Coll Cardiol 25:610–618
Maceira AM, Joshi J, Prasad SK et al (2005) Cardiovascular magnetic resonance in cardiac amyloidosis. Circulation 111:186–193
Matsunari I, Aoki H, Nomura Y et al (2010) Iodine-123 metaiodobenzylguanidine imaging and carbon-11 hydroxyephedrine positron emission tomography compared in patients with left ventricular dysfunction. Circ Cardiovasc Imaging 3:595–603

Mueller PS, Edwards WD, Gertz MA (2000) Symptomatic ischemic heart disease resulting from obstructive intramural coronary amyloidosis. Am J Med 109:181–188

Nakata T, Shimamoto K, Yonekura S et al (1995) Cardiac sympathetic denervation in transthyretin-related familial amyloidotic polyneuropathy: detection with iodine-12-MIBG. J Nucl Med 36:1040–1042

Noordzij W, Glaudemans AW, van Rheenen RWJ et al (2012) (123)I-Labelled metaiodobenzylguanidine for the evaluation of cardiac sympathetic denervation in early stage amyloidosis. Eur J Nucl Med Mol Imaging 39:1609–1617

Raffel DM, Jung YW, Gildersleeve DL et al (2007) Radiolabeled phenethylguanidines: novel imaging agents for cardiac sympathetic neurons and adrenergic tumors. J Med Chem 50: 2078–2088

Ronsyn M, Shivalkar B, Vrints CJM (2011) Cardiac amyloidosis in full glory. Heart 97:720

Sasano T, Abraham R, Chang KC et al (2008) Abnormal sympathetic innervation of viable myocardium and the substrate of ventricular tachycardia after myocardial infarction. J Am Coll Cardiol 51:2266–2275

Scholte AJHA, Schuijf JD, Delgado V et al (2010) Cardiac autonomic neuropathy in patients with diabetes and no symptoms of coronary artery disease: comparison of ^{123}I-metaiodobenzylguanidine myocardial scintigraphy and heart rate variability. Eur J Nucl Med Mol Imaging 37:1698–1705

Simões MV, Barthel P, Matsunari I et al (2004) Presence of sympathetically denervated but viable myocardium and its electrophysiologic correlates after early revascularised, acute myocardial infarction. Eur Heart J 25:551–557

Sipe JD, Benson MD, Buxbaum JN et al (2012) Amyloid fibril protein nomenclature: 2012 recommendations from the Nomenclature Committee of the International Society of Amyloidosis. Amyloid 19:167–170

Suhr OB, Anan I, Ahlström KR et al (2003) Gastric emptying before and after liver transplantation for familial amyloidotic polyneuropathy, Portuguese type (Val30Met). Amyloid 10:121–126

Tanaka M, Hongo M, Kinoshita O et al (1997) Iodine-123 metaiodobenzylguanidine scintigraphic assessment of myocardial sympathetic innervation in patients with familial amyloid polyneuropathy. J Am Coll Cardiol 29:168–174

Travin M, Anathassubramaniam K, Henzlova MJ et al (2009) Imaging of myocardial sympathetic innervation for prediction of cardiac and all-cause mortality in heart failure: analysis from the ADMIRE-HF trial. Circulation 120:S350

Tsuchimochi S, Tamaki N, Tadamura E et al (1995) Age and gender differences in normal myocardial adrenergic neuronal function evaluated by iodine-123-MIBG imaging. J Nucl Med 36: 969–974

Verberne HJ, Feenstra C, de Jong WM et al (2005) Influence of collimator choice and simulated clinical conditions on 123I-MIBG heart/mediastinum ratios: a phantom study. Eur J Nucl Med Mol Imaging 32:1100–1107

Verberne HJ, Habraken JB, van Eck-Smit BL et al (2008) Variations in 123I-metaiodobenzylguanidine (MIBG) late heart mediastinal ratios in chronic heart failure: a need for standardisation and validation. Eur J Nucl Med Mol Imaging 35:547–553

Verberne HJ, Verschure DO, Somsen GA et al (2011) Vascular time-activity variation in patients undergoing ^{123}I-MIBG myocardial scintigraphy: implications for quantification of cardiac and mediastinal uptake. Eur J Nucl Med Mol Imaging 38:1132–1138

Wixner J, Karling P, Rydh A et al (2012) Gastric emptying in hereditary transthyretin amyloidosis: the impact of autonomic neuropathy. Neurogastroenterol Motil 24:1111–e568

Yamashino S, Yamazaki J (2007) Neuronal imaging using SPECT. Eur J Nucl Med Mol Imaging 34:S62–S73

Yu M, Bozek J, Lamoy M et al (2011) Evaluation of LMI1195, a novel 18F-labeled cardiac neuronal PET imaging agent, in cells and animal models. Circ Cardiovasc Imaging 4:435–443

Autonomic Imaging in Heart Transplantation

17

Frank M. Bengel

Contents

Abstract

Sympathetic reinnervation of the transplanted heart is a unique example of the plasticity and regenerative capacity of the autonomic nervous system. Radionuclide imaging studies have played a key role in demonstrating that cardiac allografts regain catecholamine storage capacity, i.e., functional sympathetic nerve terminals after complete denervation due to transplant surgery. Since its initial demonstration, the regionally heterogeneous pattern of reinnervation, its time course and determinants, as well as its functional effects on the transplanted heart have been described in detail, as summarized in this chapter.

F.M. Bengel, MD
Department of Nuclear Medicine, Hannover Medical School,
Carl-Neuberg-Str. 1, Hannover D-30625, Germany
e-mail: bengel.frank@mh-hannover.de

R.H.J.A. Slart et al. (eds.), *Autonomic Innervation of the Heart: Role of Molecular Imaging*, DOI 10.1007/978-3-662-45074-1_17

17.1 Physiology of the Transplanted Heart

At cardiac transplantation, postganglionic sympathetic nerve fibers of the donor heart are surgically interrupted, causing rapid depletion of norepinephrine within the nerve terminal and thus resulting in complete denervation (Cooper et al. 1962). This state of denervation explains the typical hemodynamic alterations that are encountered early after successful transplantation: Baseline heart rate is increased, there is chronotropic incompetence (i.e., lack of sufficient increase of heart rate) during exercise (Quigg et al. 1989), and diastolic ventricular function is slightly reduced (Paulus et al. 1992). As a consequence, exercise capacity in transplant recipients often remains reduced compared to healthy normal subjects (Kao et al. 1994).

It has also been suggested that presynaptic denervation of the cardiac allograft influences postsynaptic adrenergic signal transduction. Increased catecholamine sensitivity has, e.g., been described, which has mainly been attributed to loss of presynaptic neuronal uptake capacity (von Scheidt et al. 1992). Overall postsynaptic ß-adrenergic receptor density has been found to be normal in allografts (Denniss et al. 1989), but a shift in subtype from β_1- to β_2-adrenoceptors has been discussed, with possible implications for the response to systemic catecholamines (Leenen et al. 1995). Because of the reliance of denervated hearts on circulating catecholamines, concerns have been raised against the therapeutic use of ß-blockers in transplant recipients (Bexton et al. 1983). Some early studies have suggested detrimental effects of ß-blockade on exercise capacity and attributed their observations to cardiac denervation (Verani et al. 1994), but other studies did not confirm negative effects (Gilbert et al. 1989; Bengel et al. 2004).

The occurrence of sympathetic reinnervation after transplantation has first been reported in various animal models (Willman et al. 1964; Norvell and Lower 1973). In humans then, initial evidence was derived from reoccurrence of anginal symptoms (Stark et al. 1991), invasive measurements of tyramine- or handgrip-induced cardiac spillover of norepinephrine (Wilson et al. 1991), electrophysiologic measurements of heart rate variability (Kaye et al. 1993), and non-invasive imaging of the myocardial uptake of radiolabeled norepinephrine analogues (Schwaiger et al. 1991; DeMarco et al. 1995). Among those techniques, non-invasive PET and SPECT imaging have been especially helpful in understanding the phenomenon of sympathetic neuronal regeneration, its pattern, determinants, and physiologic importance.

17.2 The Denervated Transplanted Heart as a Model to Test Specificity of Neuronal Imaging Agents

Before discussing the process of reinnervation in more depth, it should be noted that the denervated heart early after transplantation is a useful model to test the specificity of neuronal imaging agents. Owing to the absence of any neuronal uptake and storage sites in these hearts, any fraction of myocardial retention of a neuronal imaging agent would point towards a nonspecific mechanism. In the initial publication reporting feasibility of C-11 metahydroxyephedrine ([11C]-mHED) for PET imaging of cardiac sympathetic innervation, e.g., Schwaiger et al. used early transplant recipients to show absence of myocardial [11C]-mHED retention when compared to healthy volunteers and to thereby prove usefulness of the agent (Schwaiger et al. 1990). Likewise, the specificity of other clinical sympathetic neuronal imaging agents such as I-123 metaiodobenzylguanidine ([123I]-MIBG) (DeMarco et al. 1995) or [11C]-epinephrine (Munch et al. 2000) has also been supported by the absence of significant myocardial retention in human allografts early after transplantation.

The postsynaptic receptor side, on the other hand, may remain completely unaffected despite the absence of presynaptic nerve terminals after transplantation. This has been suggested for adrenergic receptors using tissue analysis (Denniss et al. 1989), while PET imaging with [11C]-MQNB has been used to study the parasympathetic muscarinic receptors, which also were unaffected by denervation (Le Guludec et al. 1994).

17.3 Transplant Reinnervation: Pattern, Time Course, and Determinants

The first imaging evidence of human allograft sympathetic reinnervation was obtained at >1 year after transplantation using PET with [11C]-mHED, which showed reappearance of significant regional tracer retention in basal anterior left ventricular myocardium (Schwaiger et al. 1991) (Fig. 17.1). Likewise, using [123I]-MIBG and SPECT, visible cardiac catecholamine uptake was shown in approximately 50 % of patients at 1–2 years after transplantation (DeMarco et al. 1995). Further studies have greatly improved the understanding of the reinnervation process:

Serial assessment using two [11C]-mHED PET scans within 3–4 years demonstrated a continuous increase of extent and intensity of reinnervation with time after transplantation (Bengel et al. 1999). Sympathetic nerve terminals first reappeared in the basal parts of the myocardium and then extended further into distal parts, while the apex was occasionally involved late after transplantation. This finding is consistent with growth of sympathetic fibers along arterial structures. If reinnervation occurs, basal parts are reached first. In addition to a gradient from base to apex, anterior and septal walls were reinnervated earlier, while the lateral wall was involved later. These results suggest that sympathetic nerves are first restored in the territory of the left anterior descending artery, while later the left circumflex territory is involved additionally. Complete restoration of sympathetic innervation, however, was not observed until 15 years after transplantation, because inferior myocardium consistently remained denervated (Bengel et al. 1999; Uberfuhr et al. 2000b).

Using regionally heterogeneous reinnervation as a model, several studies have validated the results of catecholamine imaging by comparison with alternative tests of sympathetic innervation. [11C]-mHED PET-derived evidence of ventricular reinnervation, e.g., correlated with invasive measurements of tyramine-induced coronary arteriovenous norepinephrine spillover (Odaka et al. 2001) and with

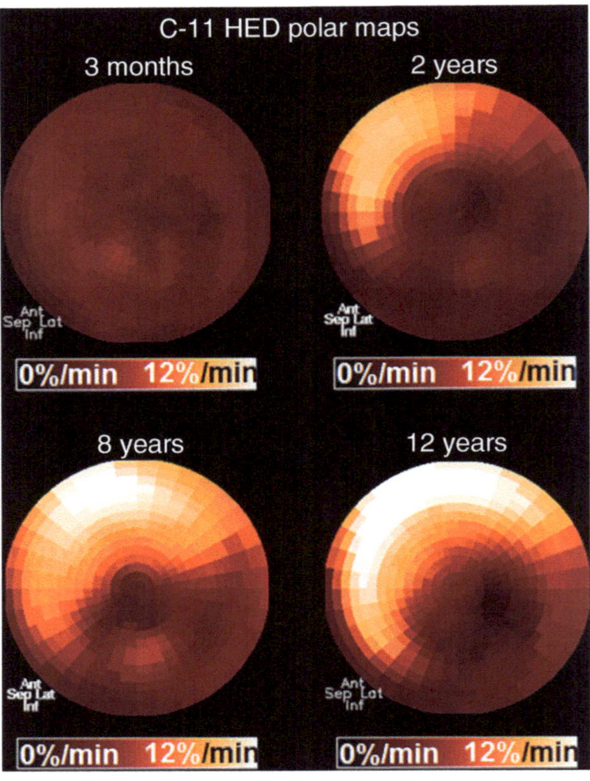

Fig. 17.1 Polar maps of myocardial retention of C-11 metahydroxyephedrine ([^{11}C]-mHED) in four cardiac transplant recipients at different times after surgery, illustrating time course and regional extent of sympathetic reinnervation (Reprinted with permission by Springer Science and Business Media, from Bengel and Schwaiger (2004))

electrophysiologic indexes of reinnervation derived from heart rate variability measurements (Ziegler et al. 1996; Uberfuhr et al. 2000a).

While time after surgery is considered a major determinant of presence and extent of reinnervation, observations of interindividual heterogeneity and the regionally incomplete pattern suggest that additional determinants are involved. This has been studied in a comparably large sample of 77 transplant recipients by a multivariate analysis. In this analysis using [^{11}C]-mHED PET, some patients remained denervated until late after transplantation, and other factors such as donor and recipient age, duration and complexity of transplant surgery, and frequency of allograft rejection were identified as independent determinants of sympathetic reinnervation (Bengel et al. 2002) (Table 17.1). Aging has been suggested to be associated with reduced availability of target-derived neurotrophic factors, which may explain reduced sympathetic reinnervation with increasing age. Reduced availability and synthesizing capacity of neurotrophins in the myocardium may also explain the lower degree of reinnervation in case of more frequent rejection episodes. Also, because surgical dissection results in axonal degeneration, sympathetic nerve fibers need to regrow along arterial structures to reach the allograft as their target organ.

Table 17.1 Parameters tested for association with cardiac transplant reinnervation

Recipient related	Donor related	Surgery related	Immunogenetical
Time after HTX[a]	*Age*[a,b]	Allograft cold ischemia	Recipient gender
Weight at HTX	Age difference		Donor gender
Height at HTX	Weight	*Aortic cross-clamp time*[a,b]	Gender mismatch
Age at HTX[a]	Height		Rhesus mismatch
Body mass at HTX	Body mass	*Perioperative aortic complications*[a]	HLA A mismatch
Ejection fraction prior to HTX	Body mass difference		HLA B mismatch
			HLA DR mismatch
Disease type[a]	CMV infection		Overall HLA mismatch
Duration of disease			Type of immunosuppression
CMV infection			
Outcome after HTX			*Rejection frequency*[a,b]

Modified from Bengel et al. (2002)
PET positron emission tomography, *HTX* heart transplantation, *CMV* cytomegalovirus, *HLA* human leukocyte antigen
[a]Significant at univariate analysis
[b]Independent at multivariate analysis

Extensive areas of scar tissue or other morphologic alterations along the path of regrowth may thus impair reappearance of nerve terminals in the myocardium. This is confirmed by less extensive reinnervation in patients with aortic complications at transplant surgery and by a significant inverse correlation with aortic cross-clamp time (Bengel et al. 2002). Hence, the surgical procedure appears to be another factor which may influence reinnervation. The observation of more intense reinnervation in patients transplanted for dilated compared to ischemic cardiomyopathy (Bengel et al. 2002) may also be explained in this context, as regrowth along sclerotic aorta and other vessels may be more difficult.

Finally, diabetes mellitus has also been shown to influence sympathetic reinnervation of the transplanted heart (Bengel et al. 2006). The regional extent of reinnervation and the regeneration rate were significantly reduced in diabetic transplant recipients compared to a matched transplant recipient group without diabetes (Fig. 17.2). The regenerative capacity of the sympathetic nervous system of the heart was reduced, but not abolished, by diabetes mellitus.

17.4 Transplant Reinnervation: Functional Effects

The pattern of regionally heterogeneous reinnervation on the one hand makes the transplanted heart a good model to determine physiologic effects of sympathetic innervation in vivo, by an intraindividual comparison of innervated and denervated myocardium. On the other hand, it also raises the general question whether this

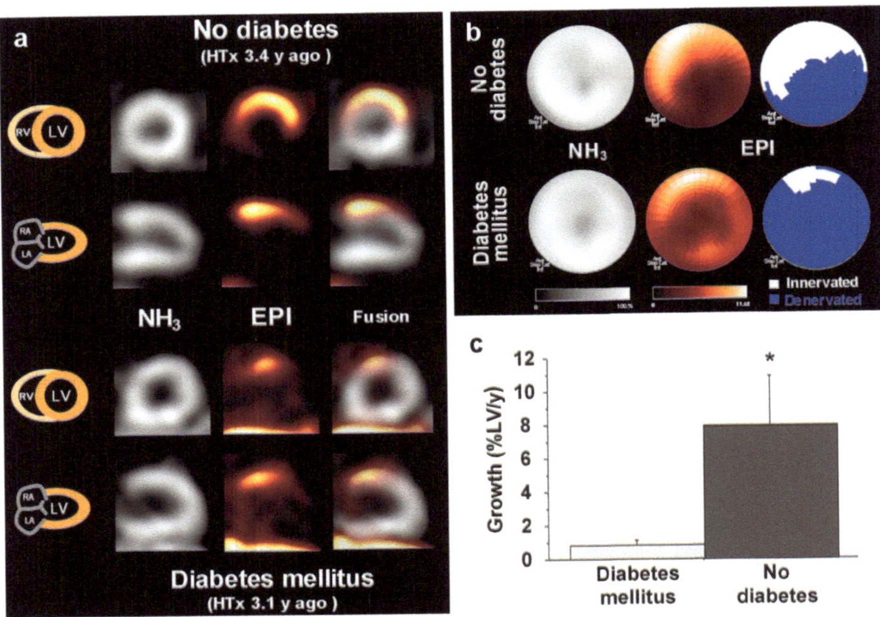

Fig. 17.2 Effect of diabetes mellitus on transplant reinnervation. Shown are representative left ventricular short- and long-axis tomographic images (**a**) and polar maps (**b**) of cardiac transplant recipient without evidence of diabetes mellitus (*top*) and another recipient with history of diabetes (*bottom*). Gray-scale images show homogeneous myocardial perfusion, determined by $[^{13}N]NH_3$. Color-scale images show regional uptake of the neurotransmitter $[^{11}C]$-epinephrine, indicating reinnervation in basal anterior wall. Extent of reinnervation was 42 % in nondiabetic recipient and 13 % in diabetic recipient. (**c**) Group results (mean ± SE) for neuronal regeneration rate. *EPI* $[^{11}C]$-epinephrine, *HTx* heart transplantation, *LA* left atrium, *LV* left ventricle, *RA* right atrium, *RV* right ventricle. $^{*}P < 0.05$ (Reprinted with permission from Bengel et al. (2006). This research was originally published in JNM. © by the Society of Nuclear Medicine and Molecular Imaging, Inc)

regenerative process, which remains incomplete, has general beneficial functional effects for the transplant recipients. Both issues have been studied in various elegant multi-tracer radionuclide imaging studies.

PET was used to determine myocardial blood flow, flow response to the cold pressor test as an index of endothelial-dependent vasodilatation, and flow response to adenosine as a composite index of endothelial-dependent and endothelial-independent vasodilatation in non-rejecting, otherwise healthy reinnervated transplant recipients. They observed a significant improvement of flow response to cold pressor in innervated compared to denervated vascular territories, while there was no difference for the response to adenosine. These results demonstrated the importance of sympathetic innervation for regulation of endothelial-dependent vascular reactivity in general, and they also supported the physiologic relevance of reinnervation for transplant recipients (Di Carli et al. 1997). Other studies focused on the effect of innervation on myocardial substrate utilization: Higher utilization of glucose were found at equal rates of overall oxidative metabolism in denervated

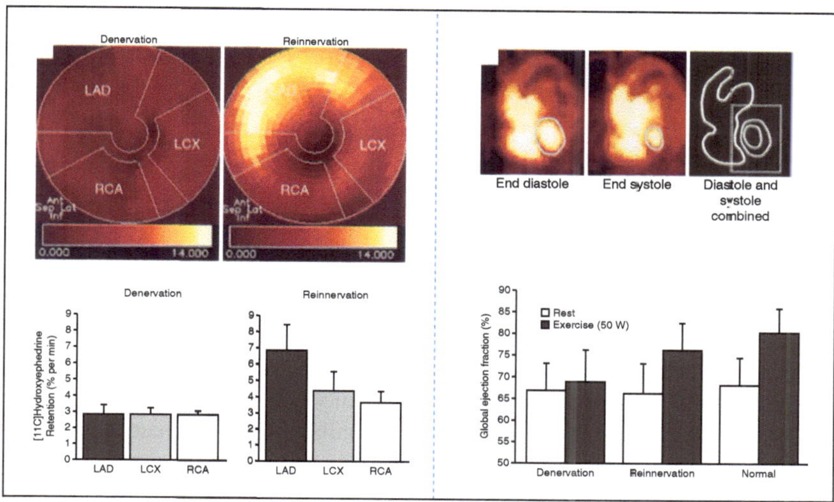

Fig. 17.3 Effect of sympathetic reinnervation on cardiac allograft performance. Left ventricular retention of the catecholamine analogue [^{11}C]-mHED (hydroxyephedrine) in transplant recipients with denervation and with reinnervation (*left*). Global left ventricular ejection fraction as determined by gated radionuclide angiography (*right*). During exercise, the ejection fraction was lower in patients with denervation than in those with reinnervation or normal subjects ($P<0.01$ for both comparisons); the ejection fraction did not differ significantly between the patients with reinnervation and the normal subjects (Reprinted with permission by Massachusetts Medical Society, from Bengel et al. (2001a). © by Massachusetts Medical Society)

compared to reinnervated myocardium of allografts, suggesting a metabolic switch from free fatty acids to glucose under conditions of denervation (Bengel et al. 2000). In another study, non-invasively determined allograft efficiency was shown to be improved in transplant recipients compared with failing hearts and was comparable to normal hearts. Differences between denervated and reinnervated allografts were not surveyed, and the dependency on loading conditions and contractility was preserved. These data suggested that normal regulatory interactions for efficiency are intact and that sympathetic tone does not play a role under resting conditions (Bengel et al. 2001b).

Finally, the effect of reinnervation on exercise performance was determined in a group of 29 transplant recipients by [^{11}C]-mHED PET and standardized exercise radionuclide angiography. Restoration of sympathetic innervation was associated with improved responses of heart rate and global as well as regional contractile function to exercise (Fig. 17.3). These results support the functional importance of reinnervation in transplanted hearts and suggest a clinical benefit for the transplant recipient through enhanced exercise capacity (Bengel et al. 2001a). A subsequent study tested the effect of acute β-adrenergic blockade on the response to exercise in denervated and reinnervated transplant recipients and showed that differences of chronotropic and inotropic response between groups were no longer present following beta-blockade. While beta-blockade was well tolerated, these results confirmed that reappearance of sympathetic nerve terminals is associated with reestablishment of intact pre-/postsynaptic interaction (Bengel et al. 2004).

17.5 Summary and Conclusions

In summary, cardiac neuronal imaging has provided unique insights into the biology of the autonomic nervous system after cardiac transplantation. Based on imaging studies, it is now well known that sympathetic reinnervation may occur later after transplantation; that presence and extent of reinnervation are determined not only by time after transplantation but also by other factors related to age, surgery, and rejection; and that reinnervation remains regionally heterogeneous but nevertheless has physiologic effects on myocardial flow regulation, metabolism, and exercise performance.

While physiologic effects of reinnervation have been consistently reported, the relevance of this phenomenon for outcome of patients after transplantation remains uncertain. To date, sample sizes in reinnervation studies have been too small, and the influence of critical issues such as rejection, allograft vasculopathy, and dysfunction as well as immunosuppression-related side effects on patient outcome is too dominant to demonstrate a survival benefit of reinnervation (Bengel et al. 2002). Given the regionally heterogeneous pattern of transplant innervation, it is notable on the other hand that coexistence of denervated and innervated viable myocardium, unlike in ischemic heart disease or cardiomyopathy (Sasano et al. 2008), is not associated with an increased arrhythmogenic risk.

Accordingly, imaging for reinnervation after transplantation has not achieved recognition in clinical practice to date. The transplanted heart, however, remains a unique and important model in cardiac neuronal imaging sciences: On the one hand, the denervated heart early after transplantation can be used to study the specificity of neuronal imaging agents. On the other hand, the reinnervating heart later after transplantation can be used to study the unique plasticity and regenerative capacity of the cardiac autonomic nervous system.

References

Bengel FM, Schwaiger M (2004) Assessment of cardiac sympathetic neuronal function using PET imaging. J Nucl Cardiol 11:603–616

Bengel FM, Ueberfuhr P, Hesse T, Schiepel N, Ziegler SI, Scholz S et al (2002) Clinical determinants of ventricular sympathetic reinnervation after orthotopic heart transplantation. Circulation 106:831–835

Bengel FM, Ueberfuhr P, Karja J, Schreiber K, Nekolla SG, Reichart B et al (2004) Sympathetic reinnervation, exercise performance and effects of beta-adrenergic blockade in cardiac transplant recipients. Eur Heart J 25:1726–1733

Bengel FM, Ueberfuhr P, Schafer D, Nekolla SG, Reichart B, Schwaiger M (2006) Effect of diabetes mellitus on sympathetic neuronal regeneration studied in the model of transplant reinnervation. J Nucl Med 47:1413–1419

Bengel FM, Ueberfuhr P, Schiepel N, Nekolla SG, Reichart B, Schwaiger M (2001a) Effect of sympathetic reinnervation on cardiac performance after heart transplantation. N Engl J Med 345:731–738

Bengel FM, Ueberfuhr P, Schiepel N, Nekolla SG, Reichart B, Schwaiger M (2001b) Myocardial efficiency and sympathetic reinnervation after orthotopic heart transplantation: a noninvasive study with positron emission tomography. Circulation 103:1881–1886

Bengel FM, Ueberfuhr P, Ziegler SI, Nekolla S, Reichart B, Schwaiger M (1999) Serial assessment of sympathetic reinnervation after orthotopic heart transplantation. A longitudinal study using PET and C-11 hydroxyephedrine. Circulation 99:1866–1871

Bengel FM, Ueberfuhr P, Ziegler SI, Nekolla SG, Odaka K, Reichart B et al (2000) Non-invasive assessment of the effect of cardiac sympathetic innervation on metabolism of the human heart. Eur J Nucl Med 27:1650–1657

Bexton RS, Milne JR, Cory-Pearce R, English TA, Camm AJ (1983) Effect of beta blockade on exercise response after cardiac transplantation. Br Heart J 49:584–588

Cooper T, Willman VL, Jellinek M, Hanlon CR (1962) Heart autotransplantation: effect on myocardial catecholamine and histamine. Science 138:40–41

DeMarco T, Dae M, Yuen GM, Kumar S, Sudhir K, Keith F et al (1995) Iodine-123 metaiodobenzylguanidine scintigraphic assessment of the transplanted human heart: evidence for late reinnervation. J Am Coll Cardiol 25:927–931

Denniss AR, Marsh JD, Quigg RJ, Gordon JB, Colucci WS (1989) Beta-adrenergic receptor number and adenylate cyclase function in denervated transplanted and cardiomyopathic human hearts. Circulation 79:1028–1034

Di Carli MF, Tobes MC, Mangner T, Levine AB, Muzik O, Chakroborty P et al (1997) Effects of cardiac sympathetic innervation on coronary blood flow. N Engl J Med 336:1208–1215

Gilbert EM, Eiswirth CC, Mealey PC, Larrabee P, Herick CM, Bristow MR (1989) ß-adrenergic supersensitivity of the transplanted human heart is presynaptic in origin. Circulation 79:344–349

Kao AC, Van TP 3rd, Shaeffer MG, Shaw JP, Kuzil BB, Page RD et al (1994) Central and peripheral limitations to upright exercise in untrained cardiac transplant recipients. Circulation 89:2605–2615

Kaye DM, Esler M, Kingwell B, McPherson G, Esmore D, Jennings G (1993) Functional and neurochemical evidence for partial cardiac sympathetic reinnervation after cardiac transplantation in humans. Circulation 88:1110–1118

Le Guludec D, Delforge J, Syrota A, Desruennes M, Valette H, Gandjbakhch I et al (1994) In vivo quantification of myocardial muscarinic receptors in heart transplant patients. Circulation 90:172–178

Leenen FH, Davies RA, Fourney A (1995) Role of cardiac beta 2-adrenergic responses to exercise in cardiac transplant patients. Circulation 91:685–690

Munch G, Nguyen NT, Nekolla S, Ziegler S, Muzik O, Chakraborty P et al (2000) Evaluation of sympathetic nerve terminals with [(11)C]epinephrine and [(11)C]hydroxyephedrine and positron emission tomography. Circulation 101:516–523

Norvell JE, Lower RR (1973) Degeneration and regeneration of the nerves of the heart after transplantation. Transplantation 15:337–344

Odaka K, von Scheidt W, Ziegler SI, Ueberfuhr P, Nekolla SG, Reichart B et al (2001) Reappearance of cardiac presynaptic sympathetic nerve terminals in the transplanted heart: correlation between PET using (11)C-hydroxyephedrine and invasively measured norepinephrine release. J Nucl Med 42:1011–1016

Paulus WJ, Bronzwaer JGF, Felice H, Kishan N, Wellens F (1992) Deficient acceleration of left ventricular relaxation during exercise after heart transplantation. Circulation 86:1175–1185

Quigg RJ, Rocco MB, Gauthier DF, Creager MA, Hartley H, Colucci WS (1989) Mechanism of the attenuated peak heart rate response to exercise after orthotopic cardiac transplantation. J Am Coll Cardiol 14:338–344

Sasano T, Abraham MR, Chang KC, Ashikaga H, Mills KJ, Holt DP et al (2008) Abnormal sympathetic innervation of viable myocardium and the substrate of ventricular tachycardia after myocardial infarction. J Am Coll Cardiol 51:2266–2275

Schwaiger M, Hutchins GD, Kalff V, Rosenspire K, Haka MS, Mallette S et al (1991) Evidence for regional catecholamine uptake and storage sites in the transplanted human heart by positron emission tomography. J Clin Invest 87:1681–1690

Schwaiger M, Kalff V, Rosenspire K, Haka MS, Molina E, Hutchins GD et al (1990) Noninvasive evaluation of sympathetic nervous system in human heart by positron emission tomography. Circulation 82:457–464

Stark RP, McGinn AL, Wilson RF (1991) Chest pain in cardiac-transplant recipients. Evidence of sensory reinnervation after cardiac transplantation. N Engl J Med 324:1791–1794

Uberfuhr P, Frey AW, Ziegler S, Reichart B, Schwaiger M (2000a) Sympathetic reinnervation of sinus node and left ventricle after heart transplantation in humans: regional differences assessed by heart rate variability and positron emission tomography. J Heart Lung Transplant 19: 317–323

Uberfuhr P, Ziegler S, Schwaiblmair M, Reichart B, Schwaiger M (2000b) Incomplete sympathic reinnervation of the orthotopically transplanted human heart: observation up to 13 years after heart transplantation. Eur J Cardiothorac Surg 17:161–168

Verani MS, Nishimura S, Mahmarian JJ, Hays JT, Young JB (1994) Cardiac function after orthotopic heart transplantation: response to postural changes, exercise, and beta-adrenergic blockade. J Heart Lung Transplant 13:181–193

von Scheidt W, Böhm M, Schneider B, Reichart B, Erdmann E, Autenrieth G (1992) Isolated presynaptic inotropic ß-adrenergic supersensitivity of the transplanted denervated human heart in vivo. Circulation 85:1056–1063

Willman VL, Cooper T, Hanlon CR (1964) Return of neural responses after autotransplantation of the heart. Am J Physiol 207:187–189

Wilson RF, Christensen BV, Olivari MT, Simon A, White CW, Laxson DD (1991) Evidence for structural sympathetic reinnervation after orthotopic cardiac transplantation in humans. Circulation 83:1210–1220

Ziegler SI, Frey AW, Uberfuhr P, Dambacher M, Watzlowik P, Nekolla S et al (1996) Assessment of myocardial reinnervation in cardiac transplants by positron emission tomography: functional significance tested by heart rate variability. Clin Sci (Lond) 91:126–128

Autonomic Imaging in Ventricular Arrhythmias

18

Alexis Vrachimis, Michael Schäfers, Lars Stegger, and Christian Wenning

Contents

Abstract

Ventricular arrhythmias may occur in cardiomyopathies, with often fatal consequences. Arrhythmias can occur during physical activity with sympathetic activation, for example, in the case of arrhythmogenic right ventricular cardiomyopathy/dysplasia (ARVC/D), or at rest with parasympathetic activation,

A. Vrachimis (✉) • M. Schäfers
Department of Nuclear Medicine, University Hospital Münster, Albert-Schweitzer-Campus 1, Building A1, Münster 48149, Germany

European Institute for Molecular Imaging, University of Münster, Mendelstraße 11, Building L1, 4th floor, Münster 48149, Germany
e-mail: vrachal@uni-muenster.de; schafmi@uni-muenster.de

L. Stegger • C. Wenning
Department of Nuclear Medicine, University Hospital Münster, Albert-Schweitzer-Campus 1, Building A1, Münster 48149, Germany
e-mail: stegger@uni-muenster.de; cwenning@uni-muenster.de

R.H.J.A. Slart et al. (eds.), *Autonomic Innervation of the Heart: Role of Molecular Imaging*, DOI 10.1007/978-3-662-45074-1_18

for example, in patients with Brugada syndrome. Medication with effect on the autonomous nervous system, most notably β-receptor blockers, can modulate the disease manifestations associated with arrhythmias such as syncopes. There is a strong clinical need to identify the optimal treatment strategy in a personalized manner. Molecular imaging of the autonomous nervous system may add valuable additional information. Radiopharmaceuticals targeting the presynaptic and postsynaptic portions of the sympathetic system for use with single-photon emission computed tomography (SPECT) and positron-emission tomography (PET) have seen the most widespread application; studies also targeting the parasympathetic function have started to appear. This chapter provides an overview over results obtained with these molecular imaging modalities so far.

Abbreviations

ARVC/D	Arrhythmogenic right ventricular cardiomyopathy/dysplasia
ARVD/C	Arrhythmogenic right ventricular dysplasia/cardiomyopathy
BS	Brugada syndrome
DCM	Dilated cardiomyopathy
ECG	Electrocardiogram
EP	Electrophysiological
HCM	Hypertrophic cardiomyopathy
HMR	Heart-to-mediastinum ratio
ICD	Implantable cardioverter–defibrillator
ILVT	Idiopathic left ventricular tachycardia
IVF	Idiopathic ventricular fibrillation
IVT	Idiopathic ventricular tachycardias
LQTS	Long QT syndrome
LV	Left ventricle
LVEF	Left ventricular ejection fraction
MQNB	Methylquinuclidinylbenzilat
PET	Positron-emission tomography
RVOT	Right ventricular outflow tract tachycardia
SPECT	Single-photon emission computed tomography
VF	Ventricular fibrillation
VT	Ventricular tachycardia

18.1 Introduction

Although less established in clinical practice than perfusion imaging, examination of the cardiac autonomous nervous system is of potential value. This may apply especially to arrhythmogenic diseases not associated with functional and anatomic changes detectable by conventional imaging. Both pre- and postsynaptic function of the sympathetic and parasympathetic nervous system are accessible by radiopharmaceutical techniques. At present, the sympathetic arm has received most attention. Presynaptic function of sympathetic innervation has been examined with the SPECT radiotracer [^{123}I]-metaiodobenzylguanidine ([^{123}I]-MIBG) and the PET radiotracer [^{11}C]-meta-hydroxyephedrine ([^{11}C]-mHED) in various ventricular disorders. (Both tracers behave similar to norepinephrine, the physiological neurotransmitter.) Whereas both, SPECT and PET, can depict regional inhomogeneities and uptake differences semiquantitatively, PEt allows for absolute quantification of presynaptic function. Many reports have shown evidence of the involvement of the sympathetic nervous system in various ventricular diseases as studied by molecular imaging.

Another objective of innervation imaging is to assess the parasympathetic arm of the autonomous nervous system. The parasympathetic nervous system uses acetylcholine as neurotransmitter with muscarinic receptors. [^{11}C]-methylquinuclidinylbenzilat ([^{11}C]-MQNB) is a radiotracer qualified to examine the parasympathetic arm of the heart nervous system.

There is increasing need for non-invasive identification of new and refinement of existing methods of risk stratification to particularly identify patients at risk for ventricular tachycardias and cardiac death. The following chapter summarizes the current knowledge about non-invasive imaging of the cardiac autonomous system in the setting of ventricular arrhythmias. A structural overview of the former and recent literature about cardiomyopathies, right and left ventricular tachycardias, Brugada syndrome, and Long QT syndrome, is given in the following chapter. Key publications concerning selected diseases are summarized in Table 18.1.

Table 18.1 Key publications concerning selected diseases

Disease	Tracer	Author
Dilated cardiomyopathy	[^{123}I]-MIBG	Zhao et al. (2001), Ohshima et al. (2005)
Hypertrophic cardiomyopathy	[^{123}I]-MIBG	Terai et al. (2003), Isobe et al. (2005)
Arrhythmogenic right ventricular dysplasia/cardiomyopathy (ARVD/C)	[^{123}I]-MIBG	Wichter et al. (1994), Paul et al. (2011)
	[^{11}C]-mHED + [^{11}C]-CGP	Wichter et al. (2000)
Right ventricular outflow tract tachycardia (RVOT)	[^{11}C]-mHED + [^{11}C]-CGP	Schäfers et al. (1998)
	[^{123}I]-MIBG	Schäfers et al. (1999)
Idiopathic ventricular tachycardias (IVT)	[^{123}I]-MIBG	Mitrani et al. (1993), Schäfers et al. (1999), Paul et al. (2006)
Brugada syndrome	[^{123}I]-MIBG	Wichter et al. (2002), Kies et al. (2004), Kawaguchi et al. (2006)
Long QT syndromes	[^{123}I]-MIBG	Chevalier et al. (2001), Kies et al. (2011)
	[^{11}C]-mHED	Mazzadi et al. (2003)

18.2 Cardiomyopathies

A cardiomyopathy is the measurable deterioration of the function of the myocardium for any reason, usually leading to heart failure; common symptoms are dyspnea (breathlessness) and peripheral edema (swelling of the legs). People with cardiomyopathy are often at risk of dangerous forms of irregular heart beat and sudden cardiac death. The most common form of inherited cardiomyopathy is dilated cardiomyopathy (DCM), while other forms like arrhythmogenic right ventricular dysplasia/cardiomyopathy (ARVD/C) are relatively rare. In the following section, we want to shine light on three major types of cardiomyopathies and to the role of imaging of cardiac sympathetic innervation and its impact in the clinical setting. Generally, cardiac [^{123}I]-MIBG uptake often decreases in patients with cardiomyopathies. This decrease could reflect abnormal cardiac sympathetic nervous function associated with cardiomyopathies (Yoshimura et al. 1998; Henderson et al. 1988). However, little is known about the relationship between cardiac autonomic disorders and the pathophysiology of cardiomyopathies, especially left ventricle (LV) function and perfusion.

18.2.1 Idiopathic Dilated Cardiomyopathy

Idiopathic DCM is characterized by left ventricular dilatation and impairment in myocardial (systolic and diastolic) function without significant coronary artery disease (Fuster et al. 1981; Kelly and Strawss 1994). Although advances in pharmacological treatments have shown beneficial effects in improving the prognosis in patients with DCM, many patients show a poor response to medical treatment; therefore, the prognosis in patients with advanced DCM is still poor. Thus, it is of particular importance to identify DCM patients with a poorer prognosis and who are, potentially, refractory to medical therapies. Imaging of the autonomous nervous system of the heart may therefore help to non-invasively identify those patients. In the following section, the most important data about cardiac autonomic imaging acquired in patients with DCM will be discussed.

Maeno et al. were one of the first who observed (with [^{123}I]-MIBG) regional sympathetic innervation defects in left ventricular myocardial regions with preserved perfusion in patients with idiopathic DCM. Moreover, they compared 11 DCM patients with a history of ventricular tachycardia (VT) with six patients without VT. Interestingly, the number of innervation defects was higher in the group of patients with VT (Maeno et al. 1993). These observations suggest a correlation between regional sympathetic denervation and the occurrence of VT in patients with DCM. Although the number of patients was very small, the authors hypothesize that cardiac sympathetic innervation imaging may help to identify patients at risk for the development of VT.

Zhao et al. studied 15 patients with DCM (and 18 patients with HCM) by cardiac [^{123}I]-MIBG and perfusion imaging. They compared parameters of [^{123}I]-MIBG imaging (uptake, washout) with LV perfusion and LV function assessed by [^{99m}]Tc-tetrofosmin SPECT imaging (Zhao et al. 2001). The study could show that washout and early uptake of [^{123}I]-MIBG were the most significant factors for predicting LV function and LV perfusion, respectively. Especially [^{123}I]-MIBG washout was closely correlated with LV function and could be a useful parameter reflecting LV function in patients with DCM. A study performed by Ohshima et al. confirmed these initial results but was especially focused on the correlation of cardiac sympathetic innervation and myocardial contractile reserve in patients with mild to moderate DCM. Twenty-four patients who showed sinus rhythm underwent echocardiography, biventricular catheterization, and myocardial [^{123}I]-MIBG scintigraphy. LV pressure was measured invasively by a micromanometer-tipped catheter and the myocardial contractile function was determined at rest and during predefined atrial pacing. Interestingly, there was a significant correlation between the delayed [^{123}I]-MIBG heart-to-mediastinum ratio (HMR) and the percentage change in LV myocardial contractile function from baseline to peak or critical heart rates. The delayed HMR was significantly lower in patients showing a worsening in LV contractile function than in those showing a favorable change (Ohshima et al. 2005). Recently, the same group postulated cardiac [^{123}I]-MIBG imaging for prediction of impairment in myocardial functional reserve in patients with DCM (Ohshima et al. 2013; Fig. 18.1). In summary, the results of all these studies consistently indicate a correlation of regional and/ or global cardiac innervation defects and poor LV function. Thus, in line with analysis of LV function, which is an important prognostic parameter by itself, imaging of the cardiac autonomous nervous system may also have an independent prognostic value with regard to the risk of VT development.

18.2.2 Hypertrophic Cardiomyopathy

Hypertrophic cardiomyopathy (HCM) is the most common genetic cardiovascular disorder. Although HCM may be asymptomatic in many cases, patients are basically at risk for the development of heart failure and sudden cardiac death. HCM is the leading cause of sudden cardiac death in young athletes in the United States (Barsheshet et al. 2011), although such events are rare with fewer than 100 deaths due to HCM in competitive athletes per year or about 1 death per 220,000 athletes (Maron et al. 2009).

Comparable to study results concerning DCM, several studies dealing with imaging of the cardiac sympathetic nervous system showed a correlation between impairment of cardiac sympathetic innervation and LV function (Matsuo et al. 2002). Nevertheless, some (distinct) differences were observed: Zhao et al. compared patients with DCM ($n=15$) and HCM ($n=18$) with healthy controls ($n=5$) (Zhao et al. 2001). The HMR (as a parameter for global cardiac innervation) in patients with HCM was significantly greater than in patients with DCM. On the contrary, no significant differences were found between normal healthy controls and HCM. On the other hand, results showed that regional [^{123}I]-MIBG washout was the most

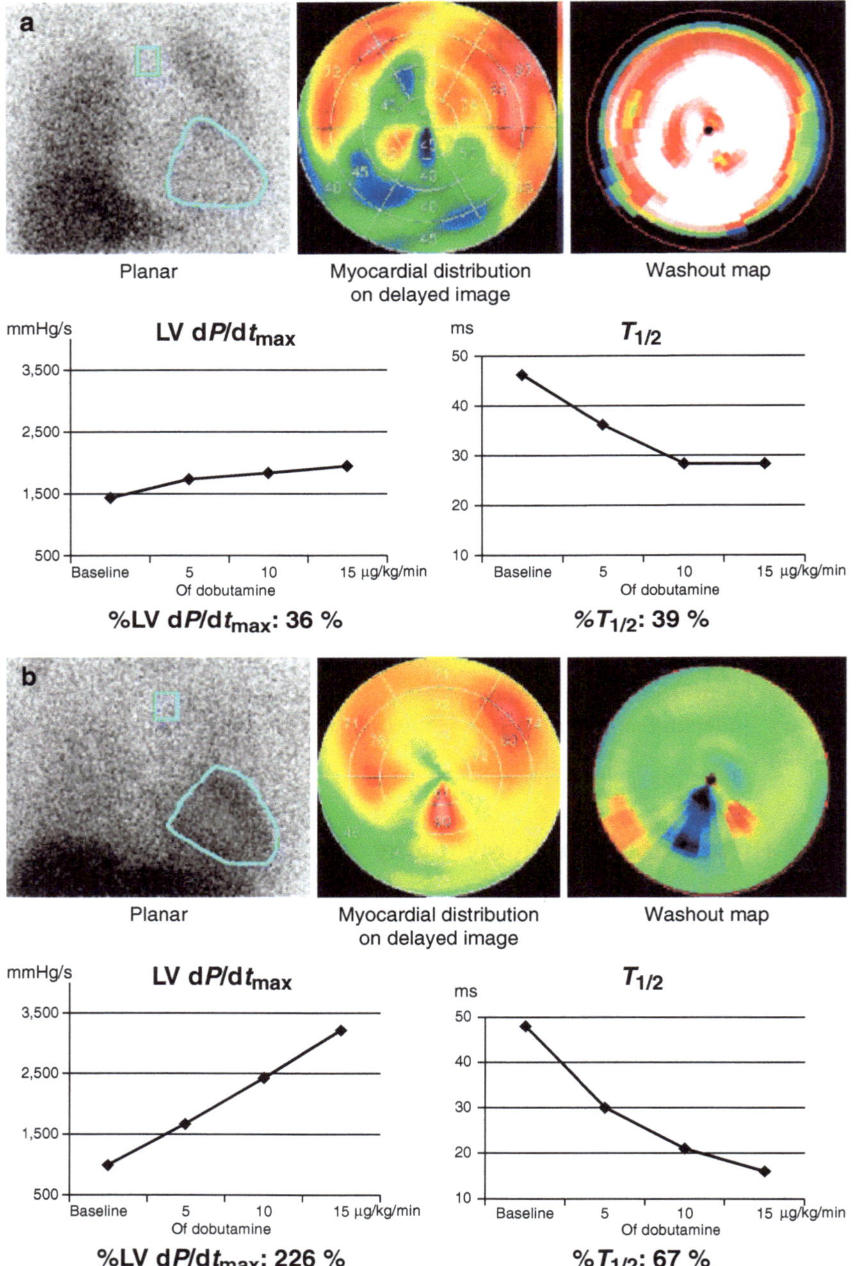

Fig. 18.1 Two typical cases of sympathetic nervous imaging in dilated cardiomyopathy. (**a**) A patient with markedly reduced cardiac uptake, globally increased washout of [^{123}I]-MIBG, and impaired inotropic, chronotropic, and lusitropic responses to β-adrenergic stimulation. (**b**) A patient with preserved cardiac uptake of [^{123}I]-MIBG shows a favorable change in heart rate and fair inotropic and lusitropic responses to β-adrenergic stimulation (Reprinted with kind permission of Springer Science and Business Media from Ohshima et al. (2013))

significant independent factor related to regional function both in DCM and HCM. These results may suggest that [^{123}I]-MIBG washout is more closely correlated with LV function and could be the more useful parameter reflecting LV function in patients with cardiomyopathies. Nevertheless, the authors stated that the relationship between [^{123}I]-MIBG imaging and LV function may vary in different diseases. Terai et al. performed cardiac [^{123}I]-MIBG SPECT in 46 patients with HCM and 18 age-matched control subjects (Terai et al. 2003). The patients were categorized into three groups: 28 patients with normal LV systolic function, 9 patients with LV systolic dysfunction, and 9 patients with LV systolic dysfunction and dilatation. The early [^{123}I]-MIBG uptake was significantly lower in the group with systolic dysfunction and dilatation than in the control group. The washout rate was progressively and significantly higher in the group with normal LV function over the group with systolic dysfunction to the group with systolic dysfunction and dilatation. Early regional uptake was found to decrease when going from the group with normal LV function to the group with dysfunction and dilatation. Especially in the latter regional [^{123}I]-MIBG uptake was significantly reduced predominantly in the interventricular septal wall, and regional washout rate was increased in the apex and lateral wall. The authors suppose that cardiac sympathetic nerve abnormalities in patients with HCM may advance with the development of LV systolic dysfunction and dilatation and that [^{123}I]-MIBG scintigraphy may be a useful tool for the evaluation of pathophysiologic changes in HCM. Another study performed by Isobe et al. showed that myocardial [^{123}I]-MIBG imaging may also non-invasively evaluate LV functional reserve in response to exercise in patients with nonobstructive HCM (Isobe et al. 2005).

Although these studies indicate a distinct correlation between findings in cardiac sympathetic innervation imaging and LV function, up to now, larger prospective studies with focus on the clinical outcome are still missing. On the basis of the currently available data, it still remains uncertain if cardiac sympathetic innervation imaging may also have a predictive value for the early detection of (functional) worsening of LV function in patients with HCM or if imaging results only reflect indirect effects caused by worsening of LV function.

18.2.3 Arrhythmogenic Right Ventricular Dysplasia/ Cardiomyopathy

Arrhythmogenic right ventricular dysplasia/cardiomyopathy (ARVD/C) is also one of the major causes of sudden death in the young. Characteristic localized or diffuse replacement of predominantly right ventricular myocardium by fibrous fatty tissue leads to global and regional right ventricular (and sometimes also left ventricular) dysfunction. Moreover, it causes a predisposition to life-threatening ventricular tachyarrhythmias (Marcus et al. 1982). The frequent provocation of ventricular tachycardia especially during exercise and the sensitivity toward catecholamines suggest an involvement of the sympathetic nervous system in the development and initiation of arrhythmias in patients with (ARVD/C). In principle, the problem is that arrhythmias originate from the right ventricle which cannot be imaged adequately by SPECT or PET. Nevertheless, cardiac imaging also revealed abnormal sympathetic innervation patterns of the left ventricle. In 1994, Wichter et al. were the first to describe an abnormal [^{123}I]-MIBG accumulation in the left ventricle (Wichter et al. 1994). Out of 48 ARVD/C patients who underwent [^{123}I]-MIBG SPECT, only 8 patients (17 %) showed a normal, homogeneous distribution of [^{123}I]-MIBG uptake, whereas 40 patients (83 %) demonstrated regional reductions or defects of tracer uptake. In 77 % of the cases, a polar map area of more than 15 % of the left ventricle was affected. In the majority (95 %) of the patients with an abnormal [^{123}I]-MIBG scan, a reduced tracer uptake was located in the basal posterior septal wall of the left ventricle. While perfusion abnormalities in the areas of [^{123}I]-MIBG defects were excluded by stress myocardial perfusion imaging and by normal coronary angiograms in all patients, the most important finding was that abnormalities in [^{123}I]-MIBG scans correlated (approximately) with the site of origin of ventricular tachycardia (=ventricular septum). The authors therefore hypothesize that cardiac sympathetic innervation imaging of the left ventricle may have implications for the early diagnosis (and for the choice of antiarrhythmic drugs in the treatment of arrhythmias) in ARVD/C patients. A few years later, the same working group also showed a reduced β-adrenergic receptor density in (8) patients with ARVD/C in comparison with (29) age-matched control subjects by PET using the tracer [^{11}C]-CGP-12177 (Wichter et al. 2000). Wichter et al. concluded that this finding is in line with their prior findings and may result from a secondary downregulation of β-adrenergic receptors after increased local synaptic norepinephrine levels caused either by increased sympathetic tone or as the result of impaired presynaptic catecholamine reuptake. On the basis of these initial findings, Paul et al. investigated 42 ARVD/C patients with [^{123}I]-MIBG SPECT and performed a clinical follow-up for 11.9 ± 4.1 years. They found that in patients with ARVD/C, an impairment of left ventricular adrenergic innervation (=abnormal left ventricular tracer uptake) was associated independently from the underlying genotype, with a higher incidence for future recurrences of ventricular tachyarrhythmias. These findings, so state the authors, may suggest a potential role of sympathetic innervation imaging for individualized risk stratification in ARVD/C patients (Paul et al. 2011; Fig. 18.2). Unfortunately, only late [^{123}I]-MIBG SPECT images 4 h post injection (p.i.) were performed, and regional washout rate (another important parameter for the appraisal of global cardiac sympathetic tone) was not assessed in this study.

Despite these promising initial results, the role of cardiac sympathetic innervation imaging and its potential implication for the arrhythmia profile among other methods of risk stratification (Sen-Chowdhry et al. 2010) in ARVD/C patients still remains to be elucidated by means of larger prospective trials.

18.2.4 Ischemic Cardiomyopathy

The role of cardiac sympathetic innervation imaging in the setting of (ischemic) heart failure is described in previous chapters. With regard to the inherited cardiomyopathies described above, a question of importance is whether patterns of cardiac sympathetic activity in ischemic and idiopathic cardiomyopathies are equal

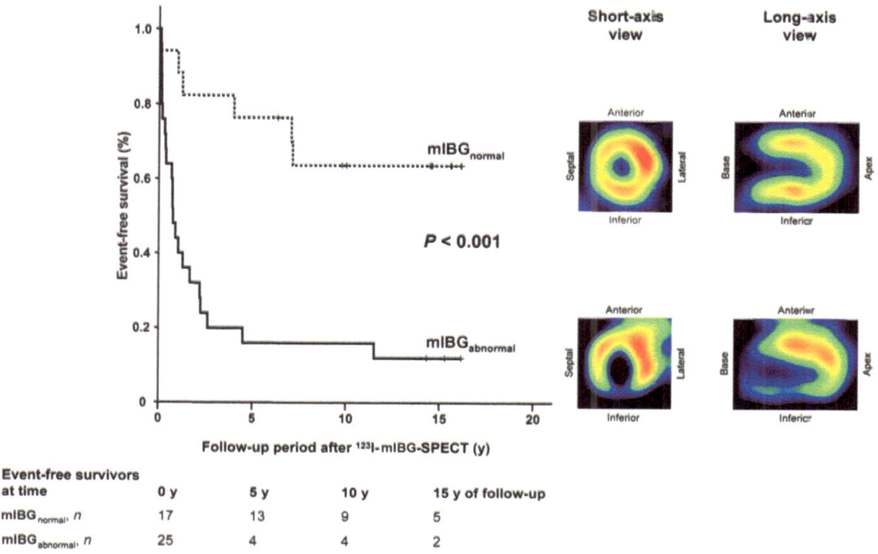

Fig. 18.2 Event-free survival (i.e., without sustained VT) during follow-up of a ARVD/C study population with normal (MIBG normal) vs. abnormal (MIBG abnormal) [^{123}I]-MIBG uptake with characteristic [^{123}I]-MIBG images (Reprinted from Paul et al. (2011))

and, if so, if they have equally prognostic value despite of the different underlying etiologies. After cardiac [^{123}I]-MIBG imaging, Wakabayashi et al. performed a prospective follow-up of 76 ischemic and 56 idiopathic cardiomyopathy patients for 54 months. Imaging data were compared with those obtained from 16 healthy volunteers (Wakabayashi et al. 2001). Late cardiac [^{123}I]-MIBG uptake (measured by HMR) turned out to be the most powerful independent predictor of a lethal clinical outcome in both ischemic and idiopathic cardiomyopathy patients, possibly indicating that both diseases have common pathophysiologic and prognostic implications of impaired cardiac sympathetic innervation, so state the authors.

In a multicenter pilot study, 50 patients with a history of myocardial infarction and left ventricular dysfunction (left ventricular ejection fraction LVEF $\leq$40 %) who were referred for a clinically indicated cardiac electrophysiological (EP) testing study because of syncope or non-sustained VT underwent cardiac [^{123}I]-MIBG (and myocardial perfusion) imaging (Bax et al. 2008). EP studies were categorized as positive (EP+) or negative (EP−) for inducibility of sustained (>30 s) ventricular tachyarrhythmias. While 30 patients were EP+ and 20 were EP−, there were no significant differences concerning global cardiac sympathetic innervation (measured by late HMR, 4-h p.i.) between the two groups. In a multivariable analysis, the only variable that showed a significant difference between EP+and EP- patients was the regional SPECT defect score (4 h p.i.), calculated semiquantitatively on the basis of a five-point scale in a 17-segment model of the left ventricle. A high defect score yielded a sensitivity of 77 % and specificity of 75 % for predicting EP results.

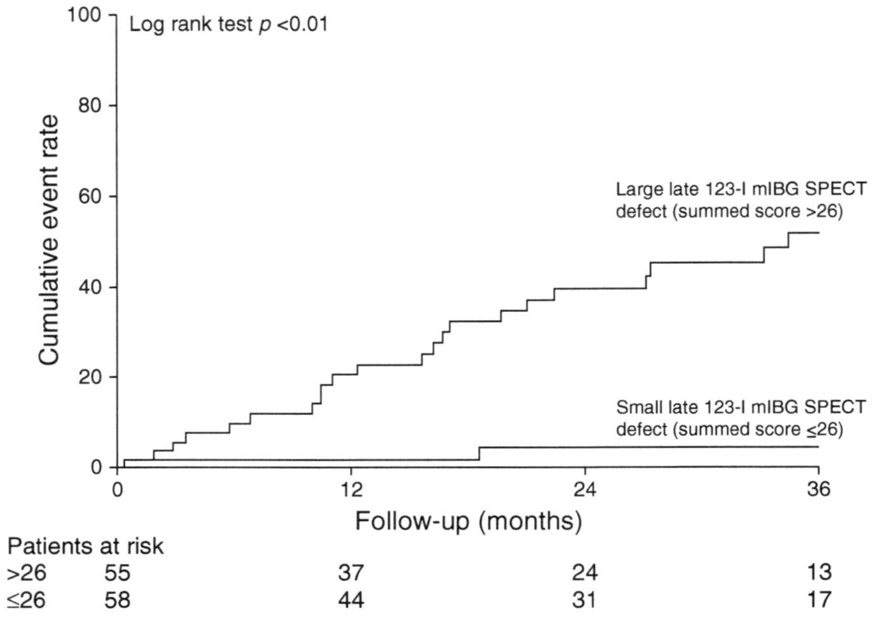

Fig. 18.3 Kaplan–Meier analysis of patients with ischemic cardiomyopathy with large or small late [^{123}I]-MIBG SPECT defects with regard to appropriate implantable cardioverter–defibrillator therapy (primary end point) (Reprinted with permission from Elsevier from Boogers et al. (2010))

Thus, the authors assume an association between [^{123}I]-MIBG SPECT defect severity and results of EP testing. Nevertheless, "classical" global parameters like HMR failed to show a correlation to EP testing.

More recently, Boogers et al. performed a study to evaluate whether cardiac [^{123}I]-MIBG imaging could predict ventricular arrhythmias causing appropriate implantable cardioverter–defibrillator (ICD) therapy and the composite of appropriate ICD therapy or cardiac death (Boogers et al. 2010). One hundred sixteen heart failure patients referred for ICD therapy were enrolled. Before ICD implantation, patients underwent [^{123}I]-MIBG (and myocardial perfusion) imaging. During a mean follow-up of 23 ± 15 months, appropriate ICD therapy (primary end point) was documented in 21 % of the patients and appropriate ICD therapy or cardiac death (secondary end point) in 28 % of the patients. Late [^{123}I]-MIBG SPECT defect score turned out to be an independent predictor for both end points. Patients with larger innervation defects showed significantly more appropriate ICD therapy and/or cardiac death than patients with smaller innervation defects (Fig. 18.3). In this context, regionally impaired sympathetic innervations (that is impaired catecholamine turnover and storage) in viable "border zones" of the myocardium after myocardial infarction may be of particular interest with regard to characterization of individual risk of ventricular arrhythmia as shown in an animal study (Sasano et al. 2008).

18.3 Arrhythmogenic Non-cardiomyopathy Diseases

18.3.1 Idiopathic Right Ventricular Outflow Tract Tachycardia

Idiopathic ventricular arrhythmias can originate in more than one area of the heart but are most common in the outflow tract area. Nearly 80 % of these arrhythmias originate from the right ventricular outflow tract and lead to right ventricular outflow tract tachycardia (RVOT) (Kim et al. 2007). Typically, RVOT occurs between the ages of 20 and 40 years and may have a slight female preponderance (Nakagawa et al. 2002). Patients may be asymptomatic but often present with palpitations, chest pain, dyspnea, pre-syncope, and even syncope. In general, outflow tract tachycardias occur more frequently with exertion or emotional stress. Long-term follow-up studies have provided evidence that the vast majority of patients do not develop structural heart disease or sudden cardiac death (Lemery et al. 1989). Typically, RVOT can be suppressed by anti-adrenergic drugs, which is suggestive of an involvement of the cardiac sympathetic nervous system in their pathophysiology (Zipes 1991). Similar to other cardiac diseases, global or regional alteration of the presynaptic function was also assumed in RVOT. On the basis of this hypothesis, Schäfers et al. studied eight patients with idiopathic RVOT and a total of 29 age-matched control subjects. Patients and control subjects were investigated by PET using [^{11}C]-meta-hydroxyephedrine ([^{11}C]-mHED) to assess presynaptic norepinephrine reuptake and [^{11}C]-CGP-12177 to measure postsynaptic β-adrenoceptor density (Schäfers et al. 1998). The major finding was that both myocardial presynaptic catecholamine reuptake and β-adrenoceptor density were significantly reduced in patients with idiopathic RVOT. These findings suggest that myocardial β-adrenoceptor downregulation in patients with RVOT occurs subsequently to increased local synaptic catecholamine levels caused by impaired catecholamine reuptake. Another study performed by the same group revealed that the majority of patients with RVOT ($n=27/45$; 60 %) presented with significant regional innervation ([^{123}I]-MIBG) defects localized in the posterior left ventricular wall, whereas patients with idiopathic left ventricular tachycardia (ILVT, $n=25$) did not (Schäfers et al. 1999). The two studies listed are initial observational studies. Up to now, no prospective studies dealing with the evaluation of a possible prognostic value of cardiac (sympathetic) innervation imaging in patients with RVOT exist.

18.3.2 Idiopathic Left Ventricular Fibrillation/Tachycardia

Idiopathic ventricular fibrillation (IVF) is defined as a VF in the absence of any identifiable structural or functional cardiac disease or laboratory findings and presents as syncope or sudden cardiac death in young people with normal hearts and no identifiable genetic syndrome. Idiopathic left ventricular tachycardias (ILVT) occur primarily due to reentry involving the fascicles of the left bundle branch, while three different subtypes exist. Patients are young, 15–40 years of age, and predominately men (>60 %). Tachycardias are usually paroxysmal, but incessant forms have also been described (Survivors of out-of-hospital cardiac arrest with apparently normal heart. Need for definition and standardized clinical evaluation 1997).

Firstly, Gill et al. described that patients with ILVT had a higher proportion of "asymmetrical" [^{123}I]-MIBG scans, particularly obvious in patients with exercise-induced VT, suggesting that patients with ILVT may have relative denervation in the septal portion of the left ventricle leading to an imbalance of the sympathetic supply/tone to the myocardium and locally imbalanced sympathetic or parasympathetic interactions (Gill et al. 1993).

In the same period, another study was published which showed that 55 % of the patients with ILVT had regional left ventricular sympathetic denervation – defined as myocardial areas having normal ^{201}Thallium uptake but reduced or absent [^{123}I]-MIBG uptake – compared with none of control patients without VT and structurally normal hearts (Mitrani et al. 1993).

In 1999, Schäfers et al. described locally reduced [^{123}I]-MIBG uptake in 33 % of ILVT patients and 68 % of IVF patients, representing a bull's-eye plot area of the left ventricle of approx. 25 and 24 %, respectively. Unlike ILVT patients, IVF patients had significantly reduced segmental [^{123}I]-MIBG uptake of the basal and midventricular parts of the posterior wall and the inferior septum compared with control patients (Schäfers et al. 1999).

In a follow-up study of the last patient cohort, the same group investigated the potential impact of sympathetic dysfunction by means of [^{123}I]-MIBG SPECT on the long-term prognosis of patients with IVF. In the follow-up scans, an abnormal [^{123}I]-MIBG uptake in 65 % of the patients with IVF was observed. Furthermore, during the follow-up time of 7.2 ± 1.5 years, 18 episodes of VF/fast polymorphic VT occurred in 30 % of the IVF patients with abnormal [^{123}I]-MIBG uptake whereas only two episodes of monomorphic ventricular tachycardia (and no VF) occurred in 14 % of IVF patients with a normal cardiac [^{123}I]-MIBG scan. Figure 18.4 shows the event-free survival in relation to the [^{123}I]-MIBG SPECT results with differences between IVF patients with normal and abnormal [^{123}I]-MIBG scans, indicating that impairment of sympathetic cardiac innervation may be a sign of a higher risk of future recurrent events in patients with IVF (Paul et al. 2006; Fig. 18.4). In this study, the patient population was small ($n = 20$), and therefore larger studies are required to validate the results with respect to event risk.

All these results suggest the involvement of the adrenergic system in the pathogenesis of these potentially life-threatening diseases and support the hypothesis that selective denervation of the human myocardium may be an important mechanism in the genesis of ventricular tachycardias in patients with "clinically normal" hearts.

18.3.3 Brugada Syndrome

The Brugada syndrome (BS) is a cardiac disorder characterized by ST-segment elevation in at least two of the leads V_1–V_3 with a typical coved morphology (referred to as type I Brugada ECG), which either arises spontaneously or is induced by administration of a sodium channel-blocking drug and is associated with an increased risk of sudden cardiac death affecting young people with structurally normal hearts (Brugada and Brugada 1992; Morita et al. 2008, Berne and Brugada 2012).

Regional sympathetic denervation or rather imbalances between the sympathetic and parasympathetic tone may play a role in the genesis of arrhythmias in BS patients. Thus, several studies have been launched to address this hypothesis.

Agostini et al. (1998) reported the first case of SPECT imaging in a patient with BS using [^{123}I]-MIBG, where innervation defects were found in the inferior, apical, and septal wall, thus providing for the first time imaging information about left ventricular dysinnervation in BS patients.

Wichter and colleagues (2002) addressed the subject once more using the same tracer. Moreover, they proceeded with a quantitative analysis. After hypothesizing that regional innervation defects may exist in patients with BS indicating cardiac autonomic dysfunction, investigation of the cardiac sympathetic innervation was performed in 17 patients with BS. They could demonstrate an abnormal [^{123}I]-MIBG uptake in 47 % of the patients, indicating presynaptic sympathetic dysfunction in the left ventricle (Fig. 18.5). In a 33-segment model of the left ventricle, [^{123}I]-MIBG uptake was reduced in the inferior and inferior septal wall. However, no correlation could be found between the results of [^{123}I]-MIBG SPECT and the clinical characteristics of the study patients (i.e., clinical events, induction of arrhythmias by the electrophysiological study, known familial predisposition, age, or gender).

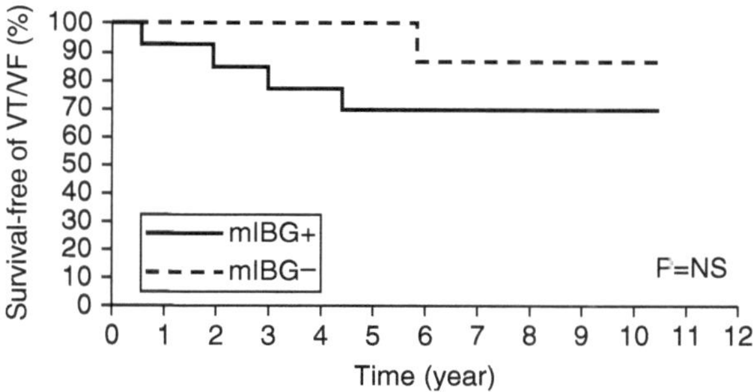

Fig. 18.4 Event-free survival after a normal (MIBG−) or abnormal (MIBG+) [^{123}I]-MIBG scan in patients with IVF. *VT* ventricular tachycardia, *VF* ventricular fibrillation, *y* years (With kind permission of Springer Science and Business Media from Paul et al. (2006))

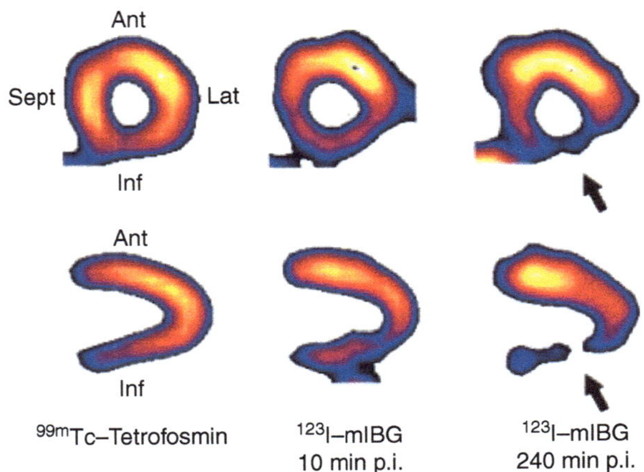

Fig. 18.5 Example of short-axis (*top*) and vertical long-axis (*bottom*) slices of cardiac [^{123}I]-MIBG SPECT (*middle and right columns*) and matching ^{99m}Tc-tetrofosmin SPECT (*left column*) in a patient with symptomatic BS. Locally reduced [^{123}I]-MIBG uptake is seen in the inferior and inferior lateral myocardial wall despite normal myocardial perfusion. *Ant* anterior, *Lat* lateral, *Inf* inferior, *Sept* septal wall (With kind permission of Wolters Kluwer Health from Wichter et al. (2002))

A Japanese group evaluated whether there are differences in cardiac [^{123}I]-MIBG scintigraphy between patients with BS divided according to the shape of their ST-segment elevation (coved type vs. saddleback type vs. controls). They observed that those patients with decreased accumulation or defects had a coved type ST-segment elevation. Moreover, the same group showed a decreased late heart-to-mediastinum ratio (3 h p.i.) and an increased washout rate (3 h vs. 15 min p.i), suggesting that the shape of the ST-segment elevation may be associated with the myocardial autonomic nervous function (Kawaguchi et al. 2006).

Kostopoulou et al. partially confirmed the results from the study of Wichter and colleagues. After quantitative analysis of the mean [^{123}I]-MIBG uptake in 13 segments of the left ventricle, they observed a lower uptake in the inferior wall. Furthermore, a lower uptake was also observed in the apical wall. On the other hand and perhaps contrary to the results from Kawaguchi, they did not find any differences regarding early and late heart-to-mediastinum ratios and washout between BS patients and controls (Kostopoulou et al. 2010).

With regard to cardiac [^{123}I]-MIBG imaging, it can be mentioned that according to the observations made, the reduction of left ventricular [^{123}I]-MIBG accumulation in BS patients can apparently be so severe that images show homogeneous absence of cardiac accumulation (Oyama et al. 2002). However, in this case report only a planar scintigraphy without SPECT technique was performed, making it practically impossible for the reader to distinguish between total absence and globally reduced myocardial uptake.

PET tracers have also been successfully applied for the investigation of the autonomous nervous system of patients with BS. In the most important study up to date,

Kies and colleagues have further investigated their previous observations made with SPECT and [^{123}I]-MIBG (Wichter et al. 2002) in patients with BS by non-invasive quantification of myocardial presynaptic and postsynaptic sympathetic function, using PET with [^{11}C]-mHED for the presynaptic norepinephrine recycling (by calculation of the volume of distribution (Vd) of [^{11}C]-mHED with the use of a single-tissue compartment model) and [^{11}C]-CGP for the myocardial adrenoceptor density (by use of a double-injection protocol) (Kies et al. 2004). They found that the volume of distribution (Vd, i.e., myocardial presynaptic catecholamine recycling) of [^{11}C]-mHED was globally increased in BS patients compared with normal control subjects, possibly due to a reduction of norepinephrine concentration in the synaptic cleft, yet without any regional differences between the four myocardial walls in the patients, who then all had significantly higher Vd values compared with control subjects. Furthermore, the myocardial adrenoceptor density in patients with BS was preserved and comparable to control subjects in all four left ventricular walls.

With regard to the regional differences, a potential limitation of this PET study and a possible explanation for the discrepancies seen between the two different acquisition techniques (PET vs. SPECT) could be the dynamic acquisition over a time period of 1 h after tracer injection, thus not being able to detect differences that would have been unmasked after a longer period of time, like, for example, 4 h p.i. due to a possible higher regional washout.

18.3.4 Long QT Syndrome

The long QT syndrome (LQTS) is characterized by abnormally prolonged repolarization that typically extends the corrected QT interval to more than 440 ms in men and 460 ms in women. At least 13 different genes involved in inherited LQTS have been identified, with the first 3 (LQT1, LQT2, and LQT3) accounting for more than 90 % of cases. Syncope, seizures, or cardiac arrest due to torsade de pointes ventricular tachycardia is the presenting symptom. In the cases of LQT1, arrhythmias typically occur during exertion and especially swimming, whereas in LQT2 they are often generated by emotional upset and acoustic stimulation. On the other hand, in cases of LQT3 events occur typically at rest or sleep (Roden 2008; Ackerman et al. 2011; John et al. 2012). In these syndromes timing and frequency of syncope, corrected QT-time prolongation, and sex were found to be predictive of risk for aborted cardiac arrest and sudden cardiac death during adolescence. Moreover β-blocker treatment was associated with a reduced risk among patients with recent syncope (Hobbs et al. 2006).

Back in 1991, Göhl and his team were the first to test the hypothesis of a specific sympathetic imbalance in members of LQTS families by means of [^{123}I]-MIBG SPECT. They found in their study population that all patients with a corrected QT time >440 ms; all who had suffered from at least one episode of torsade de pointes tachycardia, VF, or syncope; and all symptomatic patients with corrected QT-time prolongation had a reduced or abolished [^{123}I]-MIBG uptake in the inferior and inferior septal parts of the left ventricle (Göhl et al. 1991).

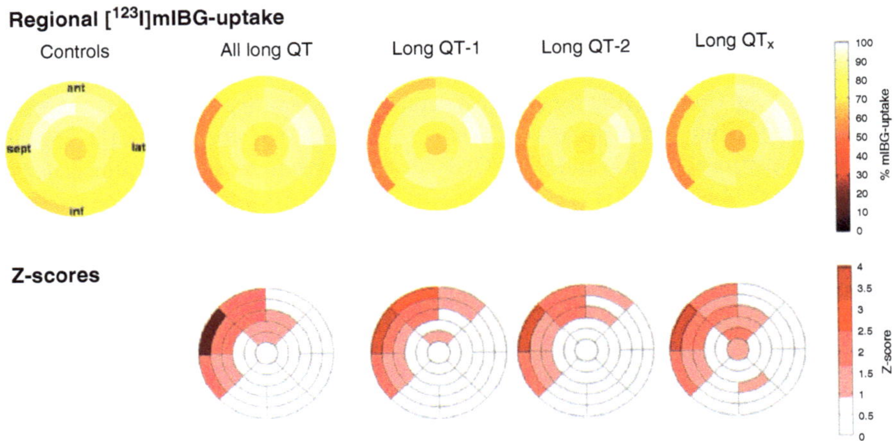

Fig. 18.6 Regional [^{123}I]-MIBG uptake in three LQTS subgroups of symptomatic patients ($n=28$) and in a healthy control group. *Upper row*: 33-segment bull's-eye display of the left ventricle showing the segmental [^{123}I]-MIBG uptake. *Lower row*: differences compared to the control group (z-score). Apical parts of the left ventricle are represented in the center whereas peripheral segments display basal regions (With kind permission of Springer Science and Business Media from Kies et al. (2011))

Chevalier et al. were able to confirm these results with regard to the regional abnormalities predominantly found in the inferior and inferior septal wall of the left ventricle. Moreover, they could demonstrate a global decrease in the sympathetic myocardial innervation with [^{123}I]-MIBG SPECT (Chevalier et al. 2001).

In a much later study with the largest number of genotyped LQTS patients, Kies et al. additionally tried to correlate the findings of cardiac [^{123}I]-MIBG scans with the underlying LQTS genotype. In this study, an abnormal [^{123}I]-MIBG scan was found in 17 of 28 (61 %) LQTS patients with a tracer reduction mainly located in the anterior septal segments of the left ventricle. This finding was independent of the genetic LQTS subtype (Fig. 18.6). In addition, no differences were found between LQTS patients with a corrected QT time >500 ms vs. <500 ms or those suffering from syncope vs. VF (Kies et al. 2011).

The herein observed anatomical location of reduced tracer uptake in the anterior septal segments of the left ventricle was quite different to that reported by Göhl and Chevalier (Göhl et al. 1991; Chevalier et al. 2001) who found a reduced tracer uptake in the inferior (septal) wall and to that by Momose et al. (1998) who could not detect any innervation defects in their cohort of 16 LQTS patients.

Furthermore, there are indications for a higher washout rate of [^{123}I]-MIBG in LQTS patients either regional (Yamanari et al. 2000) or global (as measured on planar view images) (Müller et al. 1993).

Using [^{11}C]-mHED PET, Mazzadi and coworkers detected heterogeneous tracer retention in the septal, anterior, and lateral walls of the left ventricle. The majority of LQTS patients showed a localized and decreased pattern of [^{11}C]-mHED retention (Mazzadi et al. 2003).

All of the studies listed/discussed above (either by SPECT or PET), dealing with cardiac sympathetic innervation imaging in patients with LQTS, have observational characters in rather small patient cohorts. Up to now, there is no larger clinical follow-up study investigating the clinical outcome of patients with LQTS.

References

Ackerman MJ, Priori SG, Willems S et al (2011) HRS/EHRA expert consensus statement on the state of genetic testing for the channelopathies and cardiomyopathies: this document was developed as a partnership between the Heart Rhythm Society (HRS) and the European Heart Rhythm Association (EHRA). Europace 13:1077–1109

Agostini D, Scanu P, Loiselet P et al (1998) Iodine-123-metaiodobenzylguanidine SPECT of regional cardiac adrenergic denervation in Brugada syndrome. J Nucl Med 39:1129–1132

Barsheshet A, Brenyo A, Moss AJ et al (2011) Genetics of sudden cardiac death. Curr Cardiol Rep 13:364–376

Bax JJ, Kraft O, Buxton AE et al (2008) 123 I-mIBG scintigraphy to predict inducibility of ventricular arrhythmias on cardiac electrophysiology testing: a prospective multicenter pilot study. Circ Cardiovasc Imaging 1:131–140

Berne P, Brugada J (2012) Brugada syndrome 2012. Circ J 76:1563–1571

Boogers MJ, Borleffs CJ, Henneman MM et al (2010) Cardiac sympathetic denervation assessed with 123-iodine metaiodobenzylguanidine imaging predicts ventricular arrhythmias in implantable cardioverter-defibrillator patients. J Am Coll Cardiol 55:2769–2777

Brugada P, Brugada J (1992) Right bundle branch block, persistent ST segment elevation and sudden cardiac death: a distinct clinical and electrocardiographic syndrome. A multicenter report. J Am Coll Cardiol 20:1391–1396

Chevalier P, Rodriguez C, Bontemps L et al (2001) Non-invasive testing of acquired long QT syndrome: evidence for multiple arrhythmogenic substrates. Cardiovasc Res 50:386–398

Fuster V, Gersh BJ, Giuliani ER et al (1981) The natural history of idiopathic dilated cardiomyopathy. Am J Cardiol 47:525–531

Gill JS, Hunter GJ, Gane J et al (1993) Asymmetry of cardiac [123I] meta-iodobenzyl-guanidine scans in patients with ventricular tachycardia and a "clinically normal" heart. Br Heart J 69:6–13

Göhl K, Feistel H, Weikl A et al (1991) Congenital myocardial sympathetic dysinnervation (CMSD)–a structural defect of idiopathic long QT syndrome. Pacing Clin Electrophysiol 14:1544–1553

Henderson EB, Kahn JK, Corbett JR et al (1988) Abnormal I-123 myocardial metaiodobenzylguanidine washout and distribution may reflect myocardial adrenergic derangement in patients with congestive heart cardiomyopathy. Circulation 78:1192–1199

Hobbs JB, Peterson DR, Moss AJ et al (2006) Risk of aborted cardiac arrest or sudden cardiac death during adolescence in the long-QT syndrome. JAMA 296:1249–1254

Isobe S, Izawa H, Iwase M et al (2005) Cardiac 123I-MIBG reflects left ventricular functional reserve in patients with nonobstructive hypertrophic cardiomyopathy. J Nucl Med 46:909–916

John RM, Tedrow UB, Koplan BA et al (2012) Ventricular arrhythmias and sudden cardiac death. Lancet 380:1520–1529

Kawaguchi T, Nomura M, Tujikawa T et al (2006) 123I-metaiodo-benzylguanidine myocardial scintigraphy in the Brugada-type ECG. J Med Invest 53:95–102

Kelly DP, Strawss AW (1994) Inherited cardiomyopathies. N Engl J Med 330:913–919

Kies P, Wichter T, Schäfers M et al (2004) Abnormal myocardial presynaptic norepinephrine recycling in patients with Brugada syndrome. Circulation 110:3017–3022

Kies P, Paul M, Gerss J et al (2011) Impaired cardiac sympathetic innervation in symptomatic patients with long QT syndrome. Eur J Nucl Med Mol Imaging 38:1899–1907

Kim RJ, Iwai S, Markowitz SM et al (2007) Clinical and electrophysiological spectrum of idiopathic ventricular outflow tract arrhythmias. J Am Coll Cardiol 49:2035–2043

Kostopoulou A, Koutelou M, Theodorakis G et al (2010) Disorders of the autonomic nervous system in patients with Brugada syndrome: a pilot study. J Cardiovasc Electrophysiol 21:773–780

Lemery R, Brugada P, Bella PD et al (1989) Nonischemic ventricular tachycardia: clinical course and long-term follow-up in patients without clinically overt heart disease. Circulation 79:990–999

Maeno M, Ishida Y, Shimonagata T et al (1993) The significance of 201Tl/123I MIBG (metaiodobenzylguanidine) mismatched myocardial regions for predicting ventricular tachycardia in patients with idiopathic dilated cardiomyopathy. Kaku Igaku 30:1221–1229

Marcus FI, Fontaine GH, Guiraudon G et al (1982) Right ventricular dysplasia: a report of 24 cases. Circulation 65:384–398

Maron BJ, Doerer JJ, Haas TS et al (2009) Sudden deaths in young competitive athletes: analysis of 1866 deaths in the United States, 1980–2006. Circulation 119:1085–1092

Matsuo S, Nakamura Y, Tsutamoto T et al (2002) Impairments of myocardial sympathetic activity may reflect the progression of myocardial damage or dysfunction in hypertrophic cardiomyopathy. J Nucl Cardiol 9:407–412

Mazzadi AN, André-Fouët X, Duisit J et al (2003) Cardiac retention of [11C]HED in genotyped long QT patients: a potential amplifier role for severity of the disease. Am J Physiol Heart Circ Physiol 285:1286–1293

Mitrani RD, Klein LS, Miles WM et al (1993) Regional cardiac sympathetic denervation in patients with ventricular tachycardia in the absence of coronary artery disease. J Am Coll Cardiol 22:1344–1353

Momose M, Kobayashi H, Kasanuki H et al (1998) Evaluation of regional cardiac sympathetic innervation in congenital long QT syndrome using 123I-MIBG scintigraphy. Nucl Med Commun 19:943–951

Morita H, Wu J, Zipes DP (2008) The QT syndromes: long and short. Lancet 372:750–763

Müller KD, Jakob H, Neuzner J et al (1993) 123I-metaiodobenzylguanidine scintigraphy in the detection of irregular regional sympathetic innervation in long QT syndrome. Eur Heart J 14:316–325

Nakagawa M, Takahashi N, Nobe S et al (2002) Gender differences in various types of idiopathic ventricular tachycardia. J Cardiovasc Electrophysiol 13:633–638

Ohshima S, Isobe S, Izawa H et al (2005) Cardiac sympathetic dysfunction correlates with abnormal myocardial contractile reserve in dilated cardiomyopathy patients. J Am Coll Cardiol 46:2061–2068

Ohshima S, Isobe S, Hayashi D et al (2013) Myocardial (123)I-MIBG scintigraphy predicts an impairment in myocardial functional reserve during dobutamine stress in patients with idiopathic dilated cardiomyopathy. Eur J Nucl Med Mol Imaging 40:262–270

Oyama N, Oyama N, Yokoshiki H et al (2002) Iodine-123-metaiodobenzylguanidine scintigraphy of total cardiac adrenergic denervation in Brugada syndrome. Jpn Heart J 43:183–186

Paul M, Schäfers M, Kies P et al (2006) Impact of sympathetic innervation on recurrent life-threatening arrhythmias in the follow-up of patients with idiopathic ventricular fibrillation. Eur J Nucl Med Mol Imaging 33:866–870

Paul M, Wichter T, Kies P et al (2011) Cardiac sympathetic dysfunction in genotyped patients with arrhythmogenic right ventricular cardiomyopathy and risk of recurrent ventricular tachyarrhythmias. J Nucl Med 52:1559–1565

Roden DM (2008) Clinical practice: long-QT syndrome. N Engl J Med 358:169–176

Sasano T, Abraham MR, Chang KC et al (2008) Abnormal sympathetic innervation of viable myocardium and the substrate of ventricular tachycardia after myocardial infarction. J Am Coll Cardiol 51:2266–2275

Schäfers M, Lerch H, Wichter T et al (1998) Cardiac sympathetic innervation in patients with idiopathic right ventricular outflow tract tachycardia. J Am Coll Cardiol 32:181–186

Schäfers M, Wichter T, Lerch H et al (1999) Cardiac 123I-MIBG uptake in idiopathic ventricular tachycardia and fibrillation. J Nucl Med 40:1–5

Sen-Chowdhry S, Morgan RD, Chambers JC et al (2010) Arrhythmogenic cardiomyopathy: etiology, diagnosis, and treatment. Annu Rev Med 61:233–253

Survivors of out-of-hospital cardiac arrest with apparently normal heart. Need for definition and standardized clinical evaluation. Consensus Statement of the Joint Steering Committees of the Unexplained Cardiac Arrest Registry of Europe and of the Idiopathic Ventricular Fibrillation Registry of the United States (1997). Circulation 95:265–272

Terai H, Shimizu M, Ino H et al (2003) Changes in cardiac sympathetic nerve innervation and activity in pathophysiologic transition from typical to end-stage hypertrophic cardiomyopathy. J Nucl Med 44:1612–1617

Wakabayashi T, Nakata T, Hashimoto A et al (2001) Assessment of underlying etiology and cardiac sympathetic innervation to identify patients at high risk of cardiac death. J Nucl Med 42:1757–1767

Wichter T, Hindricks G, Lerch H et al (1994) Regional myocardial sympathetic dysinnervation in arrhythmogenic right ventricular cardiomyopathy. An analysis using 123I-meta-iodobenzylguanidine scintigraphy. Circulation 89:667–683

Wichter T, Schäfers M, Rhodes CG et al (2000) Abnormalities of cardiac sympathetic innervation in arrhythmogenic right ventricular cardiomyopathy: quantitative assessment of presynaptic norepinephrine reuptake and postsynaptic beta-adrenergic receptor density with positron emission tomography. Circulation 101:1552–1558

Wichter T, Matheja P, Eckardt L et al (2002) Cardiac autonomic dysfunction in Brugada syndrome. Circulation 105:702–706

Yamanari H, Nakayama K, Morita H et al (2000) Effects of cardiac sympathetic innervation on regional wall motion abnormality in patients with long QT syndrome Heart 83:295–300

Yoshimura N, Kimura M, Ozaki T et al (1998) Two patients with hypertrophic cardiomyopathy showing regionally increased washout of 123I-MIBG from the thick myocardium. Kaku Igaku 35:315–320

Zhao C, Shuke N, Yamamoto W et al (2001) Comparison of cardiac sympathetic nervous function with left ventricular function and perfusion in cardiomyopathies by (123)I-MIBG SPECT and (99m)Tc-tetrofosmin electrocardiographically gated SPECT. J Nucl Med 42:1017–1024

Zipes DP (1991) Sympathetic stimulation and arrhythmias. N Engl J Med 325:656–657

Imaging Sympathetic Innervation of the Heart: Therapeutic Strategies SPECT/CT and PET/CT

19

Erick Alexanderson, Albert Flotats, and Luis Eduardo Juárez-Orozco

Contents

E. Alexanderson, MD (✉)
Cardiovascular Physiology, Universidad Nacional Autónoma de México, Ciudad de México, Mexico

Nuclear Cardiology Department, Instituto Nacional de Cardiología "Ignacio Chávez", Ciudad de México, Mexico
e-mail: alexandersonerick@gmail.com

A. Flotats, MD
Nuclear Medicine, Universitat Autònoma de Barcelona, Barcelona, Spain

Nuclear Medicine Department, Hospital de la Santa Creu i Sant Pau, Barcelona, Spain

L.E. Juárez-Orozco, MD
Unidad PET/CT Ciclotrón, Universidad Nacional Autónoma de México, Ciudad de México, Mexico

Department of Nuclear Medicine and Molecular Imaging, University Medical Center Groningen, University of Groningen, Groningen, The Netherlands

R.H.J.A. Slart et al. (eds.), *Autonomic Innervation of the Heart: Role of Molecular Imaging*, DOI 10.1007/978-3-662-45074-1_19

Abstract

Tracers for radionuclide imaging of cardiac neurotransmission have been developed by radiolabeling true neurotransmitters or corresponding structural analogs (false neurotransmitters). The most commonly used radiopharmaceuticals to assess cardiac neurotransmission are [^{11}C]-metahydroxyephedrine ([^{11}C]-mHED), [^{11}C]-ephedrine, [^{18}F]-dopamine, and [^{123}I]-metaiodobenzylguanidine ([^{123}I]-MIBG), which estimate neuronal presynaptic reuptake (type I uptake) and storage of norepinephrine (NE).

In heart failure (HF), there is impairment of the neuronal uptake of NE in the myocardium due to chronic sympathetic activation. Reduced myocardial uptake of these radiotracers is an indicator of poor prognosis for HF patients. Cardiac adrenergic imaging might be useful as an indicator of whether or not the HF patient's medical therapy is effective and could therefore help determine whether higher-risk and usually more expensive device therapies or cardiac transplantation is needed.

Abbreviations

ACEI	Angiotensin-converting enzyme inhibitor
ARB	Angiotensin receptor blocker
BMC	Bone marrow cell
BNP	Brain natriuretic peptide
CAD	Coronary artery disease
CRT	Cardiac resynchronization therapy
DCM	Dilated cardiomyopathy
DM	Diabetes mellitus
ECG	Electrocardiogram
EF	Ejection fraction
EPS	Electrophysiological studies
HF	Heart failure
HMR	Heart to mediastinum ratio
HRV	Heart rate variability
ICD	Implantable cardioverter defibrillator
LBBB	Left bundle branch block
LV	Left ventricular
LVEF	Left ventricular ejection fraction
MRA	Mineralocorticoid receptor antagonists
MUGA	Multiple gated acquisition
NE	Norepinephrine
NPV	Negative predictive value
NYHA	New York Heart Association
PET	Positron emission tomography
RBBB	Right bundle branch block
SCA	Sudden cardiac arrest

SCD	Sudden cardiac death
SPECT	Single-photon emission computed tomography
STEMI	ST-segment elevation myocardial infarct
VT	Ventricular tachycardia
WR	Washout rate

19.1 Introduction

The autonomic nervous system represents an important determinant of cardiac function in health and disease. There are pathological conditions such as ischemia, dilated cardiomyopathy, and heart failure that show important alterations within this system as previous and ongoing research has demonstrated.

Sympathetic innervation of the myocardium is widely distributed. Adrenergic terminals for the heart originate from the cervical ganglion and follow two main pathways. The first aims toward the atrial and ventricular "nonconducting myocardium," and the second one provides to the sinoatrial node and conduction system. Both can determine subtle changes in the myocardial performance within different segments and in a global fashion as well. Norepinephrine constitutes the main neurotransmitter within these synapses, since epinephrine acts mainly in an endocrine way.

The autonomic nervous system determines homeostatic responses to organic demands. It influences inotropism and chronotropism as noted by the heart rate variability.

Importantly, the autonomic terminals are distinctively suceptible to pathological processes. This explains the benefit of their evaluation for diagnostic and prognostic purposes (Cohn and Rector 1988; Rector et al. 1987).

Nowadays, nuclear imaging modalities such as single-photon emission computed tomography (SPECT) and positron emission tomography (PET) are able to evaluate the myocardial nervous system's regional and global distribution in vivo. This is achieved through the utilization of a number of carbon-11-, fluorine-18-, bromine-76-, and iodine-123-labeled tracers, which assess the NE uptake within the presynaptic detail. These radiotracers arise from the labeling of different catecholamines, catecholamine analogs (derived from NE or guanethidine), and receptor ligands. Some of the main advantages of catecholamine analogs are their increased metabolic stability and decreased affinity for receptor proteins. The most commonly used radiopharmaceuticals for cardiac neurotransmission are [^{123}I]-metaiodobenzylguanidine ([^{123}I]-MIBG) for SPECT and [^{11}C]-metahydroxyephedrine ([^{11}C]-mHED), [^{11}C]-ephedrine, [^{11}C]-adrenaline, and [^{18}F]-fluorodopamine for PET scanning.

The greatest experience has been obtained with the study of [^{123}I]-MIBG, which, as will be mentioned, has consistently demonstrated power to stratify risk in patients with congestive heart failure. Global cardiac uptake has shown an inverse correlation with cardiac events, yielding a high negative predictive value (NPV) with outcomes as death and arrhythmias. [^{123}I]-MIBG scans have been performed also in patients following cardiac transplantation, primary arrhythmias, coronary artery disease (CAD), diabetes mellitus (DM), and cardiotoxic chemotherapy.

PET scanning has also been established for cardiac autonomic innervation assessment. It is true that PET conveys higher methodological demands as well as less general availability. Nevertheless, high spatial and temporal resolution together with sequential attenuation correction considerably improves the quality of the scans and, therefore, of the information they provide us with. Moreover, PET radiotracers will include probably more physiologic compounds to assess presynaptic as well as postsynaptic innervation. All of this makes PET an appealing method for innervation assessment.

Adrenergic activation represents an important regulatory mechanism in cardiac function. For example, this activation serves as an initial adaptation when cardiac function decreases in heart failure of any etiology. Therefore, adrenergic function assessment can provide with earlier diagnosis over other anatomic-functional techniques. Chronic adrenergic activation conveys alterations of the NE local kinetics showing a decreased uptake of the previously mentioned radiotracers. This phenomenon is attributed to the desensitization of B_1 adrenergic receptors in heart failure (Knuuti and Sipola 2005). In the same way sympathetic tissue appears to be very sensitive to ischemia, this is suspected by observations in which patients present cardiac denervation in a more extensive area surrounding infarcted tissue, accounting for acute or chronic ischemic tissue (area at risk of myocardial ischemia) (Matsunari et al. 2000). This has been important in the increased arrhythmogenic sensibility of viable denervated myocardium.

19.2 Cardiac Adrenergic Imaging in Patients with HF

Improvement of medical therapy and outcome of HF is of main concern because of the progressive increase in its prevalence and incidence in the western world. The objectives in the management of HF are to relieve symptoms and signs, prevent hospital admission, and improve survival. The relief of symptoms and signs has not been the primary outcome in most trials because of its difficult measurement: the severity of symptoms typically fluctuates even in the absence of changes in medications. At the same time, changes in medications (Schwaiger et al. 1990) and diet can have either favorable or adverse effects on functional capacity without concomitant measurable changes in left ventricular (LV) function (Hunt et al. 2009). Moreover, some treatments previously shown to improve these outcomes also decreased survival. On the other hand, decrease in mortality and hospitalization rates reflects the ability to slow or prevent progressive worsening of HF, which is often accompanied by reverse LV remodeling and a reduction in circulating natriuretic peptide concentrations.

Two neurohumoral antagonists are critical in reducing the risk of HF hospitalizations and increasing survival, apart from improving symptoms and exercise capacity: β-blockers and angiotensin-converting enzyme inhibitors (ACEI or, if not tolerated, angiotensin receptor blockers (ARB)). They should at least be considered in every patient with HF and LV ejection fraction (EF) ≤40 %, starting as early as possible in the course of disease. ACEI are also of benefit in patients with asymptomatic LV systolic dysfunction (NYHA class I). Mineralocorticoid receptor antagonists (MRA), another type of neurohormonal antagonists, have also shown to improve symptoms, reduce the risk of HF hospitalization, and increase survival and are potentially indicated in all patients with persisting symptoms (NYHA classes II–IV) and a left ventricular ejection fraction (LVEF) ≤35 % despite treatment with β-blockers and ACEI (or ARB). Commonly, diuretics are added irrespective of LVEF to relieve the symptoms and signs of congestion, although their effects on mortality and morbidity have not been studied (McMurray et al. 2012).

19.3 Cardiac Adrenergic Imaging and Pharmacological Treatment

The benefits of treatments that ameliorate the effects of neurohumoral imbalance in patients with HF are well established. As clinical status and/or LV function improves in response to β-blockers, ACEI or ARB, and MRA, there is a parallel improvement in cardiac sympathetic nerve function as assessed by [^{123}I]-MIBG, supporting the concept that a restoration of cardiac neuronal uptake of NE is one of the beneficial effects of such a treatment in these patients (Kasama et al. 2003, 2005, 2007; Gerson et al. 2002; Agostini et al. 2000; Cohen-Solal et al. 2005; Takeishi et al. 1997; Somsen et al. 1996; Gilbert et al. 1993; Suwa et al. 1997; Fukuoka et al. 1997).

Gerson and coworkers studied the effect of chronic carvedilol treatment in patients with HF and cardiac sympathetic nerve dysfunction of varying severity due to idiopathic cardiomyopathy (Gerson et al. 2002). Most patients showed a favorable response in LV function to the treatment, regardless of the baseline level of cardiac sympathetic nervous system function, as assessed by cardiac [^{123}I]-MIBG imaging. Patients with relatively advanced cardiac sympathetic dysfunction (baseline heart to mediastinum ratio (HMR) <1.40 in [^{123}I]-MIBG studies) were the most likely to show evidence of improved cardiac sympathetic nervous system function in response to carvedilol treatment. Conversely, Suwa and coworkers showed in a study that in patients treated with bisoprolol (β_1-specific blocker), only those patients who showed a late HMR >1.7 had a significant improvement in LV size and clinical status (sensitivity of 91 % and specificity of 92 % for predicting response to β-blocker therapy) (Suwa et al. 1997). Other studies showing improvement of cardiac [^{123}I]-MIBG uptake in response to β-blocker treatment did not show any relationship between the severity of baseline cardiac [^{123}I]-MIBG uptake and subsequent improvement in adrenergic function (Rispler et al. 2013; Lotze et al. 2001). The discordance between these studies may reflect the different properties of various β-blockers.

Nakata et al. compared 88 HF patients treated with β-blockers and ACEI with 79 HF patients treated conventionally without β-blockers and ACEI during a follow-up of 43 months, with cardiac death as the primary endpoint (Nakata et al. 2005). Forty-two cardiac deaths occurred. The prevalence of cardiac death was significantly lower in patients treated with β-blockers and/or ACEI as compared with the control group (15 % vs. 37 %). After patients were divided into two groups by applying a threshold value of 1.53 for the late HMR (which was the median of the late HMR in patients with cardiac death), it was shown that treatment with β-blockers and/or ACEI significantly reduced the risk of death from 36 to 12 % if the HMR was ≥1.53. If the HMR was <1.53, the risk of death was decreased from 53 to 37 %. Survival in the patients treated with β-blockers and/or ACEI remained dependent on the severity of impairment of cardiac [^{123}I]-MIBG activity.

Aldosterone prevents the uptake of NE and promotes structural remodeling of the heart. Spironolactone, an aldosterone receptor blocker, improves LV remodeling in patients with dilated cardiomyopathy (DCM). Kasama and coworkers compared two groups of patients with DCM on ACEI and loop diuretic treatment as well as the addition of spironolactone only in one group (Kasama et al. 2003). After 6 months of treatment with spironolactone, the late HMR of [^{123}I]-MIBG and LVEF significantly increased, and the late total defect score as well as the washout rate (WR) of [^{123}I]-MIBG significantly decreased, with parallel reduction of the LV end-diastolic volume. There were no significant changes in these parameters in the group not receiving spironolactone. Moreover, a significant correlation between changes in the [^{123}I]-MIBG kinetics and changes in LV end-diastolic volume with spironolactone treatment was found. The functional class improved in both groups but was superior in the spironolactone group, which indicates the beneficial effect of spironolactone on cardiac sympathetic activity and LV remodeling.

The Task Force for the Diagnosis and Treatment of Acute and Chronic Heart Failure 2012 of the European Society of Cardiology has stated that amiodarone may be considered for controlling the ventricular rate in patients with symptomatic HF (NYHA functional classes II–IV), persistent/permanent atrial fibrillation, and no evidence of acute decompensation who are unable to tolerate a β-blocker or digoxin (class of recommendation IIb, level of evidence C). It is also recommended in HF patients with an implantable cardioverter defibrillator (ICD), who continue to have symptomatic ventricular arrhythmias or recurrent shocks despite optimal treatment and device reprogramming (class of recommendation I, level of evidence C). Moreover, amiodarone may be considered as a treatment to prevent recurrence of sustained symptomatic ventricular arrhythmias in otherwise optimally treated patients in whom an ICD is not considered appropriate (class of recommendation IIb, level of evidence C) (McMurray et al. 2012). It is unclear how amiodarone exerts its effects on LV remodeling and cardiac sympathetic nerve function in HF, but it is the only antiarrhythmic that should be used in patients with systolic HF. Toyama et al. (2004) in a prospective 1-year cohort study compared amiodarone to β-blockers in the treatment of patients with idiopathic DCM, reporting similar improvement in cardiac symptoms, function, and sympathetic nerve activity with both drugs. Tachikawa et al. reported that long-term amiodarone treatment on a rat model of DCM (healed cardiac myosin-induced autoimmune myocarditis) prevented LV remodeling, improved cardiac function, and restored cardiac sympathetic tone (late HMR increased, and WR decreased) to hold NE in the heart (Tachikawa et al. 2005).

Matsui et al. in a study of 85 consecutive patients with DCM and LVEF <45 % sought to assess whether repeated measurement of cardiac [^{123}I]-MIBG imaging before and after optimized treatment was useful for predicting prognosis (Matsui et al. 2002). Although there was no difference between the baseline HMR between survivors and nonsurvivors, the HMR was significantly decreased in nonsurvivors after 6 months. High plasma concentration of brain natriuretic peptide (BNP) after 6 months and absolute changes in the HMR were independent predictors of mortality. Likewise, Kasama and colleagues, taking into account that [^{123}I]-MIBG imaging improves by the current medical treatment for HF, analyzed the usefulness of serial [^{123}I]-MIBG studies for prognostication in 208 patients with stabilized mild-to moderate HF and LVEF <45 %, of both ischemic and nonischemic origin (Kasama et al. 2008). [^{123}I]-MIBG and echocardiographic studies were performed once patients were stabilized and after 6 months of treatment, which included ACEI, ARB, β-blockers, loop diuretics, and spironolactone. Treatment did no change during the follow-up. Fifty-six patients experienced fatal cardiac events during the study period (13 died from sudden cardiac death (SCD)). Clinical characteristics were similar in both noncardiac death and cardiac death groups, and only the use of β-blockers in the noncardiac death group was significantly higher than in the cardiac death group. The variation in the WR between the sequential [^{123}I]-MIBG studies, which was lower in the noncardiac than in the cardiac death group, was the only independent predictor of cardiac death. Therefore, it is possible that patients showing worsening of cardiac adrenergic imaging on serial studies would need additional or alternate therapies, such as devices, to improve outcome.

Despite this entire evidence showing that cardiac [^{123}I]-MIBG uptake improves in response to known effective HF medication, it remains to be proven whether such changes in populations of HF patients will be paralleled by demonstrable changes in response to drug dose changes in individual HF patients. In addition, it remains unknown whether patients with HF and LVEF ≤40 % randomized to [^{123}I]-MIBG-guided medical treatment have better outcome than patients treated following current practice guidelines.

19.4 Cardiac Adrenergic Imaging in Predicting Effect of Pharmacological Treatment

The ESC 2012 guidelines consider there is currently no potential advantage of cardiac adrenergic imaging to monitor the response to proven therapy in patients who respond well to HF therapy with full therapeutic doses of β-blockers, ACEI or ARB, and MRA (McMurray et al. 2012). However, despite that these agents have provided substantial benefits for HF patients in clinical trials, it is not clear if results would be the same when used at lower doses than those used in the major clinical trials.

Many patients with HF do not receive full, proven-to-be-effective HF drug dosing due to concerns about resultant side effects. Therefore, inadequate drug dosing may be a common problem faced when trying to optimize HF therapy. This is particularly true for agents that need to be introduced by slow up-titration aimed for target dose or, failing that, the highest tolerated dose. This suggests a potentially important role for testing that could provide a metric to determine which drug and dose are the best in a particular patient who does not tolerate full therapeutic doses.

Elevated plasma NE levels are associated with increased sympathetic nervous system function and unfavorable outcomes in HF patients (Cohn et al. 1984). Serial measurements might provide a method for assessing the response of the sympathetic nervous system to selection and dosing of HF medications, but have not entered into daily clinical practice. Plasma NE levels are altered by a wide variety of physical and emotional stimuli that affect NE release, as well as changes in cardiac output and regional blood flow that vary the rate of removal of NE from the plasma (Esler and Kaye 2000). Heart rate variability (HRV) by Holter monitoring is an indirect method for assessing cardiac sympathetic nerve activity and has been associated with HF outcomes in several studies (Nolan et al. 1998). Reduced HRV reflects sympathetic autonomic activity but requires the presence of sinus rhythm and is influenced by multiple variables including ventricular extrasystoles, parasympathetic tone, chemoreceptor function, respiratory rate and tidal volume, posture and mechanical factors (e.g., stretch of the atria from changes in cardiac filling and thoracic pressure), and level of physical activity. In addition, there are technical drawbacks in HRV measurement for its clinical adoption to adjust medical therapy. Imaging the response of cardiac sympathetic nerve function to therapy may provide this type of metric.

Furthermore, cardiac adrenergic imaging may have a role in differentiating patients likely to benefit from medical therapy from those that are likely to show poor long-term response and thus might be better candidates for nonmedical therapy (e.g., device therapy and cardiac transplantation). In addition, cardiac adrenergic imaging may help identify patients in whom aggressively increasing medical therapy despite mild side effects might produce a more favorable clinical outcome. Despite that the symptomatic response of patients is difficult to measure, it may determine the treatment endpoint in some of them but may be useless in patients who remain asymptomatic or minimally symptomatic. Cardiopulmonary exercise testing, with measurement of maximum oxygen consumption (VO_2 max), and the 6-min walk test are well-validated and accepted procedures for measuring the functional response to HF treatment and constitute important comparators for future studies to assess a potential role of serial cardiac adrenergic imaging in the assessment of clinical response to modifications in HF therapy.

19.5 Cardiac Adrenergic Imaging in Patients with HF on Nonsurgical Device Treatment

Prevention of sudden death is an important target in HF since about 50 % of mortality occurs suddenly and unexpectedly (especially in patients with milder symptoms). Mainly, mortality is related to ventricular arrhythmias (other causes may be related to bradycardia and asystole) (Francis 1986). While β-blockers, ACEI or

ARB, and MRA reduce the risk of sudden death, they do not eradicate it. In addition, specific antiarrhythmic drugs not only do not decrease this risk but also increase it. For this reason, ICD are important to reduce the risk of death from ventricular arrhythmias.

ICD reduce mortality in survivors of cardiac arrest and in patients with sustained symptomatic ventricular arrhythmias. Therefore, an ICD is recommended in the secondary prevention of such patients, irrespective of LVEF, with good functional status and a life expectancy of >1 year. An ICD is also recommended in the primary prevention of patients with symptomatic HF and good functional status (NYHA classes II–III), a life expectancy of >1 year, and LVEF ≤35 % despite ≥3 months of optimal pharmacological treatment. In these last patients, recommendations derive largely from four large randomized trials (MADIT-2, DINAMIT, DEFINITE, and SCD-HeFT) (Moss et al. 1996; Hohnloser et al. 2000; Kadish et al. 2004; Bardy et al. 2005) from which LVEF ≤30–35 % became a principal variable for deciding who should receive a device. However, >50 % of HF patients who die suddenly have a LVEF >30 % (Kelesidis and Travin 2012). Other different independent univariate predictors of SCD have been identified (low NYHA class, unsustained ventricular tachycardia (VT), and inducibility of VT in electrophysiological studies (EPS)), but their positive predictive value is low; thus, better individual risk assessment is needed to select patients with HF who are candidates for ICD placement, most of all considering that the cost for a device is about €20,000 (not including ICD follow-up costs).

An association between cardiac autonomic innervation abnormalities and SCD has been shown by different means such as the analysis of HRV and measurement of baroreflex sensitivity (Barron and Viskin 1998). The predictive value of HRV alone is modest but can improve significantly when combined with other non-invasive markers. However, the combination of additional non-invasive markers and optimal cutoff points of HRV to achieve maximum predictive capacity has yet to be defined. In addition, it remains difficult to adopt HRV in routine clinical practice mainly because of measurement reliability issues. Principal limitations of the measure of baroreflex sensitivity include the need to measure systolic blood pressure beat by beat and the difficulty of defining threshold values for use in clinical practice.

Impaired cardiac adrenergic imaging has been described in most of the disorders that result in LV dysfunction and potentially lethal ventricular arrhythmias, thus indicating its potential use to specifically predict the likelihood of fatal ventricular tachyarrhythmia, identifying those patients who would benefit most from an ICD. Although the explanation for the association between abnormalities of sympathetic innervation and the occurrence of potentially lethal ventricular arrhythmias is unclear, it is possible that denervated but still viable myocardium would either be hyperresponsive to circulating catecholamines or prone to the development of reentrant VT circuits.

Arora et al. assessed the combined predictive value of [^{123}I]-MIBG cardiac imaging and spectral analysis of HRV in predicting ICD discharges in 17 patients (Arora et al. 2003). They described more extensive [^{123}I]-MIBG defects and greater

[^{123}I]-MIBG/[^{99m}Tc]-sestamibi mismatch among patients who experienced ICD discharges. Nagahara et al. investigated during a 15-month follow-up period if cardiac [^{123}I]-MIBG imaging abnormalities were related to lethal cardiac events, defined as an appropriate ICD discharge against potentially fatal ventricular tachyarrhythmia in 54 patients who had received an ICD based on published indications (Nagahara et al. 2008). The occurrence of an ICD discharge strongly correlated with late HMR, independently of several other variables including LVEF that did not achieve statistical significance on multivariate analysis. The combination of late HMR and LVEF or BNP gave additional predictive power. From receiver-operating characteristic analysis, event predictive thresholds for late HMR (1.95), LVEF (50 %), and BNP (187 pg/mL) were obtained. Sensitivity, specificity, and positive and negative predictive values of combining the HMR and LVEF thresholds were 67, 70, 58, and 77 %, respectively. Combining the HMR and BNP thresholds, these values were of 45, 94, 82, and 73 %, respectively.

In a phase 2, open-label, multicenter study that enrolled 50 patients with LV dysfunction and previous myocardial infarction, Bax et al. found that late [^{123}I]-MIBG SPECT defect score was the only variable which showed a significant difference between patients with and without positive EPS (Bax et al. 2008). A late [^{123}I]-MIBG SPECT defect score of ≥37 yielded a sensitivity of 77 % and specificity of 75 % for predicting EPS results. The standard indices of [^{123}I]-MIBG imaging (HMR and innervation-perfusion mismatch score) were not predictive of EPS results, suggesting that such indices may not be sensitive enough to stratify the arrhythmic risk in patients with ischemic LV dysfunction. Recently, Tamaki et al. prospectively compared the predictive value of MIBG imaging for SCD with that of the signal-averaged electrocardiogram (ECG), HRV, and QT dispersion in 106 patients with chronic stable HF (LVEF <40 %) (Tamaki et al. 2009). After a follow-up of 65±31 months, 38 patients died (79 % cardiac death, 47 % SCD). Only WR and LVEF were significantly and independently associated with SCD.

In the multicenter ADMIRE-HF trial, a subgroup of 86 patients (9 %) had an arrhythmic event or SCD (12 patients had self-limited VT, 6 patients were resuscitated from cardiac arrest, 45 patients received appropriate ICD discharges, and 23 patients suffered SCD). Arrhythmia was significantly more common in patients with HMR <1.60 than in patients with HMR ≥1.60 (10.4 % vs. 3.5 %) (Jacobson et al. 2010). A very high negative predictive value of HMR was documented with respect to cardiac death or cumulative arrhythmic events, which confirmed data from previous studies in less consistent populations. Moreover, [^{123}I]-MIBG cardiac imaging confirmed an independent prognostic capability that is complementary to other commonly used markers such as LVEF and BNP.

More recently Nishisato et al. quantified cardiac [^{123}I]-MIBG uptake in 60 patients with ICD who were prospectively followed for a mean of 29 months, with endpoints of appropriate ICD shocks or cardiac death (Nishisato et al. 2010). ICD shock was documented in 30 patients (50 %); three cardiac deaths also occurred in this group of patients. Patients with a late HMR ≤1.9 and a summed score ≥12 had a significantly greater ICD discharge rate than did those who had a late HMR >1.90 and a summed score <12 (94 % vs. 18 %). This latter combination was associated with a hazard ratio of 3.8 and resulted independent and better predictor than age, sex, signal-averaged ECG, BNP, medications, inducible arrhythmias, and LVEF in predicting ICD shocks or cardiac death by Cox regression analysis. In addition, in a recent 3-year follow-up study among 116 HF patients, Boogers et al. reported that late [^{123}I]-MIBG SPECT defect score was an independent predictor for both arrhythmias causing appropriate ICD therapy as well as the composite of appropriate ICD therapy and cardiac deaths in patients referred for ICD therapy (Boogers et al. 2010). Appropriate ICD therapy was documented in 24 (21 %) patients and appropriate ICD therapy or cardiac death in 32 (28 %) patients during the follow-up. Patients with a large late [^{123}I]-MIBG SPECT defect (summed score >26) showed significantly more appropriate ICD therapy (52 % vs. 5 %) and appropriate ICD therapy or cardiac death (57 % vs. 10 %) than patients with a small defect (summed score <26). Importantly, only 2 (3 %) patients with a small late [^{123}I]-MIBG SPECT defect received appropriate ICD therapy during follow-up. Although these results significantly relate [^{123}I]-MIBG imaging to prognosis in HF patients, further studies are needed to confirm the potential use of the technique in the management of patients who are candidates to ICD implantation and to define which parameter (HMR, WR or [^{123}I]-MIBG SPECT defect score, and respective cutoff values) will be more effective in identifying patients at higher or lower risk.

To reduce the risk of HF hospitalization and the risk of premature death, current recommendations for the use of cardiac resynchronization therapy (CRT) include HF patients with NYHA functional classes II–III and a persistently reduced LVEF (≤35–30 %, respectively), despite optimal pharmacological therapy, if they are in sinus rhythm with a QRS duration of ≥120 ms, left bundle branch block (LBBB) QRS morphology (or irrespective of such morphology if QRS duration is ≥150 ms), and a life expectancy of >1 year with good functional status. There are less consensuses about patients with right bundle branch block (RBBB) or interventricular conduction delay and those in atrial fibrillation. In addition, the modus operandi in HF patients without an indication for CRT who need conventional pacemaker is still questionable. The possibility that patients with a QRS duration of <120 ms may have "mechanical dyssynchrony" (detectable by imaging) and might benefit from CRT is another area of research interest but remains to be proven.

A relationship between CRT response and effect on peripheral sympathetic nerve activity has been described (Najem et al. 2006). Recently, CRT has been shown to have a favorable effect on cardiac sympathetic innervation as reflected by improved [^{123}I]-MIBG uptake, which supports the potential value of [^{123}I]-MIBG imaging in the assessment of the efficacy of CRT in patients with HF. Higuchi et al. reported that patients who achieved resynchronization after biventricular pacing had a significant improvement in cardiac symptoms, exercise capacity, and cardiac sympathetic function by means of late HMR (Higuchi et al. 2006). Nishioka et al. reported that a decreased HMR was associated with poor response to CRT in 30 patients with HF. Moreover, they found an improvement in the HMR after CRT in responders as shown in Fig. 19.1 (Nishioka et al. 2007).

Likewise Burri et al. observed that responders to ≥6 months of CRT showed lower [^{123}I]-MIBG WR at follow-up when compared with non-responders,

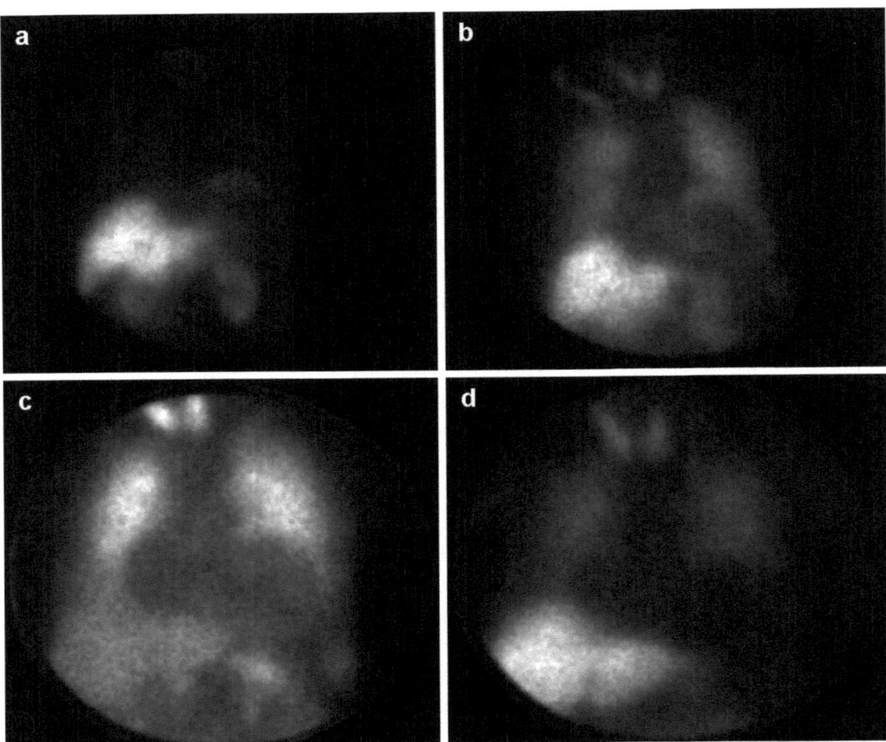

Fig. 19.1 Delayed [^{123}I]-MIBG images before (**a**, **c**) and after (**b**, **d**) CRT. Responder patient images with a HMR that improved from 1.66 to 2.01 (**a**, **b**). Non-responder patient images with a HMR that showed no difference from 0.99 to 0.98 (**c**, **d**)

indicating improvement of cardiac sympathetic nerve activity (Burri et al. 2008). The decrease in WR at follow-up was only seen in the responders and paralleled an improvement in LVEF. Subsequently, Shinohara et al. found that late HMR significantly increased 6 months after CRT in responders but not in the non-responders (Shinohara et al. 2011). Furthermore, Cha et al. reported in a prospective study that included 45 consecutive HF patients on CRT that responders (22 patients) had a significantly higher late HMR (2.11 vs. 1.48) and lower WR (37 % vs. 62 %) at baseline than non-responders (Cha et al. 2011). Recently, Tanaka et al. found that HF patients with dyssynchrony had significantly less cardiac sympathetic activity than those without dyssynchrony (late HMR 1.62 ± 0.31 vs. 1.82 ± 0.36) despite having similar LVEF (Tanaka et al. 2012). Dyssynchrony and late HMR ≥ 1.6 were associated with a high frequency of response to CRT and favorable long-term outcome over 3 years. In a recent systematic review, Scholtens et al. analyzed the available evidence regarding cardiac [^{123}I]-MIBG imaging and CRT application. Nine studies were selected from this search, including in total 225 patients. Regardless of the accounted differences between the included studies, a correlation between improvement of cardiac innervation parameters and response to CRT was evident.

Improvement of sympathetic innervations was found in patients who responded to CRT. This also strengthens the notion that diminished late HMR is related to severe heart failure without response to CRT. Nevertheless, the authors recognize the limitations in availability of data and the need for further research, standardization of the techniques, and integration of the method with other diagnostic parameters (Scholtens et al. 2013).

Ventricular assist devices for mechanical circulatory support may be used as a "bridge to decision" or longer term in selected patients presenting with end-stage HF (McMurray et al. 2012). Drakos et al. recently reported that LV assist device therapy caused clinical, functional, and hemodynamic improvements accompanied by improvements in [^{123}I]-MIBG imaging (Drakos et al. 2010). These observations might have important implications, particularly for recipients of ventricular assist devices whose native cardiac function is difficult to evaluate. Improvements in [^{123}I]-MIBG imaging could potentially identify responders to mechanical circulatory support who might become candidates for explanation of the device after the development of a potentially sustained myocardial functional recovery. Further studies are needed to determine if patients with severe HF and a poor versus favorable cardiac adrenergic imaging to maximal medical therapy have a more favorable outcome with ventricular assist devices compared to continued medical therapy alone.

19.6 PET Cardiac Innervation Studies

[^{11}C]-mHED PET is the most commonly used tracer for the assessment of cardiac sympathetic innervation activity. PET has demonstrated superior results to [^{123}I]-MIBG SPECT regarding resolution and homogeneity of tracer distribution (Bengel et al. 2009). Also PET is able to image more details by higher spatial resolution and higher signal-to-noise ratio, resulting in better regional abnormality analysis (Matsunari et al. 2010). Finally, absolute quantification by using kinetic modeling provides more accurate quantification in comparison with [^{123}I]-MIBG SPECT imaging.

An important advance in the last decade has been the organization of a first large-scale PET clinical trial (PAREPET) evaluating the viability of autonomic neuronal PET in prediction of arrhythmia (Fallavollita et al. 2006, 2014) This study included prospectively 204 patients with ischemic cardiomyopathy who were eligible for an ICD as primary prevention. [^{11}C]-mHED, [^{13}N]NH_3, and [^{18}F]-FDG PET scans were performed, and all patients were followed for sudden cardiac arrest (SCA) primarily. Interestingly, the results emphasized the importance of regional quantification of the sympathetic neuronal function. The authors concluded that sympathetic denervation predicts SCA mortality, independently from LVEF and infarct volume (Fig. 19.2). Implantation of CRT device also needs to be adapted per patient. Selection of patients that will benefit from CRT implantation is mandatory. Not all patients will experience improvement of cardiac complaints and LVEF after CRT implantation. A relationship between CRT response and effect on peripheral

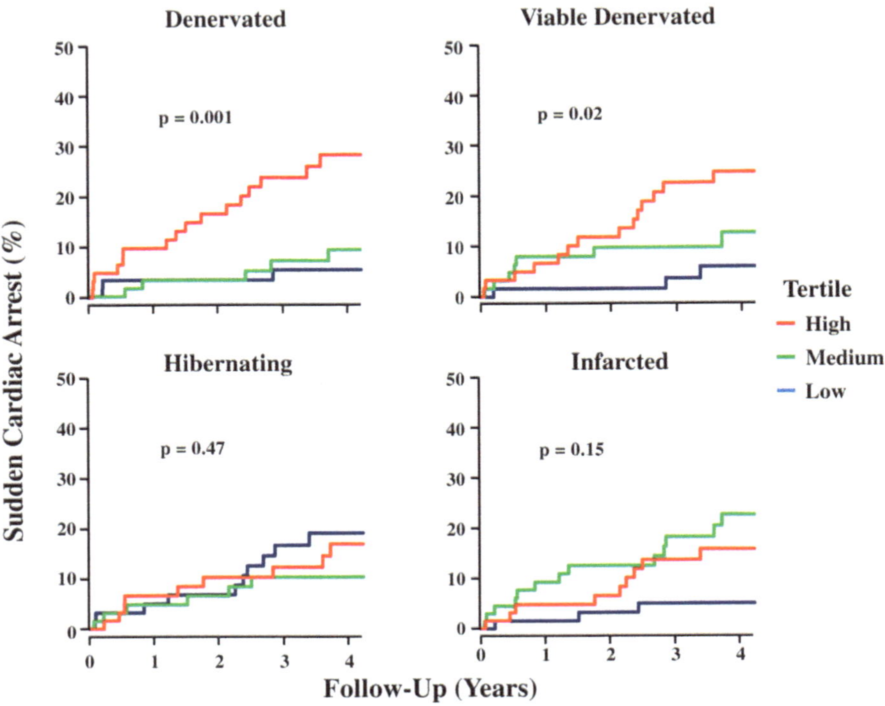

Fig. 19.2 Kaplan-Meier curves showing significantly lower survival in patients with large denervation, also in comparison with myocardial viability ([^{18}F]-FDG) and left ventricular wall hibernation (From Fallavollita et al. (2014))

sympathetic nerve activity has been described for [^{11}C]-mHED in a first study of Noordzij and coworkers (Noordzij et al. 2014). In seven heart failure patients, [^{11}C]-mHED was used for the evaluation of cardiac sympathetic innervation, before and 6 months after the treatment with cardiac resynchronization therapy (CRT). All seven patients were responders based on echocardiographic parameters (especially decrease in end-diastolic volume >10 %). Two patients showed an increase in [^{11}C]-mHED uptake after CRT implantation. Both patients also showed a significant increase in LVEF, determined with multiple gated acquisition (MUGA). The other five patients did not show a change in [^{11}C]-mHED uptake or LVEF, although they were responders to CRT (Fig. 19.3).

At the same time, imaging sympathetic innervations with PET have been useful in assessing neuronal reinnervation in patients who undergo orthotopic heart transplantation (Bengel et al. 2001a, b) (Schwaiger et al. 1991). In heart-transplant recipients, the restoration of sympathetic innervations imaged with [^{11}C]-mHED PET is associated with improved responses of the heart rate and contractile function to exercise. These results supported the functional importance of reinnervation in transplanted hearts. Mäki and coworkers studied the effect of bone marrow cell (BMC) therapy in 19 patients with acute ST-segment elevation myocardial infarct (STEMI) in a double-blind (including placebo) multicenter study (Mäki et al.

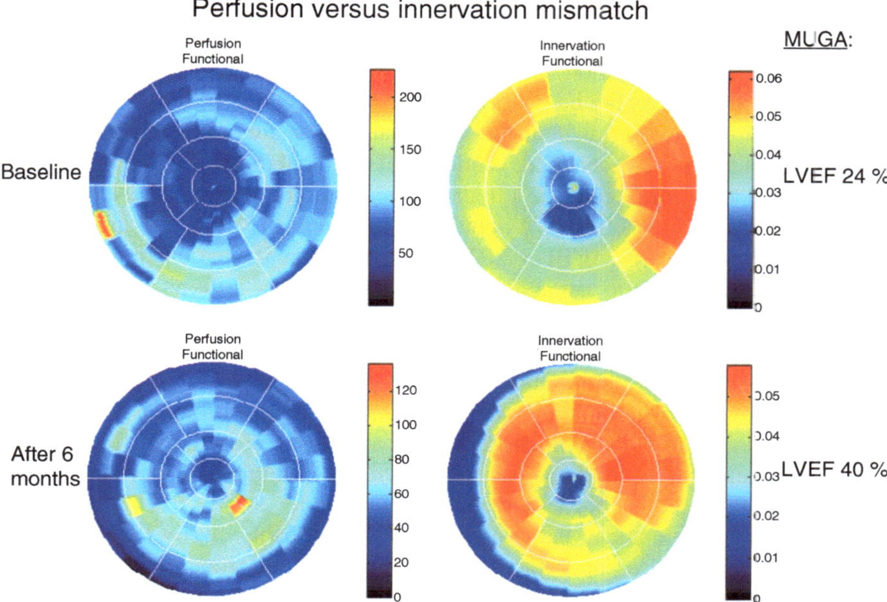

Fig. 19.3 Left polar maps indicate myocardial perfusion ([^{13}N]NH3); right polar maps indicate sympathetic innervation ([^{11}C]-mHED). Patient who showed response to the CRT scanned after 6 months. Mean [^{11}C]-mHED increased from 0.035 to 0.041 mL/min/mL after CRT application, combined with improvement of LVEF (Noordzij et al. 2014)

2012). They evaluated the feasibility of serial [^{11}C]-mHED and [^{18}F]-FDG PET and MRI studies to get more insight into the effects of BMCs on the healing process of ischemic myocardial damage. There was a decrease in [^{11}C]-mHED defect size (-4.9 ± 4.0 vs. -1.6 ± 2.2 %, $p=0.08$) and an increase in [^{18}F]-FDG uptake in the infarct area at risk (0.06 ± 0.09 vs. -0.05 ± 0.16, $p=0.07$) compared to controls, as well as less left ventricular dilatation (-4.4 ± 13.3 vs. 8.0 ± 16.7 mL/m^2, $p=0.12$) at 6-month follow-up. However, BMC treatment was inferior to placebo in terms of changes in rest perfusion in the area at risk (-0.09 ± 0.17 vs. 0.10 ± 0.17, $p=0.03$) and infarct size (0.4 ± 4.2 vs. -5.1 ± 5.9 g, $p=0.047$), and no effect was observed on ejection fraction ($p=0.37$). It was concluded that after acute phase of STEMI, BMC therapy showed only minor trends of long-term benefit in patients with rapid successful thrombolysis.

Conclusion

Cardiac autonomic innervation represents a viable target for nuclear assessment using SPECT and PET techniques. Cardiac innervation is especially susceptible to chronic and sometime subclinical damage in a variety of conditions including HF, CAD, DCM, and DM. Several SPECT and PET radiotracers have been developed to optimize and improve autonomic innervation evaluation. Still [^{123}I]-MIBG SPECT is the major player in the clinical field.

The use of cardiac adrenergic imaging may have value to risk stratify patients with HF and guided therapies. Selection of patients for ICD or CRT implantation is an important application of sympathetic innervation imaging with PET and SPECT and will possibly be cost-effective to explore.

There are many reports demonstrating that cardiac adrenergic imaging effectively monitors the effects of conventional HF medical therapies. The benefits of treatments that ameliorate the effects of neurohumoral imbalance in patients with HF are well established. As clinical status and/or LV function improves in response to β-blockers, ACEI or ARB, and MRA, there is a parallel improvement in cardiac sympathetic nerve function as assessed by radionuclide imaging. There is currently no potential advantage of cardiac adrenergic imaging to monitor the response to proven therapy in patients who respond well to conventional HF therapy with full therapeutic doses.

Cardiac adrenergic imaging might instead be more useful as an indicator of whether or not a patient's medical therapy and dosages used are effective and could therefore help determine whether higher-risk and usually more expensive device therapies or cardiac transplantation is needed.

Ongoing development and clinical trials will probably clarify PET scanning advantages as well as new tracer applications and performance including not only sympathetic neurons (Nishijima et al. 2000) but also with a new focus on receptors and parasympathetic targets.

References

Agostini D, Belin A, Amar MH et al (2000) Improvement of cardiac neuronal function after carvedilol treatment in dilated cardiomyopathy: a 123I-MIBG scintigraphic study. J Nucl Med 41:845–851

Arora R, Ferrick KJ, Nakata T et al (2003) I-123 MIBG imaging and heart rate variability analysis to predict the need for an implantable cardioverter defibrillator. J Nucl Cardiol 10:121–131

Bardy GH, Lee KL, Mark DB et al (2005) Amiodarone or an implantable cardioverter/defibrillator for congestive heart failure. N Engl J Med 352:225–237

Barron HV, Viskin S (1998) Autonomic markers and prediction of cardiac death after myocardial infarction. Lancet 351:461–462

Bax JJ, Kraft O, Buxton AE et al (2008) 123I-mIBG scintigraphy to predict inducibility of ventricular arrhythmias on cardiac electrophysiology testing: a prospective multicenter pilot study. Circ Cardiovasc Imaging 1:131–140

Bengel FM, Ueberfuhr P, Schiepel N et al (2001a) Myocardial efficiency and sympathetic reinnervation after orthotopic heart transplantation: a noninvasive study with positron emission tomography. Circulation 103:1881–1886

Bengel FM, Ueberfuhr P, Schiepel N et al (2001b) Effect of sympathetic reinnervation on cardiac performance after heart transplantation. N Engl J Med 345:731–738

Bengel FM, Higuchi T, Javadi MS et al (2009) Cardiac positron emission tomography. J Am Coll Cardiol 54:1–15

Boogers MJ, Borleffs CJ, Henneman MM et al (2010) Cardiac sympathetic denervation assessed with 123-iodine metaiodobenzylguanidine imaging predicts ventricular arrhythmias in implantable cardioverter-defibrillator patients. J Am Coll Cardiol 55:2769–2777

Burri H, Sunthorn H, Somsen A et al (2008) Improvement in cardiac sympathetic nerve activity in responders to resynchronization therapy. Europace 10:374–378

Cha Y, Chareonthaitawee P, Dong Y et al (2011) Cardiac sympathetic reserve and response to cardiac resynchronization therapy. Circ Heart Fail 4:339–344
Cohen-Solal A, Rouzet F, Berdeaux A et al (2005) Effects of carvedilol on myocardial sympathetic innervation in patients with chronic heart failure. J Nucl Med 46:1796–1803
Cohn JN, Rector TS (1988) Prognosis of congestive heart failure and predictors of mortality. Am J Cardiol 62:25A–30A
Cohn JN, Levine TB, Olivari MT et al (1984) Plasma norepinephrine as a guide to prognosis in patients with chronic congestive heart failure. N Engl J Med 311:819–823
Drakos SG, Athanasoulis T, Malliaras KG et al (2010) Myocardial sympathetic innervation and long-term left ventricular mechanical unloading. JACC Cardiovasc Imaging 3:64–70
Esler M, Kaye D (2000) Measurement of sympathetic nervous system activity in heart failure: the role of norepinephrine kinetics. Heart Fail Rev 5:17–25
Fallavollita JA, Luisi AJ Jr, Michalek SM et al (2006) Prediction of arrhythmic events with positron emission tomography: PAREPET study design and methods. Contemp Clin Trials 27:374–388
Fallavollita JA, Heavey BM, Luisi AJ Jr et al (2014) Regional myocardial sympathetic denervation predicts the risk of sudden cardiac arrest in ischemic cardiomyopathy. J Am Coll Cardiol 63:141–149
Francis GS (1986) Development of arrhythmias in the patient with congestive heart failure: pathophysiology, prevalence and prognosis. Am J Cardiol 57:3B–7B
Fukuoka S, Hayashida K, Hirose Y et al (1997) Use of iodine-123 metaiodobenzylguanidine myocardial imaging to predict the effectiveness of ß-blocker therapy in patients with dilated cardiomyopathy. Eur J Nucl Med Mol Imaging 24:523
Gerson MC, Craft LL, McGuire N et al (2002) Carvedilol improves left ventricular function in heart failure patients with idiopathic dilated cardiomyopathy and a wide range of sympathetic nervous system function as measured by iodine 123 metaiodobenzylguanidine. J Nucl Cardiol 9:608–615
Gilbert EM, Sandoval A, Larrabee P et al (1993) Lisinopril lowers cardiac adrenergic drive and increases beta-receptor density in the failing human heart. Circulation 88:472–480
Higuchi K, Toyama T, Tada H et al (2006) Usefulness of biventricular pacing to improve cardiac symptoms, exercise capacity and sympathetic nerve activity in patients with moderate to severe chronic heart failure. Circulation 70:703–709
Hohnloser SH, Connolly SJ, Kuck KH et al (2000) The defibrillator in acute myocardial infarction trial (DINAMIT): study protocol. Am Heart J 140:735–739
Hunt SA, Abraham WT, Chin MH et al (2009) Focused update incorporated into the ACC/AHA 2005 guidelines for the diagnosis and management of heart failure in adults: a report of the American College of Cardiology Foundation/American Heart Association Task Force on Practice Guidelines: Developed in Collaboration With the International Society for Heart and Lung Transplantation. Circulation 119:e391–e479
Jacobson AF, Senior R, Cerqueira MD et al (2010) Myocardial iodine-123 meta-iodobenzylguanidine imaging and cardiac events in heart failure: results of the prospective ADMIRE-HF (AdreView myocardial imaging for risk evaluation in heart failure) study. J Am Coll Cardiol 55:2212–2221
Kadish A, Dyer A, Daubert JP et al (2004) Prophylactic defibrillator implantation in patients with nonischemic dilated cardiomyopathy. N Engl J Med 350:2151–2158
Kasama S, Toyama T, Kumakura H et al (2003) Effect of spironolactone on cardiac sympathetic nerve activity and left ventricular remodeling in patients with dilated cardiomyopathy. J Am Coll Cardiol 41:574–581
Kasama S, Toyama T, Kumakura H et al (2005) Effects of candesartan on cardiac sympathetic nerve activity in patients with congestive heart failure and preserved left ventricular ejection fraction. J Am Coll Cardiol 45:661–667
Kasama S, Toyama T, Hatori T et al (2007) Evaluation of cardiac sympathetic nerve activity and left ventricular remodelling in patients with dilated cardiomyopathy on the treatment containing carvedilol. Eur Heart J 28:989–995
Kasama S, Toyama T, Sumino H et al (2008) Prognostic value of serial cardiac 123I-MIBG imaging in patients with stabilized chronic heart failure and reduced left ventricular ejection fraction. J Nucl Med 49:907–914

Kelesidis I, Travin M (2012) Use of cardiac radionuclide imaging to identify patients at risk for arrhythmic sudden cardiac death. J Nucl Cardiol 19:142–152

Knuuti J, Sipola P (2005) Is it time for cardiac innervation imaging? Q J Nucl Med Mol Imaging 49:97–105

Lotze U, Kaepplinger S, Kober A et al (2001) Recovery of the cardiac adrenergic nervous system after long-term β-blocker therapy in idiopathic dilated cardiomyopathy: assessment by increase in myocardial 123I-metaiodobenzylguanidine uptake. J Nucl Med 42:49–54

Mäki MT, Koskenvuo JW, Ukkonen H et al (2012) Cardiac function, perfusion, metabolism, and innervation following autologous stem cell therapy for acute ST-elevation myocardial infarction. A FINCELL-INSIGHT Sub-study with PET and MRI. Front Physiol 3:6

Matsui T, Tsutamoto T, Maeda K et al (2002) Prognostic value of repeated 123I-metaiodobenzylguanidine imaging in patients with dilated cardiomyopathy with congestive heart failure before and after optimized treatments – comparison with neurohumoral factors. Circulation 66:537–543

Matsunari I, Schricke U, Bengel FM et al (2000) Extent of cardiac sympathetic neuronal damage is determined by the area of ischemia in patients with acute coronary syndromes. Circulation 101:2579–2585

Matsunari I, Aoki H, Nomura Y et al (2010) Iodine-123 metaiodobenzylguanidine imaging and carbon-11 hydroxyephedrine positron emission tomography compared in patients with left ventricular dysfunction. Circ Cardiovasc Imaging 3:595–603

McMurray JJV, Adamopoulos S, Anker SD et al (2012) ESC guidelines for the diagnosis and treatment of acute and chronic heart failure 2012: the task force for the diagnosis and treatment of acute and chronic heart failure 2012 of the European Society of Cardiology. Developed in collaboration with the Heart Failure Association (HFA) of the ESC. Eur Heart J 33:1787–1847

Moss AJ, Hall WJ, Cannom DS et al (1996) Improved survival with an implanted defibrillator in patients with coronary disease at high risk for ventricular arrhythmia. N Engl J Med 335:1933–1940

Nagahara D, Nakata T, Hashimoto A et al (2008) Predicting the need for an implantable cardioverter defibrillator using cardiac metaiodobenzylguanidine activity together with plasma natriuretic peptide concentration or left ventricular function. J Nucl Med 49:225–233

Najem B, Unger P, Preumont N et al (2006) Sympathetic control after cardiac resynchronization therapy: responders versus nonresponders. Am J Physiol Heart Circ Physiol 291:H2647–H2652

Nakata T, Wakabayashi T, Kyuma M et al (2005) Cardiac metaiodobenzylguanidine activity can predict the long-term efficacy of angiotensin-converting enzyme inhibitors and/or beta-adrenoceptor blockers in patients with heart failure. Eur J Nucl Med Mol Imaging 32:186–194

Nishijima K, Kuge YF, Seki KF et al (2004) Preparation and pharmaceutical evaluation for clinical application of high specific activity S-(-)11C]CGP-12177, a radioligand for beta-adrenoreceptors. Nucl Med Commun 25:845–849

Nishioka SAD, Martinelli Filho M, Brandão SCS et al (2007) Cardiac sympathetic activity pre and post resynchronization therapy evaluated by 123I-MIBG myocardial scintigraphy. J Nucl Cardiol 14:852–859

Nishisato K, Hashimoto A, Nakata T et al (2010) Impaired cardiac sympathetic innervation and myocardial perfusion are related to lethal arrhythmia: quantification of cardiac tracers in patients with ICDs. J Nucl Med 51:1241–1249

Nolan J, Batin PD, Andrews R et al (1998) Prospective study of heart rate variability and mortality in chronic heart failure: results of the United Kingdom heart failure evaluation and assessment of risk trial (UK-heart). Circulation 98:1510–1516

Noordzij W, Tio RA, Maass AH, Willemsen ATM et al (2014) The role of 11C-mHED for sympathetic innervation in heart failure patients treated with cardiac resynchronization therapy: a pilot study. Clin Nucl Med (in press)

Rector TS, Olivari MT, Barry Levine T et al (1987) Predicting survival for an individual with congestive heart failure using the plasma norepinephrine concentration. Am Heart J 114:148–152

Rispler S, Frenkel A, Kuptzov E et al (2013) Quantitative 123I-MIBG SPECT/CT assessment of cardiac sympathetic innervation–a new diagnostic tool for heart failure. Int J Cardiol 168:1556–1558

Scholtens AM, Braat AJAT, Tuinenburg A et al (2013) Cardiac sympathetic innervation and cardiac resynchronization therapy. Heart Fail Rev. doi:10.1007/s10741C1394000

Schwaiger M, Kalff V, Rosenspire K et al (1990) Noninvasive evaluation of sympathetic nervous system in human heart by positron emission tomography. Circulation 82:457–464

Schwaiger M, Hutchins GD, Kalff V et al (1991) Evidence for regional catecholamine uptake and storage sites in the transplanted human heart by positron emission tomography. J Clin Invest 87:1681–1690

Shinohara T, Takahashi N, Saito S et al (2011) Effect of cardiac resynchronization therapy on cardiac sympathetic nervous dysfunction and serum C-reactive protein level. Pacing Clin Electrophysiol 34:1225–1230

Somsen GA, van Vlies B, de Milliano PA et al (1996) Increased myocardial 123I]-metaiodobenzylguanidine uptake after enalapril treatment in patients with chronic heart failure. Heart 76:218–220

Suwa M, Otake Y, Moriguchi A et al (1997) Iodine-123 metaiodobenzylguanidine myocardial scintigraphy for prediction of response to β-blocker therapy in patients with dilated cardiomyopathy. Am Heart J 133:353–358

Tachikawa H, Kodama M, Watanabe K et al (2005) Amiodarone improves cardiac sympathetic nerve function to hold norepinephrine in the heart, prevents left ventricular remodeling, and improves cardiac function in rat dilated cardiomyopathy. Circulation 111:894–899

Takeishi Y, Atsumi H, Fujiwara S et al (1997) ACE inhibition reduces cardiac iodine-123-MIBG release in heart failure. J Nucl Med 38:1085–1089

Tamaki S, Yamada T, Okuyama Y et al (2009) Cardiac iodine-123 metaiodobenzylguanidine imaging predicts sudden cardiac death independently of left ventricular ejection fraction in patients with chronic heart failure and left ventricular systolic dysfunction: results from a comparative study with signal-averaged electrocardiogram, heart rate variability, and QT dispersion. J Am Coll Cardiol 53:426–435

Tanaka H, Tatsumi K, Fujiwara S et al (2012) Effect of left ventricular dyssynchrony on cardiac sympathetic activity in heart failure patients with wide QRS duration Circulation 76:382–389

Toyama T, Hoshizaki H, Seki R et al (2004) Efficacy of amiodarone treatment on cardiac symptom, function, and sympathetic nerve activity in patients with dilated cardiomyopathy: comparison with β-blocker therapy. J Nucl Cardiol 11:134–141

Autonomic Imaging: The Cardiorenal Axis

20

Beata E. Chrapko and Casper F.M. Franssen

Contents

Abstract

In this chapter, we discuss the pathophysiology of the various chronic cardiorenal interactions and their consequences on the sympathetic nervous system (SNS). Increased activity of SNS is observed in all stages of chronic renal disease. The chronic elevation of SNS activity is a major contributor of the complex pathophysiology of hypertension, heart failure, insulin resistance, sleep disorders, diuretic resistance, and progressive kidney disease. Overactivity of SNS

B.E. Chrapko (✉)
Department of Nuclear Medicine, Medical University of Lublin,
Jaczewskiego 8c, Lublin 20-954, Poland
e-mail: beata.chrapko@wp.pl

C.F.M. Franssen
Division of Nephrology, Department of Internal Medicine, University Medical Center
Groningen, Hanzeplein 1, Groningen 9700 RB, The Netherlands

R.H.J.A. Slart et al. (eds.), *Autonomic Innervation of the Heart: Role of Molecular Imaging*, DOI 10.1007/978-3-662-45074-1_20

contributes to the high incidence of cardiovascular events and cardiac mortality, especially in patients with end-stage renal failure. The dysfunction of sympathetic innervation can be visualized directly by use of [^{123}I]-metaiodobenzylguanidine ([^{123}I]-MIBG) scintigraphy.

Abbreviations

[^{123}I]-MIBG	[^{123}I]-Metaiodobenzylguanidine
CKD	Chronic kidney disease
CRS	Cardiorenal syndromes
CSNS	Cardiac sympathetic nervous system
CV	Cardiovascular
ESRD	End-stage renal disease
GFR	Glomerular filtration rate
H/M	Heart to mediastinum ratio
HF	Heart failure
HRV	Heart rate variability
IDH	Intradialytic hypotension and dialytic hypotension
MBF	Myocardial blood flow
NE	Norepinephrine
NET	Norepinephrine transporter protein
RAS	Renin-angiotensin system
RRT	Renal replacement therapy
RWMA	Regional wall motion abnormality
SCD	Sudden cardiac death
WR	Washout rate

20.1 Chronic Cardiorenal Interactions

Patients with chronic kidney disease (CKD) have highly elevated cardiovascular (CV) morbidity and mortality when compared to the general population (Zuidema and Dellsperger 2012; Hause et al. 2010). Sudden cardiac death (SCD) and progressive heart failure are the major causes of death in patients with CKD (Bleyer et al. 2006; Harnett et al. 1995). Among CKD patients, many die from CV complications even before progression to end-stage renal disease (ESRD) occurs (Levin and Mendelssohn 2006). On the other hand, patients with acute and chronic heart failure frequently have acute or chronic renal dysfunction. The comorbid dysfunction of the heart and kidney is associated with a higher mortality risk compared with dysfunction of only one of these organs (Fonarow and Heywood 2006).

The cardiorenal syndrome (CRS) has been defined as "disorders of the heart and kidneys whereby acute or chronic dysfunction in one organ may induce acute or chronic dysfunction of the other" (Ronco et al. 2010). During a consensus conference, it was proposed to classify CRS into five subtypes, based on differences in

Table 20.1 Types of cardiorenal syndrome

Type of syndrome	Clinical features
Type 1 Acute cardiorenal syndrome	Acute worsening of heart function leads to acute kidney injury and/or dysfunction
Type 2 Chronic cardiorenal syndrome	Chronic abnormalities in heart function result in kidney injury and/or dysfunction
Type 3 Acute renocardiac syndrome	Acute worsening in renal function causes heart injury and/or dysfunction
Type 4 Chronic renocardiac syndrome	Chronic renal dysfunction induces heart injury and/or dysfunction
Type 5 Secondary cardiorenal syndromes	Systemic diseases (diabetes, amyloidosis, systemic lupus erythematous, sepsis) leads to simultaneous injury and/or dysfunction of heart and kidney

According to Ronco et al. (2010)

disease activity and the primary dysfunctional organ (Hause et al. 2010; Ronco et al. 2010; Pateinakis and Papagianni 2011) (Table 20.1).

It has been estimated that nearly 40 % of patients with acute heart failure also develop acute kidney injury (CRS type 1). Patients with chronic heart failure (HF) demonstrate CKD in 45–64 % of cases (Heywood et al. 2007). Of note, chronic HF and renal failure coexist in the chronic syndromes (types 2 and 4), and it is sometimes hard to distinguish the primary cause of CRS (Ronco et al. 2010). Patients may also move between the subtypes of CRS during the course of their disease (Hause et al. 2010).

In this paragraph, we focus on CRS type 2 and type 4. In the next paragraph, we discuss the derangements in the SNS in patients with various stages of CKD. Next, we review the current literature on [^{123}I]-MIBG SPECT in patients with CKD including the practical application of [^{123}I]-MIBG SPECT in CKD.

20.1.1 Chronic Cardiorenal Syndrome (CRS Type 2)

The prevalence of HF is estimated to be 2–3 % globally and increases with age. The 5-year mortality rate approximates 50 % (Dickstein et al. 2008). At the early stages of heart dysfunction, sympathetic activity increases to preserve circulatory homeostasis. This results in cardiac sympathetic stimulation and has chronotropic (increase in heart rate), inotropic (increase in contractile force), dromotropic (elevated atrioventricular conduction), and bathmotropic (increase in excitability) effects. Sympathetic activation also causes a rise in peripheral vascular resistance, sodium and water retention, and activation of other neurohormonal systems like the renin-angiotensin system (RAS) (Carrió 2001; Henneman et al. 2007; Martins da Silva et al. 2013). In patients with chronic heart failure, the sympathetic activity is up to 50 times higher than in healthy controls (Malpas 2010). The long-term stimulation of SNS has a negative impact on the CV system: the sustained sympathetic overactivity leads to changes in cardiac structure and function and contributes to the development of cardiac hypertrophy, myocyte apoptosis, fibroblastic proliferation, interstitial collagen accumulation, and myocardial fibrosis (Adameova et al. 2009; Martins da Silva et al. 2013).

Of note, the hyperactivity of SNS increases the susceptibility for arrhythmias and, thus, leads to an increased risk of cardiovascular mortality and in particular SCD (Boogers et al. 2011). [^{123}I]-MIBG imaging was also used to predict the outcome of HF (Verberne et al. 2008a). Further, it was found that an abnormal H/M ratio with [^{123}I]-MIBG imaging is an independent predictor of cardiac death, even better than impaired left ventricular ejection fraction (Merlet et al. 1999).

Hypertension and atherosclerosis are major risk factors of extensive morbidity and mortality in patients with CKD. Hypertension occurs in 80 % of patients with advanced CKD (Converse et al. 1992). The etiology of hypertension in CKD is multifactorial with hypervolemia, activation of RAS, and SNS overactivity as its major determinants (Koomans et al. 2004; Blankenstijn 2004; Kotanko 2006).

Furuhashi and Moroi analyzed the mortality rate and cardiac [^{123}I]-MIBG uptake in patients with heart failure in relation to their renal function, excluding dialysis patients (Furuhashi and Moroi 2007). They found that among patients with heart failure and a glomerular filtration rate ≥60 ml/min/1.73 m^2, the mortality rate was lower (9 %) than in patients with heart failure and a glomerular filtration rate <60 ml/min/1.73 m^2 (19 %). Interestingly, the most powerful predictor of cardiac death in the group with a glomerular filtration rate ≥60 ml/min/1.73 m^2 was a delayed H/M ratio higher than 146 %. In contrast, in patients with a glomerular filtration rate <60 ml/min/1.73 m^2, the results of [^{123}I]-MIBG myocardial imaging had no effect on the incidence of cardiac death (Furuhashi and Moroi 2007).

20.1.2 Chronic Renocardiac Syndrome (CRS Type 4)

CKD is currently defined by Kidney Disease: Improving Global Outcomes (KDIGO) as "abnormalities of kidney structure or function, present for >3 months, with implications for health" (KDIGO CKD guideline 2012). CKD is classified based on cause, GFR category, and albuminuria category (KDIGO CKD guideline 2012). CKD is a significant problem, as, since 1980, in Central Europe, the number of patients treated with renal replacement therapy has doubled every decade (Rutkowski 2006). This phenomenon is associated with a higher prevalence of risk factors for CKD such as hypertension and diabetes within the general population. Besides the 'traditional' risk factors for CKD, a kidney-specific risk factor is hyperactivity of the SNS (Blankenstijn et al. 2011).

With the onset of CKD, the likelihood of CV complications increases in both symptomatic and asymptomatic heart failure patients (Dries et al. 2000; Van Domburg et al. 2008; Schrier 2006; Caglar et al. 2006; Gansevoort et al. 2013). Dysfunction of the cardiovascular system is the cause of at least 40 % of deaths in patients with ESRD, of which one-fourth is sudden cardiac death (Zipes et al. 2006; McMahon 2003; Herzog 2007).

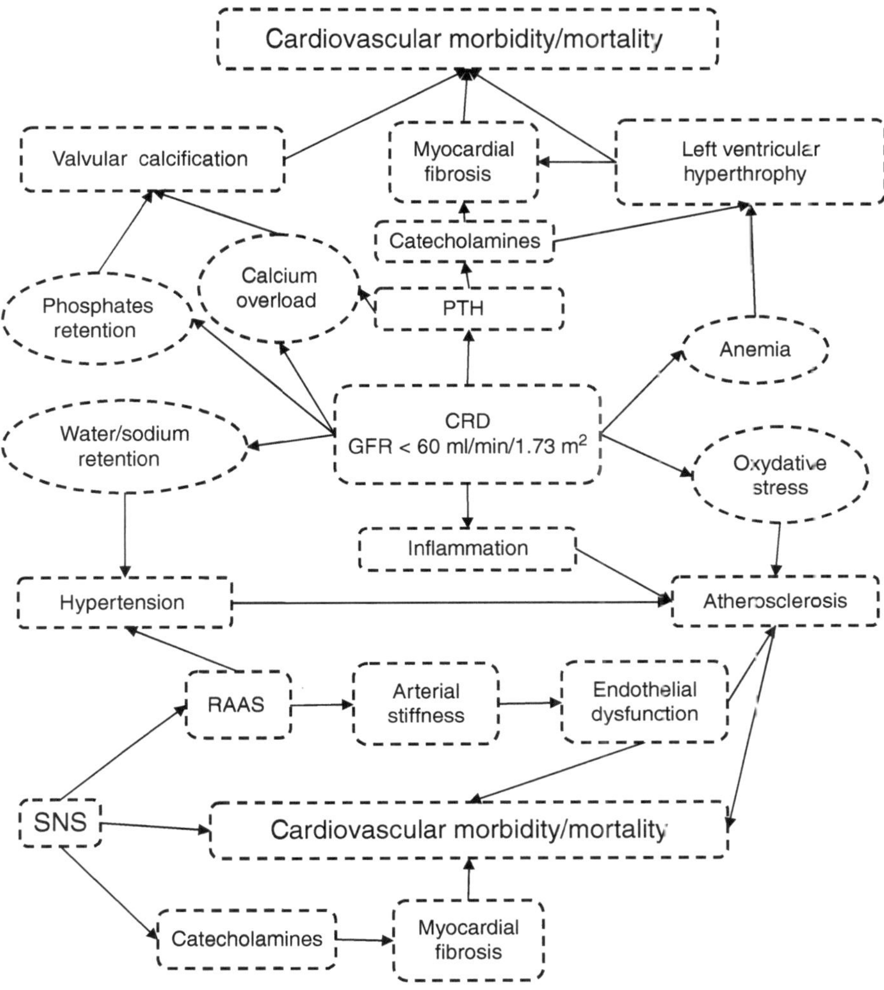

Fig. 20.1 Metabolic interactions in CKD

The main role of the kidney is the regulation of extracellular fluid volume. Renal failure is characterized by increased sodium and water retention. The subsequent increase in extracellular fluid volume leads to hypertension and excessive cardiac preload and contributes to heart enlargement and dysfunction. These changes finally lead to mitral valve insufficiency and pulmonary hypertension, as well as to right and left ventricular failure (Schrier 2006). CKD is also often associated with anemia, which, together with hypertension and increased levels of catecholamines, predisposes for the development of left ventricular hypertrophy. Systemic inflammatory reactions may also contribute to the development of atherosclerosis (Ross 1999). Moreover, increased serum levels of PTH and phosphorus are associated with increased vascular calcifications and calcification of the heart valves (Schrier 2006) (Fig. 20.1).

20.2 Hyperactivity of the Sympathetic Nervous System in CKD

As mentioned earlier, the development of chronic kidney disease is closely related to increased activation of the SNS. Kidney injury or renal ischemia is the trigger mechanism of activation of SNS and RAS (Vink and Blankenstijn 2012; Vink et al. 2013). Decreased renal oxygen supply induces adenosine release, which stimulates the rise in blood pressure, probably by afferent renal nerve activation (Katholi et al. 1984). Hyperactivity of renal SNS and RAS affects renal and vascular function (DiBona 2000, 2001). Somatic afferent impulses arising from the failing kidney cause an increase in central sympathetic drive. The kidney not only generates afferent sympathetic activity but also receives efferent sympathetic signals (Sobotka et al. 2011; Vink and Blankenstijn 2012; Vink et al. 2013). Efferent stimulation triggers a cascade of actions in the kidney. First, renal vasoconstriction leads to a reduction in renal blood flow and glomerular filtration rate. Renin is released and this stimulates angiotensin II production. This process augments the direct activation of RAS by kidney ischemia (Reid 1992). Decreases in brain nitric oxide levels and increased oxidative stress, which is characteristic of CKD, may further sensitize various organs in CRS for the damaging action of sympathetic overactivity.

The first indirect evidence that hyperactivity of SNS originates from the kidney was provided more than 40 years ago in ESRD patients, in whom hypertension and peripheral resistance were treated by bilateral nephrectomy (Kim et al. 1972). The direct evidence of hyperactivity of SNS in CKD patients was provided by muscle sympathetic nerve activity (MSNA) in microneuronography (Converse et al. 1992). In these patients, bilateral nephrectomy stopped the afferent stimulation and resulted in normalization of sympathetic activity (Converse et al. 1992; Hausberg et al. 2002). In an animal model, dorsal rhizotomy prevented elevation of blood pressure (Campese 1997). Likewise, renal denervation prevented the rise of blood pressure in animals with acute renal injury (Ye et al. 1997).

The second method of direct evaluation of cardiac SNS (CSNS) activity is myocardial scintigraphy by use of [^{123}I]-MIBG. It has been found that an extensive release of norepinephrine (NE) into the synaptic cleft reduces the production of membrane NE transporter (NET) protein and NE presynaptic reuptake (Caldwell et al. 2008). [^{123}I]-MIBG stores in the postganglionic presynaptic endings of sympathetic neuron vesicles by the same mechanism as NE and is mainly taken up by neuronal uptake-1 in membrane NET. To a lesser extent, it is taken up by a nonneuronal mechanism: a carrier-facilitated process (uptake-2) and diffusion (Henneman et al. 2008). The degree of the heart [^{123}I]-MIBG uptake, therefore, reflects the presynaptic tone of the CSNS.

The first observations of enhanced [^{123}I]-MIBG myocardial clearance in hemodialysis patients were published in 1995 by Kurata et al. They noticed that [^{123}I]-MIBG clearance was particularly rapid in hemodialysis patients that had coexisting dysfunction or hypertrophy of the left ventricle (Kurata et al. 1995). Their observations were confirmed in subsequent studies (Miyanaga et al. 1996; Kurata et al. 2000). Decreased neuronal uptake and increased myocardial clearance of [^{123}I]-MIBG in patients undergoing dialysis suggest augmented sympathetic nerve discharge due to its prolonged activation.

Diminution of excessive sympathetic activity by elimination of the renal signal could be an attractive therapeutic option. Recently, in patients with resistant hypertension, selective denervation (efferent sympathetic and afferent sensory fibers) of the kidney can be performed using endovascular radiofrequency ablation (Ahmed et al. 2012; Mahfoud and Böhm 2010). This procedure is associated with a significant fall in blood pressure. Whether renal denervation also reduces the hypertension-associated increased risk of cardiovascular events is presently unknown.

The reduction of sympathetic activity in dialysis patients could also be accomplished by increasing the frequency of the hemodialysis sessions, most likely by less fluid fluctuations (Zilch et al. 2007). Significantly lower risk of overall mortality and cardiovascular mortality in hemodialysis patient could be achieved by cold hemodialysis (Hsu et al. 2012). This procedure can also reduce the dialysis-induced LV regional wall motion abnormalities (RWMA) and in this way may improve hemodynamic stability during hemodialysis (Selby et al. 2006; Selby and McIntyre 2006).

Furthermore, inhibitors of the RAS also reduce sympathetic overactivity (Blankenstijn et al. 2011). Reduction of RAS and SNS hyperactivity are the main goals of therapy with β-blockers and angiotensin-converting enzyme inhibitors (ACEi). [^{123}I]-MIBG imaging was applied to assess the effects of these treatments – cardiac [^{123}I]-MIBG uptake improved after therapy with β-blockers (Agostini et al. 2000) and ACEi (Takeishi et al. 1997). Kasama et al. studied a group of 30 patients with dilated cardiomyopathy (DCM) before and 6 months after standard carvedilol therapy. The authors concluded that the scintigraphic parameters (H/M ratio, WR) as well echocardiographic findings (LVEF) were improved in the study group after long-term β-blocker therapy (Kasama et al. 2007). Takeishi et al. observed H/M improvement and decrease of WR in 19 NYHA class II–III patients treated by enalapril (Takeishi et al. 1997). ^{123}I-MIBG imaging was able to predict the occurrence of ventricular arrhythmias. Boogers et al. performed ^{123}I-MIBG SPECT study in 116 patients with CHF before implantable cardioverter-defibrillator (ICD) implantation. The late ^{123}I-MIBG images were independent predictive factor of appropriate ICD therapy (Boogers et al. 2010). In the ADMIRE-HF study, Jacobson et al. found that arrhythmic events were common in patients with H/M ratio <1.6 (10.4 %) compared with those with H/M ratio >1.6 (3.5 %) (Jacobson et al. 2010).

20.2.1 Intradialytic Hypotension

Intradialytic hypotension (IDH) is one of the most frequent complications of hemodialysis treatment. It is estimated to occur in 10–50 % of hemodialysis sessions (Daugirdas 2001; Orofino et al. 1990; Palmer and Henrich 2008). Dialysis hypotension can lead to serious vascular complications such as cerebral infarction and mesenteric ischemia (Schreiber 2001a, b; John et al. 2000). It is increasingly recognized that IDH may also precipitate myocardial ischemia (Zuidema and Dellsperger 2012;

McIntyre 2009). This will be discussed in the next paragraph. The pathogenesis of IDH is complex, but hypovolemia as a result of an imbalance between the ultrafiltration rate and the plasma refilling rate is generally believed to be the initiating factor (Koomans and Blankestijn 1995; van der Sande et al. 2000). Higher ultrafiltration rates (over 13 ml/h/kg) are not only associated with a greater risk of IDH but also with a significantly higher all-cause and CV mortality (Flythe et al. 2011). Importantly, frank dialysis hypotension only occurs when the CV compensatory mechanisms can no longer compensate for the reduction of blood volume (Daugirdas 2001; Palmer and Henrich 2008). Patients with autonomic insufficiency are at increased risk of IDH since an adequate cardiovascular response to hypovolemia depends on intact autonomic function (Sato et al. 2001). However, the relationship between autonomic insufficiency and the risk of IDH is not fully elucidated with some studies reporting a significant association between worse autonomic function and a higher susceptibility for IDH (Kersh et al. 1974; Enzmann et al. 1995; Sato et al. 2001), whereas other studies did not find such an association (Naik et al. 1981; Nakashima et al. 1987; Straver et al. 1998; Sapoznikov et al. 2010). Sato et al. assessed autonomic function by means of myocardial [^{123}I]-MIBG uptake and assessment of early and late H/M ratio in four groups of patients: diabetic patients with and without frequent IDH and nondiabetic patients with and without frequent IDH. Patients with frequent IDH had more severe autonomic insufficiency (the lowest H/M ratio) compared with patients without IDH, while the coexistence of diabetes enhanced this abnormality (Sato et al. 2001). The authors concluded that in patients with IDH, special attention should be given not only to dry weight but also to autonomic insufficiency. Notably, the treatment of IDH often involves reducing or withdrawing ultrafiltration, which may cause volume overload and premature stop of the dialysis session and, if repetitive, inadequate removal of uremic toxins and fluid (Palmer and Henrich 2008). In such patients, longer and/or more frequent hemodialysis sessions may be warranted to achieve adequate fluid control and removal of uremic toxins.

20.2.2 Hemodialysis-Induced Reductions in Cardiac Perfusion and Function

Although hemodialysis is a lifesaving procedure, recent studies have shown that conventional hemodialysis may have acute adverse effects on cardiac perfusion and function. McIntyre et al. (2008) studied the acute effect of hemodialysis on cardiac perfusion and left ventricular function using serial intradialytic positron emission tomography (PET) with radiolabeled water ($H_2[^{15}O]$) and echocardiography in four patients (three with diabetes) without significant coronary disease on coronary angiography. They found that global myocardial blood flow (MBF) in before dialysis was in the normal range, whereas during hemodialysis significantly fell down. All four patients developed RWMA of the left ventricle. A reduction in MBF of >30 % from baseline was significantly associated with the development of RWMA. Interestingly, the fall in segmental MBF was significantly higher in regions that developed RWMA compared with regions that preserved normal function.

At 30 min post-hemodialysis, MBF was partially recovered and most, but not all, RWMA had disappeared. Dasselaar (2009) confirmed that an uncomplicated hemodialysis procedure was associated with a significant reduction of MBF. In that study, the myocardial perfusion was evaluated by PET technique by use of radiolabeled ammonia ($[^{13}N]NH_3$) – before, in the beginning and in the end of hemodialysis session. Two of seven patients developed RWMA, and the fall in myocardial blood flow was greater in segments that developed RWMA in comparison with regions that preserved normal left ventricular function. Together, these results strongly suggest that hemodialysis is capable of inducing myocardial ischemia and cardiac stunning.

Presently, the pathogenesis of hemodialysis-induced left ventricular dysfunction is unknown. Burton et al. (2009) identified diabetes, lower albumin levels, a greater reduction in systolic blood pressure, and a higher ultrafiltration volume as risk factors for the development of hemodialysis-induced RWMA. The finding of a relationship between higher ultrafiltration volumes and hemodialysis-induced cardiac dysfunction was not found in a recent study by Assa et al. (2012a). In the study of Dasselaar et al. (2009), MBF fell significantly already early during hemodialysis when ultrafiltration volume was negligible. These studies suggest that not only hypovolemia but also other dialysis-related factors are involved in the pathogenesis of hemodialysis-induced regional left ventricular dysfunction.

Hemodialysis-induced reductions in MBF may contribute to the high mortality rates among hemodialysis patients (McIntyre 2009; Dasselaar et al. 2009). First, hemodialysis-induced cardiac ischemia may trigger arrhythmias. Indeed, the risk of sudden cardiac death is increased during and after hemodialysis session (Bleyer et al. 2006). Cardiac arrhythmias were significantly more frequent in patients with hemodialysis-induced cardiac dysfunction (Burton et al. 2008). Second, repetitive hemodialysis-induced regional ischemia may also lead to cumulative left ventricular dysfunction and eventually result in heart failure, a highly prevalent condition in hemodialysis patients. Burton et al. have shown that patients who develop RWMA during hemodialysis have a faster deterioration of left ventricular function during 1 year of follow-up in comparison with patients who do not develop hemodialysis-induced cardiac dysfunction (Burton et al. 2009).

The autonomic nervous system has an important role in the regulation of MBF. At present, however, cardiac SNS has not been compared between patients with and without cardiac ischemia during hemodialysis.

20.2.3 Hemodialysis Versus Peritoneal Dialysis

Although the nature of peritoneal dialysis and hemodialysis (HD) are essentially different, the cardiovascular outcome of both methods of RRT is comparable and unfortunately very bleak (Sato et al. 2001; Vonesh et al. 2006). However, the prevalence of myocardial stunning is substantially lower in peritoneal dialysis patients compared to HD patients (Selby and McIntyre 2011). Moreover, although hemodynamic instability can occur with peritoneal dialysis (McIntyre 2011), it is much more frequent with hemodialysis treatment than with peritoneal dialysis treatment.

This indicates that other factors than myocardial stunning and hemodynamic instability must play a role in the high all-cause and cardiovascular mortality in peritoneal dialysis patients. Several studies have demonstrated reduced heart rate variability in patients with end-stage disease. In one of these studies, a similar depression in autonomic control was demonstrated in hemodialysis ($n=8$) and peritoneal dialysis patients ($n=7$) (Axelrod et al. 1987).

20.2.4 Influence of Renal Replacement Therapy on Cardiac Adrenergic Function

Kutata et al. reported that autonomic function normalized after renal transplantation (Kurata et al. 2004). They observed a reduction of [^{123}I]-MIBG myocardial washout rate (WR), from 46±21 % before transplantation to 20±22 % after transplantation. Delayed H/M ratio also increased from 1.74±0.39 before renal transplantation to 2.06±0.39 after this procedure ($p=0.006$). Similar improvements were observed in children after renal transplantation (Parisotto et al. 2008). In that study, subjects were divided according to the following treatment strategies: conservative treatment, peritoneal dialysis, HD, and renal transplantation. The authors concluded that children undergoing dialysis had various sympathetic abnormalities, related to renal impairment, in the absence of major cardiovascular comorbidities. According to this study, cardiac adrenergic indices, like H/M ratios or WR, normalized after renal transplant, parallel to improvement of graft function, suggesting CSNS recovery (Parisotto et al. 2008).

The uremia-related toxins cannot be completely cleared, even in very effective dialysis. The efficacy of dialysis can be assessed by Kt/V, an index of fractional urea clearance. The adequacy of HD is a highly important factor in the improvement of CSNS function (Laaksonen et al. 2000). This group observed that hemodialysis patients with a Kt/V that was lower than 0.85 showed a progressive deterioration of the CSNS, whereas patients with a Kt/V higher than 1.2 had improved autonomic function, as measured by heart rate variability (HRV) (Laaksonen et al. 2000). In this respect, it is interesting that patients on overnight dialysis sessions showed an amelioration of common sympathetic uremia-related sleep breathing disorders: Chan et al. noticed that augmentation of dialysis dose and frequency in nocturnal dialysis session reduced sleep-related hypoxemia and normalized sympathetic drive as well as the heart rate variability (Chan et al. 2004).

20.3 Technical Aspects of Cardiac [^{123}I]-MIBG

The hyperactive cardiac sympathetic system is characterized by a decrease in [^{123}I]-MIBG uptake and an increase in myocardial washout of this radiotracer. The activity of CSNS can be assessed visually and semiquantitatively. The visual evaluation of regional [^{123}I]-MIBG myocardial distribution is performed by SPECT technique (Fig. 20.2) as well as planar scintigraphy, also in patients with kidney diseases (Fig. 20.3).

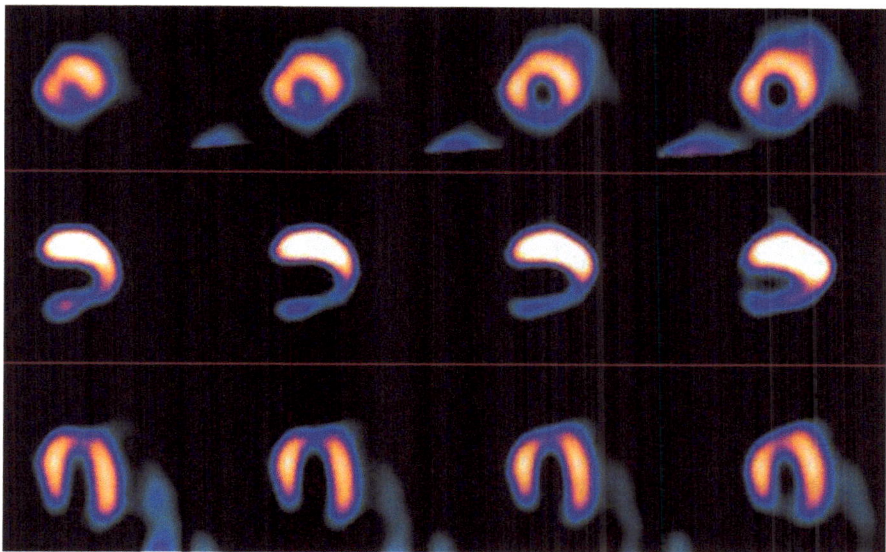

Fig. 20.2 [^{123}I]-MIBG SPECT in a 43-year-old male HD patient. Note the low activity within the inferior left ventricular wall. Low [^{123}I]-MIBG inferior wall uptake that is often seen in SPECT can be an effect of predominant parasympathetic innervation in this part of the heart. Furthermore, the low uptake in the apex can be partially due to volume effect and also to an imbalance of sympathetic and parasympathetic nerves (Scott and Kench 2004; Flotas et al. 2010; Estorch et al. 2000). In addition, the interpretation of [^{123}I]-MIBG myocardial SPECT can be difficult, especially in patients on peritoneal dialysis who show an elevated position of the diaphragm

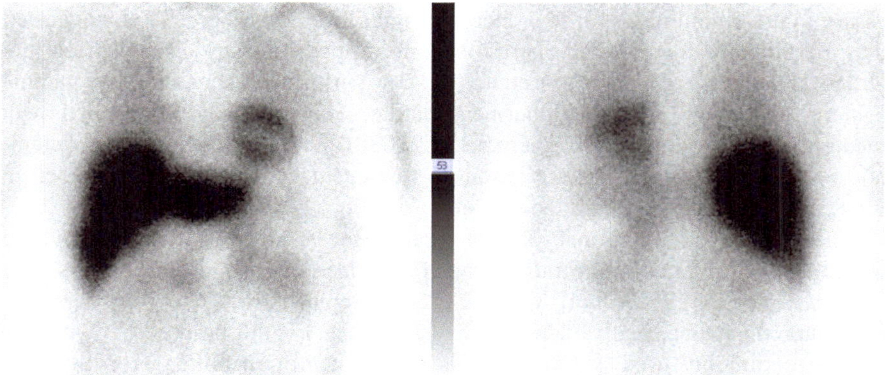

Fig. 20.3 57-year-old female patient with normal kidney function (normal eGFR) and normal activity of cardiac sympathetic nervous system. On the right planar anterior and on the left – planar posterior [^{123}I]-MIBG study. The global indices of CSNS: early H/M ratio = 3.07, delayed H/M ratio = 2.97, and WR = 30 % (Courtesy of RHJA Slart, University Medical Center Groningen, The Netherlands)

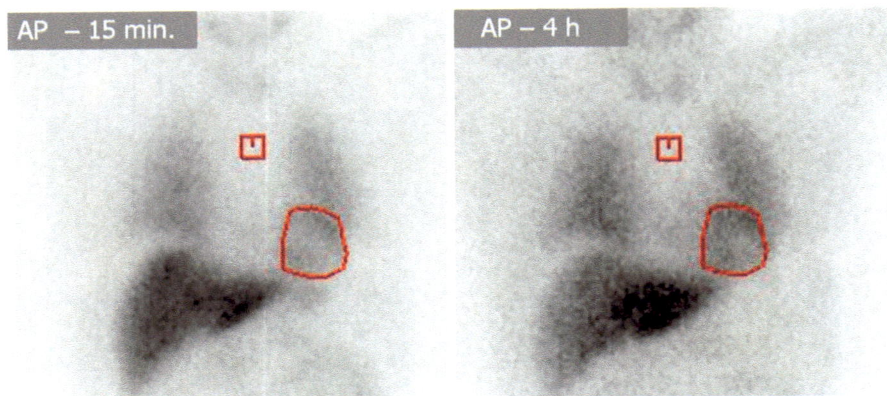

Fig. 20.4 43-year-old hemodialysed male patient, [^{123}I]-MIBG scintigraphy in planar anterior projection, performed in two point of time - 15 minutes and 4 hours post injection of radiotracer. The global indices of CSNS activity are within the normal range: early H/M = 2.15, delayed H/M = 2.12, and WR = 21.7 %. In red color the region of interest (ROI), which are needed for H/M ratio calculation, of mediastinum (*square*) and heart (*eliptic*) are defined

The quantification of cardiac adrenergic functions are more reliable than the visual SPECT evaluation (Chrapko et al. 2012) (Fig. 20.4), also in hemodialysis. Due to the excellent reproducibility of the assessment of global adrenergic function from planar [^{123}I]-MIBG cardiac images (Veltman et al. 2012), this method is the preferred method when compared with SPECT. Most authors underlined the importance of the type of collimator that is applied in achieving good quality images. Yamashina and Yamazaki (Yamashina and Yamazaki 2007) concluded that it is necessary to use a collimator for low-energy or only for ^{123}I. Verberne et al. suggested that a collimator for medium-energy is more proper, but they also reported that almost all nuclear cardiology procedures are now performed on a multi-head gamma camera, and many dedicated dual-head cardiac cameras are not supplied with medium-energy collimators (Verberne et al. 2008b) and a multicentre study, systematic review or meta-analysis are based on low-energy collimator (Agostini et al. 2008; Verberne et al. 2008a; Jacobson et al. 2010).

The sympathetic neuronal integrity can also be directly depicted by the use of positron emission tomography (PET) technique and radiotracers like [^{11}C]-*meta-hydroxyephedrine* ([^{11}C]-mHED), [^{11}C]-epinephrine, [^{11}C]-phenylephrine, [^{18}F]-fluorodopamine, and [^{18}F]-fluorobenzylguanidine. For this purpose, [^{11}C]-mHED is most commonly used. [^{11}C]-mHED is a false neurotransmitter with biodistribution and pharmacokinetics that are similar to [^{123}I]-MIBG. The quantification of [^{11}C]-mHED uptake is expressed as a retention index, the ratio of myocardial activity in the final 40 or 60 min to the integral of the arterial blood pool activity curve (Caldwell et al. 1998). There is a close relationship between [^{11}C]-mHED retention index and [^{123}I]-MIBG H/M ratio. Washout rate of both [^{11}C]-mHED and [^{123}I]-MIBG reflect sympathetic activity (Matsunari et al. 2010).

20.3.1 Some Practical Remarks

Due to the presence of radiolabeled iodine in [^{123}I]-MIBG, thyroid blocking is recommended either by oral administration of 500 mg of potassium perchlorate 30 min before or by 200 mg of potassium iodide at 1 h prior to administration of the radiopharmaceutical. However, in patients with CKD, excess potassium is poorly tolerated and can induce arrhythmias. For this reason, it is accepted to omit thyroid blocking in CKD patients (Flotas et al. 2010).

With regard to peritoneal dialysis patients, imaging procedures should be performed after draining the peritoneal cavity (empty abdomen).

Flotas et al. suggested (Flotas et al. 2010) that antihypertensive medications, such as ACEi and angiotensin receptor blockers (ARB), in patients with hypertension need not be withdrawn before [^{123}I]-MIBG scintigraphy.

In patients with normal renal function, [^{123}I]-MIBG is excreted by the kidneys. The increased sympathetic activity results in a reduction of the glomerular filtration rate and [^{123}I]-MIBG blood clearance (Kline et al. 1981). In addition, the exertion of this radiotracer also depends on tubular secretion (Blake et al. 1989). However, the residual vascular [^{123}I]-MIBG activity in renal dysfunction does not contribute to the variability of mediastinal and myocardial radiotracer uptake within the typical time frame of imaging (up to 4 h after injection) (Verberne et al. 2011). Moreover, the semiquantitative parameters of cardiac sympathetic function like the H/M ratio and washout rate are independent of estimates of renal function (Verschure et al. 2012). Furthermore, it has been shown in animal studies that vesicular uptake of [^{123}I]-MIBG is independent of blood clearance and renal function, unlike extra-vesicular functions (Arbab et al. 1996).

Besides the evaluation of the influence of uremia on CSNS, exclusion of other confounding factors is also needed. These are mainly diabetes and amyloidosis (Noordzij et al. 2012), which are frequent comorbidities in patients with CKD.

Conclusion

Chronic afferent activation of sympathetic nervous system is caused by renal dysfunction and is associated with increased efferent sympathetic drive. Sustained sympathetic overactivity is deleterious and may lead to hypertension, cardiac hypertrophy, and fibrosis. Dysfunction of the cardiovascular system is the cause of at least 40 % of deaths in patients with ESRD, of which 20 % are SCD. RRT itself, especially HD, causes also myocardial problems, such as myocardial stunning.

Nuclear medicine techniques are able to detect alterations of CSNS function. Although SNS dysfunction is recognized as an important factor in the high CV event rate, nuclear medicine procedures are not widely used in CKD patients. There is scarcity of papers on autonomic dysfunction in CKD assessed by nuclear medicine procedures, especially by the use of PET or PET/CT imaging. The majority of previous literature is focused on the abnormalities of myocardial perfusion and function of the left ventricle in CKD patients. Future studies should address the relation between alterations in sympathetic myocardial innervation and myocardial perfusion and function.

References

Adameova A, Abdellatif Y, Dhalla NS (2009) Role of the excessive amounts of circulating catecholamines and glucocorticoids in stress-induced heart disease. Can J Physiol Pharmacol 87:493–514

Agostini D, Belin A, Amar MH et al (2000) Improvement of cardiac neuronal function after carvedilol treatment in dilated cardiomyopathy: a 123I-MIBG scintigraphic study. J Nucl Med 41:845–851

Agostini D, Verberne HJ, Burchert W et al (2008) I-123-mIBG myocardial imaging for assessment of risk for a major cardiac event in heart failure patients: insights from a retrospective European multi-center study. Eur J Nucl Med Mol Imaging 35:535–546

Ahmed H, Neuzil P, Skoda J et al (2012) Renal sympathetic denervation using an irrigated radiofrequency ablation catheter for the management of drug-resistant hypertension. JACC Cardiovasc Interv 5:758–765

Arbab AS, Koizumi K, Araki T (1996) Uptake and washout of I-123-MIBG in neuronal and non-neuronal sites in rat hearts: relationship to renal clearance. Ann Nucl Med 10:211–217

Assa S, Hummel YM, Voors AA et al (2012a) Hemodialysis-induced regional left ventricular systolic dysfunction: prevalence, patient and treatment-related factors, and prognostic significance. Clin J Am Soc Nephrol 7:1615–1623

Axelrod S, Lishner M, Oz O, Bernheim J, Ravid M (1987) Spectral analysis of fluctuations in heart rate: an objective evaluation of autonomic nervous control in chronic renal failure. Nephron 45:202–206

Blake GM, Lewington VJ, Zivanovic MA, Ackery DM (1989) Glomerular filtration rate and the kinetics of 123I-metaiodobenzylguanidine. Eur J Nucl Med 15:618–623

Blankenstijn PJ (2004) Sympathetic activity in chronic renal disease. Nephrol Dial Transplant 19:1354–1357

Blankenstijn PJ, London G, Fliser D et al (2011) Major pathways of the reno-cardiovascular link: the sympathetic and renin-angiotensin system. Kidney Int Suppl 1:13–16

Bleyer AJ, Hartman J, Brannon PC et al (2006) Characteristics of sudden death in hemodialysis patients. Kidney Int 69:2268–2273

Boogers MJ, Borleffs JW, Henneman MM et al (2010) Cardiac sympathetic denervation assessed with 123-Iodine metaiodobenzylguanidine imaging predicts ventricular arrhythmias in implantable cardioverter-defibrillator patients. J Am Coll Cardiol 55:2769–2777

Boogers MJ, Fukushima K, Bengel FM, Bax JJ (2011) The role of nuclear imaging in the failing heart: myocardial blood flow, sympathetic innervations, and future applications. Heart Fail Rev 16:411–423

Burton JO, Korsheed S, Grundy BJ, McIntyre CW (2008) Hemodialysis-induced left ventricular dysfunction is associated with an increase in ventricular arrhythmias. Ren Fail 30:701–709

Burton JO, Jefferies HJ, Selby NM, McIntyre CW (2009) Hemodialysis induced cardiac injury: determinants and associated outcomes. Clin J Am Soc Nephrol 4:914–920

Caglar M, Mahmoudian B, Aytemir K et al (2006) Value of 99mTc-methoxyisobutylisonitrile (99mTc-MIBI) gated SPECT for the detection of silent myocardial ischemia in hemodialysis patients: clinical variables associated with abnormal test results. Nucl Med Commun 27:61–69

Caldwell JH, Kroll K, Li Z, Seymour K, Link JM, Krohn KA (1998) Quantitation of presynaptic cardiac sympathetic function with carbon-11-meta-hydroxyephedrine. J Nucl Med 39:1327–1334

Caldwell JH, Link JM, Levy WC, Poole JE, Stratton JR (2008) Evidence for pre- to postsynaptic mismatch of the cardiac sympathetic nervous system in ischemic congestive heart failure. J Nucl Med 49:234–241

Campese VM (1997) Neurogenic factors and hypertension in chronic renal failure. J Nephrol 10:184–187

Carrió I (2001) Cardiac neurotransmission imaging. J Nucl Med 42:1062–1076

Chan CT, Hanly P, Gabor J, Picton P, Pierratos A, Floras JS (2004) Impact of nocturnal hemodialysis on the variability of heart rate and duration of hypoxemia during sleep. Kidney Int 65:661–665

Chrapko BE, Bednarek-Skublewska A, Staśkiewicz G, Ksiażek A (2012) Relationship of haemodialysis therapy duration and cardiac adrenergic system function assessed by iodine-123 metaiodobenzylguanidine imaging in haemodialysed nondiabetic patients. Nucl Med Commun 33:155–163

Converse RL, Jacobsen TN, Toto RD, Jost CMT, Cosentino F, Fouad-Tarazi F, Victor RG (1992) Sympathetic overactivity in patients with chronic renal failure. N Engl J Med 327:1912–1918

Dasselaar JJ, Slart RHJA, Knip M et al (2009) Hemodialysis is associated with a pronounced fall in myocardial perfusion. Nephrol Dial Transplant 24:604–610

Daugirdas JT (2001) Pathophysiology of dialysis hypotension: an update. Am J Kidney Dis 38:S11–S17

DiBona GF (2000) Nervous kidney. Interaction between renal sympathetic nerves and the renin-angiotensin system in the control of renal function. Hypertension 36:1083–1088

DiBona GF (2001) Peripheral and central interactions between the renin-angiotensin system and the renal sympathetic nerves in control of renal function. Ann N Y Acad Sci 940:395–406

Dickstein K, Cohen-Solal A, Filippatos G et al (2008) ESC Guidelines for the diagnosis and treatment of acute and chronic heart failure 2008: the Task Force for the Diagnosis and Treatment of Acute and Chronic Heart Failure 2008 of the European Society of Cardiology. Developed in collaboration with the Heart Failure Association of the ESC (HFA) and endorsed by the European Society of Intensive Care Medicine (ESICM). Eur Heart J 29:2388–2442

Dries DL, Exner DV, Domanski MJ, Greenberg B, Stevenson LW (2000) The prognostic implications of renal insufficiency in asymptomatic and symptomatic patients with left ventricular systolic dysfunction. J Am Coll Cardiol 35:681–689

Enzmann G, Bianco F, Paolini F, Panzetta G (1995) Autonomic nervous function and blood volume monitoring during hemodialysis. Int J Artif Organs 18:504–508

Estorch M, Serra-Grima R, Flotas A et al (2000) Myocardial sympathetic innervations in the athlete's sinus bradycardia: is there selective inferior myocardial wall denervation? J Nucl Cardiol 7:354–358

Flotas A, Carrio I, Agostini D et al (2010) Proposal for standardization of 123-I-metaiodobenzylguanidine (MIBG) cardiac sympathetic imaging by the EANM Cardiovascular Committee and the European Council of Nuclear Cardiology. Eur J Nucl Med Mol Imaging 37:1802–1812

Flythe JE, Kimmel SE, Brunelli SM (2011) Rapid fluid removal during dialysis is associated with cardiovascular morbidity and mortality. Kidney Int 79:250–257

Fonarow GC, Heywood JT (2006) The confounding issue of comorbid renal insufficiency. Am J Med 119(Suppl 1):S17–S25

Furuhashi T, Moroi M (2007) Importance of renal function on prognostic value of cardiac iodine-123 metaiodobenzylguanidine scintigraphy. Ann Nucl Med 21:57–63

Gansevoort RT, Correa-Rotter R, Hemmelgarn BR, Jafar TH, Heerspink HJ, Mann JF, Matsushita K, Wen CP (2013) Chronic kidney disease and cardiovascular risk: epidemiology, mechanisms and prevention. Lancet 382:339–352

Harnett JD, Foley RN, Kent GM, Barre PE, Murray D, Parfrey PS (1995) Congestive heart failure in dialysis patients: prevalence, prognosis and risk factors. Kidney Int 47:884–890

Hausberg M, Kosch M, Harmelink P et al (2002) Sympathetic nerve activity in end-stage renal disease. Circulation 106:1974–1979

Hause AA, Anand I, Bellomo R et al (2010) Definition of cardio-renal syndromes: workgroup statements from the 7th ADQI Consensus Conference. Nephrol Dial Transplant 25:1416–1420

Henneman MM, Bax JJ, van der Wall EE (2007) Monitoring of therapeutic effect in heart failure patients: a clinical application of 123I-MIBG imaging? Eur Heart J. doi:10.1093/eurheartj/ehl325

Henneman MM, Bengel FM, van der Wall EE, Knuuti J, Bax JJ (2008) Cardiac neuronal imaging: application in the evaluation of cardiac disease. J Nucl Cardiol 15:442–455

Herzog CA (2007) Can we prevent sudden cardiac death in dialysis patients? Clin J Am Soc Nephrol 2:410–412
Heywood TJ, Fonarow GC, Costanzo MR, Mathu VS, Woodside JR, Wynne J (2007) High prevalence of renal dysfunction and its impact on outcome in 118,465 patients hospitalized with acute decompensated heart failure: a report from the ADHERE database. J Card Fail 13:422–430
Hsu H-J, Yen C-H, Hsu K-H et al (2012) Association between cold dialysis and cardiovascular survival in hemodialysis patients. Nephrol Dial Transplant 27:2457–2464
Jacobson AF, Senior R, Cerqueira MD et al (2010) Myocardial iodine-123 meta-iodobenzylguanidine imaging and cardiac events in heart failure: results of the prospective ADMIRE-HF (AdreView Myocardial Imaging for Risk Evaluation in Heart Failure) Study. J Am Coll Cardiol 55:2212–2221
John AS, Tuerff SD, Kerstein MD (2000) Nonocclusive mesenteric infarction in hemodialysis patients. J Am Coll Surg 190:84–88
Kasama S, Toyama T, Hatori T et al (2007) Evaluation of cardiac sympathetic nerve activity and left ventricular remodelling in patients with dilated cardiomyopathy on the treatment containing carvedilol. Eur Heart J 28:989–995
Katholi RE, Whitlow PL, Hageman GR, Woods WT (1984) Intrarenal adenosine produces hypertension by activating the sympathetic nervous system via the renal nerves in the dog. J Hypertens 2:349–359
KDIGO 2012 clinical practice guideline for the evaluation and management of chronic kidney disease (2013) Kidney Int Suppl 3:136–150
Kersh ES, Kronfield SJ, Unger A, Popper RW, Cantor S, Cohn K (1974) Autonomic insufficiency in uremia as a cause of hemodialysis-induced hypotension. N Engl J Med 290:650–653
Kim KE, Onesti G, Schwartz AB, Chinitz JL, Swartz C (1972) Hemodynamics of hypertension in chronic end-stage renal disease. Circulation. 46(3):456–464
Kline RC, Swanson DP, Wieland DM et al (1981) Myocardial imaging in man with I-123 meta-iodobenzylguanidine. J Nucl Med 22:129–132
Koomans HA, Blankestijn PJ (1995) Blood volume preservation in dialysis: tool and strategies. Nephrol Dial Translant 10:1791–1793
Koomans HA, Blankestijn PJ, Joles JA (2004) Sympathetic hyperactivity in chronic renal failure: a wake-up call. J Am Soc Nephrol 15:524–537
Kotanko P (2006) Cause and consequences of sympathetic hyperactivity in chronic kidney disease. Blood Purif 24:95–99
Kurata C, Wakabayashi Y, Shouda S et al (1995) Enhanced cardiac clearance of iodine-123-MIBG in chronic renal failure. J Nucl Med 36:2037–2043
Kurata C, Uehara A, Sugi T et al (2000) Cardiac autonomic neuropathy in patients with chronic renal failure on haemodialysis. Nephron 84:312–319
Kurata C, Uehara A, Ishikawa A (2004) Improvement of cardiac sympathetic innervation by renal transplantation. J Nucl Med 45:1114–1120
Laaksonen S, Voipio-Pulkki L, Erkinjuntti M, Asola M, Falack B (2000) Does dialysis therapy improve autonomic and peripheral nervous system abnormalities in chronic uraemia? J Intern Med 248:21–26
Levin A, Mendelssohn D (2006) Care and referral of adult patients with reduce kidney function: position paper from the Canadian Society of Nephrology. Vancouver, British Columbia: Canadian Society of Nephrology
Mahfoud F, Böhm M (2010) Interventional renal sympathetic denervation – a new approach for patients with resistant hypertension. Dtsch Med Wochenschr 135:2422–2425
Malpas SC (2010) Sympathetic nervous system overactivity and its role in the development of cardiovascular disease. Physiol Rev 90:513–557
Martins da Silva MI et al (2013) Iodine-123-metaiodobenzylguanidine scintigraphy in risk stratification of sudden death in heart failure. Rev Port Cardiol 32:509–516
Matsunari I, Aoki H, Nomura Y et al (2010) Iodine-123 metaiodobenzylguanidine imaging and carbon-11 hydroxyephedrine positron emission tomography compared in patients with left ventricular dysfunction. Circ Cardiovasc Imaging 3:595–603

McIntyre CW (2009) Effects of hemodialysis on cardiac function. Kidney Int 76:371–375
McIntyre CW (2011) Hemodynamic effects of peritoneal dialysis. Perit Dial Int 31:S73–S76
McIntyre CW, Burton JO, Selby NM et al (2008) Hemodialysis-induced cardiac dysfunction is associated with an acute reduction of global and segmental myocardial blood flow. Clin J Am Soc Nephrol 3:19–26
McMahon LP (2003) Hemodynamic cardiovascular risk factors in chronic kidney disease: what are the effects of intervention? Semin Dial 16:128–139
Merlet P, Benvenuti C, Moyse D et al (1999) Prognostic value of MIBG imaging in idiopathic dilated cardiomyopathy. J Nucl Med 40:917–923
Miyanaga H, Yoneyama S, Kamitani T, Kawasaki S, Takahashi T, Kunishige H (1996) Abnormal myocardial uptake and clearance of 123I-labeled metaiodobenzylguanidine in patients with chronic renal failure and autonomic dysfunction. J Nucl Cardiol 3:508–515
Naik RB, Mathias CJ, Wilson CA, Reid JL, Warren DJ (1981) Cardiovascular and autonomic reflexes in haemodialysis patients. Clin Sci 60:165–170
Nakashima Y, Fouad FM, Nakamoto S, Textor SC, Bravo EL, Tarazi RC (1987) Localization of autonomic nervous system dysfunction in dialysis patients. Am J Nephrol 7:375–381
Noordzij W, Glaudemans AW, van Rheenen RW et al (2012) 123I-Labelled metaiodobenzylguanidine for the evaluation of cardiac sympathetic denervation in early stage amyloidosis. Eur J Nucl Med Mol Imaging 39:1609–1617
Orofino L, Marcen R, Quereda C et al (1990) Epidemiology of symptomatic hypotension in hemodialysis: is cool dialysate beneficial for all patients? Am J Nephrol 10:177–180
Palmer BF, Henrich WL (2008) Recent advances in the prevention and management of intradialytic hypotension. J Am Soc Nephrol 19:8–11
Parisotto V, Lima EM, Silva JMP, de Sousa MR, Ribeiro AL (2008) Cardiac sympathetic dysautonomia in children with chronic kidney disease. J Nucl Cardiol 15:246–254
Pateinakis P, Papagianni A (2011) Cardiorenal syndrome type 4-cardiovascular disease in patients with chronic kidney disease: epidemiology, pathogenesis, and management. Int J Nephrol. doi:10.4061/2011/938651
Reid IA (1992) Interaction between ANG II, sympathetic nervous system, and baroreceptor reflexes in regulation of blood pressure. Am J Physiol 262:E763–E778
Ronco C, McCullough P, Anker SD, Anand I, Aspromonte N, Bagshaw SM et al (2010) Cardiorenal syndromes: report from the consensus conference of the acute dialysis quality initiative. Eur Heart J 31:703–711
Ross R (1999) Atherosclerosis-an inflammatory disease. N Engl J Med 340:115–126
Rutkowski B (2006) Highlights of the epidemiology of renal replacement therapy in Central and Eastern Europe. Nephrol Dial Transplant 21:4–10
Sapoznikov D, Backenroth R, Rubinger D (2010) Baroreflex sensitivity and sympatho-vagal balance during intradialytic hypotensive episodes. J Hypertens 28:314–324
Sato M, Horigome I, Chiba S et al (2001) Autonomic insufficiency as a factor contributing to dialysis-induced hypotension. Nephrol Dial Transplant 16:1657–1662
Schreiber MJ Jr (2001a) Clinical dilemmas in dialysis: managing the hypotensive patient. Setting the stage. Am J Kidney Dis 38:S1–S10
Schreiber MJ Jr (2001b) Clinical case-based approach to understanding intradialytic hypotension. Am J Kidney Dis 38:S37–S47
Schrier R (2006) Role of diminished renal function in cardiovascular mortality marker or pathogenetic factor? J Am Coll Cardiol 47:1–8
Scott LA, Kench PL (2004) Cardiac autonomic neuropathy in the diabetic patients: does 123I-MIBG imaging have a role to play in early diagnosis? J Nucl Med Technol 32:66–71
Selby NM, McIntyre CW (2006) A systemic review of the clinical effects of reducing dialysate fluid temperature. Nephrol Dial Transplant 21:1883–1898
Selby NM, McIntyre CW (2011) Peritoneal dialysis is not associated with myocardial stunning. Perit Dial Int 31:27–33
Selby NM, Burton JO, Chesterton LJ, McIntyre CW (2006) Dialysis-induced regional left ventricular dysfunction is ameliorated by cooling the dialysate. Clin J Am Soc Nephrol 1:1216–1225

Sobotka PA, Mahfound F, Schlaich MP, Hoppe UC, Böhm M, Krum H (2011) Sympatho-renal axis in chronic renal disease. Clin Res Cardiol 100:1049–1057

Straver B, de Vries PMJM, ten Voorde BJ, Roggekamp MC, Donker AJM, ter Wee PM (1998) Intradialytic hypotension in relation to pre-existent autonomic dysfunction in hemodialysis patients. Int J Artif Organs 21:794–801

Takeishi Y, Atsumi H, Fujiwara S et al (1997) ACE inhibitor reduces cardiac iodine-123-MIBG release in heart failure. J Nucl Med 38:1085–1089

van der Sande FM, Kooman JP, Leunissen KM (2000) Intradialytic hypotension – new concepts on an old problem. Nephrol Dial Transplant 15:1746–1748

Van Domburg RT, Hoeks SE, Welten GMJM, Chonchol M, Elhendy A, Poldermans D (2008) Renal insufficiency and mortality in patients with known or suspected coronary artery disease. J Am Soc Nephrol 19:158–163

Veltman CE, Boogers MJ, Meinardi JE et al (2012) Reproducibility of planar 123I-meta-iodobenzylguanidine (MIBG) myocardial scintigraphy in patients with heart failure. Eur J Nucl Med Mol Imaging 39:1599–1608

Verberne HJ, Brewster LM, Somsen GA, van Eck-Smit BLF (2008a) Prognostic value of myocardial 123-I metaiodobenzylguanidine (MIBG) parameters in patients with heart failure: a systemic review. Eur Heart J 29:1147–1159

Verberne HJ, Habraken JBA, van Eck-Smit BLF, Agostini D, Jacobson AF (2008b) Variations in 123I-metaiodobenzylguanidine (MIBG) late heart mediastinal ratios in chronic heart failure: a need for standarisations and validation. Eur J Nucl Med Mol Imaging 35:547–553

Verberne HJ, Verschure DO, Somsen GA, van Eck-Smit BL, Jacobson AF (2011) Vascular time-activity variation in patients undergoing ^{123}I-MIBG myocardial scintigraphy: implications for quantification of cardiac and mediastinal uptake. Eur J Nucl Med Mol Imaging 38:1132–1138

Verschure DO, Somsen GA, van Eck-Smit BLF, Verberne HJ (2012) Renal function in relation to cardiac 123I-MIBG scintigraphy in patients with chronic heart failure. Int J Mol Imaging. doi:10.1155/2012/434790

Vink EE, Blankenstijn PJ (2012) Evidence and consequence of the central role of the kidneys in the pathophysiology of sympathetic hyperactivity. Front Physiol 3:29

Vink EE, de Jager RL, Blankestijn PJ (2013) Sympathetic hyperactivity in chronic kidney disease: pathophysiology and (new) treatment options. Curr Hypertens Rep 1:95–101

Vonesh EF, Snyder JJ, Foley RN, Collins AJ (2006) Mortality studies comparing peritoneal dialysis and hemodialysis: what do they tell us? Kidney Int 103:S3–S11

Yamashina S, Yamazaki J (2007) Neuronal imaging using SPECT. Eur J Nucl Med Mol Imaging 34:62–73

Ye S, Ozgur B, Campese VM (1997) Renal afferent impulses, the posterior hypothalamus and hypertension in rats with chronic renal failure. Kidney Int 51:722–727

Zilch O, Vos PF, Oey PL, Cramer MJ, Ligtenberg G, Koomans HA, Blankestijn PJ (2007) Sympathetic hyperactivity is reduced by short daily haemodialysis. J Hypertens 25:1285–1289

Zipes DP, Camm AJ, Borggrefe M et al (2006) ACC/AHA/ESC 2006 guidelines for management of patients with ventricular arrhythmias and the prevention of sudden cardiac death- executive summary. Eur Heart J 27:2099–2140

Zuidema MY, Dellsperger KC (2012) Myocardial stunning with hemodialysis: clinical challenges of the cardiorenal patients. Cardiorenal Med 2:25–133

Imaging the Functional Brain-Heart Axis: Neurodegenerative Diseases

21

Giorgio Treglia, Antonella Stefanelli, and Ignasi Carrio

Contents

Abstract

In recent years, it has been clinically and neuropathologically revealed that some neurodegenerative diseases such as Parkinson's disease (PD), dementia with Lewy bodies (DLB), and pure autonomic failure (PAF) are overlapping diseases: Lewy body diseases (LBD) has thus become a general term for these diseases. In fact, Lewy bodies are pathologically observed in the nervous system of these

G. Treglia, MD (✉)
Department of Nuclear Medicine, Oncology Institute of Southern Switzerland, Bellinzona, Switzerland
e-mail: giorgiomednuc@libero.it

A. Stefanelli
Institute of Nuclear Medicine, Catholic University, Rome, Italy

I. Carrio
Nuclear Medicine Department, Hospital Sant Pau, Barcelona, Spain

R.H.J.A. Slart et al. (eds.), *Autonomic Innervation of the Heart: Role of Molecular Imaging*, DOI 10.1007/978-3-662-45074-1_21

neurodegenerative diseases. Since LBD may present sympathetic impairment, several studies have evaluated the role of myocardial sympathetic imaging in these diseases. LBD usually present an abnormal myocardial sympathetic imaging using iodine-123-metaiodobenzylguanidine ([^{123}I]-MIBG) scintigraphy, and this technique may be very useful in differential diagnosis between PD and other parkinsonisms such as in differential diagnosis between DLB and other dementias. PET tracers are also available to study myocardial sympathetic denervation and may help to quantify cardiac autonomic dysfunction in LBD.

Abbreviations

AADC	Aromatic amino acid decarboxylase
CBD	Corticobasal degeneration
DAT	Dopamine transporter
DLB	Dementia with Lewy bodies
FNE	Fluoronorepinephrine
FP-CIT	[123I]-N-ω-fluoropropyl-2β-carbomethoxy-3β-(4-iodophenyl)nortropan
IBZM	[123I]-(S)-2-hydroxy-3-iodo-6-methoxy-*N*-[1-ethyl-2-pyrrodinyl)-methyl]benzamide
LBD	Lewy body diseases
MSA	Multiple system atrophy
PAF	Pure autonomic failure
PD	Parkinson's disease
PET	Positron emission tomography
PSP	Progressive supranuclear palsy
SPECT	Single-photon emission computed tomography

21.1 Introduction

In recent years, it has been clinically and neuropathologically revealed that some neurodegenerative diseases such as Parkinson's disease (PD), dementia with Lewy bodies (DLB), and pure autonomic failure (PAF) are overlapping diseases: Lewy body diseases (LBD) has thus become a general term for these diseases. In fact, Lewy bodies (cytoplasmic inclusions containing alpha-synuclein protein aggregates) are pathologically observed in the nervous system of these neurodegenerative diseases (Hishikawa et al. 2003).

LBD are classified under the heading of synucleinopathies, because they are characterized by intraneuronal precipitates of alpha-synuclein protein. Multiple system atrophy (MSA) is also considered to be a form of synucleinopathy; however, alpha-synuclein deposits in MSA are localized in glial cells rather than neurons (Puschmann et al. 2012).

PD is a neurodegenerative disorder more common in the elderly. Symptoms of PD result from the death of dopamine-generating cells in the substantia nigra. Early in the course of the disease, the most obvious symptoms are movement related (including tremor, rigidity, slowness of movement, and difficulty with walking and gait). Later, cognitive and behavioral problems may arise, with dementia commonly occurring in the advanced stages of the disease. Other symptoms include sensory, sleep, and emotional problems (Jankovic 2008). Early diagnosis of PD and differential diagnosis between PD and other parkinsonisms using clinical criteria or imaging methods is often difficult. Myocardial sympathetic innervation imaging has emerged as a useful method to confirm or exclude the presence of PD (Treglia et al. 2012).

DLB is reported to be the second most common cause of degenerative dementia after Alzheimer's disease. DLB is clinically characterized by the progressive cognitive decline with fluctuations in cognition and alertness, recurrent visual hallucinations, and parkinsonism (Weisman and McKeith 2007). However, in the early disease stages, the clinical symptoms of various types of dementias largely overlap and it is difficult to distinguish between DLB and other dementias based on clinical manifestations alone. To improve the diagnosis of DLB, the latest diagnostic criteria incorporate findings from neuroimaging studies including myocardial innervation imaging (Tateno et al. 2009; McKeith 2006).

Since LBD may present sympathetic denervation, which precedes the neuronal loss in the sympathetic ganglia (Iwanaga et al. 1999; Orimo et al. 2002, 2005; Arimo et al. 2005), several studies have evaluated the role of myocardial sympathetic imaging in the early diagnosis of LBD and in the differential diagnosis between LBD and other neurodegenerative diseases (Estorch 2006; Treglia et al. 2010).

LBD are associated with imaging evidence of substantial myocardial sympathetic denervation by iodine-123-metaiodobenzylguanidine ($[^{123}I]$-MIBG) scintigraphy (Treglia et al. 2010) and by carbon-11-metahydroxyephedrine ($[^{11}C]$-mHED) and fluorine-18-fluorodopamine ($[^{18}F]$-dopamine) positron emission tomography (PET) (Bengel and Schwaiger 2004).

21.2 $[^{123}I]$-MIBG Scintigraphy

21.2.1 Rationale and Technical Aspects

Myocardial $[^{123}I]$-MIBG uptake has been shown to correlate with adrenergic innervation. Furthermore, there is evidence that $[^{123}I]$-MIBG uptake is also dependent on the functional integrity of the adrenergic system (Yamashina and Yamazaki 2007; Camacho and Carrio 2007; Treglia et al. 2010).

LBD, including PD and DLB, present an impairment of adrenergic function and consequently an abnormal innervation imaging with $[^{123}I]$-MIBG scintigraphy (Treglia et al. 2010; Nakajima et al. 2008; Rascol and Schelosky 2009). In particular, the markedly decreased $[^{123}I]$-MIBG uptake in the heart is considered to be a specific finding of LBD compared to other neurodegenerative diseases (Treglia et al. 2010). Decreased myocardial uptake of $[^{123}I]$-MIBG has been reported in the early stages of LBD; this finding suggests that degeneration of the myocardial

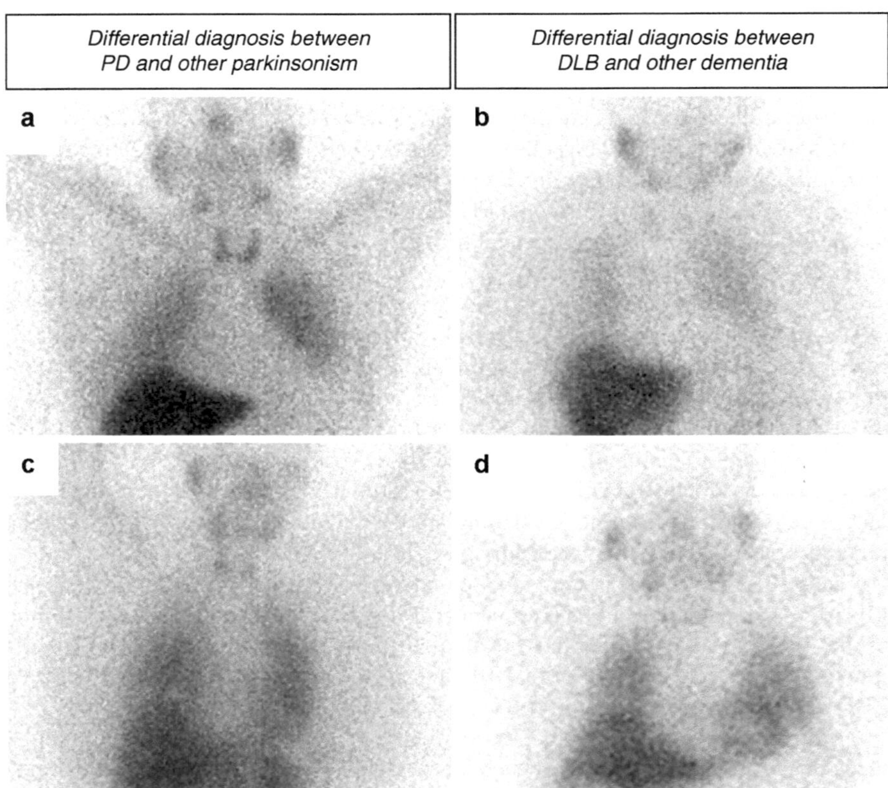

Fig. 21.1 [^{123}I]-MIBG scintigraphy (planar imaging performed at 4 h after tracer injection) showing abnormal myocardial uptake in a patient with Parkinson's disease (**a**) and in a patient with dementia with Lewy body (**b**), and normal myocardial uptake in a patient with multiple system atrophy (**c**) and in a patient with Alzheimer's disease (**d**), demonstrating myocardial sympathetic impairment in patients with Lewy body disease (**a**, **b**) and normal myocardial sympathetic innervation in other neurodegenerative diseases (**c**, **d**)

sympathetic nerves begins early in the disease process of LBD and that it occurs before neuronal cell loss (Orimo et al. 2007a).

Early and delayed planar images of the thoracic region at [^{123}I]-MIBG scintigraphy and calculation of heart to mediastinum (H/M) ratio are adequate for the evaluation of cardiac sympathetic function in LBD (Fig. 21.1). The degree of myocardial uptake is evaluated in comparison to a threshold of H/M ratio obtained from a control group (Nakajima et al. 2008; Treglia et al. 2010). One of the possible causes of false-positive and false-negative results is due to the definition of the threshold of H/M ratio. A recent publication on [^{123}I]-MIBG scintigraphy standardization showed its potential usefulness in a multicenter trial in patients with LBD (Nakajima et al. 2012).

21.2.2 [^{123}I]-MIBG Scintigraphy in Parkinson's Disease and Other Parkinsonisms

Hirayama et al. first reported a reduced myocardial uptake of [^{123}I]-MIBG in PD patients compared to normal controls (Hirayama et al. 1995). Since then, multiple clinical studies were performed showing a significant reduction in myocardial [^{123}I]-MIBG uptake in PD patients which reflected the presence of a myocardial sympathetic dysfunction in this neurodegenerative disease (Treglia et al. 2010, 2012).

[^{123}I]-MIBG scintigraphy findings showed that myocardial postganglionic sympathetic dysfunction in patients with PD is already present in early disease without clinical evidence of autonomic dysfunction. Furthermore, [^{123}I]-MIBG myocardial uptake was sometimes impaired in PD even in the absence of abnormal findings on autonomic testing, suggesting that [^{123}I]-MIBG scintigraphy is more sensitive than standard autonomic testing for the early detection of silent autonomic dysfunction (Takatsu et al. 2000; Taki et al. 2000; Oka et al. 2006). However, some studies reported a relatively lower sensitivity of [^{123}I]-MIBG scintigraphy in PD patients with early stage of disease compared to those with advanced stage (Orimo et al. 2012; Treglia et al. 2012).

Regarding the correlation between clinical subtypes of PD and myocardial [^{123}I]-MIBG uptake, conflicting results are reported in the literature: in some studies a lower myocardial [^{123}I]-MIBG uptake in the akinetic-rigid type of the disease compared to the tremor-dominant type was described (Spiegel et al. 2007; Chung et al. 2011), whereas in a recent article myocardial sympathetic innervation was found more severely impaired in the tremor-dominant type (Chiaravalloti et al. 2012).

All the major non-motor manifestations noted in PD have been reported to be associated with myocardial sympathetic denervation. These include olfactory dysfunction, REM sleep behavior disorder, dementia, visual hallucinations, and orthostatic hypotension, although literature on the latter has not been perfectly consistent (Kashihara et al. 2010; Kitayama et al. 2008; Lee et al. 2006; Miyamoto et al. 2006; Oka et al. 2007a, b; Suzuki et al. 2006; Treglia et al. 2010).

Regarding the correlation between genetic characteristics of PD and myocardial [^{123}I]-MIBG uptake, myocardial sympathetic denervation occurs less frequently in genetic PD than in idiopathic PD. In particular, myocardial [^{123}I]-MIBG uptake has a heterogeneous pattern in genetic PD, because it was differently impaired in patients with different mutations in the same gene or with the same gene mutation (Quattrone et al. 2008).

Another challenge is the presence of correlation between disease severity and myocardial uptake of [^{123}I]-MIBG. Some studies found no correlation; on the other hand, other studies reported a significant correlation between myocardial [^{123}I]-MIBG uptake and disease severity or duration, as reported by a recent systematic review (Treglia et al. 2012).

Another important issue to be clarified is the correlation between myocardial [^{123}I]-MIBG uptake and the presence of autonomic dysfunction in PD. No clear data are available whether [^{123}I]-MIBG uptake is associated with symptoms and signs of dysautonomia in PD patients. Some studies found no differences in myocardial [^{123}I]-MIBG uptake in relation to the presence and severity of clinical autonomic dysfunction or abnormal autonomic tests (Braune et al. 1999; Berganzo et al. 2012). On the other hand, de novo PD patients without clinical evidence of autonomic dysfunction showed reduced myocardial [^{123}I]-MIBG uptake suggesting that [^{123}I]-MIBG scintigraphy could be a sensitive method to detect latent subclinical autonomic dysfunction (Courbon et al. 2003; Oka et al. 2006).

However, among PD patients, the severity of myocardial sympathetic denervation does not seem to be related to the severity of loss of nigrostriatal dopaminergic neurons. For these reasons, autonomic dysfunction, as measured by sympathetic noradrenergic denervation, seems to occur independently of the dopaminergic impairment that causes the movement disorders in PD. Because of this independence, evidence of myocardial sympathetic denervation can be an early finding but may also occur after the movement disorder is overt in PD (Treglia et al. 2014).

Sequential imaging using [^{123}I]-MIBG scintigraphy revealed progressive degeneration of the cardiac sympathetic nerves in patients with PD (Watanabe et al. 2011). Therefore, [^{123}I]-MIBG scintigraphy could be a useful tool in clinical trials that intend to prove neuroprotection among patients with PD.

In the clinical practice, [^{123}I]-MIBG scintigraphy may help physicians for the differential diagnosis between PD and other parkinsonisms, in particular degenerative parkinsonisms such as MSA, corticobasal degeneration (CBD), and progressive supranuclear palsy (PSP). This differential diagnosis may be difficult using other neuroimaging methods such as striatal dopaminergic imaging (Treglia et al. 2014).

By contrast to PD, in MSA the autonomic nervous system is mainly affected in its preganglionic structures, and most MSA patients present central catecholamine deficiency but preserved myocardial sympathetic innervation showing normal myocardial [^{123}I]-MIBG uptake (Reinhardt et al. 2000; Braune et al. 1999). In PSP and CBD patients, myocardial sympathetic denervation is usually absent resulting in a normal myocardial [^{123}I]-MIBG scintigraphy compared to PD patients; few data are recorded for other parkinsonisms (Treglia et al. 2012).

Some recent meta-analyses reported the diagnostic performance of myocardial [^{123}I]-MIBG scintigraphy in the differential diagnosis between PD and other parkinsonisms (King et al. 2011; Orimo et al. 2012; Treglia et al. 2011, 2012). Although these meta-analyses showed differences in methodology, they confirmed the high sensitivity, specificity, and accuracy of [^{123}I]-MIBG scintigraphy in differentiating PD from other parkinsonisms.

Nevertheless, possible causes of false-positive and false-negative results of this scintigraphic method should be kept in mind. It should be noted that various heart diseases and diabetes may damage the postganglionic sympathetic neurons, leading to a decreased myocardial [^{123}I]-MIBG uptake and false-positive [^{123}I]-MIBG scintigraphy findings (Treglia et al. 2012). In most of the published studies, patients who had heart diseases were excluded, but in clinical setting tomographic images obtained by using single-photon emission computed tomography (SPECT) might be useful for differentiating regional defects due to heart diseases from global denervation of DLB.

Furthermore, an appropriate selection of patients taking into account drugs that may influence myocardial [^{123}I]-MIBG uptake (Solanki et al. 1992; Flotats et al. 2010) should be performed.

In comparison with PD, patients with other parkinsonisms usually show a higher myocardial [^{123}I]-MIBG uptake. Nevertheless, myocardial [^{123}I]-MIBG uptake in patients with other parkinsonisms (especially in patients with MSA and PSP) was often found slightly reduced in comparison to healthy controls, and this finding may cause false-positive results in some cases (Treglia et al. 2012). Mild degeneration of the myocardial sympathetic nervous system, as demonstrated in patients with MSA (Orimo et al. 2007b), may account for this scintigraphic finding.

False-positive results of [^{123}I]-MIBG scintigraphy may be due also to age-related and not only LBD-related postganglionic sympathetic degeneration, because myocardial [^{123}I]-MIBG uptake has significant age-related decrease (Sakata et al. 2009).

False-negative results of [^{123}I]-MIBG scintigraphy in patients with PD may be caused by early stage of disease, disease duration less than 1 year, tremor-dominant phenotypes, and some genetically determined PD (Treglia et al. 2012).

Lastly, the diagnostic accuracy of [^{123}I]-MIBG scintigraphy in patients with PD improves substantially if combined with other diagnostic tests, such as transcranial sonography, olfactory testing, or striatal dopaminergic imaging (Spiegel et al. 2005; Kajimoto et al. 2009; Izawa et al. 2012).

21.2.3 [^{123}I]-MIBG Scintigraphy in Dementia with Lewy Bodies and Other Dementias

Several single-center studies using [^{123}I]-MIBG scintigraphy have demonstrated reduced myocardial MIBG uptake in DLB, as opposed to other dementias (Treglia et al. 2010).

Estorch et al. found that myocardial [^{123}I]-MIBG uptake was significantly decreased in patients with DLB in comparison to all other neurodegenerative diseases with cognitive impairment with a sensitivity and a specificity of 94 and 96 %, respectively (Estorch et al. 2008). The same group found a high diagnostic performance of [^{123}I]-MIBG scintigraphy also at early imaging (Camacho et al. 2013).

In probable DLB, an impairment of both myocardial [^{123}I]-MIBG uptake and striatal dopaminergic imaging was found (Camacho et al. 2011; Treglia et al. 2014), suggesting that myocardial sympathetic degeneration and nigrostriatal degeneration parallel similarly in these patients.

A recent meta-analysis including eight studies found that the pooled sensitivity of [^{123}I]-MIBG scintigraphy in detection of DLB was 98 % and the pooled specificity in differential diagnosis between DLB and other dementias was 94 % (Treglia and Cason 2012).

Also striatal dopaminergic imaging has demonstrated high diagnostic accuracy in differential diagnosis between DLB and other dementias (Papathanasiou et al. 2012). An advantage of myocardial [^{123}I]-MIBG scintigraphy over other functional studies in differential diagnosis between DLB and other dementias is the short acquisition time and comfortable planar imaging, which is appreciated by patients and their caregivers (Estorch et al. 2008).

21.3 PET Tracers

[^{123}I]-MIBG is not an optimal tracer for the assessment of sympathetic myocardial innervation. To a considerable extent it is taken up also in extraneuronal structures, i.e., myocardial myocytes. The specific uptake via the neuronal norepinephrine transporter accounts for only about 50 % of uptake. Furthermore, [^{123}I]-MIBG does not allow exact quantification of myocardial innervation. PET offers higher sensitivity and more accurate measurements of tissue radioactivity concentrations than SPECT, allowing the quantification of myocardial innervation.

21.3.1 [^{11}C]-mHED

[^{11}C]-mHED is a metaraminol analog and it is a good substrate for the norepinephrine transporter. It shares the same neuronal uptake mechanism as norepinephrine and is also resistant to norepinephrine metabolism. By using [^{11}C]-mHED, the myocardial retention fraction can be calculated based on kinetic modelling (Munch et al. 2000). Further advantages of [^{11}C]-mHED in comparison with [^{123}I]-MIBG are the higher specific radioactivity and the fact that this PET tracer is primarily taken up via specific uptake (about 92 %). [^{11}C]-mHED not only provides quantitative measurements of myocardial tracer retention, reflecting sympathetic nerve density, but also allows for the detailed assessment of regional variations in left ventricular innervation (Bengel and Schwaiger 2004; Raffel and Wieland 2001; Raffel et al. 2006a, b).

Berding et al. performed a preliminary study supporting the concept that measurements of sympathetic myocardial innervation using [^{11}C]-mHED PET may contribute to the differential diagnosis of parkinsonisms. They also suggested a role for quantitative innervation imaging, particularly at early stages of PD (Berding et al. 2003).

However, Raffel et al. showed that PET with [^{11}C]-mHED detected significant losses of myocardial sympathetic nerve fibers not only in patients with PD but also in some patients with MSA and PSP. In all patients with PD and with reduced [^{11}C]-mHED retention, sympathetic denervation consistently was found to occur throughout the entire left ventricle. Although some patients with MSA also had complete left ventricular denervation, patients with MSA and PSP had mainly focal regions of denervation. In light of these findings, the scintigraphic detection of myocardial sympathetic denervation alone by [^{11}C]-mHED PET could not be used to differentiate PD from MSA and PSP. Myocardial sympathetic denervation studied by [^{11}C]-mHED PET was found not to be correlated with striatal denervation, suggesting that the neurodegenerative processes in these tissues occur independently (Raffel et al. 2006a, b).

In a recent prospective study, Wong et al. by using [^{11}C]-mHED PET in 27 PD patients demonstrated that myocardial sympathetic denervation in PD is extensive, with a segmental pattern that involves the proximal lateral left ventricular wall most severely, with relative sparing of the anterior and proximal septal walls (Wong et al. 2012).

21.3.2 [^{18}F]-dopamine

Another PET tracer used to map the regional distribution of myocardial sympathetic neurons is [^{18}F]-dopamine (Goldstein et al. 2000a, b), which is available at National Institute of Health of Bethesda (USA). This tracer is transported into sympathetic nerve ending by specific uptake then is rapidly converted to fluoronorepinephrine (FNE) by dopamine beta-hydroxylase in neuronal vesicles. Uptake of [^{18}F]-dopamine into sympathetic nerve terminals, with conversion to and storage of FNE in vesicles, would lead to more intense radioactivity signals from sympathetically innervated tissues compared to non-innervated tissues.

It was previously reported that patients with PD and orthostatic hypotension have remarkably decreased left ventricular myocardial concentrations of [^{18}F]-dopamine (Goldstein et al. 1997; Goldstein et al. 2000a, b). [^{18}F]-dopamine PET also demonstrated a reduction of myocardial uptake not only in PD patients who have orthostatic hypotension but also in one half of patients with PD without orthostatic hypotension (Goldstein et al. 2002). These findings confirmed that myocardial sympathetic denervation does not cause the orthostatic hypotension and autonomic failure in PD.

[^{18}F]-dopamine PET may be useful to study the progression of myocardial sympathetic denervation in patients with PD (Li et al. 2002). This method was also found able to differentiate PD from MSA (Goldstein et al. 2008), whereas other LBD such as PAF presented a marked myocardial sympathetic denervation similar to PD (Tipre and Goldstein 2005; Goldstein and Sewell 2009).

21.4 Comparison Between Myocardial and Brain Innervation Imaging

In LBD, progressive nigrostriatal denervation and degeneration in the peripheral autonomic nervous system are typical features.

Nigrostriatal dopaminergic system may be evaluated by using both SPECT and PET tracers. SPECT of the nigrostriatal dopaminergic system is widely used in patients with LBD. For example, imaging of dopamine transporter (DAT) binding with [^{123}I]-*N*-ω-fluoropropyl-2β-carbomethoxy-3β-(4-iodophenyl)nortropan (FP-CIT) successfully visualizes presynaptic dopaminergic degeneration of the nigrostriatal tract. This procedure allows differentiation of DLB from other dementias (Papathanasiou et al. 2012) and degenerative parkinsonism from movement disorders that are not associated with dopaminergic deficit, such as essential tremor (Treglia et al. 2014). DAT imaging alone, however, does not differentiate the various types of degenerative parkinsonism with sufficient accuracy (Südmeyer et al. 2011; Treglia et al. 2014).

In the latter regard, SPECT of dopamine D_2 receptors with radioligands such as [^{123}I]-(*S*)-2-hydroxy-3-iodo-6-methoxy-*N*-[1-ethyl-2-pyrrodinyl)-methyl]benzamide (IBZM) may be helpful, because patients with atypical parkinsonism usually display lower D_2 receptor binding than do PD patients (Südmeyer et al. 2011).

The radiopharmaceutical 3,4-dihydroxy-6-[18F]fluoro-l-phenylalanine ([^{18}F]-DOPA) is the most used PET tracer to evaluate the nigrostriatal dopaminergic system. [^{18}F]-DOPA allows to evaluate the first step in dopaminergic transmission, namely, dopamine synthesis, which takes place in the presynaptic dopaminergic neurons. [^{18}F]-DOPA is taken up into neurons by an active transport system and is converted to [^{18}F]-dopamine by aromatic amino-acid decarboxylase (AADC), which represents the rate-limiting step for dopamine synthesis in dopaminergic neurons. As such, [^{18}F]-DOPA uptake reflects the synthetic ability of dopaminergic neurons to produce dopamine through AADC. Striatal [^{18}F]-DOPA PET findings are usually impaired in patients with neurodegenerative parkinsonisms (Berti et al. 2011).

Several studies in the literature compared myocardial sympathetic with striatal dopaminergic innervation imaging by using SPECT or PET tracers in LBD.

Spiegel et al. demonstrated that in early PD patients, binding of striatal FP-CIT correlated significantly with cardiac [^{123}I]-MIBG uptake. FP-CIT SPECT and [^{123}I]-MIBG scintigraphy could contribute to the early diagnosis of PD. In addition, the functional loss of nigrostriatal and cardiac sympathetic neurons seemed to be coupled closely (Spiegel et al. 2005).

Novellino et al. reported that the combined use of both FP-CIT SPECT and [^{123}I]-MIBG scintigraphy in mixed tremors with additional extrapyramidal features could help in distinguishing patients with essential tremor from those with PD and other parkinsonism (Novellino et al. 2009).

Recent results suggested that the multidimensional combination of FP-CIT, IBZM, and [^{123}I]-MIBG scintigraphy significantly increases the diagnostic accuracy in differentiating PD from other parkinsonism (Südmeyer et al. 2011). In fact, FP-CIT SPECT showed high sensitivity in the diagnosis of LBD; [^{123}I]-MIBG scintigraphy may have a complementary role in differential diagnosis between PD and other parkinsonisms (Treglia et al. 2014).

[^{123}I]-MIBG scintigraphy and FP-CIT SPECT showed similar diagnostic accuracy in differential diagnosis between DLB and other dementias (Treglia et al. 2014). In probable DLB, myocardial [^{123}I]-MIBG uptake and FP-CIT binding in basal ganglia are reduced. The positive correlation between both measures suggests that cardiac sympathetic degeneration and nigrostriatal degeneration parallel similarly in patients with probable DLB (Camacho et al. 2011).

Conclusion

Myocardial innervation imaging by using SPECT and PET tracers provides useful information in patients with neurodegenerative diseases such as LBD.

In the clinical practice, myocardial innervation imaging by SPECT or PET tracers was found very useful in differential diagnosis of neurodegenerative diseases and, in particular, in distinguishing PD from other parkinsonisms and DLB from other dementias.

Further larger studies are required to understand whether myocardial innervation imaging by using SPECT or PET tracers is able to correlate the degree of myocardial sympathetic denervation with severity and duration of LBD and to monitor the therapy response.

References

Arimo T, Orimo S, Itoh Y et al (2005) Profound cardiac sympathetic denervation occurs in Parkinson disease. Brain Pathol 15:29–34

Bengel FM, Schwaiger M (2004) Assessment of cardiac sympathetic neuronal function using PET imaging. J Nucl Cardiol 11:603–616

Berding G, Schrader CH, Peschel T et al (2003) [N-methyl 11C]meta-Hydroxyephedrine positron emission tomography in Parkinson's disease and multiple system atrophy. Eur J Nucl Med Mol Imaging 30:127–131

Berganzo K, Tijero B, Somme JH et al (2012) SCOPA-AUT scale in different parkinsonisms and its correlation with 123I-MIBG cardiac scintigraphy. Parkinsonism Relat Disord 18:45–48

Berti V, Pupi A, Mosconi L (2011) PET/CT in diagnosis of movement disorders. Ann N Y Acad Sci 1228:93–108

Braune S, Reinhardt M, Schnitzer R et al (1999) Cardiac uptake of [123I]MIBG separates Parkinson's disease from multiple system atrophy. Neurology 53:1020–1025

Camacho V, Carrio I (2007) Targeting neuronal dysfunction and receptor imaging. Curr Opin Biotechnol 18:60–64

Camacho V, Marquie M, Lleo A et al (2011) Cardiac sympathetic impairment parallels nigrostriatal degeneration in probable dementia with Lewy bodies. Q J Nucl Med Mol Imaging 55:476–483

Camacho V, Estorch M, Marquié M et al (2013) Utility of early imaging of myocardial innervation scintigraphy in the diagnosis of Lewy body dementia. Rev Esp Med Nucl Imagen Mol 32:77–80.

Chiaravalloti A, Stefani A, Tavolozza M et al (2012) Different patterns of cardiac sympathetic denervation in tremor-type compared to akinetic-rigid-type Parkinson's disease: molecular imaging with ^{123}I-MIBG. Mol Med Rep 6:1337–1342

Chung EJ, Kim EG, Kim MS et al (2011) Differences in myocardial sympathetic degeneration and the clinical features of the subtypes of Parkinson's disease. J Cin Neurosci 18:922–925

Courbon F, Brefel-Courbon C, Thalamas C et al (2003) Cardiac MIBG scintigraphy is a sensitive tool for detecting cardiac sympathetic denervation in Parkinson's disease. Mov Disord 18:890–897

Estorch M (2006) From the heart to the brain via cardiac MIBG imaging. Eur J Nucl Med Mol Imaging 33:246–247

Estorch M, Camacho V, Paredes P et al (2008) Cardiac 123Imetaiodobenzylguanidine imaging allows early identification of dementia with Lewy bodies during life. Eur J Nucl Med Mol Imaging 35:1636–1641

Flotats A, Carrio I, Agostini D et al (2010) Proposal for standardization of 123I-metaiodobenzylguanidine (MIBG) cardiac sympathetic imaging by the EANM

Cardiovascular Committee and the European Council of Nuclear Cardiology. Eur J Nucl Med Mol Imaging 37:1802–1812

Goldstein DS, Sewell L (2009) Olfactory dysfunction in pure autonomic failure: implications for the pathogenesis of Lewy body diseases. Parkinsonism Relat Disord 15:516–520

Goldstein DS, Holmes C, Cannon RO et al (1997) Sympathetic cardioneuropathy in dysautonomias. N Engl J Med 336:696–702

Goldstein DS, Chang PC, Eisenhofer G et al (2000a) Positron emission tomographic imaging of cardiac sympathetic innervation and function. Circulation 81:1606–1621

Goldstein DS, Holmes C, Li ST et al (2000b) Cardiac sympathetic denervation in Parkinson disease. Ann Intern Med 133:338–347

Goldstein DS, Holmes CS, Dendi R et al (2002) Orthostatic hypotension from sympathetic denervation in Parkinson's disease. Neurology 58:1247–1255

Goldstein DS, Holmes C, Bentho O et al (2008) Biomarkers to detect central dopamine deficiency and distinguish Parkinson disease from multiple system atrophy. Parkinsonism Relat Disord 14:600–607

Hirayama M, Hakusui S, Koike Y et al (1995) A scintigraphical qualitative analysis of peripheral vascular sympathetic function with meta-[123I] iodobenzylguanidine in neurological patients with autonomic failure. J Auton Nerv Syst 53:230–234

Hishikawa N, Hashizume Y, Yoshida M et al (2003) Clinical and neuropathological correlates of Lewy body disease. Acta Neuropathol 105:341–350

Iwanaga K, Wakabayashi K, Yoshimoto M et al (1999) Lewy body-type degeneration in cardiac plexus in Parkinson's disease and incidental Lewy body diseases. Neurology 52:1269–1271

Izawa MO, Miwa H, Kajimoto Y et al (2012) Combination of transcranial sonography, olfactory testing and MIBG myocardial scintigraphy as a diagnostic indicator for Parkinson's disease. Eur J Neurol 19:411–416

Jankovic J (2008) Parkinson's disease: clinical features and diagnosis. J Neurol Neurosurg Psychiatry 79:368–376

Kajimoto Y, Miwa H, Okawa-Izawa M et al (2009) Transcranial sonography of the substantia nigra and MIBG myocardial scintigraphy: complementary role in the diagnosis of Parkinson's disease. Parkinsonism Relat Disord 15:270–272

Kashihara K, Imamura T, Shinya T (2010) Cardiac 123I-MIBG uptake is reduced more markedly in patients with REM sleep behavior disorder than in those with early stage Parkinson's disease. Parkinsonism Relat Disord 16:252–255

King AE, Mintz J, Royall DR (2011) Meta-analysis of 123I-MIBG cardiac scintigraphy for the diagnosis of Lewy-body-related disorders. Mov Disord 26:1218–1224

Kitayama M, Wada-Isoe K, Irizawa Y et al (2008) Association of visual hallucinations with reduction of MIBG cardiac uptake in Parkinson's disease. J Neurol Sci 264:22–26

Lee PH, Yeo SH, Kim HJ et al (2006) Correlation between cardiac 123I-MIBG and odor identification in patients with Parkinson's disease and multiple system atrophy. Mov Disord 21:1975–1977

Li ST, Dendi R, Holmes C et al (2002) Progressive loss of cardiac sympathetic innervation in Parkinson's disease. Ann Neurol 52:220–223

McKeith IG (2006) Consensus guidelines for the clinical and pathologic diagnosis of dementia with Lewy bodies (DLB): report of the Consortium on DLB International Workshop. J Alzheimer's Dis 9(3 Suppl):417–423

Miyamoto T, Miyamoto M, Inoue Y et al (2006) Reduced cardiac 123I-MIBG scintigraphy in idiopathic REM sleep behavior disorder. Neurology 67:2236–2238

Munch G, Nguyen NT, Nekolla S et al (2000) Evaluation of sympathetic nerve terminals with [11C]epinephrine and [11C]hydroxyephedrine and positron emission tomography. Circulation 101:516–523

Nakajima K, Yoshita M, Matsuo S et al (2008) Iodine-123-MIBG sympathetic imaging in Lewy-body diseases and related movement disorders. Q J Nucl Med Mol Imaging 52:378–387

Nakajima K, Okuda K, Matsuo S et al (2012) Standardization of metaiodobenzylguanidine heart to mediastinum ratio using a calibration phantom: effects of correction on normal databases and a multicentre study. Eur J Nucl Med Mol Imaging 39:113–119

Novellino F, Arabia G, Bagnato A et al (2009) Combined use of DAT-SPECT and cardiac MIBG scintigraphy in mixed tremors. Mov Disord 24:2242–2248

Oka H, Mochio S, Onouchi K et al (2006) Cardiovascular dysautonomia in de novo Parkinson's disease. J Neurol Sci 241:59–65

Oka H, Yoshioka M, Onouchi K et al (2007a) Characteristics of orthostatic hypotension in Parkinson's disease. Brain 130:2425–2432

Oka H, Yoshioka M, Onouchi K et al (2007b) Impaired cardiovascular autonomic function in Parkinson's disease with visual hallucinations. Mov Disord 22:1510–1514

Orimo S, Oka T, Miura H et al (2002) Sympathetic cardiac denervation in Parkinson's disease and pure autonomic failure but not in multiple system atrophy. J Neurol Neurosurg Psychiatry 73:776–777

Orimo S, Amino T, Itoh Y et al (2005) Cardiac sympathetic denervation precedes neuronal loss in the sympathetic ganglia in Lewy body disease. Acta Neuropathol 109:583–588

Orimo S, Takahashi A, Uchihara T et al (2007a) Degeneration of cardiac sympathetic nerve begins in the early disease process of Parkinson's disease. Brain Pathol 17:24–30

Orimo S, Kanazawa T, Nakamura A et al (2007b) Degeneration of cardiac sympathetic nerve can occur in multiple system atrophy. Acta Neuropathol 113:81–86

Orimo S, Suzuki M, Inaba A et al (2012) 123I-MIBG myocardial scintigraphy for differentiating Parkinson's disease from other neurodegenerative parkinsonism: a systematic review and meta-analysis. Parkinsonism Relat Disord 18:494–500

Papathanasiou ND, Boutsiadis A, Dickson J et al (2012) Diagnostic accuracy of ^{123}I-FP-CIT (DaTSCAN) in dementia with Lewy bodies: a meta-analysis of published studies. Parkinsonism Relat Disord 18:225–229

Puschmann A, Bhidayasiri R, Weiner WJ (2012) Synucleinopathies from bench to bedside. Parkinsonism Relat Disord 18(Suppl 1):S24–S27

Quattrone A, Bagnato A, Annesi G et al (2008) Myocardial (123)metaiodobenzylguanidine uptake in genetic Parkinson's disease. Mov Disord 23:21–27

Raffel DM, Wieland DM (2001) Assessment of cardiac sympathetic nerve integrity with positron emission tomography. Nucl Med Biol 28:541–559

Raffel DM, Chen W, Sherman PS et al (2006a) Dependence of cardiac 11C-meta-hydroxyephedrine retention on norepinephrine transporter density. J Nucl Med 47:1490–1496

Raffel DM, Koeppe RA, Little R et al (2006b) PET measurement of cardiac and nigrostriatal denervation in Parkinsonian syndromes. J Nucl Med 47:1769–1777

Rascol O, Schelosky L (2009) 123-I-Metaiodobenzylguanidine scintigraphy in Parkinson's disease and related disorders. Mov Disord 24(Suppl 2):S732–S741

Reinhardt MJ, Jóngling FD, Krause TM et al (2000) Scintigraphic differentiation between two forms of primary dysautonomia early after onset autonomic dysfunction: value of cardiac and pulmonary iodine-123 MIBG uptake. Eur J Nucl Med 27:595–600

Sakata K, Iida K, Mochizuki N et al (2009) Physiological changes in human cardiac sympathetic innervation and activity assessed by 123I-Metaiodobenzylguanidine (MIBG) imaging. Circ J 73:310–315

Solanki KK, Bomanji J, Moyes J et al (1992) A pharmacological guide to medicines which interfere with the biodistribution of radiolabelled meta-iodobenzylguanidine (MIBG). Nucl Med Commun 13:513–521

Spiegel J, Mollers MO, Jost WH et al (2005) FP-CIT and MIBG scintigraphy in early Parkinson's disease. Mov Disord 20:552–561

Spiegel J, Hellwig D, Farmakis G et al (2007) Myocardial sympathetic degeneration correlates with clinical phenotype of Parkinson's disease. Mov Disord 22:1004–1008

Südmeyer M, Antke C, Zizek T et al (2011) Diagnostic accuracy of combined FP-CIT, IBZM, and MIBG scintigraphy in the differential diagnosis of degenerative parkinsonism: a multidimensional statistical approach. J Nucl Med 52:733–740

Suzuki M, Kurita A, Hashimoto M et al (2006) Impaired myocardial 123I-metaiodobenzylguanidine uptake in Lewy body disease: comparison between dementia with Lewy bodies and Parkinson's disease. J Neurol Sci 240:15–19

Takatsu H, Nishida H, Matsuo H et al (2000) Cardiac sympathetic denervation from the early stage of Parkinson's disease: clinical and experimental studies with radiolabeled MIBG. J Nucl Med 41:71–77

Taki J, Nakajima K, Hwang EH et al (2000) Peripheral sympathetic dysfunction in patients with Parkinson's disease without autonomic failure is heart selective and disease specific. Eur J Nucl Med 27:566–573

Tateno M, Kobayashi S, Saito T (2009) Imaging improves diagnosis of dementia with Lewy bodies. Psychiatry Investig 6:233–240

Tipre DN, Goldstein DS (2005) Cardiac and extracardiac sympathetic denervation in Parkinson's disease with orthostatic hypotension and in pure autonomic failure. J Nucl Med 46:1775–1781

Treglia G, Cason E (2012) Diagnostic performance of myocardial innervation imaging using MIBG scintigraphy in differential diagnosis between dementia with Lewy bodies and other dementias: a systematic review and a meta-analysis. J Neuroimaging 22:111–117

Treglia G, Cason E, Gabellini A et al (2010) Recent developments in innervation imaging using iodine-123-metaiodobenzylguanidine scintigraphy in Lewy body diseases. Neurol Sci 31:417–422

Treglia G, Stefanelli A, Cason E et al (2011) Diagnostic performance of iodine-123-metaiodobenzylguanidine scintigraphy in differential diagnosis between Parkinson's disease and multiple system atrophy: a systematic review and a meta-analysis. Clin Neurol Neurosurg 113:823–829

Treglia G, Cason E, Stefanelli A et al (2012) MIBG scintigraphy in differential diagnosis of parkinsonism: a meta-analysis. Clin Auton Res 22:43–55

Treglia G, Cason E, Cortelli P et al (2014) Iodine-123 metaiodobenzylguanidine scintigraphy and iodine-123 ioflupane single photon emission computed tomography in Lewy body diseases: complementary or alternative techniques? J Neuroimaging 24:149–154

Watanabe M, Takeda T, Nakamagoe K et al (2011) Sequential imaging analysis using MIBG scintigraphy revealed progressive degeneration of cardiac sympathetic nerve in Parkinson's disease. Eur J Neurol 18:1010–1013

Weisman D, McKeith I (2007) Dementia with Lewy bodies. Semin Neurol 27:42–47

Wong KK, Raffel DM, Koeppe RA et al (2012) Pattern of cardiac sympathetic denervation in idiopathic Parkinson disease studied with 11C hydroxyephedrine PET. Radiology 265:240–247

Yamashina S, Yamazaki J (2007) Neuronal imaging using SPECT. Eur J Nucl Med Mol Imaging 34:939–950

Imaging the Functional Brain-Heart Axis: Mental Stress and Cardiac Dysfunction

22

Walter Noordzij, Andor W.J.M. Glaudemans, René A. Tio, Mike J.L. DeJongste, Hans C. Klein, and Riemer H.J.A. Slart

Contents

Disclosures The authors declare not having received financial support.

W. Noordzij, MD (✉) • A.W.J.M. Glaudemans, MD, PhD • R.H.J.A. Slart, MD, PhD
Department of Nuclear Medicine and Molecular Imaging,
University of Groningen, University Medical Center Groningen,
Hanzeplein 1, PO Box 30.001, 9700 Groningen, The Netherlands
e-mail: w.noordzij@umcg.nl; r.h.j.a.slart@umcg.nl

R.A. Tio, MD, PhD • M.J.L. DeJongste, MD, PhD, FESC
Department of Cardiology, University of Groningen, University Medical Center Groningen,
Groningen, The Netherlands

H.C. Klein, MD, PhD
Department of Psychiatry, University of Groningen, University Medical Center Groningen,
Groningen, The Netherlands

R.H.J.A. Slart et al. (eds.), *Autonomic Innervation of the Heart: Role of Molecular Imaging*, DOI 10.1007/978-3-662-45074-1_22

Abstract

Smoking, hypertension and diabetes mellitus are established risk factors for developing endothelial dysfunction and consequently atherosclerosis. Atherosclerosis can lead to myocardial ischemia, in response to physical exercise, change of temperature and emotional stress. Among forms of emotional stress, depression and anxiety are also associated with a higher incidence of coronary artery disease (CAD), as well as worse outcomes in patients with existing CAD. The best validated modalities for imaging myocardial ischemia are single-photon emission computed tomography (SPECT) and positron emission tomography (PET). Each imaging modality offers its own advantages. The exact pathophysiology of mental stress-induced myocardial ischemia is unclear. The cardiac-neural axis seems to play an important role, with special interest in the sympathetic nerve system and adrenomedullary hormones. This chapter describes the published literature using imaging techniques that address mental stress-induced ischemia and its relation to cardiac autonomic dysfunction. Non-invasive imaging of sympathetic and parasympathetic cardiac innervation remains a field for further exploration.

Abbreviations

ATP	Adenosine triphosphate
CAD	Coronary artery disease
CAG	Coronary angiography
CT	Computed tomography
DSM-V	The Diagnostic and Statistical Manual of Mental Disorders (version 5)
ECG	Electrocardiogram
HRV	Heart rate variability
ICN	Intracardiac neurons
LBD	Lewy body disease
LDL	Low-density lipoproteins
MI	Myocardial infarction
MPI	Myocardial perfusion imaging
MRI	Magnetic resonance imaging
MVO2	Myocardial oxygen consumption
OR	Odds ratio
PET	Positron emission tomography
PTSD	Post-traumatic stress disorders
RPP	Rate-pressure product
SPECT	Single-photon emission computed tomography
TRPV	Transient receptor potential vanilloid

22.1 Rationale

In the industrialized world, cardiovascular disease is a leading cause of morbidity and mortality, comprising a diversity of cardiac and vascular conditions. The majority of the cardiovascular morbidity and mortality results from corollaries of atherosclerotic heart disease. Many patients suffering from symptoms of ischemic heart disease have become incapacitated in their daily activities. The impact of these patients' disability on their quality of life often is accompanied by emotional changes. Conversely, patients' mental state may expose symptoms related to or have an impact on the underlying cardiovascular disease. Subsequently, indistinct symptoms such as chest pain, fatigue, dyspnoea and palpitations may indicate the presence of ischemic heart disease, heart failure or arrhythmias, respectively. Furthermore, these signs may be harbingers of an imminent disastrous event. This chapter therefore focuses on the cardiac-neural axis, with respect to mental stress-induced myocardial ischemia, and on the autonomic cardiac innervation.

Given the potential serious consequences of asymptomatic cardiovascular diseases, adequate methods are required to expose the causality and to interpret symptoms. Finally, for understanding the process, diagnosis, prevention and treatment of atherosclerosis, heart failure and arrhythmias, single-photon emission computer tomography (SPECT) and positron emission tomography (PET) have become acknowledged methods. In this chapter, we will discuss the value of PET and SPECT to study the pivotal role of the nervous system in ischemic heart diseases.

22.2 Recent Insights in the Pathophysiology of Atherosclerosis

Recent evidence suggests an association among specific bacteria, disease markers of atherosclerosis and atherosclerotic plaque formation (Koren et al. 2011). In support of recent literature on the origin of atherosclerosis is the finding that O_2, glucose and a variety of metabolites are modulating receptors of glomus cells in the gut. When oxygen tension reduces, these specialized cells activate the afferent part of the autonomic reflex system through releasing dopamine and noradrenalin and hence may alter tonic inhibition of the anti-inflammatory-cholinergic pathway, the so-called gut-brain axis (Tracey 2009). From the available evidence it is further concluded that inflammatory responses influence brain functions, via a cytokine cascade, specifically via the interleukin (IL1)-activated inflammatory-cholinergic nerves. The subsequent neuro-inflammatory status of the gut of individuals induces low-grade inflammatory responses, which ultimately may induce chronic diseases, such as atherosclerosis (McLean et al. 2012).

Following attachment of low-density lipoproteins (LDLs) to the endothelial layer of the artery, atherosclerotic plaque formation develops. Next, these LDL particles are oxidized. Oxidation of LDL is influenced among others by risk factors for coronary artery disease. Atherosclerotic plaque narrowing of a coronary artery induces myocardial ischemia when oxygen supply cannot meet the increased demand, most often resulting from an increase in heart rate and systolic blood pressure (the so-called double product), during exercise. The double product or rate-pressure product (RPP) is proportional with myocardial oxygen consumption (MVO_2).

Risk factors for developing atherosclerosis are, inter alia, aging, smoking, metabolic syndrome (high insulin resistance-induced dyslipidaemia, hypertension and diabetes mellitus), genetic abnormalities and mental stress. All these factors can affect endothelial function. To neutralize the oxidized LDL-specific cells, a subtype of lymphocytes, the so-called foam cells, induces a sequence of immune activation processes. However, foam cells are unable to metabolize the oxidized-LDL sufficiently and so are causing accumulation of oxidized cholesterol into the artery wall, creating an atheroma. According to the 'response to injury' theory following shear stress, macrophages lymphocytes are triggered to attach to the endothelial wall and so the atherosclerotic process continues (Libby et al. 2011). The atherosclerotic plaques progressively thicken, and when vulnerable the plaque may become instable and subsequently ruptures, usually at its frailest edge, the so-called shoulder. When a ruptured plaque releases its debris, this occludes a coronary artery and results in myocardial infarction. In addition, neurohumoral activation and immune activation are initiated. All this instigated processes are engaged in to limit the damage and, however, may also result in deleterious events, such as lethal arrhythmias.

22.2.1 Pathophysiology of Myocardial Ischemia

In stable coronary artery disease (CAD), the unfavourable shift in oxygen balance usually is provoked during exercise, when oxygen supply is failing to meet the increased oxygen demand. The subsequent mismatch between myocardial oxygen supply and demand induces myocardial ischemia. Myocardial ischemia provokes chemical and mechanical stimulation of sensory afferent nerve endings both in the coronary vessels and in the myocardium and so induces feelings of discomfort in specific brain centres of the individual. The successively induced vague and uneasy sensations are most often located at the chest, with or without radiation towards jaws, shoulders, back and arms and are coined as angina pectoris. In stable situations, symptoms of angina increase as a consequence of physical or emotional stress and decrease at rest or after administration of nitroglycerin. With respect to emotional stress specifically rage, anxiety and depression are considered as both triggers and predisposing causes of angina pectoris (Soufer and Burg 2007; Crea et al. 1992). Finally, in addition to physical and mental triggers for angina, all causes for myocardial ischemia, such as anaemia, apnoea, spasm and a sudden decrease in temperature, may provoke angina in patients with known CAD.

Myocardial ischemia, the consequence of the imbalance between myocardial blood supply and oxygen demand, usually arises when an obstruction in one or more coronary arteries exceeds >70 % (Abrams 2005). The oxygen demand is related to heart rate, contractility and systolic wall stress, while the blood supply is based on coronary flow and oxygen-carrying capacity of blood. Myocytes are heavily dependent on oxidative metabolism; their demand must be covered entirely by increased blood flow. Myocardial ischemia therefore alters, within a certain timeframe, the mitochondrial metabolism of the myocytes, first resulting in diastolic dysfunction. Systolic dysfunction, electrocardiogram (ECG) changes and angina are subsequent events.

22.2.2 Pathophysiology of Angina Pectoris

Angina is induced following complex neurochemical cascades initiated by myocardial ischemia. Initiated through myocardial ischemia, acidosis develops and a variety of chemical substances are released, including lactate, serotonin, bradykinin, histamine, reactive oxygen species and adenosine (Benson et al. 1999; Longhurst et al. 2001). A consequence of the release of adenosine into the vessel is that formation of energy storage of adenosine triphosphate (ATP) in the myocyte decreases. In addition to the subsequent reduction in performance of myocytes, these released substance initiate stimulation of receptors of unmyelinated nerve cells found within cardiac muscle fibres and around the coronary vessel (Foreman 1999). Adenosine has been found to induce angina via stimulation of the A1 adenosine receptor (Crea et al. 1999; Gaspardone et al. 1995).

Numerous psychological characteristics, and most notably anxiety and depression, are strong correlates of recent angina and angina in the presence of ischemia provoked by treadmill testing (Ketterer et al. 2011). In a large recently published worldwide study, 11,119 patients with a first myocardial infarction were compared with 13,648 age-matched control subjects (Rosengren et al. 2004). The incidence of reported stress at work and at home, financial stress and major life events in the past year was higher in patients than in controls. Depression was more frequent in patients with a myocardial infarction than in controls (odds ratio (OR) 1.55). Odds ratios for permanent stress at work or at home were also high: 2.14 and 2.12, respectively. Depression and anxiety are also associated with worse outcome of CAD, i.e. higher mortality and more often ventricular dysrhythmias (Frasure-Smith and Lesperance 2008; Watkins et al. 2006). In case of depression and comorbid anxiety, the prevalence of cardiac events (defined as stroke, myocardial infarction, heart failure and CAD-related mortality) is even higher (Rutledge et al. 2009).

Several studies have shown that the distressed (type D) personality can be considered as a risk marker for poor health outcomes in patients with cardiovascular disease, including CAD (OR 1.54) (Beutel et al. 2012). Moreover, type D personality was associated negatively with health-related quality of life, in a meta-analysis of 15 separate studies (O'Dell et al. 2011). Albeit that the pathway through which personality D induces cardiac disorders is largely unravelled, interest is growing to study different forms of mental stress, specifically since mental stress may induce myocardial ischemia in patients not familiar with CAD.

22.3 Neural Hierarchy in Cardiac Control

When the coronary atherosclerotic process gives rise to myocardial ischemia, this eventually may result in derailments like myocardial infarction, heart failure and lethal arrhythmias. With respect to the latter two, the nervous system plays a vital role. In addition to the efferent (sympathetic) nervous system, the nervous system also controls the heart via a humoral pathway, among others through the release of catecholamines. Recently, it was hypothesized that along with the nervous and humoral pathway from brain to heart and a nervous route from heart to brain, there also is evidence for a humoral route from both heart (DeJongste et al. 2009) and periphery to brain (Zhao et al. 2012). Zhao et al. suggested that stimulation of the cholinergic anti-inflammatory pathway may play an additional role in the treatment of cardiac diseases.

These reciprocal links in transmission between heart and brain have become increasingly important topics to study neurocardiological interactions. Furthermore, since cardiac function is continuously under the auspice of the neurocardiac axis, knowledge of the hierarchically entailed neurohumoral control of the heart is essential, because the onset of neurohumoral remodelling often starts before cardiac symptoms become clear. In addition, knowledge on the neurocardiac axis helps to improve diagnostic procedures and develop newer therapies (Lathrop and Spooner 2001). In this regard, the use of imaging techniques is often a prerequisite for clinical studies on neurocardiac interactions.

22.3.1 Peripheral Afferent Nervous Relay of Cardiac Function

Afferent nerves from the heart contain the vasoactive neuropeptides substance P and calcitonin gene-related peptide. These compounds are capable to increase, through a so-called neurogenic inflammation, vascular permeability and also may induce vasoconstriction in atherosclerotic coronary segments. These afferent nerves are identified as the transient receptor potential vanilloid (TRPV) channels type 1. Stimuli such as high temperatures, stretch, pharmacologic and endogenous ligands may activate the TRPV1 channel. Therefore, it is suggested that TRPV1 plays a pivotal role in chest discomfort following myocardial ischemia (Robbins et al. 2013). After the ischemic cardiac event, activated cardiac TRPV1 receptors propagate sensory information from the heart to lamina II–IV of Lissauer in the spinal cord (Foreman 1999). Sensory information from the visceral innervated heart is then further relayed via the hypothalamic nuclei and limbic system to the frontal visceral cortex, via afferent pathways of the neuroaxis. The nerve fibres travel along the sympathetic afferent pathways from the heart and enter the sympathetic ganglia in lower cervical and upper thoracic spinal cord (C7-T4).

22.3.2 Higher Brain Centres for Cardiac Control

Through the spinal thalamic tracts impulses are then transmitted via ascending spinal pathways to thalamic and hypothalamic parts of the limbic system and further projected onto the frontal cerebral cortex, where the angina is ultimately ‘felt’. The limbic system is considered as a relay station, participating in integration of emotional and motor information. A variety of cortical sites presides over the limbic system and additionally exerts strong tonic control over descending information via direct connections to the spinal cord. So, in similarity to brain damage, for instance, as a consequence of stroke, a variety of behavioural and emotional factors enables the initiation of deleterious cardiovascular conditions. The outcome of the nervous derailments is among others ventricular arrhythmias, sudden death (Fleet et al. 2000; Tsuchihashi et al. 2001), myocytolysis and stress cardiomyopathy, also known as Tako Tsubo (Kurisu et al. 2002).

In summary, central autonomic control may be considered as the result of higher-level integration influencing descending pathways that project to intrathoracic neurons controlling among others heart rate and contractility. Depending on the site in the cortex where the commotion takes place, the result of perturbation may be more or less deleterious (Cechetto 2004).

22.3.3 Final Common Pathway of Neural Hierarchy in Cardiac Control

Intracardiac neurons (ICNs) are highly specified ganglionated plexi localized in the fatty patches on the heart. The ICN, considered as 'little brain of the heart', have mutual communications within the neural hierarchy to maintain adequate efferent neural output to cardiomyocytes and to process cardiovascular sensory information to cardiac motor neurons. Though under control of higher brain centres, the ICN may act independently. The nine identified ICNs are controlling all cardiac functions and are containing sympathetic, parasympathetic neurons and interneurons. The ICNs govern among others the β-receptors and muscarine receptors of the heart and so are capable to protect the integrity of the myocyte. Neurohumoral remodelling of the neurocardiac axis, occurring before a cardiac disease is recognized, influences both prognosis and clinical management (Foreman et al. 2004).

22.4 Effects of Mental Stress on Cardiac Performance

22.4.1 Emotions and the Nervous System

Especially depression, hostility (type A behaviour), vital exhaustion and anxiety are forms of mental stress associated with a higher incidence of CAD, as well as with a worse outcome in patients with already present CAD. In addition, a variety of mental stress conditions are linked with cardiovascular disorders, such as the association between depression and heart failure or impetuous exaggeration with stress cardiomyopathy or occurrence of arrhythmias.

The exact pathophysiology of mental stress-induced myocardial ischemia remains still indistinct. However, it is evident that psychological stress induces physiological changes through a rise of the sympathetic tone. This increase in activity within the cardiac-neural axis induces the release of adrenomedullary hormones, augments blood pressure, heart rate, myocardial ischemia and thrombosis tendency and may further provoke (fatal) arrhythmias. Further, interfering in the neurocardiac axis with pharmacotherapeutical agents or through electrical stimulation are both methods that can be used to improve our understanding of the underlying mechanisms in processing information from brain to heart and vice versa.

The most valid modalities for imaging myocardial ischemia are SPECT and PET, each modality with its own advantages. The following section therefore emphasizes the existing literature using imaging techniques to elucidate the pathophysiology of mental stress-induced ischemia and its relation to cardiac autonomic dysfunction. Imaging of sympathetic and parasympathetic cardiac innervation is still a field needing further exploration.

22.5 Imaging Techniques for Neurocardiological Interactions

PET and SPECT are both radionuclide methods used to construct a three-dimensional image of a series of (metabolic) actions of a living creature, through analysing differences in tracer (uptake) concentrations. To date these techniques can be combined with others, like computed tomography (CT). Though many radionuclide tracers can be used, glucose analogues are the most common employed energy source constituents for tracking of metabolic processes. More specifically, radionuclide techniques may be applied to investigate both dynamic processes in metabolic active organs, such as heart and brain, and to study interactions between these organs.

Several tests are available to demonstrate the presence of myocardial ischemia, i.e. exercise treadmill, stress echocardiography or nuclear myocardial perfusion imaging (MPI), either with SPECT or PET (Fig. 22.1), with or without the combination of CT. In SPECT, radioactive (technetium-99m ([^{99m}Tc])-labelled) tracers are used which disintegrate by emitting single gamma rays. SPECT has become a widely available and a thoroughly validated, non-invasive method for imaging of myocardial perfusion defects (Underwood et al. 2004). Myocardial perfusion imaging with SPECT is able to detect obstructive CAD with a sensitivity and specificity >85 %, only slightly less than the test characteristics of PET (using rubidium-82 ([^{82}Rb]), nitrogen-13 ammonia ([^{13}N]NH_3) or oxygen-15 water (H_2[^{15}O])), with sensitivity and specificity >90 % (Machac 2005; Di Carli and Hachamovitch 2007). Furthermore, both early and late stress myocardial perfusion SPECT have superior prognostic value, when compared to visually analysed coronary angiography (Sobic-Saranovic et al. 2013).

Recent developments in both soft- and hardware led to the implementation of hybrid systems, combining SPECT and PET myocardial perfusion imaging with CT. Contrast-enhanced angiography using CT can be an attractive alternative to (invasive) coronary angiography (CAG), also providing anatomical information (Schroeder et al. 2008). In addition, the quantity of coronary artery calcium load, as determined with CT, coined as 'Agatston' or 'calcium score', is used for risk stratification for future cardiac events (Greenland et al. 2007). The clinical use of hybrid imaging (either myocardial perfusion imaging with calcium score or CT angiography with calcium score) provides higher accuracy and faster diagnosis of CAD, especially in cases with equivocal results of separate tests (Flotats et al. 2011).

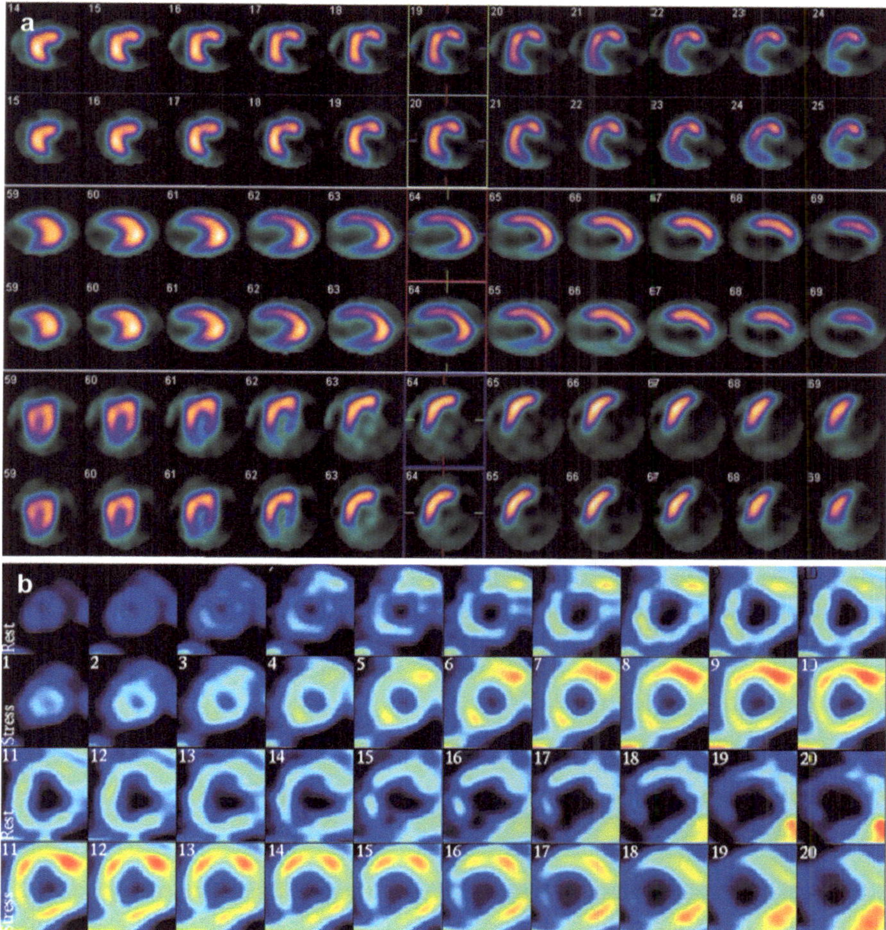

Fig. 22.1 Irreversible defect in the infero-postero-lateral wall on a [^{99m}Tc]-tetrofosmin myocardial perfusion SPECT scan (**a**), indicating myocardial infarction. Infarction in the inferior wall and basal infero-septal region on a [^{13}N]NH_3 PET scan but preserved global perfusion reserve in the remaining tissue (**b**)

22.5.1 Imaging of Effects of Emotional of Stress Responses on Myocardial Ischemia and Autonomic Function, Using PET and SPECT

An early report on imaging techniques to assess nervous control over myocardial ischemia studied the effect of mental arithmetic tasks on myocardial perfusion (Deanfield et al. 1984). During the mental stress tasks, executed in patients with CAD, size and location of perfusion defects on myocardial perfusion scintigraphy were comparable to perfusion defects induced during an exercise performance. Patients with CAD suffered from mental stress more often than patients without

CAD; especially, they may suffer from hostility, depression and anxiety, psychological conditions that all are capable to induce myocardial infarction (MI) (Das and O'Keefe 2008). In this respect, it is worth notifying that depression is an independent risk factor for mortality (Serrano et al. 2011).

Actually, it is reported that various types of anxiety disorders have different impact on the outcomes after MI. In this regard, a generalized anxiety disorder appears to predict a superior 5-year outcome after MI. The authors hypothesized that these patients are expected to seek early help after the manifestation of somatic symptoms and are also more willing to participate in rehabilitation programmes (Parker et al. 2011). On the other hand, panic disorders often co-occur with CAD (Soh and Lee 2010; Fleet et al. 2000). Post-traumatic stress disorders (PTSD) – which is no longer classified as an anxiety disorder but according to the Diagnostic and Statistical Manual of Mental Disorders (DSM-V, American Psychiatric Association 2013) criteria considered to be a 'trauma- and stressor-related disorder' – has also been associated with CAD (Ahmadi et al. 2011). The underlying mechanism of the association of panic disorder with CAD is not yet clear. Reduced heart rate variability (HRV), which is common in both panic disorder and PTSD patient groups, was not significantly different in CAD populations with and without panic disorder. This suggests that reduced HRV may not be the underlying explanation of increased cardiovascular morbidity and mortality in panic disorder patients (Lavoie et al. 2004). Other anxiety disorders, according to the recent DSM-V including inter alia social anxiety disorder, separation anxiety disorder and selective mutism, are not associated with CAD.

22.5.2 Imaging Myocardial Ischemia in Patients with Mental Stress

Myocardial perfusion imaging is often used in patients with mental stress (Fig. 22.2). In fact, the early studies using PET were designed to identify mental stress-induced ischemia (Deanfield et al. 1984). In the latter study, myocardial perfusion imaging with PET showed signs of ischemia in 12 out of 16 patients, though perfusion defects induced by mental stress (arithmetic task) were less pronounced when compared to perfusion defects following physical exercise.

As mentioned before, myocardial perfusion imaging can be performed after physical exercise as well as with pharmacological stress. However, neither of the two methods can be considered to represent emotional or mental stress. In the setting of a laboratory, several mentally demanding and emotionally provocative tasks for inducing stress have been evaluated. The best reproducibility results were observed during anger recall and speaking in public (Burg et al. 1993; Kim et al. 2003). Still, no major clinical trial has been performed to investigate which method to stress is the most reliable to demonstrate mental stress-induced myocardial ischemia.

Mental stress tests activate the sympathetic nervous system which is known to cause vasodilatation in healthy coronary arteries and vasoconstriction in case of endothelial dysfunction. Comparison with other sympathetic tests should, however,

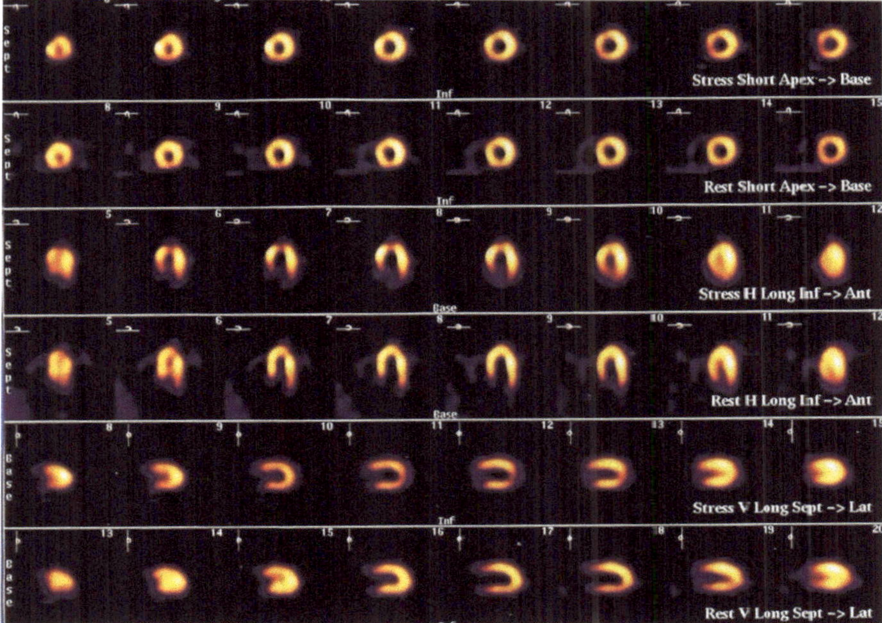

Fig. 22.2 Reversible defect in the apex on a [^{99m}Tc]-tetrofosmin myocardial perfusion scan, consistent with mental stress-induced ischemia (Reprinted from Vashist et al. (2004) with permission from Elsevier)

be interpreted with caution since different responses between the tests have been described (Monnink et al. 2002). Still, at the cardiac level, mental stress causes an increased coronary vascular resistance and ensuing myocardial ischemia (Arrighi et al. 2002). The latter was reported in a study in which ten patients and five control subjects underwent both a CAG and a myocardial perfusion imaging using [^{13}N]NH_3 PET scans. PET was performed at rest, during mental stress and during pharmacological stress with dipyridamole. Coronary flow reserve was calculated as the ratio of stress to rest blood flow. A narrowing of >50 % in a coronary artery revealed by CAG was considered significant. As expected, during dipyridamole infusion myocardial blood flow and coronary flow reserve were less in the regions with significant CAD, when compared to the regions without disease. However, during mental stress the opposite pattern was found: coronary flow reserve was less in regions without significant stenosis, than in those with significant stenosis. Even after correction for individual rate-pressure products, this was present in regions without narrowing of a coronary artery, when compared to regions with stenosis (0.8 ± 0.3 vs 1.1 ± 0.3, $p = 0.001$). The authors hypothesize that during mental stress, regions with significant stenosis show an increase in absolute myocardial blood flow, which increase is not found in regions without coronary artery stenosis. Also, the regions with lower flow reserve during mental stress showed a paradoxical increase in coronary microvascular resistance. In the control subjects, myocardial blood flow increased during both mental and pharmacological stress. Furthermore, coronary flow reserve in the controls was higher than in patients with CAD, also when normalized for rate-pressure products.

This study demonstrates reduction of myocardial blood flow during mental stress in regions without significant coronary artery stenosis. The investigators therefore conclude that microvascular endothelial dysfunction has a crucial role in this form of ischemia. Their findings were confirmed by others (Schöder et al. 2000). In the latter study, 17 patients with documented stable CAD and a comparable number of age-matched healthy control subjects underwent myocardial perfusion imaging with PET, using [^{13}N]NH_3. After acquiring images in rest, all participants were encouraged to relax during 45 min. Thereafter, mental stress was induced by asking each participant to perform arithmetic tasks. Every 2 min the tasks became more difficult, until a plateau in increased heart rate and blood pressure was established. At that time a second scan was performed. In both patients and healthy controls, the increase in rate-pressure product was similar (2,760 ± 794 vs 2,391 ± 1,196), as was the increase in serum epinephrine and norepinephrine blood levels. However, the increase in myocardial blood flow during mental stress was less in patients with known CAD than in healthy controls (14 ± 17 % vs 29 ± 14 %, $p = 0.01$).

Finally, other cofactors contributing to the relationship between mental stress and myocardial ischemia are probably a misbalance in sympathetic and parasympathetic tone (leading to diminished heart rate variability), changes in platelet activation and high levels of cortisol (Serrano et al. 2011).

22.5.3 Imaging of the Cardioneural Axis

Making use of [^{15}O]-labelled water as a tracer for PET, regional cerebral blood flow changes were studied in 12 patients with significant coronary artery disease, following dobutamine-induced angina, for the first time about two decades ago (Rosen et al. 1994). Since cortical activation is required for the awareness of pain, the investigators proposed that the changes in blood flow in the lower brain areas represent pathways for perception of angina. Furthermore, the authors suggest that with H_2[^{15}O] labelling, PET research can be executed to study inconsistencies in visceral pain perception, such as during silent myocardial ischemia and cardiac syndrome X. And indeed this group and others performed PET studies in patients with cardiac syndrome X and showed that chest pain and ECG changes, not accompanied with left ventricular dysfunction on echocardiography; however, they reported changes in neural processing of afferent signals, specifically in the right insula (Rosen et al. 2002). In addition, in patients with cardiac syndrome X, high trait anxiety was shown to be associated with an increase in myocardial ischemia on myocardial perfusion imaging (Vermeltfoort et al. 2009).

In another study cortical evoked potentials were recorded, following peripheral stimulation in 16 patients with cardiac syndrome X, and the outcomes were compared to matched controls with and without coronary artery disease. A reduced habituation to repetitive noxious stimuli was observed in the patients with cardiac syndrome X, which reduction is thought to be responsible for the altered clinical characteristics of angina in these patients (Valeriani et al. 2005). Electrical neurostimulation has been demonstrated to normalize this disturbed abnormal cortical processing of pain (Sestito et al. 2008). Using PET and [^{15}O]-labelled water, we reported on regional cerebral flow changes following electrical neuromodulation (Hautvast et al. 1997). Our findings corroborate the earlier study by Rosen et al. in identifying corresponding areas in the brain associated with cardiovascular control as Rosen et al. reported, following active electrical neuromodulation. Finally, to study the neurocardiac axis at the cardiac level and unravel the underlying mechanism of electrical neuromodulation, we have performed a PET study comparing active electrical neuromodulation with PET tracings after withholding neurostimulation. We found a more homogeneous distribution of perfusion, following active neuromodulation (Hautvast et al. 1996).

22.6 Conclusions

As mentioned previously, anxiety should be distinguished from emotional disorders. It is known that different forms of mental disorders, especially panic disorder and PTSD, are associated with a worse outcome of comorbid CAD. In subjects with a general anxiety disorder, this association was not found. Furthermore, mental and emotional stress can provoke myocardial ischemia and myocardial infarction. The role of heart rate variability is not yet clear but may not be as important as thought before. Finally, PET has been found to be a very relevant and reliable tool in the assessment of both, unravelling and understanding the underlying mechanism in the field of neurocardiology.

22.7 Future Perspectives

In the last three decades, many studies have been performed concerning mental stress-induced ischemia. Especially anxiety and depressive disorders seem to be associated with activation of cardioneural sympathetic pathways, resulting in myocardial ischemia, in patients with and without known CAD. Furthermore, the approach of these patients is different from those with conventional inducible ischemia. Still the exact pathophysiology needs further investigations.

The introduction of hybrid camera systems combining PET with magnetic resonance imaging (MRI) provides the clinician with additional information on perfusion and functional parameters of the heart (Slart et al. 2012). PET-MRI is a powerful tool for the evaluation of regional changes in perfusion and contractility after myocardial infarction. However, the combined use of these modalities in patients with mental stress-induced myocardial ischemia has not been reported. PET-MRI of the heart may be able to provide additional insight in its pathophysiology.

A novel field of interest concerns the use of SPECT and PET tracers for cardiac sympathetic and parasympathetic innervation imaging. Especially iodine-123-labelled metaiodobenzylguanidine ([^{123}I]-MIBG) and carbon-11-labelled meta-hydroxyephedrine ([^{11}C]-mHED) are established tracers for imaging cardiac sympathetic innervation. These analogues of norepinephrine bind to adrenergic receptors. Myocardial [^{123}I]-MIBG uptake is diminished in patients with autonomic failure. For example, [^{123}I]-MIBG can be used to discriminate idiopathic Parkinson's disease from multisystem atrophy. Also in patients with Lewy body disease (LBD), myocardial [^{123}I]-MIBG uptake is low (Suzuki et al. 2006). Therefore, the presence of cardiac sympathetic innervation abnormalities is able to distinguish LBD from fronto-temporal dementia (Novellino et al. 2010). However, [^{123}I]-MIBG uptake levels in patients with LBD were not associated with a clinical profile of depression and anxiety (Kobayashi et al. 2010). This would still be an interesting field to explore, despite the fact that sympathetic tone appeared not to change in patients with stable CAD with and without concurrent diabetes (Fricke et al. 2007, 2008).

Finally, the therapeutic options in patients suffering from conventional myocardial ischemia are well established. However, the effect of calcium-channel blockers and ß-blockers in patients with mental stress-induced myocardial ischemia is limited (Andersson et al. 2011; Bairey et al. 1991). Therefore, future treatments may focus on behavioural intervention, either with or without antidepressant drugs such as dual-action antidepressant (e.g. mirtazapine). These interventions may improve outcome after myocardial infarction, possibly by reducing the stress-related induction of myocardial ischemia. However, major trials thus far consistently suggest no outcome benefits from depression treatment. Future studies should focus more in depth on monitoring treatment response, for example, in a subpopulation of patients that experience reductions in stress-induced myocardial ischemia. Furthermore, little is known about receptor expression and ligand binding during mental stress-induced myocardial ischemia and after successful treatment of this ischemic response. Also little information is available on the biological variability based on genetic polymorphisms. Myocardial perfusion imaging with SPECT or PET has the potential to develop into a helpful tool in treatment monitoring and may differentiate responders from non-responders.

References

Abrams J (2005) Clinical practice: Chronic stable angina. N Engl J Med 352:2524–2533

Ahmadi N, Hajsadeghi F, Mirshkarlo HB et al (2011) Post-traumatic stress disorder, coronary atherosclerosis, and mortality. Am J Cardiol 108:29–33

American Psychiatric Association (2013) Diagnostic and statistical manual of mental disorders, 5th edn. American Psychiatric Publishing, Arlington

Andersson KE, Campeau L, Olshansky B (2011) Cardiac effects of muscarine receptor antagonists used for voiding dysfunction. Br J Clin Pharmacol 72:186–196

Arrighi JA, Burg M, Cohen IS et al (2002) Myocardial blood-flow response during mental stress in patients with coronary artery disease. Lancet 356:310–311

Bairey CN, Krantz DS, Dequattro V et al (1991) Effect of beta-blockade on low heart rate–related ischemia during mental stress. J Am Coll Cardiol 17:1388–1395

Benson CJ, Eckert SP, McCleskey EW (1999) Acid-evoked currents in cardiac sensor neurons: a possible mediator of myocardial ischemic sensation. Circ Res 84:921–928

Beutel ME, Wiltink J, Till Y et al (2012) Type D personality as a cardiovascular risk marker in the general population: results from the Gutenberg health study. Psychother Psychosom 81:108–117

Burg MM, Jain D, Soufer R et al (1993) Role of behavioral and psychological factors in mental stress-induced silent left ventricular dysfunction in coronary artery disease. J Am Coll Cardiol 22:440–448

Cechetto DF (2004) Forbrain control of healthy and diseased hearts. In: Eds Armour JA, Ardell JL (eds) Basic and clinical neurocardiology, 1st edn. Oxford University Press Inc, New York

Crea F, Gaspardone A, Kaski JC et al (1992) Relation between stimulation site of cardiac afferent nerves by adenosine and distribution of cardiac pain: results of a study in patients with stable angina. J Am Coll Cardiol 20:1498–1502

Crea F, Gaspardone A, Versaci F et al (1999) Algogenic effects of the proximal and distal intracoronary infusion of adenosine. Pathophysiological implications on the mechanisms of ischemic cardiac pain. Cardiol 44:835–839

Das S, O'Keefe JH (2008) Behavioral cardiology: recognizing and addressing the profound impact of psychosocial stress on cardiovascular health. Curr Hypertens Rep 10:374–381

Deanfield JE, Shea M, Kensett M et al (1984) Silent myocardial ischaemia due to mental stress. Lancet 2:1001–1005

DeJongste MJ, TerHorst GJ, Foreman RD (2009) Basic research models for the study of underlying mechanisms of electrical neuromodulation and ischemic heart-brain interactions. Cleve Clin J Med 76:S41–S46

Di Carli MF, Hachamovitch R (2007) New technology for noninvasive evaluation of coronary artery disease. Circulation 115:1464–1480

Fleet R, Lavoie K, Beitman BD (2000) Is panic disorder associated with coronary artery disease? A critical review of the literature. J Psychosom Res 48:347–356

Flotats A, Knuuti J, Gutberlet M et al (2011) Hybrid cardiac imaging: SPECT/CT and PET/CT. A joint position statement by the European Association of Nuclear Medicine (EANM), the European Society of Cardiac Radiology (ESCR) and the European Council of Nuclear Cardiology (ECNC). Eur J Nucl Med Mol Imaging 38:201–212

Foreman RD (1999) Mechanisms of cardiac pain. Annu Rev Physiol 61:143–167

Foreman RD, DeJongste MJL, Linderoth B (2004) Integrative control of cardiac function by cervical and thoracic spinal neurons. In: Armour JA, Ardell JL (eds) Basic and clinical neurocardiology, 1st edn. Oxford University Press Inc, New York

Frasure-Smith N, Lesperance F (2008) Depression and anxiety as predictors of 2-year cardiac events in patients with stable coronary artery disease. Arch Gen Psychiatry 65:62–71

Fricke E, Fricke H, Eckert S et al (2007) Myocardial sympathetic innervation in patients with chronic coronary artery disease: is the reduction in coronary flow reserve correlated with sympathetic denervation? Eur J Nucl Med Mol Imaging 34:206–211

Fricke E, Eckert S, Dongas A et al (2008) Myocardial sympathetic innervation in patients with symptomatic chronic coronary artery disease: follow-up after 1 year with neurostimulation. J Nucl Med 49:1458–1464

Gaspardone A, Crea F, Tomai F et al (1995) Muscular and cardiac adenosine-induced pain is mediated by A1 receptors. J Am Coll Cardiol 25:251–257

Greenland P, Bonow RO, Brundage BH et al (2007) ACCF/AHA 2007 clinical expert consensus document on coronary artery calcium scoring by computed tomography in global cardiovascular risk assessment and in evaluation of patients with chest pain: a report of the American College of Cardiology Foundation Clinical Expert Consensus Task Force (ACCF/AHA Writing Committee to Update the 2000 Expert Consensus Document on Electron Beam Computed Tomography) developed in collaboration with the Society of Atherosclerosis Imaging and Prevention and the Society of Cardiovascular Computed Tomography. J Am Coll Cardiol 49:378–402

Hautvast RW, Blanksma PK, De Jongste MJ (1996) Effect of spinal cord stimulation on myocardial blood flow assessed by positron emission tomography in patients with refractory angina pectoris. Am J Cardiol 77:462–467

Hautvast RW, Ter Horst GJ, DeJong BM et al (1997) Relative changes in regional cerebral blood flow during spinal cord stimulation in patients with refractory angina pectoris. Eur J Neurosci 9:1178–1183

Ketterer MW, Bekkouche NS, Goldberg AD et al (2011) Symptoms of anxiety and depression are correlates of angina pectoris by recent history and an ischemia-positive treadmill test in patients with documented coronary artery disease in the Pimi study. Cardiovasc Psychiatry Neurol 2011:134040

Kim CK, Bartholomew BA, Mastin ST et al (2003) Detection and reproducibility of mental stress-induced myocardial ischemia with Tc-99m sestamibi SPECT in normal and coronary artery disease populations. J Nucl Cardiol 10:56–62

Kobayashi K, Sumiya H, Nakano H et al (2010) Detection of Lewy body disease in patients with late-onset depression, anxiety and psychotic disorder with myocardial meta-iodobenzylguanidine scintigraphy. Int J Geriatr Psychiatry 25:55–65

Koren O, Spor A, Felin J et al (2011) Human oral, gut, and plaque microbiotica in patients with atherosclerosis. Proc Natl Acad Sci U S A 108:4592–4598

Kurisu S, Sato H, Kawagoe T (2002) Tako-tsubo-like left ventricular dysfunction with ST-segment elevation: a novel cardiac syndrome mimicking acute myocardial infarction. Am Heart J 143:448–455

Lathrop DA, Spooner PM (2001) On the neural connection. J Cardiovasc Electrophysiol 12:841–844

Lavoie KL, Fleet RP, Laurin C et al (2004) Heart rate variability in coronary artery disease patients with and without panic disorder. Psychiatry Res 128:289–299

Libby P, Ridker PM, Hansson GK (2011) Progress and challenges in translating the biology of atherosclerosis. Nature 473:317–325

Longhurst JC, Tjen ALS, Fu LW (2001) Cardiac sympathetic afferent activation provoked by myocardial ischemia and reperfusion. Mechanisms and reflexes. Ann N Y Acad Sci 940:74–95

Machac J (2005) Cardiac positron emission tomography imaging. Semin Nucl Med 35:17–36

McLean PG, Bergonzelli GE, Collins SM et al (2012) Targeting the microbiota-gut-brain axis to modulate behavior: which bacterial strain will translate best to humans? Proc Natl Acad Sci U S A 109:E174

Monnink SHJ, van Haelst PL, van Boven AJ et al (2002) Endothelial dysfunction in patients with coronary artery disease: a comparison of three frequently reported tests. J Investig Med 50:19–24

Novellino F, Bagnato A, Salsone M et al (2010) Myocardial (123)I-MIBG scintigraphy for differentiation of Lewy bodies disease from FTD. Neurobiol Aging 31:1903–1911

O'Dell KR, Masters KS, Spielmans GI et al (2011) Does type-D personality predict outcomes among patients with cardiovascular disease? A meta-analytic review. J Psychosom Res 71:199–206

Parker G, Hyett M, Hadzi-Pavlovic D et al (2011) GAD is good? Generalized anxiety disorder predicts a superior five-year outcome following an acute coronary syndrome. Psychiatry Res 188:383–389

Robbins N, Koch SE, Rubinstein J (2013) Targeting TRPV1 and TRPV2 for potential therapeutic interventions in cardiovascular disease. Transl Res 161:469–476

Rosen SD, Paulescu E, Frith CD et al (1994) Central nervous pathways mediating angina pectoris. Lancet 344:147–150

Rosen SD, Paulesu E, Wise RJ et al (2002) Central neural contribution to the perception of chest pain in cardiac syndrome X. Heart 87:513–519

Rosengren A, Hawken S, Ounpuu S et al (2004) Association of psychosocial risk factors with risk of acute myocardial infarction in 11119 cases and 13648 controls from 52 countries (the INTERHEART study): case-control study. Lancet 364:953–962

Rutledge T, Linke SE, Krantz DS et al (2009) Comorbid depression and anxiety symptoms as predictors of cardiovascular events: results from the NHLBI-sponsored Women's Ischemia Syndrome Evaluation (WISE) study. Psychosom Med 71:958–964

Schöder H, Silverman DH, Campisi R et al (2000) Effect of mental stress ischemia on myocardial blood flow and vasomotion in patients with coronary artery disease. J Nucl Med 41:11–16

Schroeder S, Achenbach S, Bengel F et al (2008) Cardiac computed tomography: indications, applications, limitations, and training requirements: report of a Writing Group deployed by the Working Group Nuclear Cardiology and Cardiac CT of the European Society of Cardiology and the European Council of Nuclear Cardiology. Eur Heart J 29:531–556

Serrano CV, Setani KT, Sakamoto E et al (2011) Association between depression and development of coronary artery disease: pathophysiologic and diagnostic implications. Vasc Health Risk Manag 7:159–164

Sestito A, Lanza GA, Le Pera D et al (2008) Spinal cord stimulation normalizes abnormal cortical pain processing in patients with cardiac syndrome X. Pain 139:82–89

Slart RH, Glauche J, Golestani R et al (2012) PET and MRI for the evaluation of regional myocardial perfusion and wall thickening after myocardial infarction. Eur J Nucl Med Mol Imaging 39:1065–1069

Sobic-Saranovic DP, Bojic L, Petrasinovic Z et al (2013) Diagnostic and prognostic value of gated SPECT MIBI early post-stress imaging in patients with intermediate Duke Treadmill Score. Clin Nucl Med 38:784–978

Soh KC, Lee C (2010) Panic attack and its correlation with acute coronary syndrome – more than just a diagnosis of exclusion. Ann Acad Med Singapore 39:197–202

Soufer R, Burg MM (2007) The heart-brain interaction during emotionally provoked myocardial ischemia: implications of cortical hyperactivation in CAD and gender interactions. Cleve Clin J Med 74 Suppl 1:S59–62

Suzuki M, Kurita A, Hashimoto M et al (2006) Impaired myocardial 123I-metaiodobenzylguanidine uptake in Lewy body disease: comparison between dementia with Lewy bodies and Parkinson's disease. J Neurol Sci 240:15–19

Tracey KJ (2009) Reflex control of immunity. Nat Rev Immunol 9:418–428

Tsuchihashi K, Ueshima K, Uchida T et al (2001) Transient left ventricular apical ballooning without coronary artery stenosis: a novel heart syndrome mimicking acute myocardial infarction. J Am Coll Cardiol 38:11–18

Underwood SR, Anagnostopoulos C, Cerqueira M et al (2004) Myocardial perfusion scintigraphy: the evidence. Eur J Nucl Med Mol Imaging 31:261–291

Valeriani M, Sestito A, Le Pera D et al (2005) Abnormal cortical pain processing in patients with cardiac syndrome X. Eur Heart J 26:975–982

Vashist A, Arrighi JA, Soufer R (2004) Mechanistic and methodological consideration for the imaging of mental stress ischemia. In: Zaret BL, Beller GA (eds) Clinical nuclear cardiology: state of the art and future directions, 3rd edn. Elsevier Mosby, St Louis

Vermeltfoort IA, Raijmakers PG, Odekerken DA et al (2009) Association between anxiety disorder and the extent of ischemia observed in cardiac syndrome X. J Nucl Cardiol 16:405–410

Watkins LL, Blumenthal JA, Davidson JR et al (2006) Phobic anxiety, depression, and risk of ventricular arrhythmias in patients with coronary heart disease. Psychosom Med 68:651–656

Zhao M, Sun L, Liu JJ et al (2012) Vagal nerve modulation: a promising new therapeutic approach for cardiovascular diseases. Clin Exp Pharmacol Physiol 39:701–705

Autonomic Imaging Cardiotoxicity with [^{123}I]-MIBG: The Effects of Chemotherapy, Monoclonal Antibody Therapy, and Radiotherapy

23

L.P. Salm, B.F. Bulten, H.W.M. Van Laarhoven, and L.F. De Geus-Oei

Contents

Abstract

Anticancer therapy has led to prolonged survival and better quality of life of cancer patients. However, some treatments may have significant adverse cardiotoxic side effects. The current gold standard to evaluate cardiac function in relation to cardiotoxicity is the assessment of the left ventricular ejection fraction, which is reduced only after a certain critical mass of cell damage has occurred. [^{123}I]-labeled metaiodobenzylguanidine ([^{123}I]-MIBG) scintigraphy images the efferent sympathetic nervous innervation of the heart and has successfully been applied for risk stratification, prognosis assessment, and treatment monitoring in patients with congestive heart failure and to predict ventricular arrhythmias. [^{123}I]-MIBG scintigraphy is a promising novel approach for early assessment of cardiotoxicity induced by certain anticancer treatment regimens but still warrants further research. This chapter focuses on the evaluation of the autonomic heart

L.P. Salm (✉)
Nuclear Medicine, Medical Spectrum Twente, Enschede, The Netherlands
e-mail: liesbeth.salm@gmail.com

B.F. Bulten • L.F. De Geus-Oei
Nuclear Medicine, Radboud University Nijmegen Medical Center, Nijmegen, The Netherlands

H.W.M. Van Laarhoven
Medical Oncology, Academic Medical Center Amsterdam, Amsterdam, The Netherlands

R.H.J.A. Slart et al. (eds.), *Autonomic Innervation of the Heart: Role of Molecular Imaging*, DOI 10.1007/978-3-662-45074-1_23

function by [^{123}I]-MIBG for the assessment of cardiotoxicity induced by chemotherapy, monoclonal antibody therapy, or radiotherapy.

Abbreviations

[^{123}I]-MIBG	[^{123}I]-labeled metaiodobenzylguanidine
BNP	B-type natriuretic peptide
CHF	Congestive heart failure
EANM	European Association of Nuclear Medicine
HER2	Human epidermal growth factor receptor type 2
H/L	Heart to lung
H/M	Heart to mediastinum
LVEF	Left ventricular ejection fraction
MUGA	Multi-gated radionuclide ventriculography
PET	Positron emission tomography
SPECT	Single-photon emission computed tomography
WR	Washout rate

23.1 Introduction

Improvements in the treatment of cancer have led to prolonged survival and better quality of life of cancer patients. However, some anticancer regimens may have significant adverse cardiotoxic side effects, including left ventricular dysfunction, ischemia, thromboembolism, and arrhythmias (Shaikh and Shih 2012). Mostly, these side effects are transient, but irreversible cardiac damage does occur in a subgroup of patients, up to 26 % at high cumulative doses, and may cause clinically overt congestive heart failure (CHF) (Swain et al. 2003). Non-invasive imaging prior to treatment may assist in identifying patients at risk for acquiring cardiotoxicity, in monitoring patients during anticancer regimens with known cardiotoxic side effects, and in identifying patients who are likely to develop irreversible damage (Gillespie et al. 2011).

The current gold standard to evaluate cardiac function in relation to cardiotoxicity is the assessment of left ventricular ejection fraction (LVEF) by multi-gated radionuclide ventriculography (MUGA) (de Geus-Oei et al. 2011). This technique makes use of labeling [^{99m}Tc] to erythrocytes, either in vivo or in vitro, which enables the cardiac blood pool to be visualized with a gamma camera in multiple views. After the acquisition, the data is gated to the simultaneously acquired patient's heartbeat to obtain different images of 16 or 32 stages of the cardiac cycle. Using a count-based method LVEF is derived from the ventricular time-activity curves. This approach is independent of geometric considerations and permits the use of automatic edge detection programs to compute LVEF from left anterior oblique images with high reproducibility and low intra- and interobserver variability (Heidendal et al. 1983; Rocco et al. 1989). Guidelines to monitor patients who are to receive doxorubicin chemotherapy include a baseline MUGA (Schwartz et al. 1987). If baseline is normal (≥50 %), a repeat study should be performed after a dose of 250–300 mg/m^2 and thereafter prior to each dose. If baseline is abnormal (<50 %), sequential studies should be obtained prior to each dose. Therapy should not be initiated if baseline LVEF is below 30 %. Discontinuation of therapy is recommended if there is an absolute decrease in LVEF ≥10 % associated with a decline to a level ≤50 %. Implementation of these guidelines leads to a fourfold reduction in the incidence of CHF in the 80s. Alternative methods to obtain LVEF include cardiac magnetic resonance and two- or three-dimensional echocardiography (Altena et al. 2009; Walker et al. 2010). However, LVEF will only decrease after a certain critical mass of cell damage has occurred (Bristow et al. 1981). Several studies have demonstrated a poor correlation between LVEF at rest and early myocardial damage after doxorubicin therapy, verified by endomyocardial biopsy (Druck et al. 1984; Ewer et al. 1984). The compensatory reserve of the myocardium enables sufficient ventricular output, even when structural damage to the myocytes had occurred. Therefore, LVEF may underestimate actual cardiac injury (Altena et al. 2009; Bristow et al. 1981).

A non-invasive approach which accurately identifies cardiotoxicity already in a subclinical stage, before decline of LVEF, is preferable. Sympathetic nervous innervation imaging of the heart with PET or SPECT is a promising tool in providing such an approach. Various PET tracers for imaging the cardiac autonomic nervous system have been developed, including [^{11}C]-metahydroxyephedrine ([^{11}C]-mHED), [^{11}C]-epinephrine, [^{11}C]-phenylephrine, and [^{18}F]-fluorodopamine (Lautamaki et al. 2007). An overview of the physiological mechanisms of these tracers is provided in Chap. 9. Due to the complex synthesis and radiolabeling process, PET imaging of the cardiac autonomic nervous system is restricted to few, highly specialized centers and has not gained wide attention. Studies using PET tracers to evaluate the cardiac autonomic nervous system after different chemotherapeutic regimens or radiotherapy are lacking. In contrast, several studies have evaluated the use of [^{123}I]-labeled metaiodobenzylguanidine ([^{123}I]-MIBG) scintigraphy in cardiotoxicity induced by chemotherapy, monoclonal antibody therapy, or radiotherapy.

This chapter focuses on the evaluation of the autonomic heart function by [^{123}I]-MIBG for the assessment of cardiotoxicity induced by chemotherapy, monoclonal antibody therapy, or radiotherapy.

23.2 [^{123}I]-Labeled Metaiodobenzylguanidine ([^{123}I]-MIBG) Scintigraphy

MIBG, labeled with radioactive iodine [^{123}I], is a guanethidine analogue which is taken up, concentrated, and stored in the presynaptic nerve terminals of the sympathetic nervous system in a manner similar to norepinephrine (Chirumamilla and Travin 2011). In contrast with norepinephrine, [^{123}I]-MIBG is not catabolized but retained in the sympathetic nerve endings after reuptake at a sufficient concentration to be imaged with a gamma camera. The background, procedure, and image analysis of [^{123}I]-MIBG scintigraphy are discussed in detail in Chap. 6. [^{123}I]-MIBG scintigraphy of the heart can be used for risk stratification, prognosis assessment, and treatment monitoring in patients with CHF, to predict ventricular arrhythmias and to detect CHF in an early stage in patients with hypertrophic cardiomyopathy (Boogers et al. 2010; Carrio et al. 2010; Hiasa et al. 2004). Decrease of LVEF is a relatively late sign of CHF. The neurohumoral response to the presence of dysfunctional myocytes results in a compensatory sympathetic drive, which increases the contractility, conduction, and heart rate. [^{123}I]-MIBG can be used to generate a scintigraphic image of the efferent sympathetic nervous innervations of the heart before left ventricular function is reduced.

23.2.1 Effects of Chemotherapy

Many chemotherapeutic agents have a spectrum of cardiotoxic effects (Table 23.1) (Panjrath and Jain 2006; Yeh et al. 2004). These effects vary from mild, transient changes in cardiac function during or immediately after treatment to more serious complications at a later stage, which may result in irreversible cardiac dysfunction or CHF.

Table 23.1 Cardiotoxicity profiles of chemotherapeutic agents

Drug class/generic name (brand)	Cardiac adverse events	Relative frequency of adverse effect[a]	Relative frequency of therapeutic use
Anthracyclines/anthraquinones			
Doxorubicin (Adriamycin)	CHF/LV dysfunction	Common	Very frequent
Daunorubicin (Cerubidine)	CHF/LV dysfunction	Common	Very frequent
Epirubicin (Ellence, Pharmorubicin)	CHF/LV dysfunction	Common	Very frequent
Idarubicin (Idamycin)	CHF/LV dysfunction	Common	Very frequent
Mitoxantrone (Novantrone)	CHF/LV dysfunction	Uncommon	Infrequent
Alkylating agents			
Busulfan (Myleran)	Endomyocardial fibrosis	Rare	Infrequent
	Cardiac tamponade	Rare	
Cisplatin (Platinol)	Ischemia	Uncommon	Very frequent
	Hypertension	Frequent	
	CHF	Uncommon	
Cyclophosphamide (Cytoxan)	Pericarditis/myocarditis	Rare	Very frequent
	CHF	Uncommon	
Ifosfamide (Ifex)	CHF	Uncommon	Common
	Arrhythmias	Uncommon	
Mitomycin (Mutamycin)	CHF	Uncommon	Infrequent
Antimetabolites			
Capecitabine (Xeloda)	Ischemia	Rare	Very frequent
Cytarabine, Ara-C (Cytosar)	Pericarditis	Rare	Very frequent
	CHF	Rare	
Fluorouracil (Adrucil)	Ischemia	Uncommon	Very frequent
	Cardiogenic shock	Rare	

Table 23.1 (continued)

Drug class/generic name (brand)	Cardiac adverse events	Relative frequency of adverse effect[a]	Relative frequency of therapeutic use
Antimicrotubules			
Paclitaxel (Taxol)	Sinus bradycardia, AV block	Rare	Very frequent
	Ventricular tachycardia	Rare	
	Hypotension	Rare	
	CHF	Uncommon	
Vinca alkaloids	Ischemia	Uncommon	Common
Biological agents			
Monoclonal antibodies			
Alemtuzumab (Campath)	Hypotension	Common	Infrequent
	CHF	Rare	
Bevacizumab (Avastin)	Hypertension	Common	Common
	CHF	Uncommon	
	Deep venous thrombosis	Rare	
Cetuximab (Erbitux)	Hypotension	Rare	Common
Rituximab (Rituxan)	Hypotension, angioedema	Uncommon	Common
	Arrhythmias	uncommon	
Trastuzumab (Herceptin)	CHF/LV dysfunction	uncommon	Common
Interleukins			
IL-2	Hypotension	Frequent	Infrequent
	Arrhythmias	Uncommon	
Denileukin diftitox (Ontak)	Hypotension	Frequent	Infrequent
Interferon-α	Hypotension	Common	Very frequent
	Ischemia	Uncommon	
	LV dysfunction	Rare	
Miscellaneous			
All-*trans* retinoic acid (tretinoin)	CHF	Uncommon	Infrequent
	Hypotension	Uncommon	
	Pericardial effusion	Rare	
Arsenic trioxide (Trisenox)	QT prolongation	Frequent	Infrequent
Imatinib (Gleevec)	Pericardial effusion	Uncommon	Very frequent
	CHF, edema	Common	
Pentostatin (Nipent)	CHF	Uncommon	Infrequent
Thalidomide (Thalomid)	Edema	Uncommon	Infrequent
	Hypotension	Rare	
	Deep venous thrombosis	Uncommon	
	Bradycardia	Uncommon	
Etoposide (Vepesid)	Hypotension	Uncommon	Common

CHF congestive heart failure

[a]Relative frequency of adverse effect: rare indicates <1 %; uncommon indicates 1–5 %; common indicates 6–10 %; frequent indicates >10 %

Anthracyclines, such as doxorubicin, are most commonly associated with cardiotoxicity. The anticancer effects of anthracyclines are mediated primarily through inhibition of DNA synthesis, transcription, and replication (Smith et al. 2010). Simultaneously, oxygen-derived free radicals are formed, causing direct damage to proteins, lipids, and DNA, which may lead to myocyte apoptosis in the heart. This process is thought to be the key mechanism in anthracycline cardiotoxicity. Alternate hypotheses include calcium overload of myocytes, alterations in adrenergic function, and inhibition of protein synthesis (Panjrath and Jain 2006). A meta-analysis of 55 randomized controlled trials demonstrated an increased risk of clinical cardiotoxicity by anthracycline-based regimens by 5.43 fold, subclinical cardiotoxicity by 6.25 fold, and cardiac death by 4.94 fold compared with non-anthracycline regimens (Smith et al. 2010). Risk factors for developing cardiotoxicity comprise a high cumulative anthracycline dose, mediastinal radiation therapy, combination chemotherapy, combination chemotherapy with monoclonal antibody therapy, preexisting cardiovascular disease, emphysema, diabetes, female sex, and very young or older age (Panjrath and Jain 2006; Yeh et al. 2004). Toxic effects on the myocardium due to anthracyclines may occur early, during or immediately after infusion, or late, after months up to 20 years after therapy. Toxic effects on the myocardium during or immediately after infusion are usually self-limiting with discontinuation. Chronic effects may persist after discontinuation of therapy, or may present after months or years, and can progress to overt cardiac dysfunction or CHF. Therefore, early detection before irreversible functional cardiac impairment has occurred is crucial.

[^{123}I]-MIBG scintigraphy was investigated as an early marker for cardiotoxicity after anthracycline therapy. In a rat model, a clear dose-dependent reduction in MIBG uptake was demonstrated after doxorubicin therapy (Wakasugi et al. 1992). The reduction in MIBG uptake was larger and more linear dose-dependent than impairment of LVEF. Furthermore, MIBG uptake was significantly reduced after 6 weeks of therapy with only mild myocyte damage at histopathological examination, whereas LVEF decreased only slightly after 7 weeks and showed a remarkable decrease after 8 weeks of therapy, suggesting MIBG to be a sensitive biomarker for early detection of doxorubicin-induced cardiomyopathy (Wakasugi et al. 1993). The subendocardial layer appeared to be more vulnerable to doxorubicin than the subepicardium (Jeon et al. 2000). Congestive heart failure due to Adriamycin in an early stage in a rat model was found to accelerate exocytotic release of norepinephrine from cardiac adrenergic neurons, rather than disturb the neuronal uptake function (Wakasugi et al. 1995). In an advanced stage, nonexocytotic metabolic release is induced due to energy depletion, increasing norepinephrine release. Both mechanisms lead to a reduction of myocardial MIBG uptake.

In a case report, [^{123}I]-MIBG scintigraphy with SPECT of a patient after doxorubicin therapy without cardiac symptoms and normal LVEF was described, showing reduced uptake in several segments and a high washout rate (WR) (Takano et al. 1995). After 10 months the patient died of CHF, and at necropsy structural changes, corresponding to the impaired segments at the [^{123}I]-MIBG, were found in a dilated left ventricle (Figs. 23.1 and 23.2). Conversely, in segments with preserved [^{123}I]-MIBG uptake, myocardial nerve fibers had a normal aspect.

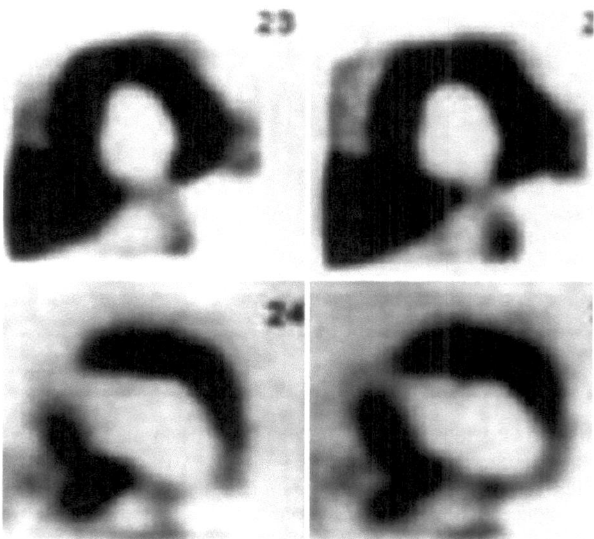

Fig. 23.1 A 52-year-old female patient, treated with doxorubicin for malignant lymphoma, had no cardiac symptoms, and a LVEF of 52 % was obtained by echocardiography. Illustration of [^{123}I]-MIBG scintigraphy, delayed images, performed 2 weeks after the last chemotherapy treatment. [^{123}I]-MIBG uptake was markedly reduced in the apical anterior, inferior, and lateral walls of the left ventricle. Delayed H/M ratio was reported to be 1.12 % with a WR of 49.5 %. ^{201}Thallium uptake was normal in all segments, indicating normal cardiac perfusion (Reproduced with permission from Takano et al. (1995))

In patients receiving doxorubicin therapy, the dose-dependent reduction in [^{123}I]-MIBG uptake (heart/mediastinum ratio (H/M ratio)) was confirmed in several studies (Lekakis et al. 1996; Takano et al. 1996; Takeishi et al. 1994; Valdes Olmos et al. 1995). Even at low dosage, the H/M ratio showed a decline, whereas LVEF derived by echocardiography or multi-gated radionuclide ventriculography was preserved. The 4-h WR tended to increase but did not reach statistical significance in a small, proof-of-concept study (Valdes Olmos et al. 1995). Complementary SPECT examinations to identify segment abnormalities were of good quality in patients with normal H/M ratio, though 4-h SPECT images of patients with abnormal tracer retention were of poorer quality and needed a longer acquisition time.

When [^{123}I]-MIBG scintigraphy was compared with [^{111}In]-antimyosin scintigraphy in the evaluation of cardiotoxicity after doxorubicin therapy, [^{111}In]-antimyosin detected early myocardial damage at intermediate doses of doxorubicin, whereas H/M ratio was only impaired at high cumulative doses (Carrio et al. 1995). In four patients with symptomatic anthracycline-induced cardiomyopathy, [^{123}I]-MIBG and [^{111}In]-antimyosin scintigraphy was performed 2–116 months after the onset of CHF, showing a persistent decreased H/M ratio in [^{123}I]-MIBG and an increased heart-to-lung ratio (H/L ratio) in [^{111}In]-antimyosin scintigraphy in all patients, suggesting permanent damage to the cardiac adrenergic nerve endings and myocytes

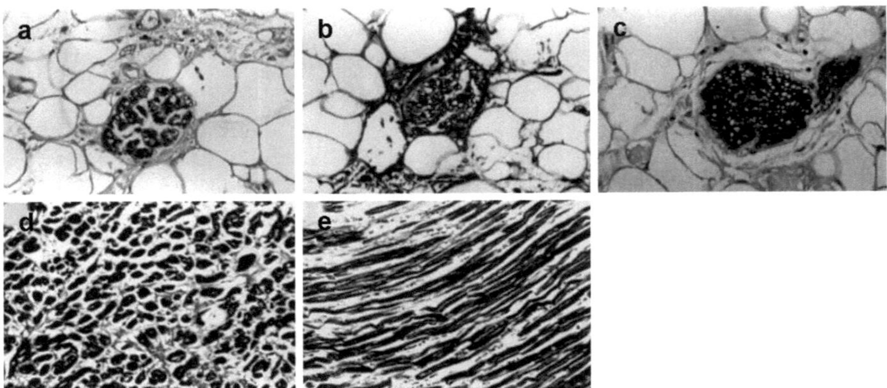

Fig. 23.2 Histology of the left ventricle after the patient had died from doxorubicin-induced cardiomyopathy 10 months after the performance of [^{123}I]-MIBG scintigraphy. (**a**) S-100 stained section of the inferior wall, showing markedly atrophic nerve fibers. Prior [^{123}I]-MIBG uptake herein was clearly reduced. (**b**) Azan-stained section of the inferior wall, showing atrophic and fibrotic nerve fibers. (**c**) S-100 stained section of the septum, depicting normal nerve fibers. The septum displayed normal [^{123}I]-MIBG uptake. (**d**) Azan-stained section of the inferior wall, confirming atrophic myocytes and remarkable interstitial fibrosis, whereas the septum revealed a normal myocyte structure (**e**) (Reproduced with permission from Takano et al. (1995))

(Nousiainen et al. 2001). H/M and heart/lung (H/L) ratios remained impaired even in patients who had recovered clinically, and LVEF had returned to near normal.

All of these studies included only a limited number of patients and lacked appropriate follow-up. No studies have been performed yet for other chemotherapeutic agents, such as alkylating agents or antimetabolites, using [^{123}I]-MIBG scintigraphy as a biomarker to evaluate cardiotoxicity.

23.2.2 Effects of Monoclonal Antibody Therapy

Several monoclonal antibody therapeutic agents may have cardiovascular side effects, such as hyper- and hypotension, CHF, and arrhythmias (Table 23.1). Trastuzumab is a humanized monoclonal antibody against human epidermal growth factor receptor type 2 (HER2), which may be overexpressed in several cancer types and is at present frequently used as targeted therapy for breast cancer and esophagogastric cancer.

Trastuzumab is known to cause a (mostly) transient, asymptomatic decline in LVEF, but patients may develop CHF years after therapy (Di Cosimo 2011). Patients receiving a combination chemotherapeutic regimen including trastuzumab are at highest risk to present a cardiac event, CHF, or cardiac death (Russell et al. 2010; Tan-Chiu et al. 2005). The mechanism of trastuzumab-related cardiac toxicity is still largely unclear, though it is now considered a dual-step process. First, the expression of HER2 is increased or the HER2/HER4 signaling is activated in myocytes due to cardiac stress by chemotherapy. Then, the inhibition of HER2 by trastuzumab impairs the response to myocardial damage, which may provoke the development of cardiac dysfunction (Di Cosimo 2011). The pooled incidence of trastuzumab-related cardiotoxicity, obtained from 15 randomized controlled trials and case control studies, was reported to be 10 %, whereas the pooled incidence of cardiotoxicity in studies with a non-trastuzumab comparator arm was 2 % (Panjrath and Jain 2007).

In a preliminary study, the detection of trastuzumab-related cardiotoxicity with an asymptomatic, confirmed LVEF decrease in nine patients was evaluated by [^{123}I]-MIBG scintigraphy (Stokkel et al. 2013). Patients who showed an impairment in H/M ratio <1.6 and WR >25 % did not demonstrate a recovery of LVEF in a 13-month follow-up, whereas patients with normal H/M ratio and (near) normal WR revealed an improvement in LVEF, suggesting that [^{123}I]-MIBG scintigraphy can be used for risk stratification and disease monitoring during trastuzumab therapy.

Larger studies with follow-up or exploring different monoclonal antibody therapies with [^{123}I]-MIBG scintigraphy are absent.

23.2.3 Effects of Radiotherapy

Radiotherapy to the chest may also induce a variety of cardiovascular complications, such as myocardial injury or fibrosis, diastolic dysfunction, pericarditis, coronary artery disease, valvular abnormalities, and conduction disturbances (Bovelli et al. 2010; Hull et al. 2003). The cardiotoxic mechanism relies on direct injury from the high-energy radiation beam. Risk factors for radiation-associated cardiovascular side effects include a radiation dose >30 Gy, dose per fraction >2 Gy, large volume of irradiated heart, younger age, longer time since exposure, use of concomitant cytotoxic chemotherapy, endocrine therapy or trastuzumab, and presence of other cardiovascular risk factors, e.g., diabetes, hypertension, dyslipidemia, obesity, and smoking.

Cardiac morbidity and mortality associated with the use of chest radiotherapy was demonstrated to be increased in several large, multicenter registries (Early Breast Cancer Trialists' Collaborative Group 2000; Paszat et al. 1998; Rutqvist and Johansson 1990). In one study the relative risk of cardiovascular mortality in patients treated with thoracic radiotherapy was reported to be 1.27 (Clarke et al. 2005). Radiotherapy for left-sided breast cancer was found to induce volume-dependent myocardial perfusion defects with [^{99m}Tc]-tetrofosmin or sestamibi scintigraphy in approximately 40 % of patients (Marks et al. 2005). The perfusion defects were associated with corresponding wall motion abnormalities. The long-term clinical consequences of these findings are unknown.

With the development of modern radiotherapy techniques, such as three-dimensional treatment planning, linear accelerator photons or multiple-field conformal or intensity modulation, postradiation cardiotoxicity has already shown a declining trend (Bovelli et al. 2010).

In only one study, [¹²³I]-MIBG scintigraphy was used to evaluate cardiotoxicity in cancer patients treated with anthracyclines with or without chest radiotherapy, or chest radiotherapy alone, describing significantly reduced H/M ratio and increased WR in all treatment groups (Valdes Olmos et al. 1996). An example of [^{123}I]-MIBG examinations from a patient in the control group and from a patient after radiotherapy from this study is displayed in Fig. 23.3. The study was, however, too small to analyze the different treatment groups separately, and patient outcome was not evaluated.

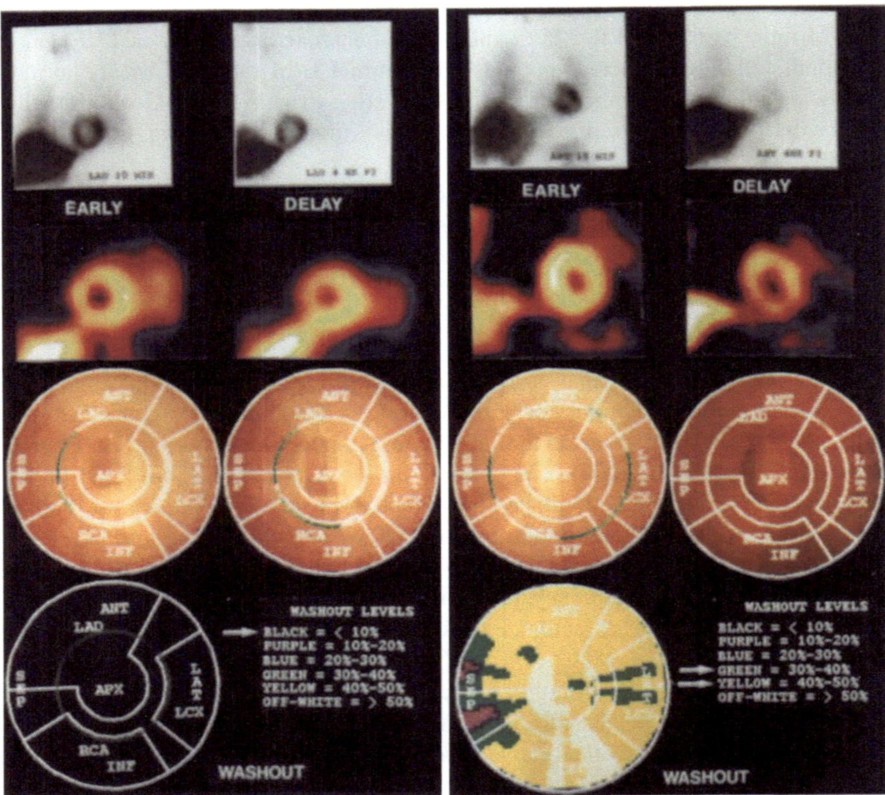

Fig. 23.3 The *left panel* displays planar images (*top*), SPECT (*second row*), and polar map distribution (*third row*) of the early and delayed [^{123}I]-MIBG studies showing a normal pattern of myocardial uptake and washout in a patient of the control group. Note on the polar washout distribution (*bottom*) that 4-h myocardial washout was less than 10 % in all segments. The *right panel* displays planar images, SPECT, and polar map distribution of the early and late [^{123}I]-MIBG scintigrams showing an abnormal pattern of myocardial washout and uptake after 4 h in a patient investigated 13 years after radiotherapy of the left breast and the internal mammary chain. Note on the washout distribution diagram that 4-h washout varied between 30 % and 50 % for the various myocardial segments. LVEF was normal (56 %) at the time of [^{123}I]-MIBG examination (Reproduced with permission from Valdes Olmos et al. (1996))

23.3 Considerations and Future Perspectives

[^{123}I]-MIBG scintigraphy displayed a clear dose-dependent uptake reduction after anthracycline therapy, even at low dosage, and the reduction appeared earlier than a decrease in LVEF. In trastuzumab-related cardiotoxicity, myocardial [^{123}I]-MIBG scintigraphy was able to predict LVEF recovery in a short follow-up period. After chest radiotherapy [^{123}I]-MIBG scintigraphy showed impairment. Despite these promising results of [^{123}I]-MIBG to evaluate and monitor early cardiotoxicity after anticancer therapy, large prospective trials with long-term follow-up are lacking. And despite well-known cardiotoxic effects of several monoclonal antibody agents, large [^{123}I]-MIBG studies are missing.

A major consideration is the fact that delayed cardiotoxicity may present up to 10 years. This may lead to false-negative results in studies with a limited follow-up. No accurate surrogate markers for clinical outcome have yet been identified. In addition, since [^{123}I]-MIBG is thought to be a more sensitive marker to detect cardiotoxicity in an early stage than LVEF assessment, there is no adequate, non-invasive gold standard of cardiotoxicity to compare with, other than long-term follow-up. Furthermore, standardization of the imaging protocol and formulation of reference values for [^{123}I]-MIBG parameters, H/M ratio and WR, is warranted. In the past decade, several acquisition protocols have been conducted, varying, for instance, in patient preparation, collimators used, and time to scan after injection. In 2010 the EANM Cardiovascular Committee and the European Council of Nuclear Cardiology proposed a standard acquisition protocol for cardiac [^{123}I]-MIBG imaging, yielding, e.g., the use of a medium-energy collimator, acquisition 15 min and 4 h after injection, and discontinuation of a list of interfering medications (Flotats et al. 2010). Following this detailed imaging protocol, reference values for H/M ratio and WR in a normal population may be formulated, possibly corrected for age.

Another consideration is radiation burden, especially when a baseline and several follow-up examinations are required, such as in cancer patients. It should be noted, however, that for cardiac [^{123}I]-MIBG imaging the reported effective dose is 0.013 mSv/MBq (de Geus-Oei et al. 2011; Flotats et al. 2010). In comparison, the effective dose for multi-gated radionuclide ventriculography is similar, but a five-fold higher administered activity is needed for an adequate acquisition. Thus, patients would benefit from undergoing serial [^{123}I]-MIBG examinations instead of multi-gated radionuclide ventriculography examinations.

Several other radionuclide tracers have been evaluated in the detection of cardiotoxicity, e.g., [^{111}In]-antimyosin, [^{99m}Tc]-annexin, and [^{111}In]-trastuzumab (de Geus-Oei et al. 2011). [^{111}In]-antimyosin is a marker for myocardial cell injury and necrosis and demonstrated high sensitivity for the detection of cardiotoxicity; however, myocardial uptake remained even after recovery of LVEF (Nousiainen et al. 2001). [^{99m}Tc]-annexin is used to image cell death and apoptosis. Although promising results were shown in an animal model (Bennink et al. 2004), both tracers are no longer commercially available. [^{111}In]-trastuzumab was hypothesized to directly visualize trastuzumab-induced cardiotoxicity. Since the cardiotoxic mechanism of trastuzumab in combination with anthracyclines is a two-step process, studies assessing [^{111}In]-trastuzumab showed conflicting results (de Korte et al. 2007; Perik et al. 2006). Further research is needed to evaluate the clinical usefulness of [^{111}In]-trastuzumab.

Modalities without ionizing radiation to measure LVEF include cardiac magnetic resonance and echocardiography. However, cardiac magnetic resonance yields several contraindications, e.g., implanted medical devices and claustrophobia, and echocardiography is highly user dependent. Three-dimensional echocardiography has been shown to slightly underestimate LVEF, as compared with MUGA, although they display a strong correlation (Walker et al. 2010). A novel technique is echocardiography with strain imaging, which depicts myocardial muscle deformation by speckle tracking. It captures both regional and global assessment of cardiac function and does not rely on assumptions about cardiac geometry. Preliminary results suggest that echocardiography with strain imaging can detect cardiotoxicity due to cancer therapy at an early stage (Stoodley et al. 2011). In a study of 56 asymptomatic pediatric patients 2–15 years after anthracycline treatment, a significant decrease of strain measurements was observed, whereas LVEF remained normal (Ganame et al. 2007). Further research and follow-up is warranted for this technique.

Also, different biomarkers were investigated in the early detection of anthracycline cardiotoxicity, mainly in childhood cancer survivors. In several studies a significant correlation of cardiac dysfunction (by echocardiography) with elevated B-type natriuretic peptide (BNP), N-terminal pro-BNP, and troponin T was found, but other reports failed to confirm these results (Mavinkurve-Groothuis et al. 2008). No elevation of troponin I was observed after anthracycline therapy.

A novel [^{18}F]-based PET tracer, LMI1195, is being developed for cardiac sympathetic neuronal imaging and has finished a phase 1 trial. LMI1195 is a noradrenaline transporter substrate, and preliminary results show that it has favorable safety, dosimetry, and tolerability profiles. In addition, LMI1195 provided high-quality, well-defined three-dimensional images of the autonomic nervous system of the heart (Yu et al. 2011, 2012). In the near future, this tracer may be researched to evaluate cardiotoxicity in patients undergoing anticancer therapy.

For [^{123}I]-MIBG scintigraphy, future studies should focus on early recognition of cardiotoxicity with [^{123}I]-MIBG and formulate cutoff values for H/M ratio and WR. When subclinical cardiotoxicity is recognized, patients can be monitored more closely, and if necessary, another chemotherapeutic regimen may be chosen, or therapy may be temporarily discontinued to observe heart function. Irreversible damage to the myocardium may be prevented or treated at an early stage to avoid further harm. Standard treatment for heart failure is advised in chemotherapy-induced cardiomyopathy, including angiotensin-converting enzyme inhibitors, β-blockers, and/or angiotensin receptor blockers, but this is not based on large randomized clinical trials (Shaikh and Shih 2012). Furthermore, studies investigating late cardiotoxicity with [^{123}I]-MIBG with a long-term follow-up, preferably up to 10 years, are warranted.

Conclusion

Of the radionuclide tracers imaging the cardiac autonomic nervous system, most research focused on [^{123}I]-MIBG. In evaluating early cardiotoxicity, [^{123}I]-MIBG holds promising results in patients who received anthracycline chemotherapy, adjuvant trastuzumab, and/or chest radiotherapy. No studies have been performed yet focusing on other potential cardiotoxic anticancer regimes, or with long-term follow-up. Developments in PET tracers may provide new insights into the cardiac autonomic nervous system.

References

Altena R, Perik PJ, van Veldhuisen DJ et al (2009) Cardiovascular toxicity caused by cancer treatment: strategies for early detection. Lancet Oncol 10:391–399

Bennink RJ, van den Hoff MJ, van Hemert FJ et al (2004) Annexin V imaging of acute doxorubicin cardiotoxicity (apoptosis) in rats. J Nucl Med 45:842–848

Boogers MJ, Borleffs CJ, Henneman MM et al (2010) Cardiac sympathetic denervation assessed with 123-iodine metaiodobenzylguanidine imaging predicts ventricular arrhythmias in implantable cardioverter-defibrillator patients. J Am Coll Cardiol 55:2769–2777

Bovelli D, Plataniotis G, Roila F (2010) Cardiotoxicity of chemotherapeutic agents and radiotherapy-related heart disease: ESMO clinical practice guidelines. Ann Oncol 21(Suppl 5):v277–v282

Bristow MR, Mason JW, Billingham ME et al (1981) Dose-effect and structure-function relationships in doxorubicin cardiomyopathy. Am Heart J 102:709–718

Carrio I, Cowie MR, Yamazaki J et al (2010) Cardiac sympathetic imaging with mIBG in heart failure. JACC Cardiovasc Imaging 3:92–100

Carrio I, Estorch M, Berna L et al (1995) Indium-111-antimyosin and iodine-123-MIBG studies in early assessment of doxorubicin cardiotoxicity. J Nucl Med 36:2044–2049

Chirumamilla A, Travin MI (2011) Cardiac applications of 123I-mIBG imaging. Semin Nucl Med 41:374–387

Clarke M, Collins R, Darby S et al (2005) Effects of radiotherapy and of differences in the extent of surgery for early breast cancer on local recurrence and 15-year survival: an overview of the randomised trials. Lancet 366:2087–2106

de Geus-Oei LF, Mavinkurve-Groothuis AM, Bellersen L et al (2011) Scintigraphic techniques for early detection of cancer treatment-induced cardiotoxicity. J Nucl Med 52:560–571

de Korte MA, de Vries EG, Lub-De Hooge MN et al (2007) 111Indium-trastuzumab visualises myocardial human epidermal growth factor receptor 2 expression shortly after anthracycline treatment but not during heart failure: a clue to uncover the mechanisms of trastuzumab-related cardiotoxicity. Eur J Cancer 43:2046–2051

Di Cosimo S (2011) Heart to heart with trastuzumab: a review on cardiac toxicity. Target Oncol 6:189–195

Druck MN, Gulenchyn KY, Evans WK et al (1984) Radionuclide angiography and endomyocardial biopsy in the assessment of doxorubicin cardiotoxicity. Cancer 53:1667–1674

Early Breast Cancer Trialists' Collaborative Group (2000) Favourable and unfavourable effects on long-term survival of radiotherapy for early breast cancer: an overview of the randomised trials. Early Breast Cancer Trialists' Collaborative Group. Lancet 355:1757–1770

Ewer MS, Ali MK, Mackay B et al (1984) A comparison of cardiac biopsy grades and ejection fraction estimations in patients receiving Adriamycin. J Clin Oncol 2:112–117

Flotats A, Carrio I, Agostini D et al (2010) Proposal for standardization of 123I-metaiodobenzylguanidine (MIBG) cardiac sympathetic imaging by the EANM Cardiovascular Committee and the European Council of Nuclear Cardiology. Eur J Nucl Med Mol Imaging 37:1802–1812

Ganame J, Claus P, Uyttebroeck A et al (2007) Myocardial dysfunction late after low-dose anthracycline treatment in asymptomatic pediatric patients. J Am Soc Echocardiogr 20:1351–1358

Gillespie HS, McGann CJ, Wilson BD (2011) Noninvasive diagnosis of chemotherapy related cardiotoxicity. Curr Cardiol Rev 7:234–244

Heidendal GA, Bezemer PD, Koopman PA et al (1983) Reproducibility of ejection fraction measurements by gated equilibrium blood pool scintigraphy. Eur J Nucl Med 8:467–470

Hiasa G, Hamada M, Saeki H et al (2004) Cardiac sympathetic nerve activity can detect congestive heart failure sensitively in patients with hypertrophic cardiomyopathy. Chest 126:679–686

Hull MC, Morris CG, Pepine CJ et al (2003) Valvular dysfunction and carotid, subclavian, and coronary artery disease in survivors of hodgkin lymphoma treated with radiation therapy. JAMA 290:2831–2837

Jeon TJ, Lee JD, Ha JW et al (2000) Evaluation of cardiac adrenergic neuronal damage in rats with doxorubicin-induced cardiomyopathy using iodine-131 MIBG autoradiography and PGP 9.5 immunohistochemistry. Eur J Nucl Med 27:686–693

Lautamaki R, Tipre D, Bengel FM (2007) Cardiac sympathetic neuronal imaging using PET. Eur J Nucl Med Mol Imaging 34(Suppl 1):S74–S85

Lekakis J, Prassopoulos V, Athanassiadis P et al (1996) Doxorubicin-induced cardiac neurotoxicity: study with iodine 123-labeled metaiodobenzylguanidine scintigraphy. J Nucl Cardiol 3:37–41

Marks LB, Yu X, Prosnitz RG et al (2005) The incidence and functional consequences of RT-associated cardiac perfusion defects. Int J Radiat Oncol Biol Phys 63:214–223

Mavinkurve-Groothuis AM, Kapusta L, Nir A et al (2008) The role of biomarkers in the early detection of anthracycline-induced cardiotoxicity in children: a review of the literature. Pediatr Hematol Oncol 25:655–664

Nousiainen T, Vanninen E, Jantunen E et al (2001) Anthracycline-induced cardiomyopathy: long-term effects on myocardial cell integrity, cardiac adrenergic innervation and fatty acid uptake. Clin Physiol 21:123–128

Panjrath GS, Jain D (2006) Monitoring chemotherapy-induced cardiotoxicity: role of cardiac nuclear imaging. J Nucl Cardiol 13:415–426

Panjrath GS, Jain D (2007) Trastuzumab-induced cardiac dysfunction. Nucl Med Commun 28:69–73

Paszat LF, Mackillop WJ, Groome PA et al (1998) Mortality from myocardial infarction after adjuvant radiotherapy for breast cancer in the surveillance, epidemiology, and end-results cancer registries. J Clin Oncol 16:2625–2631

Perik PJ, Lub-De Hooge MN, Gietema JA et al (2006) Indium-111-labeled trastuzumab scintigraphy in patients with human epidermal growth factor receptor 2-positive metastatic breast cancer. J Clin Oncol 24:2276–2282

Rocco TP, Dilsizian V, Fischman AJ et al (1989) Evaluation of ventricular function in patients with coronary artery disease. J Nucl Med 30:1149–1165

Russell SD, Blackwell KL, Lawrence J et al (2010) Independent adjudication of symptomatic heart failure with the use of doxorubicin and cyclophosphamide followed by trastuzumab adjuvant therapy: a combined review of cardiac data from the National Surgical Adjuvant breast and Bowel Project B-31 and the North Central Cancer Treatment Group N9831 clinical trials. J Clin Oncol 28:3416–3421

Rutqvist LE, Johansson H (1990) Mortality by laterality of the primary tumour among 55,000 breast cancer patients from the Swedish Cancer Registry. Br J Cancer 61:866–868

Schwartz RG, McKenzie WB, Alexander J et al (1987) Congestive heart failure and left ventricular dysfunction complicating doxorubicin therapy. Seven-year experience using serial radionuclide angiocardiography. Am J Med 82:1109–1118

Shaikh AY, Shih JA (2012) Chemotherapy-induced cardiotoxicity. Curr Heart Fail Rep 9:117–127

Smith LA, Cornelius VR, Plummer CJ et al (2010) Cardiotoxicity of anthracycline agents for the treatment of cancer: systematic review and meta-analysis of randomised controlled trials. BMC Cancer 10:337

Stokkel MP, de Wit-van der Veen LJ, Boekhout A (2013) I-123-MIBG myocardial imaging in trastuzumab-based cardiotoxicity: the first experience. Nucl Med Commun 34:19–24

Stoodley PW, Richards DA, Meikle SR et al (2011) The potential role of echocardiographic strain imaging for evaluating cardiotoxicity due to cancer therapy. Heart Lung Circ 20:3–9

Swain SM, Whaley FS, Ewer MS (2003) Congestive heart failure in patients treated with doxorubicin: a retrospective analysis of three trials. Cancer 97:2869–2879

Takano H, Ozawa H, Kobayashi I et al (1995) Atrophic nerve fibers in regions of reduced MIBG uptake in doxorubicin cardiomyopathy. J Nucl Med 36:2060–2061

Takano H, Ozawa H, Kobayashi I et al (1996) Myocardial sympathetic dysinnervation in doxorubicin cardiomyopathy. J Cardiol 27:49–55

Takeishi Y, Sukekawa H, Sakurai T et al (1994) Noninvasive identification of anthracycline cardiotoxicity: comparison of 123I-MIBG and 123I-BMIPP imaging. Ann Nucl Med 8:177–182

Tan-Chiu E, Yothers G, Romond E et al (2005) Assessment of cardiac dysfunction in a randomized trial comparing doxorubicin and cyclophosphamide followed by paclitaxel, with or without trastuzumab as adjuvant therapy in node-positive, human epidermal growth factor receptor 2-overexpressing breast cancer: NSABP B-31. J Clin Oncol 23:7811–7819

Valdes Olmos RA, ten Bokkel Huinink WW, ten Hoeve RF et al (1995) Assessment of anthracycline-related myocardial adrenergic derangement by [123I]metaiodobenzylguanidine scintigraphy. Eur J Cancer 31A:26–31

Valdes Olmos RA, ten Bokkel Huinink WW, Dewit LG et al (1996) Iodine-123 metaiodobenzylguanidine in the assessment of late cardiac effects from cancer therapy. Eur J Nucl Med 23:453–458

Wakasugi S, Wada A, Hasegawa Y et al (1992) Detection of abnormal cardiac adrenergic neuron activity in adriamycin-induced cardiomyopathy with iodine-125-metaiodobenzylguanidine. J Nucl Med 33:208–214

Wakasugi S, Fischman AJ, Babich JW et al (1993) Metaiodobenzylguanidine: evaluation of its potential as a tracer for monitoring doxorubicin cardiomyopathy. J Nucl Med 34:1283–1286

Wakasugi S, Inoue M, Tazawa S (1995) Assessment of adrenergic neuron function altered with progression of heart failure. J Nucl Med 36:2069–2074

Walker J, Bhullar N, Fallah-Rad N et al (2010) Role of three-dimensional echocardiography in breast cancer: comparison with two-dimensional echocardiography, multiple-gated acquisition scans, and cardiac magnetic resonance imaging. J Clin Oncol 28:3429–3436

Yeh ET, Tong AT, Lenihan DJ et al (2004) Cardiovascular complications of cancer therapy: diagnosis, pathogenesis, and management. Circulation 109:3122–3131

Yu M, Bozek J, Lamoy M et al (2011) Evaluation of LMI1195, a novel 18F-labeled cardiac neuronal PET imaging agent, in cells and animal models. Circ Cardiovasc Imaging 4:435–443

Yu M, Bozek J, Lamoy M et al (2012) LMI1195 PET imaging in evaluation of regional cardiac sympathetic denervation and its potential role in antiarrhythmic drug treatment. Eur J Nucl Med Mol Imaging 39:1910–1919

Index

R.H.J.A. Slart et al. (eds.), *Autonomic Innervation of the Heart: Role of Molecular Imaging*, DOI 10.1007/978-3-662-45074-1

Q

R

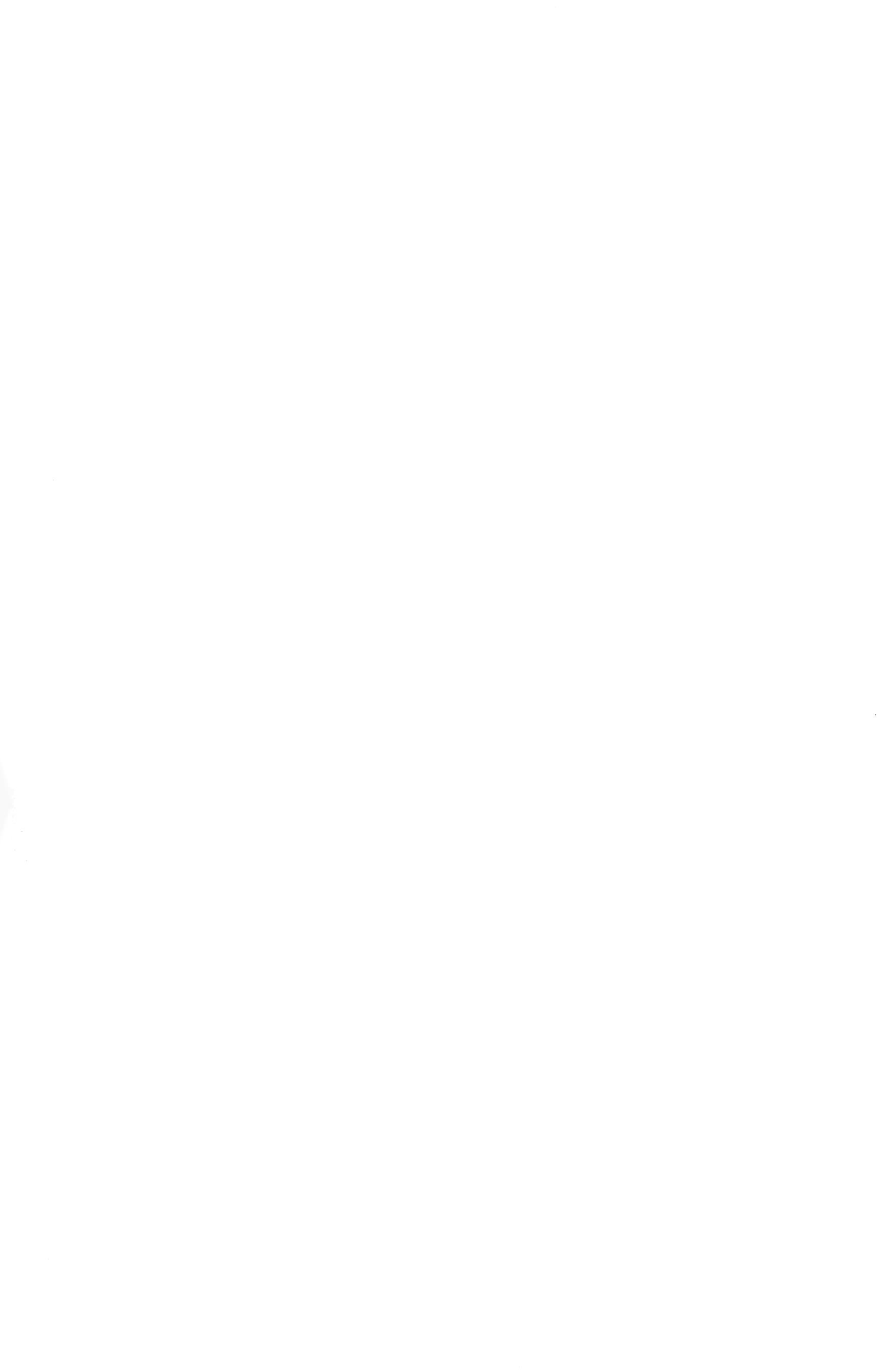

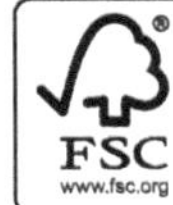

MIX
Papier aus verantwortungsvollen Quellen
Paper from responsible sources
FSC® C105338

If you have any concerns about our products, you can contact us on
ProductSafety@springernature.com

In case Publisher is established outside the EU, the EU authorized representative is:
Springer Nature Customer Service Center GmbH
Europaplatz 3, 69115 Heidelberg, Germany

Printed by Libri Plureos GmbH
in Hamburg, Germany